Neurotransmitters and their Receptors

Based on a Workshop
Sponsored by the European Molecular Biology Organisation
and The Weizmann Institute of Science, Rehovot
February 1980

Edited by

U. Z. Littauer, Y. Dudai, I. Silman, V. I. Teichberg and Z. Vogel

Department of Neurobiology, The Weizmann Institute of Science, Rehovot

A Wiley–Interscience Publication

JOHN WILEY & SONS

Chichester · New York · Brisbane · Toronto

British Library Cataloguing in Publication Data

Neurotransmitters and their Receptors
1. Drug receptors – Congresses
I. Littauer, U Z, Dudai Y, Silman I,
Teichberg V I and Vogel Z
596'.01'88 RM301 80-41130

ISBN 0-471-27893-9

CONTENTS

PREFACE

Studies of neurotransmitters and neuromodulators, their metabolism and their interactions with receptors, comprise a cornerstone of modern neurobiological research. The immense amount of data accumulated in this fast-growing field during recent years has led to the formation of novel concepts and has shed new light on the complex and delicate mechanisms by which chemical signals mediate and modulate the flow of information in the nervous system. Some highlights of trends and developments in the study of neurotransmission are presented in this volume, based on lectures presented at and EMBO workshop which was held in Israel at Ein Bokek by the Dead Sea in February 1980, in which some of the leading figures in the field participated.

The majority of the contributions to this book are grouped in chapters which bear the titles of known or putative neurotransmitters, e.g. catecholamines or acetylcholine. Nevertheless, several themes, which time and again cross the borders of the various subfields of neurotransmitter research, emerge again and again from the studies presented here on the different neurotransmitter systems. They characterize recent developments in the field. Among them:

- The diversity and complexity of the mechanisms which control the efficacy of neurotransmission. Such control can be implemented, for example, by modulating release, by modulating the sensitivity of post-synaptic receptors or receptor-ionophore complexes, or by regulating degradative mechanisms. It is now evident that both coarse and fine tuning of various neurotransmitter systems is possible, e.g. by short term desensitization of receptors or by ligand-induced long-term alterations in the number of receptor molecules. Whereas the former processes may be involved in tuning the response of a cell to an incoming signal, the latter processes may play an important role in adaptive processes and in the etiology of various pathological conditions.

- The heterogeneity of neurotransmitter systems. An increasing number of studies indicate that classes of receptors for neurotransmitters that were regarded until recently as homogeneous, can, in fact, be divided into subclasses. In some cases. this heterogeneity can be ascribed to the presence of both post- and pre-synaptic receptors; in other cases a multiplicity of post-synaptic receptor classes has been invoked, the detailed physiological significance of which is not yet understood. It thus appears that the same chemical signal may evoke either a feedback response in its releasing cell or different responses in various target cells, depending on the type of receptor occupied.

• In spite of the complexity and heterogeneity revealed by receptor binding studies, some mechanisms of signal transduction, e.g. via ionophores or cyclases, seem to be common to many systems. Detailed studies of relatively simple model systems (e.g. giant mollusc cells or neuronal cells in culture) may therefore shed light on basic receptor-mediated events in more complex tissues.

• The arsenal of neurotransmitters and neuromodulators is diverse, and, in spite of the major advances in the field, is only partially known. As yet unidentified natural ligands seem to exist in our brain for receptors that interact with important classes of drugs, e.g. benzodiazepines or barbiturates. The discovery of the enkephalins and the endorphins seems thus to represent only the first step into a fascinating field, the clinical importance of which cannot be underestimated. Moreover, many peptides have been identified in the brain whose physiological function has not yet been fully elucidated, e.g. cholecystokinin and substance P.

Examples stressing the above mentioned themes are interwoven in the following chapters with an abundance of recently acquired data on catecholamines, acetylcholine, excitatory amino acids, GABA, benzodiazepines, neuropeptides and ion channels. The function of cytoskeletal proteins and other elements in neurite outgrowth as well as the introduction of new research methods to probe neuronal development and activity are also presented. The latter are of special interest since the more precise and sophisticated our probes, the more insight we gain in the intricate chemical language by which nerve cells communicate with each other. It is our hope that this volume will prove of value to those engaged in efforts to decipher the various dialects of this language.

The workshop at Ein Bokek was attended by about 100 scientists from 14 countries, and supported by the European Molecular Biology organisation (EMBO), the Weizmann Institute of Science, the Centre for Neurosciences and Behavioral Research of the Weizmann Institute of Science, the Israel Academy of Sciences and Humanities, the Israeli Center for Psychobiology - Charles Smith Family Foundation, and the British Council. Their support is gratefully acknowledged.

The workshop was organized by the Department of Neurobiology at the Weizmann Institute of Science with the assistance of the Conference Unit of the Weizmann Institute. Special thanks are due to Ms. Chava Bohak and Mr. Itzhak Berman for their crucial role in organizing the workshop, to Ms. Chava Bohak and Ms. Neta Shalit for typing part of the manuscripts, and to Ms. Miriam Balaban for seeing to the publication of this volume.

Rehovot

July 1980

U.Z. Littauer, Y. Dudai, I. Silman
V.I. Teichberg and Z. Vogel.

B I O G E N I C   A M I N E S

Neurotransmitters and their Receptors
Edited by U.Z. Littauer, Y. Dudai, I. Silman,
V.I. Teichberg and Z. Vogel

Autoregulation of Noradrenaline and Dopamine Release Through Presynaptic Receptors

S. Z. Langer, S. Arbilla and L. Kamal

Biology Department Synthélabo-LERS,

58, rue de la Glacière, 75013 Paris, France

ABSTRACT

In peripheral tissues, presynaptic inhibitory α-adrenoceptors are involved in a negative feed back mechanism for noradrenaline released by nerve stimulation. These presynaptic receptors correspond to the pharmacological profile of the α_2-adrenoceptor subtype. In addition, presynaptic β-adrenoceptors facilitate the release of neurotransmitter elicited by low frequencies of stimulation.

In the central nervous system, similarly to peripheral tissues, the calcium dependent release of noradrenaline is modulated through a negative feed-back mechanism mediated by presynaptic α-adrenoceptors. However there is as yet no evidence for the presence of facilitatory β-adrenoceptors for the release of noradrenaline.

In the corpus striatum, presynaptic inhibitory dopamine receptors modulate the calcium dependent release of dopamine through a negative feed-back mechanism. Presynaptic dopamine receptors located in the corpus striatum do not modulate the calcium-independent release of dopamine elicited by amphetamine or tyramine.

Activation of inhibitory α-adrenoceptors or dopamine autoreceptors with somato dendritic localization leads to a reduction of neuronal firing with a concomitant reduction in transmitter release.

Regulation of the release of noradrenaline in peripheral tissues by presynaptic inhibitory α-adrenoceptors.

Evidence accumulated during recent years clearly demonstrate in peripheral tissues that agonists and antagonists possessing affinity for α-adrenoceptors modulate the electrically evoked release of noradrenaline, thus α-agonists inhibit noradrenaline release during nerve stimulation while α-adrenoceptor blocking agents enhance the stimulation evoked release of neurotransmitter (1, 2, 3, 4, 5, 6, 7, 8).

In figure 1 is shown schematically the involvment of presynaptic α-adrenoceptors in the negative feed-back mechanism for the autoregulation of the release of noradrenaline during nerve stimulation.

The effects of α-adrenoceptor agonists and antagonists on noradrenaline release are observed irrespective of the α or β type of postsynaptic adrenoceptor that mediates the response of the effector organ (2,5,6,7,8).

Evidence in favor of the presynaptic localization of the inhibitory α-adrenoceptors involved in the regulation of noradrenergic neurotransmission are given by the fact that the increase in the stimulation evoked release of noradrenaline obtained by α-adrenoceptor blocking agents is not affected by the atrophy of the postsynaptic effector cell as demonstrated after duct ligation of the rat submaxillary gland. (9). In addition, α-adrenoceptor blockade enhances ^{3}H-noradrenaline release induced by potassium depolarization from recently formed nerve endings in cultured rat cervical ganglion under conditions of absence of postsynaptic effector cells (10).

The following features characterize the regulation of noradrenaline release mediated by presynaptic α-adrenoceptors.

a) Regulation of noradrenaline release through presynaptic α-adrenoceptors is only observed when the release of neurotransmitter is elicited by a calcium dependent mechanism, as nerve stimulation, or potassium depolarization. The calcium independent release of noradrenaline induced by tyramine is not modified by α-adrenoceptor agonists or antagonists (11, 12, 13).

b) The magnitude of the reduction in the stimulation evoked release of noradrenaline obtained with α-adrenoceptor agonists is more pronounced the lower the frequency of nerve stimulation (14, 15, 16). In fact, α-adrenoceptor agonists fail to reduce the release of noradrenaline elicited by high frequency of nerve stimulation (17, 18).

c) The inhibition of noradrenergic neurotransmission by α-adrenoceptor agonists of the catecholamine type can only be demonstrated when neuronal uptake of noradrenaline is inhibited by cocaine or desipramine. (18,19,20). On the other hand the inhibition of noradrenergic neurotransmission by α-adrenoceptor agonists of the imidazoline type like clonidine or oxymetazoline is reduced by cocaine or desipramine (13,19).

d) The negative feed back mechanism for noradrenaline release during nerve stimulation appears to operate most effectively when the transmitter released by nerve impulses reaches a threshold concentration in the synaptic gap. Evidences in support of this view are given by the lack of effectiveness of phenoxybenzamine to increase transmitter or dopamine β-hydroxylase release in tissues pretreated with reserpine or when electrically induced release of noradrenaline is elicited by a single pulse. (21,22,23).

More recently, it has been postulated that in addition to the presynaptic negative feed-back mechanism for noradrenaline released by nerve stimulation which is mediated by presynaptic α-adrenoceptors, a positive feed-back mechanism exists in noradrenergic nerve terminals that is triggered through the activation of presynaptic β-adrenoceptors (Fig.1). This hypothesis is based on the fact that exposure to low concentrations of the β-adrenoceptor agonist, isoproterenol, enhances the release of noradrenaline during nerve stimulation at low frequencies in several noradrenergically inervated organs : guinea pig atria, cat thoracic aorta and perfused cat spleen, rat pineal gland and portal vein, human oviduct and vasoconstrictor nerves (12,24,25,26,27,28). Similar findings are also reported under in vivo conditions in the anaesthetized dog by stimulation of the right cardioacelerator nerve using low frequencies of stimulation (29).

The increase in stimulation-evoked release of noradrenaline by isoproterenol is antagonized by preincubation with 0.1 μM propanolol (24,25). However, propranolol by itself does not reduce the stimulation-evoked release of the neurotransmitter in most tissues studied so far small reductions or lack of effects of propanolol on transmitter release elicited by nerve stimulation are reported in several preparations (12,24,25,30,31). When high concentrations of propranolol are used a reduction of noradrenaline release is obtained in several tissues. However, this effect appears to be related to local anaesthetic properties rather than to blockade of presynaptic β-adrenoceptors (32,33). Under in vivo conditions, it was reported that sotalol reduces significantly the release of noradrenaline induced at low frequencies of stimulation (29).

The β_1 or β_2 nature of the presynaptic β adrenoceptors is not entirely clarified yet. Evidence in favor of β_1 type is given by the fact that these receptors are blocked by metoprolol (30). However, most of the evidence supports the view that the presynaptic β-adrenoceptor is of the β_2 type since terbutaline and salbutamol enhance the stimulation-evoked transmitter release under conditions in which H 110/38 is without affect (31). More recently, it was found that terbutaline enhanced the potassium evoked release of ^{3}H-noradrenaline from the rat pineal gland (12).

It is possible that the different results reflect species and tissue differences. It is also possible that the presynaptic β-adrenoceptors which mediate the facilitation of transmitter release during low frequency nerve stimulation differ from the classical β_1 and β_2 postsynaptic adrenoceptors which mediate the responses of the effector organ.

It is likely that presynaptic facilitatory β-adrenoceptors are mainly activated by circulating adrenaline to enhance noradrenergic neurotransmission (Fig.1). In support of this view is the fact that propanolol becomes more effective in reducing noradrenergic neurotransmission when peripheral noradrenergic nerve terminals are labelled with adrenaline (34,35).

The presynaptic β-adrenoceptor appears to be stereospecific, (-) isoproterenol enhances, while (+) isoproterenol fails to modify transmitter release in the perfused cat spleen (25).

The presynaptic localization of β-adrenoceptors is supported by results obtained in recently formed noradrenergic nerve endings when rat superior cervival ganglion are cultured (36).

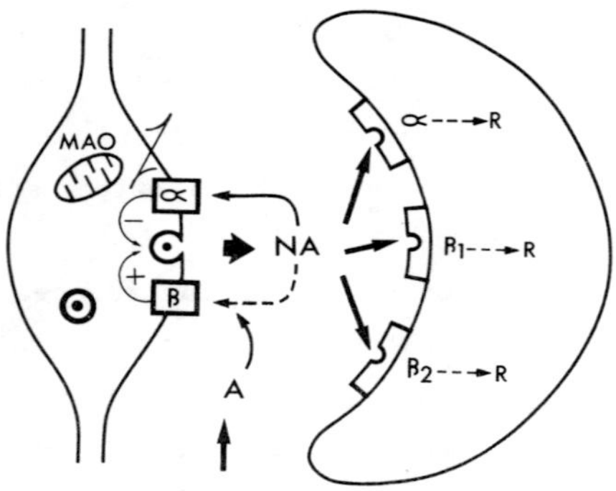

Figure 1 : Presynaptic α and β-adrenoceptors on peripheral noradrenergic nerve terminals.

Presynaptic inhibitory α-adrenoceptors activated by released noradrenaline (NA) inhibit further release of the neurotransmitter. Presynaptic facilitatory β-adrenoceptors activated by circulating adrenaline (A) increase the release of noradrenaline. The responses (R) of the efector organ are mediated through α, β_1 or β_2 adrenoceptors of the effector cell MAO : monoamine oxidase.

Modulation of the release of noradrenaline in the central nervous system by presynaptic autoreceptors.

Like in the peripheral nervous system, presynaptic α-adrenoceptors possibly located on noradrenergic nerve endings of the central nervous system appear to modulate the release of noradrenaline. The evidence available supports the view that presynaptic inhibitory α-adrenoceptors exist on the noradrenergic nerve endings of several brain regions. It was reported that α-adrenoceptor agonists inhibit while α-antagonists enhance the electrically or potassium induced release of noradrenaline in the rat cerebral cortex (8,37,38,39,40) and guinea pig hypothalamus (41,42). These results were obtained in superfused brain slices, and similar results have been reported in synaptosomes (43). The modulation of noradrenaline release by alpha-adrenoceptor agonists and antagonists in synaptosomal preparations support the view that the α_2-release modulating adrenoceptor is located presynaptically in the central nervous system.

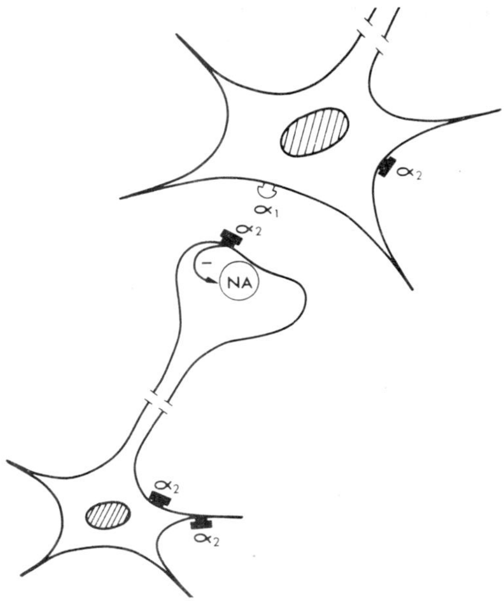

Figure 2 : Schematic representation of a central noradrenergic neuron.

Somato dendritic inhibitory α_2 adrenoceptors are present in addition to the presynaptic inhibitory α_2 adrenoceptors on the noradrenergic nerve terminal. Postsynaptic adrenoceptors are of the α_1 as well as the α_2 type.

It is of interest to note that clonidine and oxymetazoline but not methoxamine reduce the potassium evoked release of ^{3}H-noradrenaline from slices of rat occipital cortex (38). On the other hand yohimbine and phentolamine but not prazosin or WB4101 increase the potassium induced release of ^{3}H-noradrenaline from rat occipital cortex slices (38,39). These findings are well correlated with the relative order of potency of these drugs to modulate noradrenaline release in peripheral tissues (6). These pharmacological characteristics would indicate that presynaptic α-adrenoceptors in the central nervous system are of α_2 type. As shown in Fig. 2, in addition to the presynaptic, release modulating α_2-adrenoceptors in the central nervous system, there is evidence for the presence of somato-dentritic inhibitory α_2-adrenoceptors in the locus coeruleus (44). Additional evidence originating from receptor binding studies indicate that both the α_1 and α_2 type of adrenoceptors are present in the central nervous system with postsynaptic localization (45,46).

In contrast to the presynaptic inhibition of noradrenaline release mediated through α_2 adrenoceptors which are present in peripheral as well as in central noradrenergic nerve endings, there is as yet no evidence for the presence of presynaptic facilitatory β-adrenoceptors in areas of the central nervous system containing noradrenergic nerve terminals.

<u>Modulation of the release of dopamine through presynaptic autoreceptors</u>.

The existence of autoreceptors in nerve terminals of central dopaminergic neurons was first suggested by Carlsson and co-workers (47) in *in vivo* experiments, which showed that ongoing dopamine release control the rate of dopamine synthesis.

Later on, the presence of presynaptic inhibitory dopamine receptors for the release of dopamine on the dopaminergic nerve endings of the rat striatum was postulated. This suggestion was based on the inhibition by apomorphine and the enhancement by chlorpromazine of the stimulation evoked release of tritium from slices of rat corpus striatum prelabelled with ^{3}H-dopamine (48). Attemps to reproduce these findings have given contradictory results (49,50). While the question of presynaptic inhibitory dopamine receptors in the rat striatum remains controversial.

The dopaminergic neuron contains autoreceptors which regulate either electrical firing on these cells in the somato-dendritic area or tyrosine hydroxylase activity and dopamine release in the nerve terminals. It is possible that dopamine autoreceptors are of DA_2 type, while dopamine receptors in the effector cell are of DA_1 and DA_2 type.

Convincing experiments for the presence of presynaptic inhibitory dopamine receptors were reported using superfused slices of the rabbit caudate nucleus (51,52). In this structure, it was clearly shown that apomorphine dopamine and bromocriptine, three dopaminergic agonists

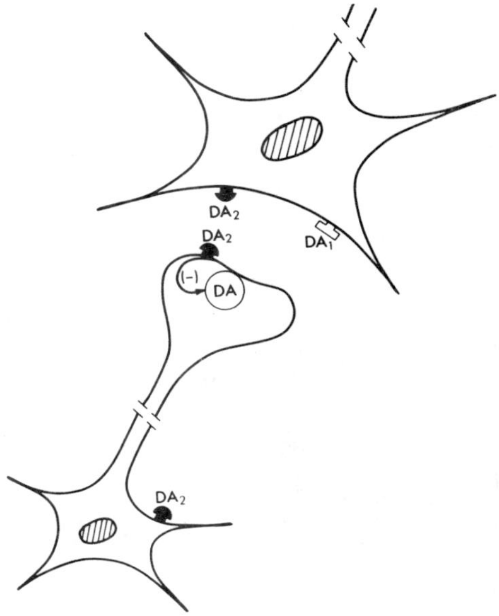

Figure 3 : Schematic representation of a nigro-striatal dopaminergic neuron.

from different chemical structures inhibited while phenotiazine and butyrophenone neuroleptics increased the stimulation evoked release of dopamine. These results support the presence of a negative feed-back mechanism regulating the release of dopamine by electrical stimulation. Recent results obtained in the cat caudate nucleus demonstrate the existence of a negative feed-back mechanism for the stimulation-evoked release of dopamine (Lehmann, Arbilla and Langer, unpublished observations).

Low doses of apomorphine have been reported to improve the psychotic symptoms in schizophrenic patients (53). It is likely that this effect is linked to the activation of presynaptic dopamine receptors which decrease synthesis and release of dopamine.

Pharmacological and biochemical evidences suggest that dopamine receptors in dopaminergic nerve terminals are probably of the DA_2 type (Fig.3). Studies on rat striatal DA sensitive adenylate cyclase have povided evidence that this enzyme is not located on terminals of dopaminergic neurons (54). Thus, the presynaptic inhibitory autoreceptors in the dopaminergic nerve terminals which modulate the release of the transmitter appear to be functionally unrelated to the activation of the dopamine sensitive adenylate cyclase. In support of this view, sulpiride, a dopaminergic antagonist which does not block dopamine receptors linked to dopamine sensitive adenylate cyclase enhances ^{3}H-dopamine release in the rabbit caudate nucleus and blocks stereospecifically the inhibitory effects of apomorphine (Fig. 4).

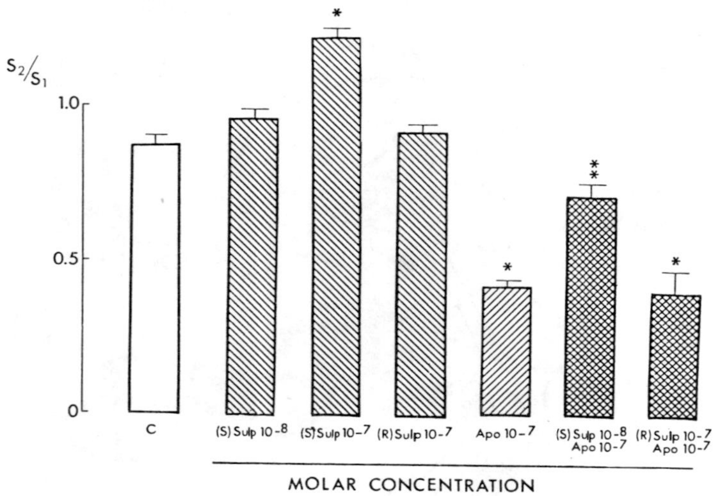

<u>Figure 4 : Stereospecific effect of sulpiride on the electrical stimulated release of ^{3}H-DA from slices of rabbit caudate nucleus.</u>
<u>Ordinate</u> : ratio of fractional release (S_2/S_1) of total tissue radioactivity released from slices of rabbit caudate nucleus prelabeled with ^{3}H-DA ; S_1 corresponds to the first period of electrical stimulation (3 Hz, 2 msec, 2 min) and S_2 to the second one obtained 44 min later. Sulpiride was added 24 min and apomorphine 20 min before S_2.

C : controls ; Sulp : sulpiride ; Apo : apomorphine.

The values shown are the means ± S.E.M. of 6-20 experiments per group.

* $p < 0.0002$ when compared to the untreated group.

** $p < 0.0002$ when compared to the apomorphine 0.1 μM group (Mann-Whitney two-tailed test).

The existence of dopamine autoreceptors on the dentrites of the dopaminergic neurons has been postulated on the basis of electrophysiological studies. Sistemic and iontophoretic application of dopaminergic agonists decreases the electrical activity of units of dopaminergic cells in the zona compacta in the sustantia nigra. The depression is blocked by local injection of neuroleptic drugs (55,56,57). Dopamine can be released by depolarizing stimuli from dendrites in the substantia nigra through a calcium dependent process (58,59). It is possible that dopamine released from dendrites autoinhibits dopaminergic activity by acting on cell body dopamine autoreceptors. Inhibitory dopamine receptors located in the somato dentritic area of the dopaminergic neuron (Fig.3) appear to be of the DA_2 type (60,61,62). Furthermore, sulpiride was shown to be a potent antagonist of the physiological response to dopamine of individual neurons in the rat substantia nigra (63).

	S_1	S_2/S_1		
		Control	Apomorphine 10^{-6} M	Haloperidol 10^{-8} M
Electrical stimulation (3 Hz, 2 min)	4.07 ± 0.19	0.90 ± 0.02	0.10 ± 0.01**	1.32 ± 0.01**
Amphetamine 10 µM, 2 min	4.03 ± 0.19	0.83 ± 0.03	0.82 ± 0.02	0.94 ± 0.04
Tyramine 5 µM, 2 min	4.44 ± 0.30	0.78 ± 0.02	0.74 ± 0.03	0.88 ± 0.04*

Table 1 : Presynaptic autoregulation of the electrically but not the amphetamine or tyramine induced release of ^{3}H-DA from slices of rabbit caudate nucleus.

S_1 corresponds to the percent of total tissue radioactivity released by the first period of either electrical stimulation (3 Hz, 2 msec, 2 min), amphetamine (10 µM, 2 min) or tyramine (5 µM, 2 min) and S_2 to the second period of stimulation obtained 44 min later. Drugs were added 20 min before S2.

$^*p < 0.05$: $^{**}p < 0.0002$ when compared against the control group (Mann-Whitney, two-tailed test).
Shown are mean values ± S.E.M. of 6 to 22 experiments per group.

Similarly to the regulation of noradrenaline release through presynaptic inhibitory α-adrenoceptors, the modulation of dopamine release through presynaptic inhibitory dopamine receptors has certain characteristics features :

a) The inhibition of ^{3}H-dopamine release by dopamine agonists and the enhancement by antagonists was described in the rabbit caudate nucleus for the calcium dependent electrical stimulated release of neurotransmitter (51,52). On the other hand, in the same tissue, the calcium independent release of neurotransmitter elicited by exposure to amphetamine or tyramine (64) is not modified by concentrations of apomorphine or haloperidol which significantly modify the electrically induced release of dopamine (Table 1). Thus, presynaptic inhibitory dopamine receptors modulate only the calcium-dependent induced release of neurotransmitter.

b) The magnitude of the reduction of the stimulation evoked release of dopamine from slices of rabbit caudate nucleus is more pronounced the lower the frequency of nerve stimulation. Thus, a more pronounced inhibition by apomorphine or enhancement by haloperidol of the release of dopamine was obtained when slices of rabbit caudate nucleus were stimulated at 3Hz than at 10 Hz. (Kamal, Arbilla and Langer, unpublished observations).

CONCLUSIONS

In peripheral tissues as well as in the central nervous system, presynaptic α-adrenoceptors modulate the stimulation-evoked release of noradrenaline through a negative feed-back mechanism. Presynaptic release modulating α-adrenoceptors correspond to the α_2-subtype of receptor. In peripheral tissues, presynaptic β-adrenoceptors facilitate noradrenergic neurotransmission but the presence of these receptors in the central nervous system remains an open question.

Presynaptic inhibitory dopamine receptors regulating the release of dopamine are present in the caudate nucleus of the rabbit. There is as yet not enough information as to whether the presynaptic inhibitory receptors that modulate the release of dopamine are similar or different from the postsynaptic dopamine receptors.

Finally, it is well established that presynaptic inhibitory autoreceptors for noradrenaline or dopamine release regulate only the calcium dependent release of neurotransmitter through a mechanism which operates most effectively for the low and intermediate frequencies of nerve stimulation.

REFERENCES

1 Langer, S.Z.: The regulation of transmitter release elicited by nerve stimulation through a presynaptic feed-back mechanism. In "Frontiers in Catecholamine Research", ed. Usdin, E. & Synder, S., pp 543-549, New York : Pegamon Press, 1973.

2 Langer, S.Z. : Presynaptic regulation of catecholamine release. Biochem. Pharmac., 23, 1793-1800, 1974.

3 Langer, S.Z. : Presynaptic receptors and their role in the regulation of transmitter release. Sixth Gaddum Memorial Lecture. Br. J. Pharmac. 60, 481-497, 1977.

4 Langer, S.Z. : Modern concept of adrenergic transmission. In "Neurotransmitter Systems and their Clinical Disorders". Ed. N.J. Legg, Academic Press, pp 29-51, 1978.

5 Langer, S.Z. : Physiological and pharmacological role of presynaptic receptor systems in neurotransmission. In : "Presynaptic Receptors", eds. S.Z. Langer, K. Starke and M.L. Dubocovich, Pergamon Press, Oxford, pp 13-22, 1979.

6 Langer, S.Z. : Presynaptic adrenoceptors and regulation of release. "The Release of Catecholamines from Adrenergic Neurons". ed. D.M. Paton, Pergamon Press, pp 59-85, 1979.

7 Langer, S.Z. : Presynaptic receptors and the regulation of transmitter release in the peripheral and central nervous system : Physiological and pharmacological significance. In : "Catecholamines : Basic and Clinical Frontiers", ed. Usdin, E., Pergamon Press (New York), Vol.I, pp 387-391, 1979.

8 Starke, K. : Regulation of adrenaline release by presynaptic receptor systems. Rev. Physiol. Biochem. Pharmac. 77, 3-124, 1977.

9 Filinger, E.J., Langer, S.Z., Perec, C.J., and Stefano, F.J.E. : Evidence for the presynaptic location of the alpha-adrenoceptors which regulate noradrenaline release in the rat submaxillary gland. Naunyn-Schmiederberg's Arch. Pharmac. 304, 21-26, 1978.

10 Vogel, S.A., Silberstein, S.D., Berv, K.R., and Kopin, I.J. : Stimulation-induced release of norepinephrine from rat superior cervical ganglion in vitro. Eur. J. Pharmac. 20, 308-311, 1972.

11 Starke, K and Montel, H. : Influence of drugs with affinity for α-adrenoceptors on noradrenaline release by potassium, tyramine and dimethylphenylpiperazinium. Eur. J. Pharmacol. 27, 273-280, 1974.

12 Pelayo, F., Dubocovich, M.L., and Langer, S.Z. : Regulation of noradrenaline release from the rat pineal through presynaptic adrenoceptors : possible involvement of cyclic nucleotides. Nature 274, 76-78, 1978.

13 Pelayo, F., Dubocovich, M.L. and Langer, S.Z. : Inhibition of neuronal uptake reduces the presynaptic effects of clonidine but not of α-methylnoradrenaline on the stimulation-evoked release of ^{3}H-noradrenaline from rat occipital cortex slices. Eur. J. Pharmacol. 64, 143-155, 1980.

14 Dubocovich, M.L., and Langer, S.Z. : Negative feed-back regulation of noradrenaline release by nerve stimulation in the perfused cat's spleen : differences in potency of phenoxybenzamine in blocking the pre- and postsynaptic adrenergic receptors. J. Physiol., Lond., 237, 505-519, 1974.

15 Dubocovich, M.L., and Langer, S.Z. : Influence of the frequency of nerve stimulation on the metabolism ^{3}H-noradrenaline released from the perfused cat spleen : differences observed during and after the period of stimulation. J. Pharmac. Exp. Ther., 198, 83-101, 1976.

16 Langer, S.Z., Dubocovich, M.L. and Celuch, S.M. : Prejunctional regulatory mechanisms for noradrenaline release elicited by nerve stimulation. In "Chemical Tools in Catecholamine Research II". ed. Almgren, O., Carlsson, A. and Engel, J., pp 183-191, Amsterdam : Elsevier, North-Holland, U.S.A., 1975.

17 Armstrong, J.M., and Boura, A.L.A. : Effects of clonidine and guanethidine on peripheral sympathetic nerve function in the pithed rat. Br. J. Pharmac., 47, 850-852, 1973.

18 Langer, S.Z., Enero, M.A., Adler-Graschinsky, E., Dubocovich, M.L. and Celuch, S.M. : Presynaptic regulatory mechanisms for noradrenaline release by nerve stimulation. Proceeds. Symposium on "Central Action of Drugs in the Regulation of Blood Pressure". ed. Davies, D.S. & Reid, J.L., pp 133-151, London, Pitman Medical, 1975.

19 Langer, S.Z. and Dubocovich, M.L. : Cocaine and amphetamine antagonize the decrease of noradrenergic neurotransmission elicited by oxymetazoline but potentiate the inhibition by alpha-methyl norepinephrine in the perfused cat spleen. J. Pharmac. Exp. Ther. (submitted).

20 Dubocovich, M.L., Langer, S.Z., and Moret, C. : Antagonism by α-amphetamine of the inhibition of ^{3}H-noradrenaline overflow obtained by alpha-adrenoceptor agonists or bretylium in the perfused cat spleen. Br. J. Pharmac. 66, 460P, 1979.

21 Enero, M.A. and Langer S.Z. : Influence of reserpine-induced depletion of noradrenaline on the negative feed-back mechanism for transmitter release during nerve stimulation. 49, 214-225, 1973.

22 Cubeddu, L.X. and Weiner, N. : Nerve-stimulation mediated overflow of norepinephrine and dopamine β-hydroxylase. III. Effects of norepinephrine depletion on the alpha-presynaptic regulation of release. J. Pharmac. Exp. Ther. 192, 1-14, 1975.

23 Rand, M.J., Story, D.F., Allen, G.S., Glover, A.B., and McCulloch, M.W. : Pulse-to-pulse modulation of noradrenaline release through a prejunctional receptor auto-inhibitory mechanism. In " Frontiers in Catecholamine Research", eds. E. Usdin and S.H. Snyder, pp 579-581, Pergamon Press, New York, 1973.

24 Adler-Graschinsky, E., and Langer, S.Z. : Possible role of a β-adrenoceptor in the regulation of noradrenaline release by nerve stimulation through a positive feed-back mechanism. Br. J. Pharmac. 53, 43-50, 1975.

25 Celuch, S.M., Dubocovich, M.L. and Langer, S.Z. : Stimulation of presynaptic β-adrenoceptors enhances ^{3}H-noradrenaline release during nerve stimulation in the perfused cat spleen. Br. J. Pharmac. 63, 97-108, 1978.

26 Dahlöf, C., Ljung, B., and Ablad, B. : Increased noradrenaline release in the rat portal vein during sympathetic nerve stimulation due to activity of presynaptic β-adrenoceptors by noradrenaline and adrenaline. Eur. J. Pharmac. 50, 75-78, 1978.

27 Westfall, T.C., Peach, M.J., and Titermary, V. : Enhancement of the electrically induced release of norepinephrine from the rat portal vein : mediation by β_2-adrenoceptors. Eur. J. Pharmac. 58, 67-74, 1974.

28 Hedqvist, P., and Moawad, A. : Presynaptic α- and β-adrenoceptor mediated control of noradrenaline release in human oviduct. Acta Physiol. Scand., 95, 494-496, 1975.

29 Yamaguchi, N., De Champlain, J., and Nadeau, R.A. : Regulation of norepinephrine release from cardiac sympathetic fibers in the dog by presynaptic alpha and beta-receptors. Circulation Res. 41, 108-117, 1977.

30 Dahlöf, C., Åblad, B., Borg, K.O., EK, L., and Waldeck, B. : Prejunctional inhibition of adrenergic nervous vasomotor control due to β-receptor blockade. Proceeds. Symposium on "Chemical Tools in Catecholamine Research. Vol.II, pp 201-210, eds. Almgren, O., Carlsson, A. and Engel, J. Amsterdam : North-Holland Publishing Company, 1975.

31 Stjärne, L., and Brundin, J. : Dual adrenoceptor-mediated control of noradrenaline secretion from human vasoconstrictor nerves : facilitation by β-receptors and inhibition by α-receptors.. Acta Physiol. Scand., 94, 139-141, 1975.

32 Barret, A.M., and Nunn, B. : Adrenergic neuron blocking properties of (±)-propranolol and (+)-propranolol. J. Pharm. Pharmac., 22, 806-810, 1970.

33 Hughes, I.E., and Kneen, B. : The effect of propranolol on sympathetic nerve stimulation in isolated vasa deferentia. J. Pharm. Pharmac., 28, 200-205, 1976.

34 Guimaraes, S., Brandao, F., and Paiva, M.Q. : A study of the adrenoceptor-mediated feedback mechanisms by using adrenaline as a false transmitter. Naunyn-Schmiedeberg's Arch. Pharmacol. 305, 185-188, 1978.

35 Rand, M.J., Majewski, H., Mc Culloch, M.W. and Story, D.F. : An adrenaline-mediated positive feedback loop in sympathetic transmission and its possible role in hypertension. In "Presynaptic receptors, eds. S.Z. Langer, K. Starke and M.L. Dubocovich, Pergamon Press, Oxford, pp 263-269, 1979.

36 Weinstock, M., Thoa, N.B., and Kopin, I.J. : β-adrenoceptors modulate noradrenaline release from axonal sprouts in cultured rat superior cervical ganglia. Eur. J. Pharmacol, 47, 297-302, 1978.

37 Dismukes, K., Mulder, A.H.: Cyclic AMP and α-receptor-mediated modulation of noradrenaline release from rat brain slices. Eur. J. Pharmac. 39, 383-388, 1976.

38 Dubocovich, M.L. : Pharmacological differences between the alpha-presynaptic adrenoceptors in the peripheral and the central nervous system. In : "Presynaptic Receptors", eds. S.Z. Langer, K. Starke and M.L. Dubocovich, Pergamon Press, Oxford, pp 29-36,1979.

39 Galzin, A.M., Dubocovich, M.L., and Langer, S.Z. : Presynaptic inhibitory receptors are present on the noradrenergic nerve terminals of the rabbit hypothalamus. Eur. J. Pharmac., submitted.

40 Baumann, P.A. and Koella, W.P. : Feed-back control of noradrenaline release as a function of noradrenaline concentration in the synaptic cleft in cortical slices of the rat. Brain Research 189, 437-448, 1980.

41 Bryant, B.J., McCulloch, M.W., Rand, M.J. and Story, D.F. : Release of ^{3}H-noradrenaline from guinea-pig hypothalamic slices : effects of adrenoceptor agonists and antagonists. Br. J. Pharmacol. 53, 454P, 1975.

42 Rand, M.J., Mc Culloch, M.W. and Story, D.F. : Prejunctional modulation of noradrenergic transmission by noradrenaline, dopamine and acetylcholine. In "Central action of drugs in blood pressure regulation" (eds) D.S. Davis and J.L. Reid, Pitman Medical Publishing, Townbridge Wells, pp.94-132, 1975.

43 De Langen, C.D.J., Hogenboom, F. and Mulder, A.H. : Presynaptic noradrenergic α-receptors and modulation of ^{3}H-noradrenaline release from rat brain synaptosomes. Eur. J. Pharmacol. 60, 79-89, 1979.

44 Svensson, T.H., Bunney, B.S. and Aghajanian, G.K. : Inhibition of both noradrenergic and serotoninergic neurons in brain by the α-adrenergic agonist clonidine. Brain Res. 92, 291-306, 1975.

45 Miach, P.J., Dausse, J.P., and Meyer, P. : Direct biochemical demonstration of two types of α-adrenoceptor in rat brain. Nature 274, 492-494, 1978.

46 U'Prichard, D.C. and Snyder, S.H. : Distinct α-noradrenergic receptors differenciated by binding and physiological relationship. Life Sciences 24, 79-88, 1979.

47 Kehr, W., Carlsson, A., Lindqvist, M., Magnusson, T and Atack, C. : Evidence for a receptor-mediated feedback control of striatal tyrosine hydroxylase activity. J. Pharmacol, 24, 744-747, 1972.

48 Farnebo, L.O., and Hamberger, B. : Drug-induced changes in the release of ^{3}H-monoamines from field stimulated rat brain slices. Acta Physiol. Scand., Suppl. 35-44, 1971.

49 Raiteri, M., Cervoni, A.M., and Del Carmine, R. : Do presynaptic autoreceptors control dopamine release ? Nature 274, 706-708, 1978.

50 Raiteri, M., Cervoni, A.M., Del Carmine, R., and Levi, G. : Lack of presynaptic autoreceptors controlling dopamine release in striatal synaptosomes. In : "Presynaptic Receptors", eds. S.Z. Langer, K.Starke and M.L. Dubocovich, Pergamon Press, Oxford, pp 225-230, 1979.

51 Starke, K., Reimann, W., Zumstein, A., and Hertting, G. : Effect of dopamine receptor agonists and antagonists on the release of dopamine in the rabbit caudate nucleus in vitro. Naunyn-Schmiedeberg's Arch. Pharmac. 305, 27-36, 1978.

52 Reimann, W., Zumstein, A., Jackisch, R. Starke, K. and Hertting, G. : Effect of extracellular dopamine on the release of dopamine in the rabbit caudate nucleus : evidence for a dopaminergic feed-back inhibition. Naunyn-Schmiedeberg's Arch. Pharmacol. 306, 53-40, 1979.

53 Tamminga, C.A., Schaffer, M.H., Smith, R.C. and Davis, J.M. : Schizophrenic symptoms improve with apomorphine. Science 200, 567-568, 1978.

54 DiChiara, G., Porceddu, M.L., Spano, P.F. and Gessa, G.L. : Haloperidol increases and apomorphine decreases striatal dopamine metabolism after destruction of striatal dopamine-sensitive adenylate cyclase by kainic acid. Brain Research 130, 374-382, 1977.

55 Aghajanian, G.K., and Bunney, B.S. : Central dopaminergic neurons : Neurophysiological identification and responses to drugs. In : "Frontiers in Catecholamine Research" (ed.E. Usdin and S.M. Snyder), pp 643-648, Pergamon Press, Oxford, 1973.

56 Aghajanian, G.K. and Bunney, B.S. : Dopamine "autoreceptors" : Pharmacological characterization by microiontophonetic single cell recordings studies. Arch. Pharcol, 297, 1-7., 1977.

57 Dray, A. and Straughan, D.W. : Synaptic mechanisms in the substantia nigra. J. Pharmacol. 28, 400-405, 1976.

58 Arbilla, S. and Langer, S.Z. : Influence of monoamine oxidase inhibition on the release of ^{3}H-dopamine elicited by potassium and by amphetamine from the rat substantia nigra and corpus striatum. Naunyn-Schmiedeberg's Arch. Pharmacol. 311, 45-52, 1980.

59 Geffen, L.B., Jessel, T.M., Cuello, A.C. and Iversen, L.L. : Release of dopamine from dendrites in the rat substantia nigra. Nature 260, 258-260, 1976.

60 Gale, K., Guidotti, A. and Costa, E. : Dopamine sensitive adenylate cyclase : location in the substantia nigra. Science, 195, 503-505, 1977.

61 Kebabian, J.W. and Saavedra, J.M. : Dopamine sensitive adenylate cyclase occurs in a region of substantia nigra containing dopaminergic dendrites. Science 193, 683-685, 1976.

62 Kebabian, J.W and Calne, D.B. : Multiple receptors for dopamine. Nature 277, 93-96, 1977.

63 Pinnock, R.D., Woodruff, G.N. and Turnbull, M.J. : Sulpiride blocks the action of dopamine in the rat substantia nigra. Eur. J. Pharmacol. 56, 413-414, 1979.

64 Arbilla, S., Kamal, L.A. and Langer, S.Z. : Presynaptic dopamine receptors modulate electrical stimulation but not amphetamine-evoked release of ^{3}H-dopamine from the rabbit caudate nucleus. Br. J. Pharmacol. (in press).

Neurotransmitters and their Receptors
Edited by U.Z. Littauer, Y. Dudai, I. Silman,
V.I. Teichberg and Z. Vogel

Mechanism of Alpha-adrenergic Inhibition of Catecholamine Secretion

Yehuda Gutman

Department of Pharmacology, The Hebrew University-Hadassah Faculty of Medicine, Jerusalem

ABSTRACT

Activation of alpha adrenergic receptors inhibits the secretion of catecholamines (CA) in adrenergic nerve endings and in chromaffin cells of the adrenal medulla. This effect could be shown in CA secretion induced by acetylcholine (10^{-4}M) or by high potassium (56mM). Both of these stimuli cause exocytotic secretion and are totally dependent on calcium. Tyramine-induced CA secretion, which is not exocytotic, was not affected by alpha adrenergic agonists. Secretion of CA induced by ouabain or by omission of potassium from the medium was also not affected by adrenergic agonists or antagonists. Under these conditions the sodium potassium pump is inactivated.

Alpha-adrenergic agonists increased Na,K-ATPase activity in membrane fractions of adrenal medulla, as well as of the submaxillary gland, which is richly supplied with adrenergic nerve endings. The effect of alpha agonists on Na,K-ATPase in the salivary gland was increased after ligation of the excretory duct (which results in involution of glandular cells without affecting nerve endings). After sympathetic denervation of the submaxillary gland the effect of alpha adrenergic agonists on Na,K-ATPase was abolished. This suggested that alpha agonists cause reduced CA release through activation of the sodium pump.

Calcium efflux from adrenal medulla and from submaxillary glands was studied in vitro. Alpha adrenergic agonists enhanced calcium efflux from both tissues after preloading with ^{45}Ca. Alpha antagonists abolished this effect on calcium efflux. After sympathetic denervation of the submaxillary gland the effect of alpha agonists on calcium efflux was abolished. It is suggested that activation of the sodium pump by alpha adrenergic agonists results in enhancement of calcium efflux and a decrease of free intracellular calcium, thus causing inhibition of the exocytotic release of CA.

INTRODUCTION

The secretion of noradrenaline (=NA) from sympathetic nerve endings can be modulated in several ways. The frequency of nerve impulses at the nerve terminal determines the amount of NA released into the synaptic area. However, reuptake of NA into the terminal can affect the overflow of the transmitter following stimulation (1). More recently it has been shown that various modulators can act on the membrane of adrenergic nerve endings and affect secretion: alpha adrenergic agonists, beta-adrenergic agonists, dopamine, prostaglandins (PGE) (2). Of particular interest are alpha-adrenergic agonists since their action may indicate a physiologic mechanism, i.e. - that the endogenous transmitter, NA, acts as a negative feedback regulator of its own release. This possibility is supported by the finding that alpha adrenergic antagonists increase the release of NA following stimulation of sympathetic nerves (3).

However, the mechanism underlying the inhibition of NA secretion by activation of presynaptic alpha adrenergic receptors deserves some exploration. The presynaptic alpha receptors regulate exocytotic release of NA. This is indicated by the simultaneous inhibition of NA and dopamine-beta-hydroxylase (=DBH) secretion (4,5), while non-exocytotic release of catecholamines (CA), induced by tyramine, is not affected by alpha adrenergic agonists (6,7).

Adrenal medulla chromaffin cells secrete CA, in a process similar to that of adrenergic terminals. The secretion of CA by these cells has been shown to be modulated by the same agents as in sympathetic nerve endings (7), in particular-inhibition of exocytotic secretion by alpha agonists (5,7).

The effect of alpha agonists on presynaptic terminals has been suggested to be on a different receptor type (alpha-2) than that on post-synaptic receptors (alpha-1) (8). This assumption is based mainly on differences in potency of a series of alpha agonists and antagonists when pre- and post-synaptic effects are compared (8). However, a more basic difference between pre- and post-synaptic effects may be discerned: Activation of post-synaptic alpha-receptors causes smooth muscle contraction (spleen, vascular muscle, nictitating membrane) or induces secretion in exocrine glands (salivary glands). In all these cases the effects induced by alpha receptor activation are mediated by increased intra-cellular calcium and can be mimmicked by application of a calcium ionophore (provided calcium is present extracellularly).

On the other hand, the presynaptic action of alpha agonists causes inhibition of exocytotic NA secretion and could imply reduced intra-cellular calcium concentration, although other mechanisms for inhibiting Na release may be formulated.

MATERIALS AND METHODS

Experiments were carried-out on bovine adrenal medulla, rat adrenal glands and the submaxillary glands of rats. Bovine adrenals were obtained from the slaughterhouse, placed on ice and immediately brought to the laboratory. The adrenal medulla was separated from the cortex by dissection. Slices of adrenal medulla (10-20 mg each) were incubated in Locke's solution or modified solutions, as specified. Rat adrenal glands were taken out through a mid-abdominal incision, following dislocation of the neck. Submaxillary glands were obtained through a midline incision in the neck of rats under ether anesthesia. Sympathetic denervation of the submaxillary glands was achieved by superior cervical ganglionectomy three weeks prior to the experiments. Submaxillary duct ligation was performed through a midline incision in the neck in rats under ether anesthesia. This procedure was also carried out three weeks prior to experiment.

The secretion of CA from adrenals was studied in rat adrenals and bovine adrenal medulla slices by incubation at $37^{o}C$ for 10 min, with constant shaking. At the end of incubation the medium was separated from the slice, acidified with $HClO_4$ (0.4M final concentration) and the amount of adrenaline (A) and noradrenaline (NA) was assayed by the trihydroxyindole method, as described previously (9).

For studies on calcium fluxes slices of adrenal medulla were incubated in Locke's solution containing 0.1 uCi/ml of $^{45}CaCl_2$. The incubation was carried out for 20 min. at $37^{o}C$. For study of the influx of ^{45}Ca, the slices were separated at the end of incubation, blotted on filter paper, weighed and then each slice was extracted overnight in 2 ml of distilled water in a thermostatic bath with constant shaking. The amount of ^{45}Ca was then determined in an aliquot of 0.2 ml of the extraction medium. Preliminary experiments have shown that no further extraction of ^{45}Ca was obtained by more prolonged incubation.

For the study of ^{45}Ca efflux, the slices were first loaded with ^{45}Ca, as described. Following the loading, each slice was blotted on filter paper, rinsed shortly in ice-cold solution (of the same composition to be used for superfusion) blotted again on filter paper and then placed on a funnel. Superfusion of the slice was then started, at the rate of 0.2 ml/min, for 30 min. The effluent fluid was collected in samples of

2 min. At the end of superfusion each slice was extracted, as described above. The total amount of ^{45}Ca at the beginning of the superfusion was calculated as the sum of the ^{45}Ca in the effluent during superfusion and that found in the slice at the end of superfusion. The amount of ^{45}Ca present in the slice at each time during the superfusion was then expressed as per-cent of that present at time 0 (beginning of superfusion) and plotted against time.

For assay of Na, K-Activated ATPase a membrane fraction was isolated from homogenates of adrenal medulla and submaxillary glands, as previously described (10). Total ATPase activity was assayed by incubation in a medium consisting of 100 mM NaCl, 10 mM KCl, 4 mM $MgCl_2$, 4 mM ATP and 33 mM Tris buffer (pH 7.4). Mg-ATPase was assessed either by omission of KCl or by addition of ouabain (10^{-3}M) and the difference between total ATPase and Mg ATPase was calculated as Na,K-ATPase activity.

RESULTS AND DISCUSSION

Addition of alpha adrenergic agonists (phenylephrine, naphazoline, clonidine) caused significant inhibition of CA secretion from the adrenal glands induced either by the addition of acetyl-choline (ACh) or by incubation in a high potassium (56 mM K^+) Locke's medium (11). This effect was found also in human adrenal medulla in vitro (12). Injection of NA to rats in vivo also inhibited the release of CA from the adrenal medulla of rats induced by insulin hypoglycemia (13).

Furthermore, in the presence of alpha-adrenergic antagonists (phentolamine, phenoxybenzamine) CA release from the adrenal medulla was increased (11). Thus, the same modulatory effect on CA secretion seems to be effective in adrenal medulla as in adrenergic nerve terminals.

CA secretion from adrenal medulla can be stimulated by incubation in a potassium-free medium or in Locke's medium with ouabain (10^{-3}M). However, under these two conditions addition of either alpha adrenergic agonists or alpha antagonists had no significant effect on CA secretion (11). Since both of these conditions cause inhibition of the sodium pump, the effect of alpha agonists was next studied on the activity of Na,K-ATPase. Various alpha adrenergic agonists (NA, naphazoline, phenylephrine) caused significant activation of Na,K-ATPase in a membrane preparation of adrenal medulla _in vitro_ (7, 11).

A membrane preparation of submaxillary glands was prepared from the duct-ligated gland. This procedure, induces degeneration of glandular cell while preserving adrenergic nerve endings, as can be seen in Table 1. In a membrane preparation of the duct-ligated submaxillary gland alpha-adrenergic agonists (clonidine, naphazoline, phenylephrine) caused activation of Na,K-ATPase but had no effect on Mg-ATPase (14). This activation was inhibited by alpha antagonists (Fig. 1) and was abolished after aympathetic denervation of the submaxillary gland. This would indicate that the effect of the alpha-agonists was on Na,K-ATPase activity in sympathetic nerve endings and not in glandular tissue.

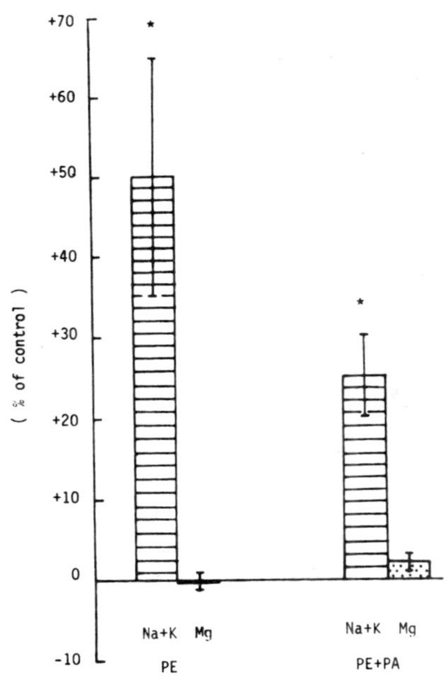

Fig. 1. Effect of phentolamine on phenylephrine stimulation of Na,K-ATPase activity in the submaxillary gland.

Na + K - Effect on Na,K-ATPase activity; Mg - Effect on Mg-ATPase activity. PE - Effect of 10^{-5}M phenylephrine (N=31); PE + PA - Phenylephrine (10^{-5}M) and phentolamine (10^{-5}M) present simultaneously (N=25). Vertical bars - s.e. mean $*p < 0.01$.

It has been previously reported that very low concentrations of cardiac glycosides cause an increase rather than inhibition of Na,K-ATPase activity in kidney (15). When the effect of low concentration of ouabain was studied on a membrane fraction of adrenal medulla we observed activation of Na,K-ATPase at concentrations of 10^{-9}M - 10^{-11}M (14). The effect of 10^{-10}M ouabain was then studied on the release of CA from adrenal medulla in vitro. This low concentration of ouabain caused in fact inhibition of CA secretion (16). This experiment further supports the possibility that activation of the sodium pump causes inhibition of CA secretion. Furthermore, when CA secretion was induced by a potassium-free medium (i.e. - by causing inactivation of the sodium pump) the inhibitory effect of low concentrations of ouabain on CA secretion was abolished (16).

Table 1. Effect of various surgical procedures on noradrenaline content and Na,K - ATPase activity of submaxillary gland.

	Control	Denervated	Ligature	Ligature & Denervation
Noradrenaline (μg/gland)	0.19±0.01 (N=11)	0.04±0.006 (N=6)	0.18±0.01 (N=8)	0.07±0.006 (N=3)
Na,K - ATPase (μmole Pi/mg prot. x hr)	28.6±1.4 (N=28)	34.6±2.6 (N=28)	10.3±0.8 (N=34)	6.1±0.4 (N=38)

N - number of experiments. Results expressed as mean ± s.e. mean. Ligature - submaxillary glands taken three weeks after ligation of the major salivary duct. Denervated - sympathetically denervated glands by superior cervical ganglionectomy. For noradrenaline content - "denervated" compared to "control" and "denervation + ligature" compared to "ligature" $p < 0.01$. For Na,K - ATPase activity - ligature vs. control, ligature + denervation vs. ligature $p < 0.01$.

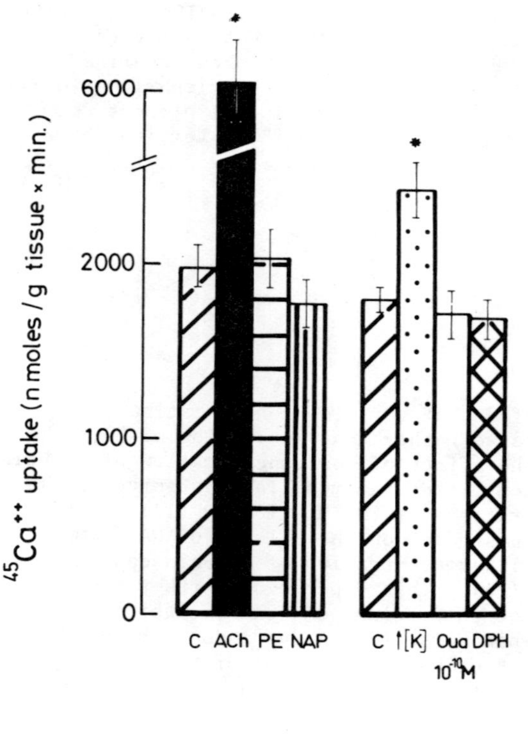

Fig. 2 Effect of various agents on ^{45}Ca uptake by slices of adrenal medulla in vitro.

For each column of the group on the left side of the figure - N=20; for each column of the group on the right side of the figure - N=10. Vertical bars - s.e. mean C - uptake of ^{45}Ca by control slices; ACH - uptake of ^{45}Ca in the presence of 10^{-4}M acetylcholine; PE - uptake of ^{45}Ca in the presence of 10^{-5}M phenylephrine; Nap. - uptake of ^{45}Ca in the presence of 10^{-5}M naphazoline. ↑[K] - uptake of ^{45}Ca in the presence of 56mM K^+; Oua 10^{-10}M - uptake of ^{45}Ca in the presence of 10^{-10}M ouabain; DPH - uptake of ^{45}Ca in the presence of 10^{-4}M diphenylhydantoin. *$p<0.01$ compared to control (C).

The inhibition of CA secretion by alpha adrenergic agonists concerns exocytotic secretion. Since exocytotic secretion depends on an increase of free intracellular calcium concentration (Ca_i) one possibility for the mechanism of action of alpha-adrenergic agonists could be an effect on Ca_i. Reduction of Ca_i will inhibit exocytosis. This could be achieved either by inhibition of calcium influx or by acceleration of calcium removal from the cytoplasm. The latter could be caused by binding of calcium to intracellular organelles or by calcium efflux from the cell.

Fig. 2 shows that alpha-agonists (as well as low ouabain concentrations) which inhibited CA secretion had no significant effect on ^{45}Ca influx, while ACh or high potassium (56 mM)enhanced ^{45}Ca uptake.

On the other hand, alpha-adrenergic agonists had a pronounced effect on ^{45}Ca efflux from adrenal medulla slices, i.e. - acceleration of efflux (14). A similar phenomenon was observed on ^{45}Ca efflux from slices of submaxillary glands (with excretory ducts ligated 3 weeks prior to the experiment) (14). Furthermore, this enhancement of ^{45}Ca efflux was abolished by the addition of an alpha-adrenergic antagonist (phentolamine) as well as by sympathetic denervation of the submaxillary gland. Thus, alpha adrenergic agonists enhance efflux of ^{45}Ca from adrenergic nerve endings but not from other components of the gland.

The finding that alpha adrenergic agonists increase Na,k-ATPase activity has been reported in muscle and brain (17,18). On the other hand enhancement of calcium efflux by alpha adrenrgic agonists has been reported in liver (19) and muscle (20). Can these two phenomena be related as cause and effect, i.e. : can enhancement of the sodium pump induce calcium efflux? Sodium and calcium movement have been suggested to be associated by a common carrier system. This has been suggested for heart (21) and for other tissues (22). It has been suggested that this carrier exchanges sodium for calcium. Thus, intracellular sodium would move out and cause influx of calcium into the cell whereas movement of extracellular sodium into the cell would cause calcium extrusion simultaneously. In this Na,Ca - antiporter system the concentration gradient of sodium could, therefore, determine the direction of calcium movement and would potentially contribute to the calcium gradient. A similar Na,Ca anti-porter system has also been suggested in membranes of heart mitochondria (23), thus an increase of Na_i could cause release of calcium from the mitochondria while a fall of Na_i would decrease release of calcium and thus reduce free Ca_i.

Recently such a system has been described in vesicles formed of heart muscle cell membrane fragments. These sarcolemmal vesicles showed Na,Ca anti-porter flow and a sodium pump (inhibited by ouabain) (24).

If a Na,Ca carrier of similar nature acts in adrenergic nerve endings and adrenal chromaffin cells, one would expect that an increased activity of the sodium pump (caused by alpha-adrenergic agonists) would result in lowering of Na_i and, therefore, increased sodium gradient. This should enhance the exchange extracellular sodium-intracellular calcium and thus accelerate calcium efflux, as observed experimentally in adrenal medulla and submaxillary gland slices (14).

The generalized scheme of alpha adrenergic inhibition of CA secretion would, therefore, be as follows:

1. Alpha agonists → Na,K-ATPase ⟶ $\overset{Na_o}{\underset{Na_i}{\uparrow}}$
2. $\begin{matrix} Na_o & & Ca_o \\ \downarrow & \times & \uparrow \\ Na_i & & Ca_i \end{matrix}$ ← Na,Ca antiporter system
3. ↓ Ca_i → reduced exocytosis

Interestingly, a very similar sequence of events has been recently suggested for the relaxation of smooth muscle by CA (25). The only difference is that the initial step in this case is activation of adenylate cyclase by beta-adrenergic agonists. The increased level of cAMP serves in this case to activate Na,K-ATPase and the rest of the sequence follows the same steps (25). The reduced Ca_i (due to increased calcium efflux) in the smooth muscle would when inhibit contraction.

It is also of interest that by increasing Na_i we could induce enhanced secretion of CA from chromaffin cells. This experiment was carried out in calcium-free medium. Thus, only intracellular calcium stores could be involved. The increase of Na_i was induced by incubating the chromaffin cells in the presence of liposomes loaded with sodium. Fusion of the liposomes with the cells resulted in release of CA. If EGTA was incorporated in the liposomes together with sodium the release of CA was blocked (26). Thus it seems that sodium may affect both intracellular calcium stores in adrenal medulla as well as calcium efflux through the cell membrane.

REFERENCES

1. IVERSEN, L.L. Br. J. Pharmacol. 41, 571, 1971.

2. STARKE, K., TAUBE, H.D. and BOROWSKI, E. Biochem. Pharmacol. 26, 259, 1977.

3. LANGER, S.Z., ADLER-GRASCHINSKY, E. and GIORGI, O. Nature 265, 648, 1977.

4. DE POTTER, W.P., CHUBB, I.W., PUT, A. and DE SCHAEPDRYVER, A.F. Arch. Int. Pharmacodyn. Ther. 193, 191, 1971.

5. BOONYAVIROJ, P., SEIDEN, A. and GUTMAN, Y. Biochem. Pharmacol. 26, 351, 1977.

6. STARKE, K. and MONTEL, H. Eur. J. Pharmacol. 27, 273, 1974.

7. GUTMAN, Y. in: Advances in Pharmacology and Therapeutics, Ed. SIMON P. Pergamon Press, Oxford, 2, 217, 1978.

8. LANGER, S.Z. Biochem. Pharmacol. 23, 1973, 1974.

9. FEUERSTEIN, G., BOONYAVIROJ, P. and GUTMAN, Y. Eur. J. Pharmacol. 44, 131, 1977.

10. GUTMAN, Y., HOCHMAN, S. and WALD, H. Biochim. Biophys. Acta. 298, 284, 1973.

11. GUTMAN, Y. and BOONYAVIROJ, P. J. Neural Trans. 40, 245, 1977.

12. BOONYAVIROJ, P. and GUTMAN, Y. Eur. J. Pharmacol. 41, 73, 1977.

13. GUTMAN, Y. and BOONYAVIROJ, P. Eur. J. Pharmacol. 22, 384, 1974.

14. COHEN, J., ECKSTEIN, L. and GUTMAN, Y. Br. J. Pharmac. (in press).

15. PALMER, P.F. and NECHAY, B.R. J. Pharmacol. Exp. Ther. 146, 92, 1969.

16. GUTMAN, Y. and BOONYAVIROJ, P. Naunyn-Schmiedeberg's Arch. Pharmacol. 296, 293, 1977.

17. BRESSLER, B.H., PHILLIS, J.W. and KOZACHUK, W. Eur. J. Pharmacol. 33, 208, 1975.

18. LEE, S.K. and PHILLIS, J.W. Can. J. Physiol. Pharmacol. 55, 961, 1977.

19. BLACKMORE, P.F., ASSIMACOPOULOS-JEANNET, F., CHAN, T.M. and EXTON, J.H. J. Biol. Chem. 254, 2828, 1979.

20. ISSEBAH, A.H., CLARKE, P., VYDELINGUM, N., HOPE-GILL, H., TULLOCH, B. and FRASER, T.R. Eur. J. Clin. Invest. 5, 339, 1975.

21. LANGER, G.A. Circ. Res. 17, 78, 1965.

22. BLAUSTEIN, M.P. Rev. Physiol. Biochem. Pharmacol. 70, 33, 1974.

23. CROMPTON, M., CAPANO, M. and CARAFOLI, E. Eur. J. Biochem. 69, 453, 1976.

24. PITTS, B.J. J. Biol. Chem. 254, 6232, 1979.

25. SCHEID, R.C., HONEYMAN, T.W. and FAY, F.S. Nature 277, 32, 1979.

26. GUTMAN, Y., LICHTENBERG, D., COHEN, J. and BOONYAVIROJ, P. Biochem. Pharmacol. 28, 1209, 1979.

Neurotransmitters and their Receptors
Edited by U.Z. Littauer, Y. Dudai, I. Silman,
V.I. Teichberg and Z. Vogel

In Vivo and In Vitro Studies on the Presynaptic Control of Dopamine Release from Nerve Terminals of the Nigrostriatal Dopaminergic Neuron

M.F. Giorguieff-Chesselet, A. Chéramy and J. Glowinski

Groupe MB, Inserm U. 114, Collège de France, 75231 Paris 5, France

ABSTRACT

Two complementary approaches were used to study the role of neurotransmitters present in striatal nerve endings on the regulation of the release of dopamine (DA) from terminals of the nigrostriatal dopaminergic neurons. Their effects, those of their agonists or antagonists were examined both *in vitro* on rat striatal slices and *in vivo* on the cat caudate nucleus using push pull cannulae, by measuring changes in the spontaneous release of ^{3}H-DA continuously synthetized from ^{3}H-tyrosine.

Acetylcholine (ACh), oxotremorine and nicotine, GABA and GABA related compounds, L-glutamic acid, glycine and angiotensin II enhanced the release of newly synthetized ^{3}H-DA from striatal slices. These effects which could be direct or indirect involved specific receptors since they were reduced in all cases by respective antagonists. Curiously, in agreement with results of others, morphine was without effect on ^{3}H-DA release.

Both ACh and GABA stimulated the release of newly synthetized ^{3}H-DA from the caudate nucleus of halothane anesthetized cats. By contrast to that observed *in vitro*, morphine enhanced the *in vivo* release of ^{3}H-DA. The electrical stimulation of cortico-striatal fibers, thought to be glutamatergic, enhanced the release of ^{3}H-DA. Finally, it was shown that the presynaptic regulation of DA release could be dependent on the activity of nigral DA cells since the stimulatory effect of ACh on ^{3}H-DA release in the caudate nucleus was not seen any more after activation of these neurons induced by the local application of substance P in the substantia nigra.

I - INTRODUCTION

It is well known that the amount of neurotransmitter released from nerve terminals is dependent on nerve impulse flow. However, this mechanism is not the only one involved since the release process can also be regulated by presynaptic influences. Via presynaptic receptors located on nerve terminals, various neurotransmitters or pharmacological agents can modulate the release of the neurotransmitter. This phenomenon has been demonstrated, in particular, on peripheral noradrenergic neurons, which possess not only noradrenergic presynaptic receptors but also several other receptors including those of the muscarinic and nicotinic varieties (1). Thus, the release of noradrenaline may be increased or reduced by drugs interacting with these receptors. Presynaptic regulation of the release process may also intervene in physiological condition. For example, in peripheral organs innervated both by noradrenergic and cholinergic neurons, the stimulation of the cholinergic neurons was shown to reduce the release of noradrenaline (2).

Our interest in studying presynaptic modulations in the control of neurotransmitter release from central neurons began several years ago when we observed that ACh could evoke the release of ^{3}H-DA previously synthetized from ^{3}H-tyrosine in the isolated rat striatum(3).This structure is devoid of catecholaminergic cell bodies but is densely innervated by dopaminergic arborizations originating from cells grouped in the mesencephalon and contains relatively few noradrenergic terminals (4). For these anatomical reasons, the nigrostriatal dopaminergic system is thus highly appropriate for such studies.

2) Methodological considerations

Two approaches were used. The first one consisted in measuring the release of DA from striatal slices superfused with a physiological medium. This study was complemented by *in vivo* experiments in the cat, where the caudate nucleus was superfused originally with a cup and more recently with a push-pull cannula. In both cases, we measured the release of ^{3}H-DA continuously synthetized from L-3,5-^{3}H-tyrosine of high specific activity (5Ci/mM,50 μCi/ml), the ^{3}H-amine being isolated from its ^{3}H-precursor and ^{3}H-metabolites by ion-exchange chromatography on Amberlite CG50 and adsorption on alumina (5,6). This method has several advantages:1) it ensures specificity since tyrosine hydroxylase is only contained in catecholaminergic neurons (7) ; 2) it is possible to detect changes in the release of the newly synthetized ^{3}H-neurotransmitter which is preferentially involved in the release process (8); 3) it is much more sensitive than all other techniques presently available since as little as 10 fentomoles of ^{3}H-DA can be acurately measured in superfusates, this allowing the estimation of the spontaneous release of the ^{3}H-amine not only *in vivo* but also *in vitro* ; 4) finally,since one molecule of ^{3}H-H_2O is formed during the conversion of 3,5-^{3}H-tyrosine into ^{3}H-DOPA, information about the rate of ^{3}H-DA synthesis can be simultaneously obtained by measuring ^3H-H_2O in superfusates. Even in striatal slices, the spontaneous release of newly synthetized ^{3}H-DA can be regarded as a physiological process since it is reduced in the presence of a calcium-free medium or of tetrodotoxin (5). The *in vitro* and *in vivo* approaches offer complementary advantages. Results obtained with slices reveal events that are intrastriatal since exogenous neurotransmitters or pharmacological agents act directly or indirectly on dopaminergic nerve terminals. By contrast, the relationships between presynaptic regulations and nerve activity can be studied *in vivo* since the integrity of the dopaminergic neurons is preserved. Moreover, in these experiments, striatal afferent pathways which may interact with dopaminergic terminals can be stimulated.

3) *In vitro studies*

Several neurotransmitters or putative neurotransmitters present in the striatum stimulated the spontaneous release of endogenously synthetized ^{3}H-DA in striatal slices of the rat. This was the case for ACh, GABA, L-glutamic acid, glycine and angiotensin which were used in rather low concentrations (between 10^{-6} and 5.10^{-5}M) (Table 1, fig.1). Although no comparative analysis was made, the increase in ^{3}H-DA release induced by these compounds reached an additional 70 to 150% of the spontaneous release value. These stimulatory effects appear to be mediated by specific receptors: the ACh (10^{-5}M) evoked release of ^{3}H-DA was antagonized either by muscarinic and nicotinic blockers such as atropine (10^{-6}M) or pempidine (10^{-5}M) respectively. Oxotremorine (10^{-5}M) and nicotine (10^{-6}M) mimicked the effect of ACh and were selectively blocked by their respective antagonists (5). The increased release of ^{3}H-DA induced by GABA (5.10^{-5}M) was partially prevented by picrotoxin (10^{-5}M) (9). Muscimol (10^{-5}M) and 3-amino propane sulfonic acid (5.10^{-5}M) drugs which are known to act on some GABAergic receptors also enhanced ^{3}H-DA release (10). The L-form of glutamic acid (5.10^{-5}M) stimulated the release of ^{3}H-DA but the D-form, used at the same concentration, was without effect (11). Strychnine reduced the glycine-evoked release of ^{3}H-DA (12). Finally, Sar^1, Ileu^8 angiotensin (5.10^{-5}M), a potent blocker of peripheral angiotensin receptors prevented the stimulatory effect of angiotensin (5. 10^{-5}M) on ^{3}H-DA release (13).

Table 1

Agonists	Conc.(M)	Stim. %	Antagonists	Conc.(M)	Inhib.%
ACh	10^{-5}	125	Atropine	10^{-6}	50
"	"	"	Pempidine	10^{-5}	50
"	"	"	Atropine + Pempidine	10^{-6} 10^{-5}	100
Oxo.	"	59	Atropine	10^{-6}	100
"	"	"	Pempidine	10^{-5}	0
Nic.	10^{-6}	72	Atropine	10^{-6}	0
"	"	"	Pempidine	10^{-5}	100
GABA	5.10^{-5}	80	Picrotoxin	10^{-5}	50
Glycine	5.10^{-5}	56	Strychnine	10^{-5}	40
L-GLU	"	62			
A II	"	50	Sar^{1}-Ileu-A II	5.10^{-5}	100

Effects of various neurotransmitters or agonists on the release of newly synthetized ^{3}H-DA in absence or in presence of antagonists in striatal slices of the rat.

Striatal slices were continuously superfused with a physiological medium containing L-3,5-^{3}H-tyrosine and ^{3}H-DA was estimated in successive superfusate fractions(2.5 min each). Neurotransmitters or their agonists were added for at least 7.5 min in the superfusion medium 22.5 min after the beginning of the superfusion. When antagonists were used they were added during all the superfusion. The stimulatory effect of each neurotransmitter or agonist corresponds to the mean changes in ^{3}H-DA release detected during 7.5 min expressed in percent of the spontaneous release. The inhibitory effect of antagonists was estimated by measuring the reduction of ^{3}H-DA release expressed in percent of the changes in ^{3}H-DA release induced by the neurotransmitters or agonists alone. The detailed analysis of these results can be found in previous published articles (5,9-13). (ACh = acetylcholine ; Oxo. oxotremorine ; Nic. = Nicotine; L-GLU = L-glutamic acid ; A II = angiotensin II).

In some experiments, the effects of ACh (10^{-5}M)(5), GABA(5. 10^{-5}M)(9) and angiotensin (10^{-6}M)(13) on ^{3}H-DA synthesis and release were studied simultaneously. In all cases the changes in ^{3}H-DA release were not associated with modifications of ^{3}H-DA synthesis.

Measuring changes in the release of ^{3}H-DA previously taken up in striatal slices other authors have also obtained indications of the existence of various striatal receptors involved

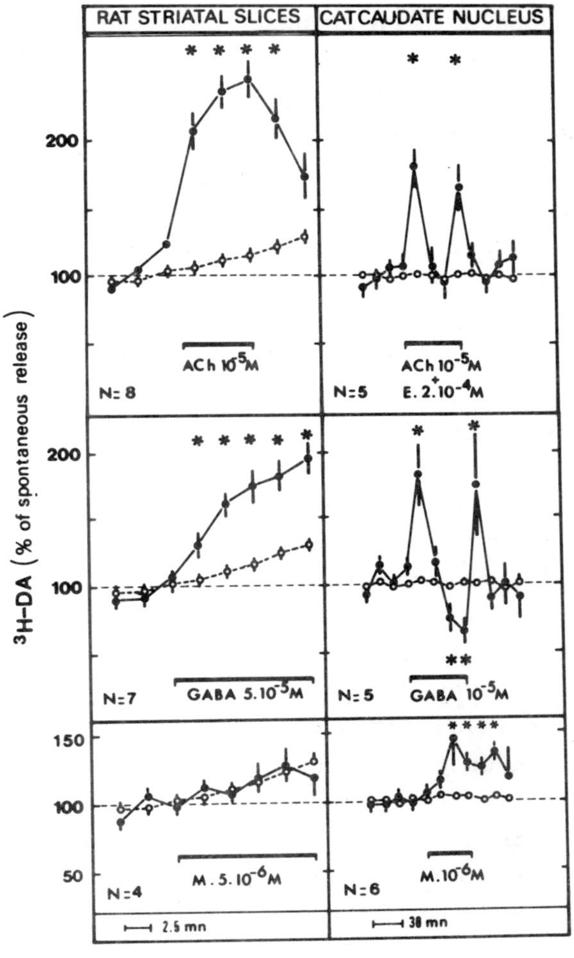

Fig. 1

Comparison of the in vitro and in vivo effects of ACh, GABA and morphine (M) on the spontaneous release of newly synthetized ^{3}H-DA

In vitro studies were made by superfusing rat striatal slices with L-3,5-^{3}H-tyrosine as described in table 1. In vivo studies were made in cats implanted with a push-pull cannula, ^{3}H-DA being estimated in superfusates during the continuous delivery of L-3,5-^{3}H-tyrosine. ACh was applied in presence of eserine(E). Results are expressed in percent of the spontaneous release of ^{3}H-DA estimated in 3 to 5 fractions just before the drug application.

* $p < .05$ when compared with results obtained with control slices or control cats (-o-).

in the control of DA release. ACh or metacholine reduced the release of exogenous ^{3}H-DA induced either by potassium, field stimulation or a high concentration of nicotine (10^{-3}M) and these effects were antagonized by atropine (14). Although GABA stimulated the potassium-evoked release of exogenous ^{3}H-DA, this effect was neither calcium-dependent, nor sensitive to picrotoxin nor mimicked by muscimol and 3-amino-propane sulfonic acid (15). Recently, however it has also been reported that GABA stimulates the spontaneous release of ^{3}H-DA ; this effect was inhibited by both picrotoxin and strychnine (16). A calcium-dependent stimulatory effect of L-glutamic acid on ^{3}H-DA release has also been observed, which could be antagonized by diethyl ester glutamic acid, one of the few drugs known to act as an antagonist of glutamatergic receptors. Surprisingly, however D-glutamic acid was as effective as L-glutamic acid in enhancing the spontaneous release of exogenous ^{3}H-DA (17). An efflux of the ^{3}H-amine was also shown to occur in the presence of glycine : it could be blocked by strychnine (16). As far as we know the effect of angiotensin II on the release of exogenous ^{3}H-DA has not yet been studied.

The receptors involved in the changes in DA release induced by ACh or other neurotransmitters or agonists might be located on dopaminergic terminals or on other neurons interacting with these terminals, ie the effects observed could be direct or indirect. Three procedures have been used to determine the location of some of these receptors:1) the first approach consists of studying the effects of neurotransmitters on the release of newly taken up or endogenously synthetized ^{3}H-DA from striatal synaptosomes. This method has only been used to test the effect of ACh which was shown to influence the potassium-evoked release of DA through muscarinic and nicotinic receptors (18); 2) the second method actually used in our own studies, was to examine the effects of neurotransmitters on the spontaneous release of newly synthetized ^{3}H-DA in the presence of tetrodotoxin. By blocking sodium channels, this neurotoxin should interrupt nerve activity and exclude indirect effects. However, care should be taken in interpreting the results since it must be remembered that tetrodotoxin is without effect on calcium spikes and that some sodium channels are resistant to the compound (19). In the presence of tetrodotoxin (5.10^{-7}M), ACh (10^{-5}M), oxotremorine (10^{-5}M), nicotine (10^{-6}M)(5) and L-glutamic acid (5.10^{-5}M)(11) still enhanced the release of ^{3}H-DA while GABA (5.10^{-5}M)(10) and glycine (5.10^{-5}M)(12) no longer exerted their stimulatory effects. These results favour the existence of muscarinic, nicotinic and L-glutamatergic presynaptic receptors on dopaminergic terminals and may suggest that this is not the case for the GABAergic and glycinergic receptors; 3) finally, attempts to localize presynaptic receptors on dopaminergic terminals can be made by measuring the reduction of binding of appropriate ligands after 6-hydroxydopamine-induced degeneration of the nigrostriatal dopaminergic neurons. This approach has also some limitations since a significant decrease in binding sites can hardly be detected if a large number of the same type of receptors is also located on striatal cells or fibers other than the dopaminergic terminals. Furthermore, the destruction of the dopaminergic neurons may induce changes in activity of striatal neurons and thus indirectly reduce the number of a population of striatal receptors. Thus, although we observed a decreased specific binding of ^{3}H-atropine on striatal membranes after selective destruction of the dopaminergic neurons, this effect was reversible and could not be attributed to the disappearance of muscarinic receptors located on dopaminergic terminals (20). Using ^{3}H-QNB, other authors also failed to detect a significant reduction of muscarinic receptors a long time after the degeneration of the dopaminergic neurons (21,22). As previously mentioned, due to the large number of muscarinic striatal binding sites, those which may be associated with dopaminergic nerve terminals could be difficult to identify with this approach. Similarly, no modification in the number of ^{3}H-muscimol binding sites was observed in 6-hydroxydopamine lesioned rats (22). In fact, at the moment binding studies combined with lesions of the dopaminergic neurons have demonstrated the presence of only nicotinic (21) and opiate receptors on dopaminergic terminals (22,23). This latter result prompted various authors to investigate the possible effect of morphine or enkephalines on DA release in striatal slices. Some groups reported that morphine and enkephalines reduced the potassium-evoked release of exogenous ^{3}H-DA (24,25) but others were unable to reproduce these findings although they could show the inhibitory effect of morphine on the potassium-evoked release of ^{3}H-noradrenaline in cortical slices (26). In our own experiments, morphine (5.10^{-6}M) did not modify the spontaneous release of endogenously synthetized ^{3}H-DA. These contradictory results may indicate that appropriate conditions, such as a critical state of depolarization of the membrane are a requisite for the detection of the presynaptic influence of opioid compounds on DA release from nerve terminals.

Wherever the location of the receptors by which neurotransmitters or agonists influence the release of DA is, these interactions may intervene *in vivo* and have a function. Indeed, the striatum is rich in cholinergic interneurons (27) and also receives cholinergic afferent inputs from the thalamus (28). GABA is not only contained in collaterals of the striato-nigral GABAergic neurons but also in interneurons (29). Numerous enkephalinergic neurons are also located in the striatum and a striato-pallidal projection has even been described. Lesion and biochemical studies have revealed the presence of striatal glutamatergic terminals originating from the anterior cortex (30). More recently, the angiotensin I converting enzyme has been visualized in striatal terminals with immuno-histochemical techniques (31) and results obtained in rats with striatal kainic acid lesions have suggested the existence of a striato-nigral angiotensin containing pathway (32). Finally, a specific high affinity uptake of glycine was demonstrated in striatal slices (33) and it has also been shown that the release of ^{3}H-glycine is evoked in slices of rat neonatal striatum by potassium through a calcium-dependent process (16). This could suggest the presence of glycinergic terminals in the striatum.

4) *In vivo studies*

The first experiments in cats with intact dopaminergic neurons consisted of reproducing some of the results obtained *in vitro* ie the determination of the local effects of exogenous neurotransmitters or agonists on ^{3}H-DA release. This has already been achieved for ACh, GABA and morphine (fig.1).

In the presence of eserine (2.10^{-4}M), ACh (10^{-5}M) stimulated the *in vivo* release of ^{3}H-DA endogenously synthetized from ^{3}H-tyrosine in the caudate nucleus of cats implanted with a cup (34) or a push-pull cannula (35). However, this effect was more complex than that observed *in vitro* since it did not last throughout the entire period of application of ACh (30 minutes) and a second prolonged increase of ^{3}H-DA release occurred after the removal of ACh from the superfusion fluid. Complex changes in ^{3}H-DA release were also seen with the delivery of GABA (10^{-5}M) (60 minutes) to the push-pull cannula (36). In this case, during the course of application of the amino-acid a stimulation followed by an inhibition of ^{3}H-DA release were observed. As seen following administration of ACh, a second increased release of ^{3}H-DA occurred at the end of the GABA application. Finally, in contrast to that observed *in vitro*, morphine (10^{-6}M) stimulated significantly the release of endogenously synthetized ^{3}H-DA *in vivo*. This effect differed from those induced by ACh or GABA since it was less pronounced and last during all the drug application.

Several factors could be responsible for the complexity of the *in vivo* effects of ACh and GABA on ^{3}H-DA release or for the difference in the *in vitro* and *in vivo* results obtained with morphine:1) variations between species, 2) indirect effects mediated by extrastriatal neuronal loops, 3) changes in the activity of dopaminergic cells which could influence presynaptic mechanisms.

To determine the influence of the activity of the dopaminergic neurons on presynaptic regulations, we examined the effect of the local application of ACh on the release of ^{3}H-DA during activation of nigral dopaminergic cells.Since we have shown that the striato-nigral substance P neurons exerts a tonic excitatory influence on dopaminergic neurons (38) we delivered substance P into the substantia nigra using cats implanted with a second push pull cannula. As expected the nigral application of substance P induced a prolonged increased release of ^{3}H-DA in the ipsilateral caudate nucleus which was reversed when the nigral substance P transmission was interrupted by the local application of a substance P antibody. In contrast to that observed in controls, the stimulatory effect of ACh on ^{3}H-DA release from nerve terminals was no longer detected during the activation of dopaminergic cells by substance P (35). Thus, the state of membrane polarization seems to be critical for the efficiency of presynaptic regulations. This is also supported by recent *in vivo* results obtained in the rat since it was shown that the intrastriatal injection of morphine stimulates DA turnover after interruption of the nigrostriatal pathway but is without effect in animals with intact dopaminergic neurons (38). This role of nerve activity on presynaptic regulations could also explain some of the differences seen in the *in vitro* effects of transmitters or agonists on the spontaneous or potassium-induced release of DA.

As discussed earlier, *in vivo* studies are an essential requisite for the demonstration of a physiological role of presynaptic mechanisms in the regulation of DA release from nerve terminals. The most convenient approach is to stimulate striatal afferents. Since the motor cortex sends a massive bilateral glutamatergic projection to the caudate nuclei we have investigated the effects of the unilateral electrical stimulation of the motor cortex on ^{3}H-DA release in the two caudate nuclei in cats implanted with two push-pull cannulae. This stimulus evoked the release of newly synthetized ^{3}H-DA in both structures (6). Furthermore, the contralateral effect was abolished after transection of the corpus callosum which is in agreement with the involvement of the cortico-striatal projection. Considering these results and the fact that L-glutamic acid stimulates ^{3}H-DA release from rat striatal slices (11) through a tetrodotoxin sensitive process we concluded that the cortico-striatal glutamatergic projection was implicated in a functional presynatpic regulation of DA release from the terminals of the nigrostriatal dopaminergic neurons. In order to establish more conclusively the existence of this regulation we are now reproducing the *in vivo* experiments in animals with acute transection of the nigrostriatal dopaminergic pathway.

5) CONCLUDING REMARKS

Several neurotransmitters or putative neurotransmitters present in the striatum stimulate the spontaneous release of endogenously synthetized ^{3}H-DA from striatal slices of the rat. As revealed by the blocking effects of respective antagonists, these changes in ^{3}H-DA release are mediated by receptors which may or may not be located on dopaminergic terminals. There is already evidence that the ACh and L-glutamic acid induced stimulation of ^{3}H-DA release are mediated by presynaptic receptors distributed on dopaminergic terminals. The exact localization of the GABA, glycine and angiotensin receptors involved in the intrastriatal regulation of DA release has yet to be determined. Although binding studies have clearly established the presence of presynaptic enkephalinergic receptors on dopaminergic terminals, the stimulatory effect of morphine on the spontaneous release of ^{3}H-DA has only been shown *in vivo* but not *in vitro* in our experimental conditions. From results obtained in *in vivo* experiments in cats implanted with push-pull cannulae it has been already possible to demonstrate that the ACh stimulatory effect on ^{3}H-DA release in the caudate nucleus was dependent on the firing rate of nigral dopaminergic cells. Moreover, evidence has been acquired suggesting a functional presynaptic regulation of DA release from striatal terminals by the cortico-striatal glutamatergic projection.

One of our working hypotheses is that the two forms of regulation of DA release from nerve terminals ie nerve activity and presynaptic neuronal influences, are interdependent processes. For example, presynaptic neuronal excitatory influences could predominate when nerve activity is reduced in dopaminergic cells and vice versa. This situation would explain the surprising results obtained in recent studies where we observed an enhanced release of ^{3}H-DA in the ipsilateral caudate nucleus during the nigral application of tetrodotoxin, a treatment which should interrupt the propagation of nerve impulse flow in dopaminergic neurons. If such events occur they will have important consequences and care should be taken in the interpretation of electrophysiological studies. The amount of neurotransmitter which is released from DA nerve terminals should not be directly deduced from the firing rate of dopaminergic cells. Complex interneuronal feedback processes would have to be taken into consideration in order to understand how the flow of messages leaving the striatum is regulated by the dopaminergic neurons.

ACKNOWLEDGEMENTS

This study was supported by grants from INSERM (ATP 58.78.90) DRET (n° 79.077) and Rhône-Poulenc S.A.

REFERENCES

1 WESTFALL, T.C.: Local regulation of adrenergic neurotransmission. Physiol. Rev. 57: 660-728 (1977)

2 LAVALLEE,M., DE CHAMPLAIN, J., NADEAU, R.A., YAMAGUCHI, N.: Muscarinic inhibition of endogenous myocardial catecholamine liberation in the dog. Can.J.Physiol.Pharmacol. 56: 642-649 (1978)

3 BESSON, M.J., CHERAMY, A., FELTZ, P., GLOWINSKI, J.: Release of newly synthetized dopamine from dopamine containing nerve terminals in the striatum of the rat. Proc.Nat.Acad.Sci. (USA) 62: 741-748 (1969)

4 SPECIALE, S.G., CROWLEY, W.R., O'DONOHUE, T.L., JACOBOWITZ, D.M.: Forebrain catecholamine projections of the A5 cell group. Brain Res. 154: 128-133 (1978)

5 GIORGUIEFF, M.F., LE FLOC'H, M.L., GLOWINSKI, J., BESSON,M.J.: Involvement of cholinergic presynaptic receptors of nicotinic and muscarinic types in the control of the spontaneous release of DA from striatal dopaminergic terminals in the rat. J.Pharmacol.exp.Ther. 200: 535-544 (1977)

6 NIEOULLON, A., CHERAMY, A., GLOWINSKI, J.: Release of dopamine evoked by electrical stimulation of the motor and visual areas of the cerebral cortex in both caudate nuclei and in the substantia nigra in the cat. Brain Res. 145: 69-83 (1978)

7 POIRIER, L.S.,MC GEER, E.G., LAROCHELLE, L., MC GEER, P.L., BEDARD, P., BOUCHER, R.: The effect of brain stem lesions on tyrosine and tryptophan hydroxylases in various structures of the telencephalon of the cat. Brain Res. 14: 147-155 (1969)

8 BESSON, M.J., CHERAMY, A., GAUCHY, C., GLOWINSKI, J.: In vivo continuous estimation of ^{3}H-dopamine synthesis and release in the cat caudate nucleus. Effect of α-methyl-p-tyrosine and of transection of the nigro-neostriatal pathway. Naunyn Schmiedeberg's Arch.Pharmacol. 278: 101-105 (1973)

9 GIORGUIEFF, M.F., KEMEL, M.L., GLOWINSKI, J.: Stimulation of dopamine release by GABA in rat striatal slices. Brain Res. 139: 115-130 (1978)

10 GIORGUIEFF-CHESSELET, M.F., KEMEL, M.L., WANDSCHEER, D., GLOWINSKI, J.: Attempts to localize the GABA receptors involved in the GABA-induced release of newly-synthetized ^{3}H-dopamine in rat striatal slices. Brain Res. 175: 383-386 (1979)

11 GIORGUIEFF, M.F., KEMEL, M.L., GLOWINSKI, J.: Presynaptic effect of L-glutamic acid on the release of dopamine in rat striatal slices. Neurosci.Lett. 6: 73-77 (1977)

12 GIORGUIEFF-CHESSELET, M.F., KEMEL, M.L., WANDSCHEER, D., GLOWINSKI, J.: Glycine stimulates the spontaneous release of newly synthetized ^{3}H-dopamine in rat striatal slices. Eur.J.Pharmacol. 60: 101-104 (1979)

13 SIMONNET, G., GIORGUIEFF-CHESSELET, M.F.: Stimulating effect of angiotensin II on the spontaneous release of newly synthetized ^{3}H-dopamine in rat striatal slices. Neurosci.Lett. 15: 153-158 (1979)

14 WESTFALL, T.C.: The effect of cholinergic agents on the release of ^{3}H-dopamine from the rat striatal slices by nicotine, potassium and electrical stimulation. Fed.Proc. 33: 524 (1974)

15 STARR, M.S.: GABA-mediated potentiation of amine release from nigrostriatal dopamine neurons in vitro. Eur. J. Pharmacol. 53: 215-226 (1979)

16 KERWIN, R., PYCOCK, C.: Effects of ω-amino acids on tritiated dopamine release from rat striatum : evidence for a possible glycinergic mechanism. Biochem.Pharmacol. 28: 2193-2197 (1979)

17 ROBERTS, P.J., SHARIF, N.A.: Effects of L-glutamate and related amino acids upon the release of ^{3}H-dopamine from rat striatal slices. Brain Res. 157: 391-395 (1978)

18 DE BELLEROCHE, J., BRADFORD, H.F.: Biochemical evidence for the presence of presynaptic receptors on dopaminergic nerve terminals. Brain Res. 142: 53-68 (1978)

19 FUKUDA, J., KAMEYAMA, M.: Tetrodotoxin-sensitive and tetrodotoxin-resistant sodium channels in tissue-cultured spinal ganglion neurons from adult mammals. Brain Res. 182: 191-197 (1980)

20 KATO, G., CARSON, S., KEMEL, M.L., GLOWINSKI, J., GIORGUIEFF, M.F.: Changes in striatal specific ^{3}H-atropine binding after unilateral 6-hydroxydopamine lesions of nigrostriatal dopaminergic neurons. Life Sci. 22: 1607-1614 (1978)

21 MC GEER, P.L., MC GEER, E.G., INNANEN, V.T., Dendroaxonic transmission.I.Evidence from receptor binding of dopaminergic and cholinergic agents. Brain Res. 169: 433-441 (1979)

22 REISINE, T.D., NAGY, J.I., BEAUMONT, K.,FIBIGER, H.C., YAMAMURA, H.I.: The localization of receptor binding sites in the substantia nigra and striatum of the rat. Brain Res. 177: 241-252 (1979)

23 POLLARD, H., LLORENS, C., SCHWARTZ, J.C., GROS, J.C., DRAY, F.: Localization of opiate receptors and enkephalins in the rat striatum in relationship with the nigral-striatal dopaminergic system: lesion studies. Brain Res. 151: 392-398 (1978)

24 LOH, H.H., BRASE, D.A., SAMPATH-KHANNA, S., MAR, J.B., WAY, E.L.: β-Endorphin in vitro inhibition of striatal dopamine release. Nature, 264: 567-568 (1976)

25 SUBRAMAMIAN, N., MITZNEFF, P., SPRUGEL, W., DOMSCHKE, W., DOMSCHKE, S., WUNSCH, E.: Influence of enkephalin on K^+ evoked efflux of putative neurotransmitters in rat brain. Naunyn Schmiedeberg's Arch.Pharmacol. 299:163-165 (1977)

26 ARBILLA, S., LANGER, S.Z.: Morphine and β-endorphin inhibit release of noradrenaline from cerebral cortex but not of dopamine from rat striatum.Nature 271: 559-561 (1978)

27 HATTORI, T., SINGH, V.K., MC GEER, E.G., MC GEER, P.L.: Immunohistochemical localization of choline acetyl transferase containing neostriatal neurons and their relationship with dopaminergic synapses. Brain Res. 102:164-173 (1976)

28 WAGNER, A., HASSLER, R., KIM, J.S.: Striatal cholinergic enzyme activities following discrete centro-median nucleus lesion in the cat thalamus.Trans.Int.Soc.Neurochem. Abst. 59, 116 (1975)

29 MC GEER, P.L., MC GEER, E.G.: Evidence of glutamic acid decarboxylase-containing interneurons in the striatum. Brain Res. 91:331-335 (1975)

30 DIVAC, I., FONNUM, F., STORM-MATHISEN, J.: High affinity uptake of glutamate in terminals of cortico-striatal axons. Nature, 266: 377-378 (1977)

31 FUXE, K., GANTEN, D., HÖKFELT, T., BALME, P.: Immunohistochemical evidence for the existence of angiotensin II containing nerve terminals in the central nervous system of the rat.In:J.P. Buckley, C.H. Ferrario (eds.), Central action of angiotensin and related hormones, Pergamon Press, Oxford pp.515-518 (1977)

32 ARREGUI, A., EMSON, P.C., SPOKES, E.G.: Angiotensin-converting enzyme in substantia nigra: reduction of activity in Huntington's disease and after intrastriatal kainic acid in rats. Eur.J.Pharmacol. 52: 121-124 (1978)

33 ROBERTS, P.J., ANDERSON, S.D.: Stimulatory effect of L-glutamate and related amino-acids on ^{3}H-dopamine release from rat striatum: an in vitro model from glutamate action. J. Neurochem. 32: 1539-1545 (1979)

34 GIORGUIEFF, M.F., LE FLOC'H, M.L., WESTFALL, T., GLOWINSKI, J., BESSON, M.J.: Nicotinic effect of ACh on the release of newly synthetized ^{3}H-DA in rat striatal slices and cat caudate nucleus. Brain Res. 106:117-131 (1976)

35 GIORGUIEFF-CHESSELET, M.F., KEMEL, M.L., GLOWINSKI, J.: The presynaptic stimulating effect of acetylcholine on dopamine release is suppressed during activation of nigro-striatal dopaminergic neurons in the cat. Neurosci. Lett. 14: 177-182 (1979)

36 CHERAMY, A., NIEOULLON, A., GLOWINSKI, J.: GABAergic processes involved in the control of dopamine release from nigro-striatal dopaminergic neurons in the cat. Eur.J.Pharmacol. 48: 281-295 (1978)

37 CHERAMY, A., MICHELOT, R., NIEOULLON, A., LEVIEL, V., KERDELHUE, B. : Effect of a nigral application of substance P and of anti-substance P serum on dopamine release from dendrites and nerve terminals of the nigrostriatal dopaminergic neurons in the cat. In: E. Usdin, E., Kopin, J., Barchas, P. (eds), Catecholamines: basic and clinical frontiers, Pergamon Press, pp.1098-1100 (1979)

38 MOLEMAN, P., BRUINVELS, J.: Morphine-induced striatal dopamine efflux depends on the activity of nigrostriatal dopamine neurons. Nature 281: 686-687 (1979)

Neurotransmitters and their Receptors
Edited by U.Z. Littauer, Y. Dudai, I. Silman,
V.I. Teichberg and Z. Vogel

Noradrenergic Regulation of Dopaminergic Neurotransmission in Rat CNS

F. Ponzio

Istituto di Ricerche Farmacologiche "Mario Negri", Via Eritrea, 62, 20157-Milan, Italy

and

G. Jonsson

Karolinska Institute, Department of Histology, S-10401 Stockholm 60, Sweden

ABSTRACT

Systemic treatment of newborn rats with 6-hydroxydopamine (6-OHDA) or with [β-chloroalkylamine-N-(2-chloroethyl)-N-ethyl-2-bromobenzylamine; DSP_4] selectively alters postnatal development of the central noradrenaline (NA) neurons, leaving dopamine (DA) neurons apparently unaffected from a structural viewpoint. The present study was undertaken to investigate whether neonatal 6-OHDA or DSP_4 treatment produces any functional changes in DA neurons of striatum, cerebral cortex and pons-medulla. Endogenous DA levels were not significantly changed. The α-methyl-p-tyrosine induced depletion of DA was reduced in 12-day-old animals compared to controls, but no clear-cut change was observed in adults, indicating that neonatal 6-OHDA or DSP_4 treatment causes a transient reduction in DA turnover. Pretreatment with the NA uptake blocker desipramine to prevent the action of 6-OHDA on NA neurons abolished the changes in DA neurons in the neostriatum, cerebral cortex and pons-medulla of 12-day-old rats.
The present results indicate that NA neurons may be involved in the regulation of dopaminergic neurotransmission.

The early postnatal period is critical for the outgrowth of axons and terminals from cell bodies and for the development of mechanisms regulating monoamine synthesis and storage. It is also a vulnerable period for the functional maturation of the central dopaminergic systems, may be more than for the central noradrenergic system which is relatively mature at birth (1,2). Previous studies (3,4) have shown that systemic treatment of newborn rats with the catecholamine neurotoxin 6-hydroxydopamine (6-OHDA) preferentially alters postnatal development of the central noradrenergic neurons belonging to the *locus coeruleus* system, leaving dopaminergic neurons structurally unaffected, as evaluated by neurochemical techniques. The treatment leads to permanent denervation of distant NA nerve terminal projections, and permanent iper-innervation of areas near to the *locus coeruleus*: a "pruning effect" (5,6).
This effect favors the view that postnatal development of monoamine neurons is rigidly ordered with respect quantity of axonal nerve terminals. In fact, total ^{3}H-NA uptake is not changed (4) but ^{3}H-NA uptake is reduced in the cortex and increased in the pons-medulla, indicating a nerve-terminal rearrangement. Since earlier studies indicated a functional interaction

between NA and DA neurons in adult rats (7,8), the present study was undertaken to investigate whether or not neonatal 6-OHDA treatment produces any functional change in DA neurons.

MATERIALS AND METHODS

Animals and drug treatments

Litters of albino rats (Sprague-Dawley obtained from Anticimex, Stockholm) were treated with 6-OHDA (100 mg/kg s.c.) within 6 h of birth. They received an additional 6-OHDA injection 24 h later. In most experiments tha animals were treated with the tyrosine-hydroxylase inhibitor, α-methyl-p-tyrosine (250 mg/kg i.p. 2h). In some experiments newborn rats were treated with β-chloroalkylamine-N-(2-chloroethyl)-N-ethyl-2-bromobenzyl-amine (DSP_4) (50 mg/kg s.c.), a new neurotoxin selective for NA neurons (9,10,11). In other experiments newborn rats received the NA uptake blocker desipramine (DMI, 25 mg/kg s.c.) 30 min before each 6-OHDA injection. Controls were treated with an equal amount of the vehicle.

The animals were killed by decapitation at either 12 days (Y) or 3 months (A) and brain areas were rapidly dissected out, frozen on dry ice and kept at -80°C for biochemical determinations.

Catecholamine assay

Endogenous catecholamines were determined using the LCEC-technique described by Keller et al. (12). The values obtained were expressed as percentages of control values.

Monoamine metabolite assay

Endogenous monoamine metabolites were determined using the LCEC-technique described by Ponzio and Jonsson (13). The values were expressed as nanograms per gram weight of tissue.

RESULTS AND DISCUSSION

Neonatal 6-OHDA treatment produced marked, permanent changes in NA levels consistent with the "pruning effect" concept (Fig. 1) while this treatment does not significantly affect the DA levels in adult rats. The exact reason for the resistance of the DA system towards 6-OHDA treatment is not yet known.

In line with findings in the striatum, DA metabolites homovanillic acid (HVA) and dihydroxyphenylacetic acid (DOPAC) were significantly reduced 12 days after 6-OHDA, though unchanged in adults (Fig. 2).

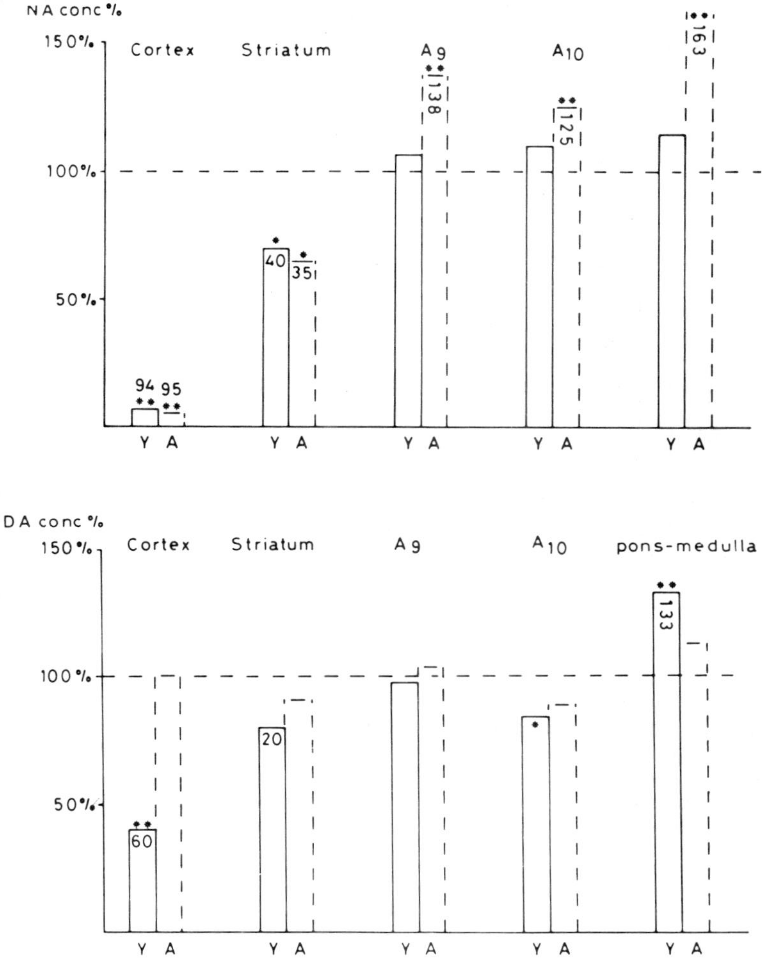

Regional changes in NA and DA levels in young and adult animals after 6-OH-DA treatment

Fig. 1 - Effect of neonatal 6-OHDA treatment (2 x 100 mg/kg s.c. 6 and 30 h after birth) on NA and DA levels in various brain regions of 12-day-old (Y) and adult (3-month-old) (A) rats.
Endogenous NA levels are affected by the treatment in both young (Y) and adult (A) rats. Endogenous DA levels are slightly changed in young rats but are unchanged in adults. The column heights represent percentages of controls. The values in the columns show the percentage changes in NA or DA levels after 6-OHDA treatment compared to control values.
Statistical significance: Student's "t" test
$^{*}p < 0.05$; $^{**}p < 0.01$ versus controls.

The tyrosine-hydroxylase (TH) inhibition model was used to evaluate changes in depletion of NA and DA endogenous levels after neonatal treatment with 6-OHDA or DSP_4 (Fig. 3 and 5). There was a marked reduction in α-methyl-p-tyrosine induced depletion of NA in all regions 12 days after 6-OHDA or DSP_4 treatment, indicating reduced NA turnover (Fig. 3 and 5). The situation in the adult stage is somewhat more complex (Fig. 4 and 6), with indications of both increases (pons-medulla) and decreases (cortex and striatum) in NA turnover.

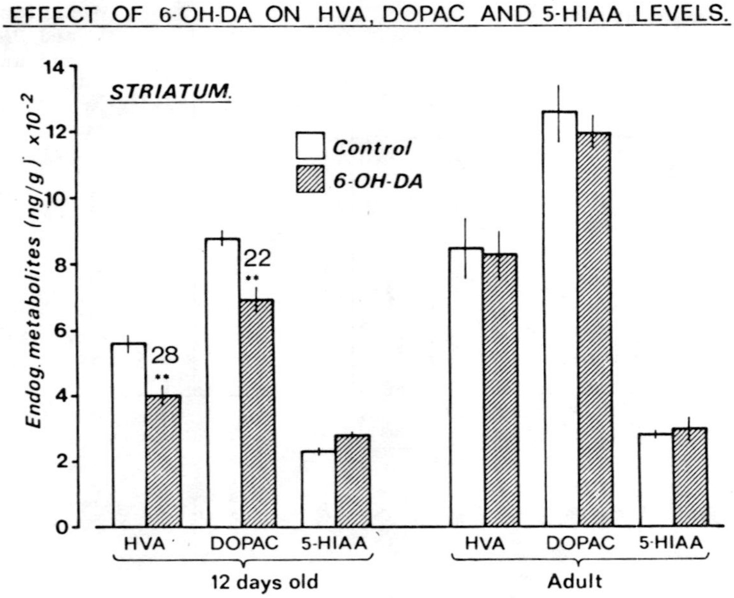

Fig. 2 - Effect of neonatal 6-OHDA treatment (see Fig. 1) on striatal HVA, DOPAC and 5HIAA.
Endogenous HVA and DOPAC levels are slightly reduced in 12-day-old rats, but are unaffected in the adults. The column heights represent ng per gram of tissue. The values in the columns show the percentage changes in NA or DA levels after 6-OHDA treatment compared to control values.
Statistical significance Student's "t" test.
** $p < 0.01$ versus controls.

α -methyl-p-tyrosine induced depletion of DA (Fig. 3 and 5) was reduced in the cerebral cortex and striatuam at 12 days suggesting reduced DA turnover (Fig. 3 and 5). These changes were largely absent in the adults (Fig. 4 and 6), in which both endogenous DA levels and turnover were normal. However 6-OHDA or DSP_4 neonatal treatment changed endogenous NA levels in young and adult rats and changed NA turnover in young rats.
In young animals, NA alteration seemed to affect the DA system, proportionally changing endogenous DA levels and turnover; the situation was normal in adult animals. Pretreatment with the uptake blocker desipramine (DMI), which prevents 6-OHDA neurotoxic action on NA neurons, left endogenous NA levels unaffected and abolished 6-OHDA's effect on NA turnover (Fig. 7). Similarly endogenous DA levels and turnover in young and adult animals were unaffected (Fig. 7).

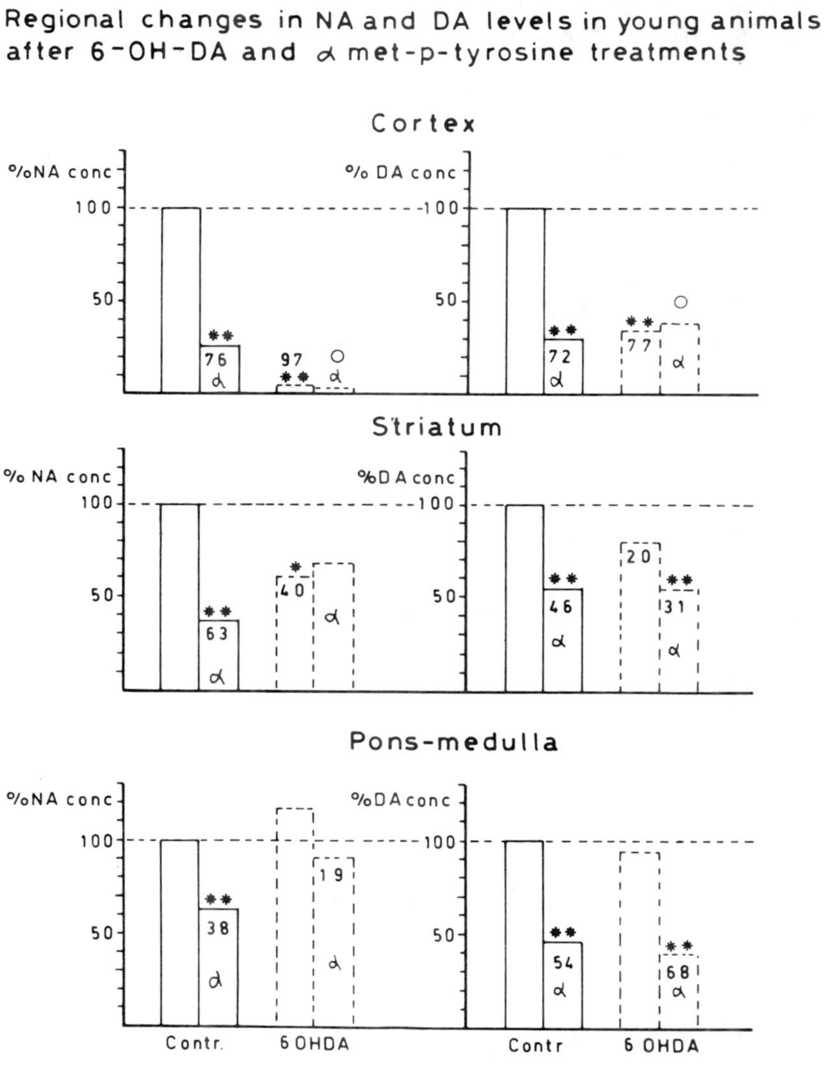

Fig. 3 - Effect of α methyl-p-tyrosine (α) treatment (250 mg/kg i.p. 2 h) on NA and DA levels in brain regions of young rats after neonatal 6-OHDA treatment (see Fig. 1). The column heights indicate NA and DA levels (as a percentage of controls) before and after α-methyl-p-tyrosine (α) treatment in controls and 6-OHDA treated rats. 6-OHDA neonatal treatment significantly changes endogenous NA and DA levels and reduces the depletion due to α treatment.
The values in the columns show the percentage changes in NA and DA levels after 6-OHDA or 6-OHDA + α treatment.
Statistical significance:

*$p < 0.05$
**$p < 0.01$ versus controls by Duncan's new multiple range test

°$p < 0.05$ versus controls by F. interaction

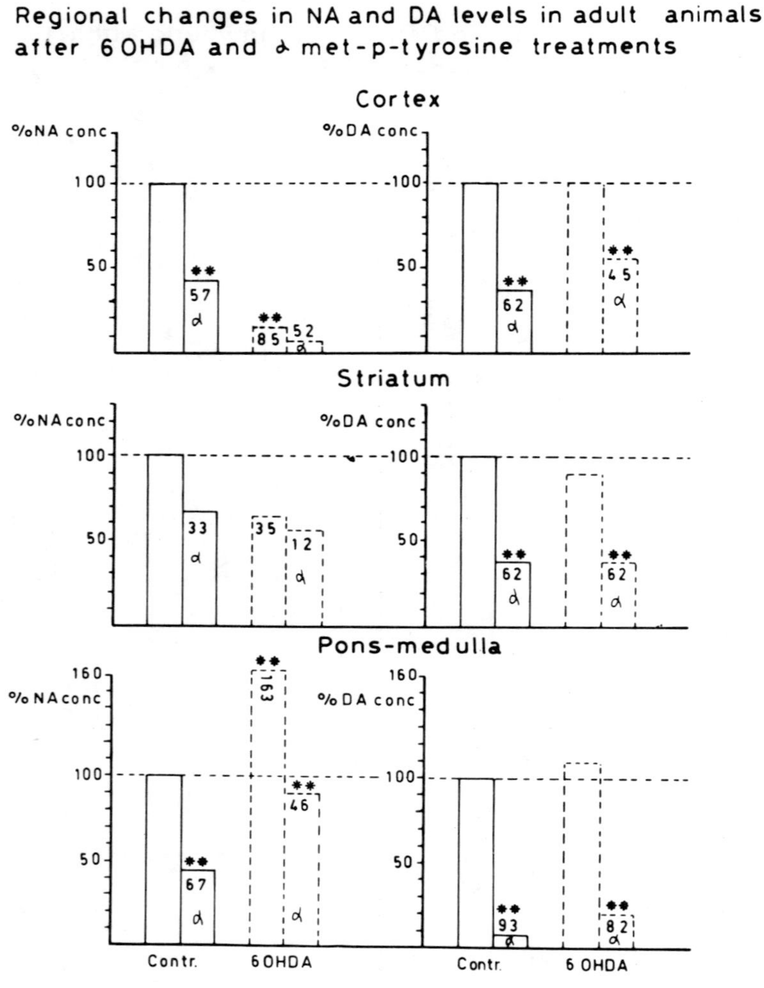

Fig. 4 - Effect of α methyl-p-tyrosine (α) treatment (250 mg/kg i.p. 2 h) on NA and DA levels of 3-month-old rats after neonatal 6-OHDA treatment (see Fig.1) The column heights indicate the NA and DA levels (as percentage of controls) before and after α methyl-p-tyrosine (α) treatment of controls and 6-OHDA treated rats. 6-OHDA neonatal treatment significantly changes endogenous NA levels in adult rats, but the percent of NA depletion due to α treatment is unchanged. 6-OHDA neonatal treatment in adult rats does not affect endogenous DA levels and the depletion induced by α treatment.
The values in the columns show the percentage changes in NA and DA levels after α, 6-OHDA or 6-OHDA +α treatments.
Statistical significance:

** $p < 0.01$ versus controls by Duncan's new multiple range test.

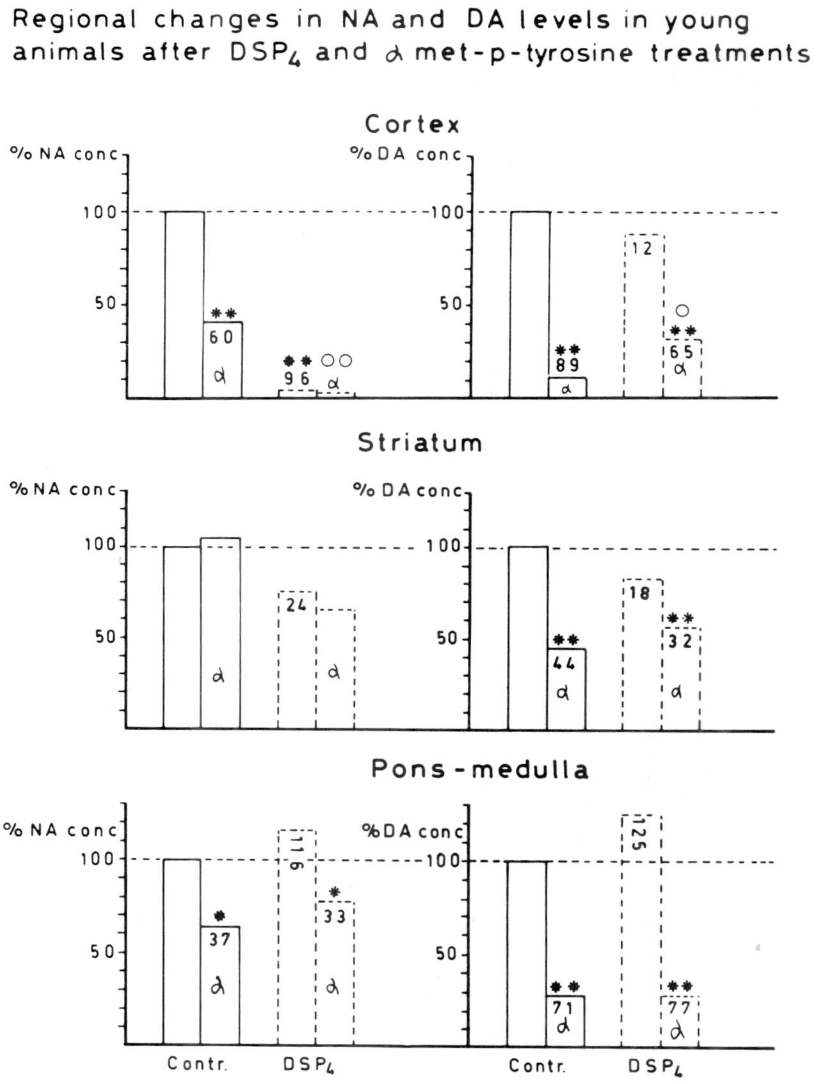

Fig. 5 - Effect of α methyl-p-tyrosine (α) treatment (250 mg/kg i.p. 2 h) on NA and DA levels of young rats after neonatal DSP_4 treatment (50 mg/kg s.c. 6 h after birth).
The column heights indicate the NA and DA levels (as a percentage of controls) before and after α methyl-p-tyrosine (α) treatment of controls and DSP_4 treated rats. DSP_4 neonatal treatment significantly changes endogenous NA and DA levels and reduces the depletion due to α treatment.
The values in the columns show the percentage changes in NA and DA levels after α, DSP_4 or DSP_4 + α treatments.
Statistical significance:

* $p < 0.05$
** $p < 0.01$ versus controls by Duncan's new multiple range test

° $p < 0.05$
°° $p < 0.01$ versus controls by F. interaction.

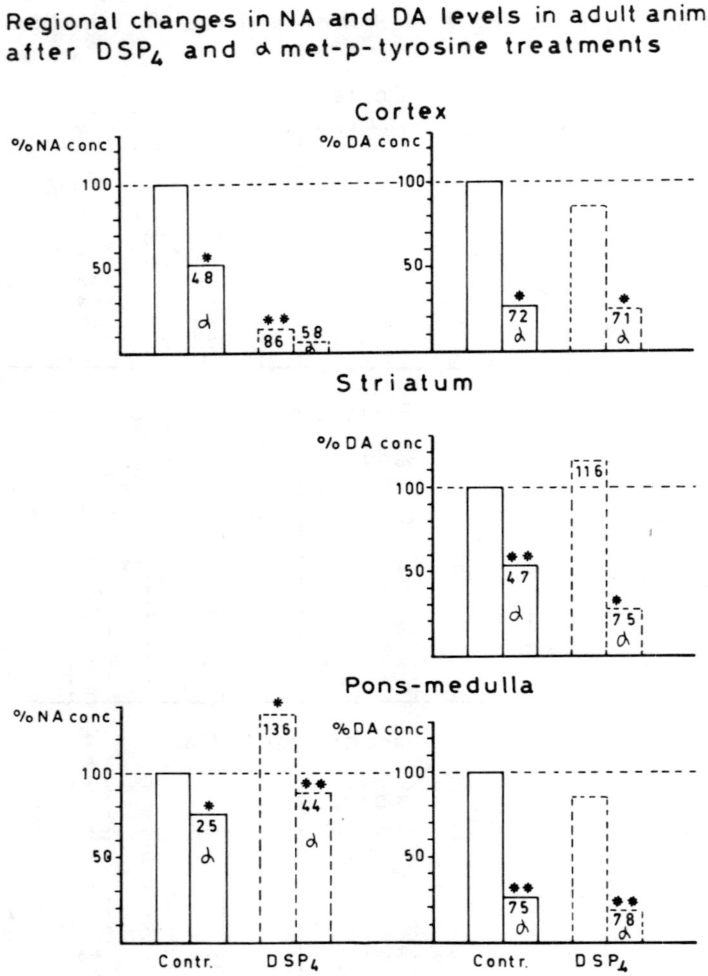

Fig. 6 - Effect of α methyl-p-tyrosine (α) treatment (250 mg/kg i.p. 2 h) on NA and DA levels of 3-month-old rats after neonatal DSP_4 treatment (see Fig. 5).
The column heights indicate the NA and DA levels (as a percentage of controls) before and after α methyl-p-tyrosine (α) treatment of controls and DSP_4 treated rats. DSP_4 neonatal treatment significantly changes endogenous NA levels, in adult rats, but NA depletion due to α treatment is unchanged. DSP_4 neonatal treatment in adult rats does not affect endogenous DA levels or the depletion induced by α treatment. The values in the columns show the percentage changes in NA and DA levels after α, DSP_4 or DSP_4 + α treatments.
Statistical significance:

* $p < 0.05$
** $p < 0.01$ versus controls by Duncan's new multiple range test

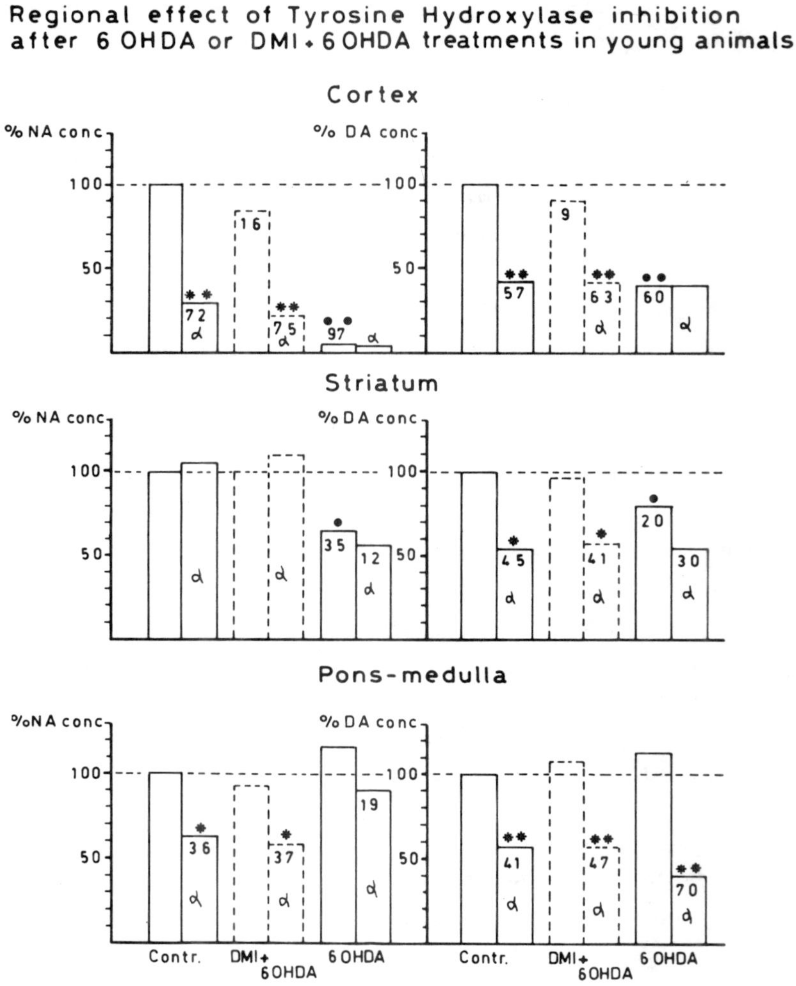

Fig. 7 - Effect of α methyl-p-tyrosine (α) treatment (250 mg/kg i.p. 2 h) on NA and DA levels of young rats after neonatal 6-OHDA or DMI + 6-OHDA treatments.

DMI (2 x 25 mg/kg i.p.) was injected 30 min before each 6-OHDA dose. The column heights indicate the NA and DA levels (as a percentage of controls) before and after α methyl-p-tyrosine (α) treatment of controls, DMI + 6-OHDA and 6-OHDA treated rats. 6-OHDA neonatal treatment significantly changes endogenous NA and DA levels and reduces the depletion due to α treatment, while the NA reuptake blocker DMI protects the neurons against the effect of 6-OHDA and in DMI + 6-OHDA treated animals the levels of NA and DA and the depletion induced by α treatment is similar to the controls. The values in the columns show the percentage changes in NA and DA levels after α, DMI + 6-OHDA, DMI + 6-OHDA + α, 6-OHDA and 6-OHDA + α treatments.

Statistical significance:

* $p < 0.05$
** $p < 0.01$ versus controls by Duncan's new multiple range test

° $p < 0.05$
°° $p < 0.01$ versus controls by F. interaction.

These results support the view that the changes in DA turnover seen in young animals after neonatal 6-OHDA treatment are related to 6-OHDA induced alteration of postnatal development of NA neurons. They indicate that NA neurons are involved in the regulation of DA neurotransmission in the cerebral cortex and in the striatum, this regulation occurring early in development.

It remains to be clarified wheather NA modulates dopaminergic system directly or indirectly.

ACKNOWLEDGEMENTS

The present study was partially supported by a CNR grant, contract number 79.01815.04.

We are grateful to the ETP twinning program for support for living and travel expenses.

REFERENCES

1. Engel J., Ahlenius S, Brown R. and Lundborg P. in: Experimental Model Systems in Toxicology and Their Significance in Man, Vol. XV p.20, Excerpta Medica, Amsterdam (1973).
2. Coyle J.T. and Molliver M.E. : Science 196: 444 (1977).
3. Sachs Ch. and Jonsson G. in: Chemical Tools in Catecholamine Research I, p. 163, Jonsson G., Malmfors T., Sachs Ch. eds., North Holland, Amsterdam (1975).
4. Jonsson G. and Sachs Ch.: Med.Biol. 54: 286 (1976).
5. Jonsson G. : Exp.Neurol. 53: 801 (1976).
6. Jonsson G. and Hallman H. : Neurosci.Lett. 9: 27 (1978).
7. Donaldson I.MacG., Dolphin A., Jenner P., Marsden C.D. and Pycock C. J.Pharm.Pharmacol. 28: 329 (1976).
8. Braestrup C. : Psychopharmacology 51: 199 (1977).
9. Ross S.B. : Br.J.Pharmacol. 58: 521 (1976).
10. Jonsson G., Ponzio F., and Ross S. in : Abstracts 7th. Int. Congress of Pharmacology Paris July 16-21, p.926 (1978).
11. Jaim-Etcheverry G. and Zieher L.M. : Brain Res. 188: 513 (1980).
12. Keller R., Oke A., Mefford I. and Adams R.N. : Life Sci. 19: 995 (1976).
13. Ponzio F. and Jonsson G. : Dev.Neurosci. 1: 80 (1978).

Neurotransmitters and their Receptors
Edited by U.Z. Littauer, Y. Dudai, I. Silman,
V.I. Teichberg and Z. Vogel

Displacement from α - noradrenergic Binding Sites by Clonidine Analogues Using [^{3}H] clonidine and [^{3}H] WB 4101 as Ligands

J. Mierau and W.D. Bechtel

Department of Biochemistry, C.H. Boehringer Sohn, 6507 Ingelheim, Germany

Abstract

The specific α-noradrenergic binding using [^{3}H]WB 4101 and [^{3}H]clonidine was measured and the displacement by clonidine and structurally related compounds from these binding sites determined using rat cerebral cortex homogenates. The results demonstrate that the in vivo blood pressure lowering activity of the clonidine analogues tested does not parallel the in vitro affinity to specific [^{3}H]WB 4101 binding sites. In contrast to these findings recently a statistically significant correlation could be found between the blood pressure lowering activity and the affinity to specific [^{3}H]clonidine binding sites studying the same compounds. Thus, the results agree well with the α-receptor subclassification into α_1 for WB 4101 and α_2 for clonidine activity.

Introduction

The mode of action of the antihypertensive clonidine (Catapres®) is thought commonly to be central α-adrenergic (Reviewed by SCHMITT). The high affinity to α-adrenergic binding sites which is shown using [^{3}H]clonidine and the receptor binding technique (GREENBERG et al., U'PRICHARD et al.) is in good agreement with this view. Furthermore, a good correlation could be demonstrated comparing the blood pressure lowering efficacy in rabbits of clonidine and analogue compounds and the specific [^{3}H]clonidine receptor binding to rat cortex membranes in vitro (BECHTEL & MIERAU).

Based on pharmacological studies in vivo (BERTHELSON & PETTINGER) and in vitro (WOOD et al.) a subclassification of α-adrenergic receptors into α_1 and α_2 was introduced. [^{3}H]clonidine and [^{3}H]WB 4101 are known to be selective α_2 and α_1 receptor ligands, respectively.

The purpose of the present study was to demonstrate whether or not a comparison of the blood pressure lowering effect and the displacement of [^{3}H]WB 4101 from its specific binding sites by some clonidine analogues reflects the α_1/α_2 differentiation.

Material and Methods

[^{3}H]WB 4101 had a specific radioactivity of 23 Ci/mmole (Amersham-Buchler, Braunschweig, Germany). Phentolamine was obtained from Ciba. ST and STH compounds were synthetized by Dr. Stähle, Dept. of Chemistry, Boehringer-Ingelheim. All other chemicals were purchased from Merck (Darmstadt, Germany) in their analytical pure form.

Tissue preparation from rat cortex and standard binding assays were performed exactly as described by GREENGERG et al. A 0.2 nM [^{3}H]WB 4101 concentration was used.

Radioactivity was measured by liquid scintillation counting using a toluene containing cocktail. Counting efficiency was between 35 and 37 %.

The specific [^{3}H]WB 4101 binding equalled the total binding minus blank which was obtained in the presence of 10^{-4} M phentolamine.

Results and Discussion

The displacement of [^{3}H]WB 4101 from its specific binding sites by clonidine (=ST 155) and 26 structurally related compounds was measured. In figure 1 a couple of typical displacement curves is shown using phentolamine and some ST compounds. From these curves the specific [^{3}H]WB 4101 binding of approximately 93 % (= 3200 dpm) of the total binding (= 3450 dpm) can be calculated. Figure 2 shows displacement curves from recent [^{3}H]clonidine receptor binding studies (BECHTEL & MIERAU).

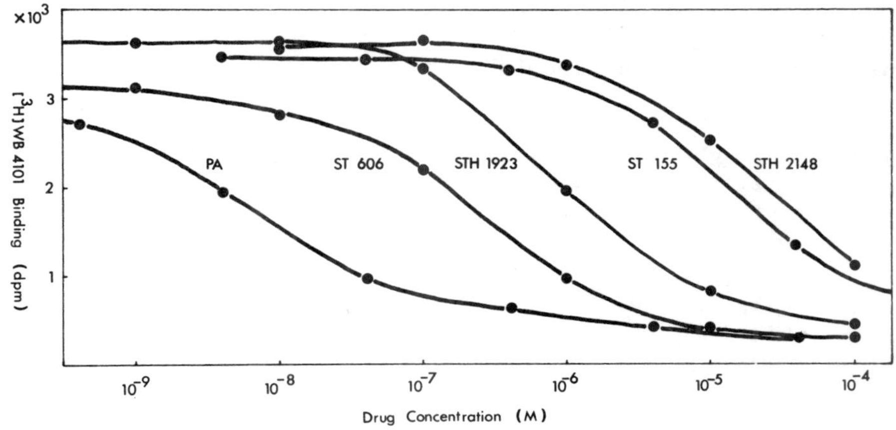

Fig. 1. Displacement of [^{3}H]WB 4101 from binding sites by phentolamine (PA) and some ST compounds. Means of triplicates ofsingle experiments.

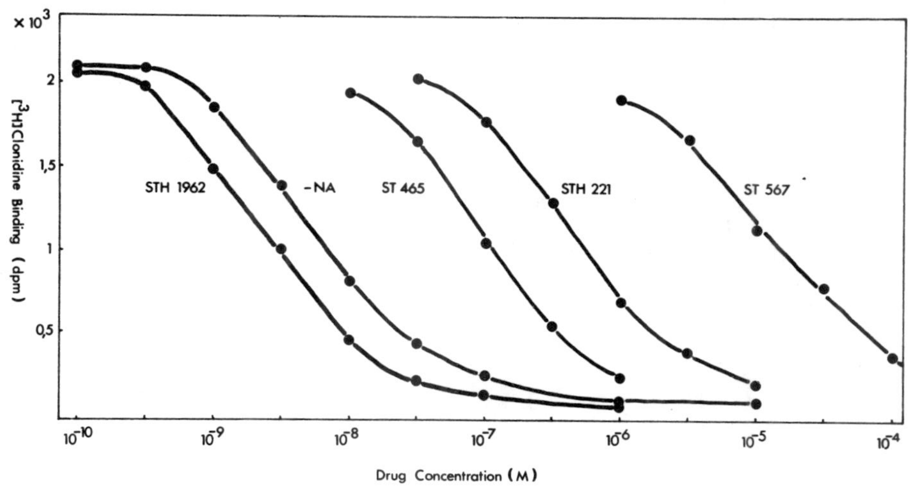

Fig. 2. Displacement of [^{3}H]clonidine from its binding sites by l-noradrenaline and some ST compounds. Mean of triplicates of single experiments.

Displacement of [^{3}H]clonidine and [^{3}H]WB 4101 from specific binding sites by clonidine analogues compared to blood pressure lowering activities and lipophilic properties.

Substance	Aryl-substitution	N-substit.	log P	ED 20	[^{3}H]CLO IC 50	[^{3}H]WB IC 50
ST 91	2,6 diEt	-	-1,22	>3	19	866
ST 93	2-Cl,6-Me	-	-0,52	0,05	3,1	380
ST 95	2,6-diMe	-	-1,40	>3	2,5	637
ST 155	2,6-diCl	-	0,48	0,01	2,6	3600
ST 341	2-Me,4-Cl	-	-0,66	0,1	1,5	440
ST 375	2-Cl,4-Me	-	-0,96	0,014	3,1	387
ST 450	2-Me,3-Cl	-	-0,79	0,1	2,1	353
ST 464	2,6-diBr	-	1,17	0,045	6,3	457
ST 465	H	-	-1,92	>3	440	4700
ST 473	3,4-diCl	-	0,33	>3	21	1470
ST 474	3,5-diCl	-	1,08	3,0	93	1370
ST 476	2,3-diCl	-	0,53	0,03	2,3	360
ST 567	2,6-diCl	allyl	-1,66	3,0	144000	51300
ST 606	2-Me,3-Br	-	-0,2	0,01	2,2	247
ST 608	2-Cl,3-Me	-	-0,57	0,45	6,3	413
ST 615	2-Br,3-Me	-	-0,15	>3	1300	
ST 666	2,6-diCl,4-OH	-	-0,46	>1	50	1570
ST 732	2,4,6-triCl	-	1,44	0,09	7,7	
ST 871	2,6-diCl,4-Br	-	1,76	0,035	7,4	463
ST 1912	2,6-diF	-	-0,35	>3	26	5370
ST 1923	2-Cl,6-F	-	0,02	0,04	7,4	1170
ST 1962	2-Br,6-Cl	-	0,98	0,1	4,0	493
ST 1988	2,4,6-triF	-	-0,12	1,0	62	8170
STH 2073	3-Cl,4-OH	-	-1,75	>1	160	4700
STH 2100	2-Cl,3-Br	-	0,67	0,01	2,5	320
STH 2148	2,6-diBr	cycloprop. methyl	-1,12	>2	8600	27500
STH 2169	2-Br,3-F	-	-0,02	0,1	36	610
STH 2210	2,6-diBr	methyl	-1,71	>2	900	4800
STH 2224	2,3-diBr	-	0,89	0,006	1,5	233

IC 50: Drug concentration in nM which reduced specific [^{3}H]clonidine and [^{3}H]WB 4101 binding by 50 %. Values are means of at least 3 separate experiments, each performed in triplicate.

ED 20: I.v. dose in mg/kg causing a blood pressure decrease in anaesthetized rabbits of 20 %.

log P: Logarithm of distribution of drugs between octanol and phosphate buffer, pH 7,4.

All substances studied with their exact chemical structure are summarized in the table. Also the results of the displacement studies are given in this table as IC 50's, i.e. that drug concentration which displaced 50 % of the specific [^{3}H]WB 4101 binding. Moreover, the table contains a) logarithms of the distribution between octanol and phosphate buffer, pH 7.4, b) the intravenous doses which led to a blood pressure decrease of 20 mm Hg in anaesthetized rabbits and c) the IC 50's of [^{3}H]clonidine displacement from its specific binding sites.

Comparing the blood pressure lowering activity and the affinity to the specific [^{3}H]WB 4101 binding sites no correlation could be found (Figure 3: n = 17, r = 0.30). Omitting weak lipophilic compounds of log P < -0.50 the correlation coefficient calculated was even worse (n = 12, r = 0.28).

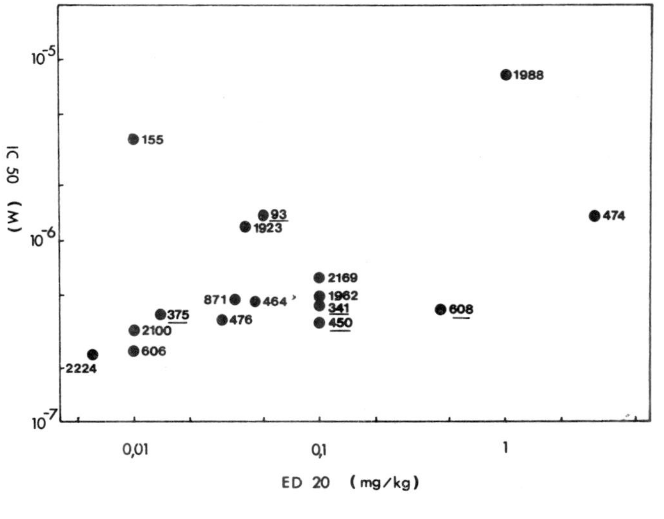

Figure 3

Correlation between the affinity for [^{3}H]WB 4101 binding sites in vitro and the blood pressure lowering activities in rabbits in vivo of clonidine analogues.

Correlation coefficient calculated
using all compounds: r = 0.30, n = 17
without compounds underlined (log P < -0.50): = 0.28, n = 12

This result is in contrast to recent findings measuring displacement of [^{3}H]clonidine from its specific binding sites by clonidine and analogue compounds. Those data correlated well with the blood pressure lowering activity (Figure 4: n = 13, r = 0.92, P < 0.001).

The affinities to the central α-adrenergic [^{3}H]clonidine binding sites of clonidine and its analogues agree well with the generally accepted central mode of action of these drugs. High in vitro activity associated with low in vivo efficacy might be due to a weak permeation of the blood brain barrier. Moreover, the good correlation of the blood pressure lowering activity and the affinity to specific [^{3}H]clonidine binding sites let assume a close relationship between these two actions.

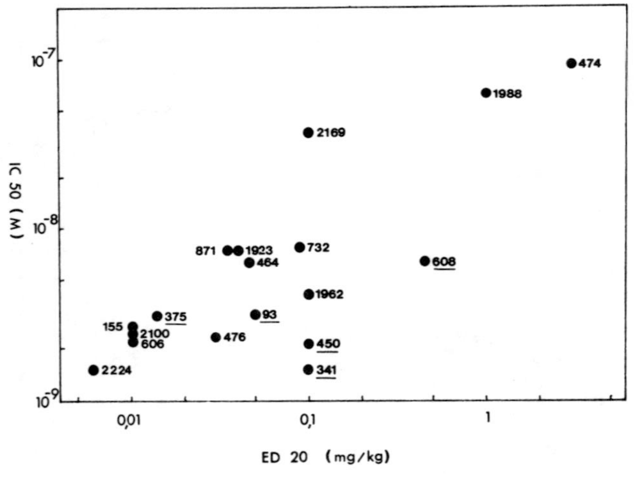

Figure 4

Correlation between the affinity for specific [^{3}H]clonidine binding sites in vitro and the blood pressure lowering activity in rabbits in vivo of clonidine analogues.

Correlation coefficient calculated
using all compounds: r = 0.91, P < 0.001, n = 18

without compounds underlined (log P_i < -0.50): r = 0.92, P <0.001, n = 13

In contrast to this the lack of correlation of blood pressure lowering activity and the affinity to the specific [^{3}H]WB 4101 binding sites showed the non relationship of these actions. However, [^{3}H]WB 4101 rather than [^{3}H]clonidine binding seems to characterize that type of sympatholytic activity according CREESE & SNYDER which occurs as unwanted side effects giving antipsychotics.

In conclusion, it could be clearly demonstrated that the blood pressure lowering activity of clonidine type drugs parallels not the affinity to [^{3}H]WB 4101 but to [^{3}H]clonidine binding sites. The result is in agreement with the α-receptor subclassification into α_1 for WB 4101 and α_2 for clonidine activity.

Acknowledgement

The authors thank Dr. W. Hoefke, Department of Pharmacology, for giving the ED 20 values and Dr. K. Brandt, Department for Analytical Development, Boehringer-Ingelheim, for the log P values.

References

W.D. BECHTEL a. J. MIERAU, Naunyn-Schmiedeberg's Arch. Pharmacol. 307, Suppl. R59 (1979)

S. BERTHELSON a. W.A. PETTINGER, Life Sci. 21, 595-606 (1977)

I. CREESE a. S.H. SNYDER, Ann. Rep. Med. Chem. 12, 249-259 (1977)

D.A. GREENBERG, D.C. U'PRICHARD a, S.H. SNYDER, Life Sci. 19, 69-76 (1976)

H. SCHMITT, in Handbook exp. Pharmacol., Vol. 39, p. 299-396, F. Gross (Ed.), Springer, Berlin 1977

D.C. U'PRICHARD, D.A. GREENBERG a. S.H. SNYDER, Mol. Pharmacol. 13, 454-473 (1977)

C.L. WOOD, C.D. ARNETT, W.R. CLARKE, B. SHUNG TSAI a. R.J. LEFKOWITZ, Biochem. Pharmac. 28, 1277-1282 (1979)

Neurotransmitters and their Receptors
Edited by U.Z. Littauer, Y. Dudai, I. Silman,
V.I. Teichberg and Z. Vogel

In vivo ^{3}H-Spiroperidol Binding:Characterization of Dopamine and Serotonin Receptors in Different Areas of the Rat Central Nervous System

H. Bittiger and S. Bischoff

Research Department, Pharmaceuticals Division, CIBA-GEIGY Ltd., 4002 Basle, Switzerland

ABSTRACT

Specific in vivo binding of ^{3}H-Spiroperidol has been demonstrated in the corpus striatum, frontal cortex, mesolimbic system, hippocampus, cerebellum and the retina of the rat central nervous system. The density of binding sites and the kinetics of binding differed in these areas. The study of the inhibition of ^{3}H-spiroperidol binding by spiroperidol, haloperidol, pipamperone, dipropyl-ATN [5,6-dihydroxy-2(di-n-propylamino)-1,2,3,4-tetrahydro-naphthalin hydrochloride], methysergide, cinanserine, cyproheptadine, metergoline, clozapine and GP 50 302 [2-methyl-2,3-dihydro-1 H-dibenzo (2,3:6,7) thiepino (4,5-c) pyrrol-methansulfonate] revealed widely differing inhibition characteristics of the drugs from brain area to brain area. The results obtained suggest, that in corpus striatum, mesolimbic system, hippocampus and retina, dopamine receptors predominate whereas in the frontal cortex at least 60 % of the binding sites can be ascribed to serotonin receptors; of the remaining sites a majority seem to be dopamine receptors.

AIM OF WORK

It has been shown by in vitro radioreceptor assays, that ^{3}H-spiroperidol binds to different types of receptors in specific brain areas (1,2,3). This study extends to in vivo radioreceptor assays (4,5) in order to evaluate differential receptor interactions.

Parts of the CNS studied were: Cerebral cortex, cerebellum, corpus striatum, mesolimbic system, hippocampus and retina.

Drugs used: mianserin, cinanserine, methysergide, metergoline, cyproheptadine, GP 50 302 (experimental compound of CIBA-GEIGY, 2-methyl-2,3-dihydro-1 H-dibenzo (2,3:6,7)thiepino(4,5-c)pyrrol-methansulfonate), thioridazine, clozapine, chlorpromazine, pipamperone, haloperidol, spiroperidol, dipropyl- ATN (5,6-dihydroxy-2(di-n-propylamino)-1,2,3,4-tetrahydronaphthalin hydrochloride).

In order to be able to study brain areas with low receptor densities, a filtration method was employed to reduce unspecific binding.

EXPERIMENTAL

Male rats (Tif: RAI f (SPF) 150-200 g body weight were injected i.v. with 12 or 36 µCi of ^{3}H-spiroperidol (NEN, 25.6. Ci/mmole). The animals were decapitated at various time intervals after ^{3}H-spiroperidol (10 min to 8 h). Brain areas were rapidly dissected according to Glowinski and Iversen and immediately frozen on dry ice and kept at -20°C overnight. Eyes were rapidly removed, the lens was discarded and the remaining tissue frozen and processed as brain tissue. The tissues were thawed and homogenized in 1.5 ml ice-cold 50 mM Tris/HCl buffer, pH 7.7 with a mini-Polytron (position 0.5, 4 sec) and aliquots of 300 µl were immediately filtered on Whatman GF/B glass fibre filters in duplicate. The filters were washed twice with 5 ml ice-cold Tris buffer and transferred into scintillation vials. Filter bound tissue was dissolved in 1 ml Soluene and scintillator added after one hour. Unspecific binding was determined in animals pretreated with 3mg/kg i.p. spiroperidol; only rats showing pronounced catalepsy were used.
For inhibition studies drugs were given 30 min before ^{3}H-spiroperidol and the animals decapitated 2 h after the label. ^{3}H-spiroperidol is not metabolized within this time period. Protein according to Lowry.

RESULTS

Technical aspects. By the filtration method unspecific binding (pretreatment with 3 mg/kg i.p. spiroperidol) was reduced by 50 - 80 % whereas specific binding was not changed.
Kinetics of binding. Binding characteristics differed very much from brain area to brain area. Whereas amount of bound radioactivity and time course of unspecific binding were practically the same in all brain areas at 12 µCi and 36µCi, total binding differed very much. In the striatum with highest binding the peak was only reached after 3 h whereas in the hippocampus with lowest binding capacity maximum binding was achieved within less than one hour. Radioactivity disappeared also very slowly from the striatum, whereas in other areas the rate was faster.
In all brain areas unspecific binding was low, in the striatum only a few percent of total binding.
Inhibition of binding by drugs (Figures 1,2,3). The inhibition curves of selected compounds differ very much from brain area to brain area. Pipamperone, clozapine, GP 50 302 inhibited most potently in the frontal cortex, much less in the hippocampus and most weakly in the striatum. Dipropyl-

Fig. 1

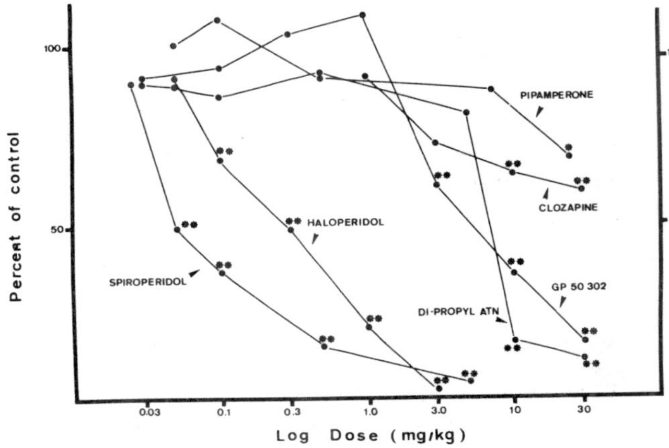

Fig. 2

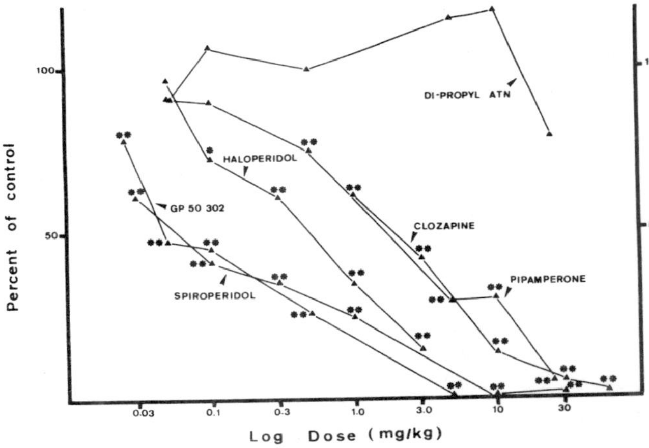

Fig. 3

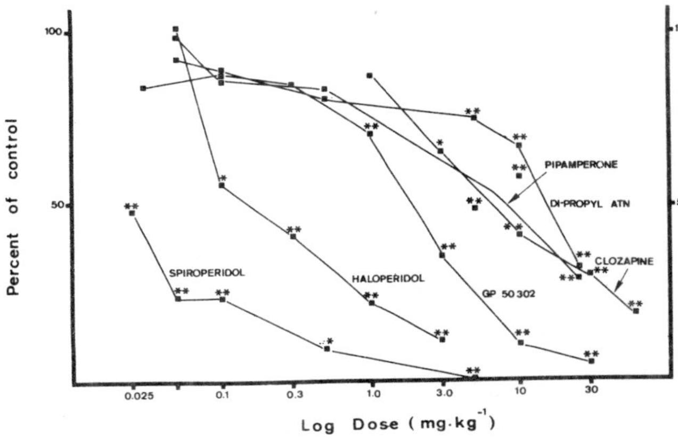

Inhibition of <u>in vivo</u> ^{3}H-spiroperidol binding Doses in mg/kg i.p. Figure 1: Striatum, Fig. 2: Frontal cortex, Fig. 3: Hippocampus

ATN, a specific dopamine agonist, appears inactive in the frontal cortex and about equally potent in the striatum and in the hippocampus. Haloperidol and spiroperidol are about equally potent in all three brain areas. These differential effects of drugs become even more impressive in the Table, where a larger series of compounds has been compiled and where the retina as a substrate has also been included. Typical serotonin antagonists like mianserin and cinanserine are only active in the frontal cortex. Drugs considered to interact specifically with serotonin receptors like methysergide, metergoline and cyproheptadine inhibited ^{3}H-spiroperidol binding also in other parts of the CNS, but only at higher concentrations. These compounds, however, exhibited dopaminergic activity in psychopharmacological and biochemical test systems. The series of thioridazine, clozapine, chlorpromazine and pipamperone were about equally potent in the frontal cortex and in hippocampus, but much weaker in the striatum. Haloperidol and spiroperidol inhibited the binding about equally in all brain areas, and the specific dopamine agonist dipropyl-ATN was inactive in the frontal cortex.

CONCLUSIONS

In vivo radioreceptor assays with ^{3}H-spiroperidol allow the characterization of serotonin and dopamine receptors in different brain areas. In the frontal cortex the majority of binding sites appear to be serotonin receptors, a minority dopamine receptors. In all other parts of the CNS studied ^{3}H-spiroperidol seems to bind to dopamine receptors. The presence of serotonin receptors, which are not labelled by ^{3}H-spiroperidol, cannot be excluded. It appears as if dopamine receptors in different brain areas differ in their properties. This study is the first direct demonstration in *in vivo* of dopamine receptors in rat hippocampus.

TABLE

Inhibition of in vivo ^{3}H-spiroperidol binding
(ID_{50} in mg/kg i.p.)

Class 1	Hippocampus	Frontal cortex	Striatum	Retina
mianserin	-35% at 30	1.2	30 Ø	30 Ø
cinanserin	100 Ø	17	100 Ø	100 Ø
Class 2				
methysergide	-25% at 30	30	100 Ø	30
metergoline	4.8	0.48	-35% at 30	2.5
cyproheptadine	3.4	0.40	27	22.5
GP 50 302	1.9	0.04	4.4	1.7
Class 3				
thioridazine	7	6.2	100	
clozapine	6.5	1.9	-40% at 30	
chlorpromazine	4	3.5	20	
pipamperone	8	1.6	-30% at 25	
Class 4				
haloperidol	0.15	0.4	0.24	0.14
spiroperidol	0.024	0.046	0.05	0.026
dipropyl-ATN	15.5	Ø	7	

Class 1: Drug acting only on 5-HT receptors
Class 2: Drugs acting preferentially on 5-HT receptors
Class 3: Drugs acting preferentially on non-striatal DA receptors
Class 4: Drugs acting on hippocampal and striatal DA receptors

References

1. Creese, I., and Snyder, S.H., Eur.J.Pharmac. 49, 201 (1978)

2. Leysen, J., Niemegeers, C., Tollenaere, J., and Laduron, P., Nature 272, 168 (1978)

3. Quick, M., Iversen, L.L., Larder, A., and Mackay, A.V.P., Nature 274, 513, (1978)

4. Laduron, P. and Leysen, J., Biochem. Pharmac. 26, 1003 (1977)

5. Hoellt, V., Czlonkowski, A. and Herz, A., Brain Res. 130, 176 (1977)

Neurotransmitters and their Receptors
Edited by U.Z. Littauer, Y. Dudai, I. Silman,
V.I. Teichberg and Z. Vogel

Sites of Action of Monamine Oxidase Inhibitors

M.B.H. Youdim and J. Finberg

Technion, Faculty of Medicine, Department of Pharmacology, Haifa, Israel

ABSTRACT

Although the differentiation of CNS and peripheral monoamine oxidase (MAO) into types A and B has serious limitations, it is a useful model for the biochemical characterization of the oxidase and its inhibitors. There is abundant evidence that MAO inhibitors benefit certain types of depression and can act as adjuncts to L-Dopa therapy of Parkinson's disease. Understanding of the biochemical and pharmacological basis of the action of irreversible inhibitors on uptake and release of biogenic monoamines together with their action at the enzyme active site is necessary for the synthesis of therapeutically useful selective MAO inhibitors. Highly purified mitochondrial MAO from beef and rat has been compared with regard to the presence of A and B type enzymes. Substrate specificity studies have shown that in beef liver only type B enzyme is present, while in contrast, rat liver contains both A and B type MAO in a 1:1 ratio. (^{14}C)-labelled deprenyl and pargyline (type B) inhibitors are stoichiometrically bound to the beef and rat liver enzymes (1 mol. inhibitor/mol. enzyme mol. wt. 150,000) but clorgyline (selective type A inhibitor) is bound to beef enzyme in amounts in considerable stoichiometric excess indicating non-specific binding. The enzyme from both sources binds the acetylenic "suicide" inhibitors at N-5 of the covalently bound flavin co-factor in a flavocyanine linkage. SDS-polyacrylamide gel-electrophoresis of (^{14}C)-inhibitor-labelled MAO indicates that the subunit structures of A and B enzymes are different. No conversion of the A to the B type of enzyme on extraction of the enzyme from the membrane and removal of lipid has been noted. It is apparent that the differences in the behaviour of MAO from rat and beef liver are not artifacts but reflect a genuine biological divergence. As a result of their irreversible enzyme inhibitory action, most acetylenic "suicide" inhibitors of MAO (clorgyline, pargyline, AGN 1133, J-508, U-1424) potentiate the effects of indirectly acting sympathomimetic amines, e.g. tyramine. However, the potent selective type B inhibitors deprenyl and AGN 1135 are devoid of such effects in isolated pharmacological preparations and *in vivo*. Their usefulness as drugs is discussed.

INTRODUCTION

The physiological function of the ubiquitous mitochondrial monoamine oxidase (MAO) (monoamine: O_2 flavin-oxido reductase (deaminating) EC 1.4.3.4.) can be summarized in the following manner: (a) it plays a crucial role in the intraneuronal inactivation and regulation of catecholamines and 5-hydroxytryptamine (1, 2, 3); (b) intestinal MAO inactivates the pressor amines e.g. tyramine, L-Dopa of foodstuff (4); (c) the enzyme in the liver may control blood levels of the pressor amines and (d) blood vessels and the lung MAO could have a crucial role in protecting the organs from the toxic effect of circulating vasoactive monoamines (5).

The discovery in 1951 of iproniazid, a potent irreversible inhibitor of MAO, with mood elevating effects in depressed patients led to the development of other drugs with similar actions and their introduction into psychiatry for the treatment of depression (6). However, one of the main pharmacological consequences of irreversible MAO inhibition in man is the increased entry into the circulation of indirectly acting vasoactive amines, e.g. tyramine, which is produced in the gut from decarboxylation of dietary tyrosine (4). Such amines can provoke a marked rise in blood pressure, which has on occasion had fatal consequences. This action of MAO inhibitors, known as the "cheese effect" is one of the major limitations to the clinical use of these drugs (14).

The electrophoretic separation of highly purified MAO into active bands (7) together with chemical differentiation of the oxidase into type A and type B forms having different substrate specificity and inhibitor sensitivity (8) has prompted many investigators to search for selective MAO inhibitors without the "cheese effect". Of the drugs so far described to date, deprenyl, a selective inhibitor of type B (9) is best known since this drug has been successfully used both as an antidepressant as well as an adjunct to L-Dopa in the treatment of Parkinson's disease without exhibiting any side effect in the peripheral sympathomimetic nervous system (10,11,12). This paper will deal with the molecular aspect of MAO type A and type B active sites and the pharmacological action of selective inhibitors on the sympathomimetic nervous system in relation to their ability to inhibit MAO A or B.

SUBSTRATE SPECIFICITY OF MAO TYPES A AND B

The classification of MAO into types A and B activity was originally proposed by Johnston (8), however, this differentiation may not be universally applicable (13). MAO A is responsible for the oxidative deamination of hydroxylated amines, e.g. 5-hydroxytryptamine, adrenaline, noradrenaline and octopamine and is selectively inhibited by clorgyline (8) and tryptolines (14); while MAO type B deaminates non-hydroxylated amines such as benzylamine, iodo-benzylamine, tryptamine and phenylethylamine and is selectively inactivated by deprenyl, pargyline, des-methylpargyline, AGN 1133, AGN 1135 (15) and U-1424 (16). Tyramine and dopamine are substrates for both forms of the enzyme. However, the Km of type A MAO for hydroxylated amines is significantly higher than is the Km of the type B species for non-hydroxylated amines (5,17). This would suggest that the amine binding sites of the two species are different (18). However, monoamine substrate deamination by each MAO species, and inhibition of each form by the above drugs, is not absolutely selective. For example, beef liver and human platelet MAO which are purely type B, also deaminate hydroxylated amines although at a relatively much lower rate than non-hydroxylated amines and are inhibited by high concentrations of clorgyline (18,19). There is no MAO which inactivates one amine only and is specifically inactivated by only one drug. These results led us to examine the inhibitor binding sites of MAO more closely.

THE BINDING SITES OF SELECTIVE AND NON-SELECTIVE MAO INHIBITORS

(a) Selective acetylenic inactivators

The present investigation was prompted by the development of a rapid and relatively mild procedure for purifying MAO from beef and rat liver (18) and human placenta (20,21) and a chemical procedure for measuring MAO content regardless of the form or degree of inactivation of the enzyme, based on the analysis of the covalently bound MAO prosthetic group, cysteinyl-flavin (22). The aim was to compare the inhibitory effects and binding capacity of (^{14}C)-pargyline, (^{14}C)-clorgyline, (^{14}C)-deprenyl and (^{14}C)-phenylethylhydrazine in the above enzyme preparations and confirm our expectation that these inhibitors bind to the enzyme active center (18,20).

All three enzyme preparations were compared with regard to the presence of MAO types A and B. Human placenta enzyme oxidizes A (5-hydroxytryptamine, epinephrine, norepinephrine) and A-B type substrates (tyramine and dopamine) rapidly and B type substrates (benzylamine and phenylethylamine) slowly (20,21). Beef liver enzyme has substrate specificity opposite to that of the human placenta enzyme while MAO from rat liver oxidizes both A and B type substrates relatively rapidly (5,17,18). Clorgyline inhibited the soluble human placenta enzyme at very low concentrations and the I_{50} for inhibition with A and A-B substrates was $\approx 10^{-7}M$, while deprenyl inhibited the enzyme only at very much higher concentrations ($I_{50} \approx 10^{-5}M$). With beef liver MAO, deprenyl ($I_{50} \approx 10^{-7}M$) was the selective inhibitor and a higher concentration of clorgyline ($I_{50} \approx 10^{-5}M$) was needed to inhibit the enzyme. With neither preparations were biphasic curves noted with A-B substrates as would be expected if both forms of the enzyme were present. In contrast, rat liver contains both A and B types of MAO (18) in equal amounts, and biphasic inhibition curves were obtained with clorgyline and deprenyl using A-B substrates (tyramine and dopamine). In conclusion, human placenta, beef liver and rat liver MAO satisfy the criteria of MAO types A, B and A-B respectively.

The acetylenic (clorgyline, deprenyl, pargyline, AGN 1133, AGN 1135 and U-1424) and hydrazine (phenylethylhydrazine) inhibitors are considered to be "suicide" irreversible inactivators of MAO (23). These compounds structurally resemble substrates of the oxidase. Enzyme inhibition by these compounds is time dependent, and as expected, substrate protects from inhibition, suggesting that inhibitor binding and substrate deamination sites are either close to each other or identical.

Although most studies of the action of acetylenic and hydrazine suicide inhibitors on MAO have been conducted with pargyline, clorgyline, deprenyl and phenylethylhydrazine, the structure of the adducts formed with the enzyme and their stoichiometry were not elucidated until very recently. In our studies we have shown that (^{14}C)-deprenyl and (^{14}C)-pargyline are stoichiometrically bound (1 mole/mole enzyme) to the beef and rat liver MAO with complete inhibition of the enzyme. However, (^{14}C)-clorgyline is bound to the beef liver enzyme in amounts in considerable stoichiometric excess (4 fold) with partial inhibition of MAO, indicating non-specific binding (18). Recently Salach et al. (20) have observed that human placenta MAO, which is solely type A, binds (^{14}C)-clorgyline stoichiometrically with complete inhibition of the enzyme .

It is known that N, N-dimethylpropargylamine, an irreversible acetylenic inhibitor of MAO, forms a flavocyanine with the covalently bound cysteinyl-flavin co-factor of MAO. Binding occurs at N-5 of the flavin (24). Since clorgyline, deprenyl, pargyline, AGN 1133 and AGN 1135 share the same mechanism of action as that of N,N-dimethylpropargylamine, it is concluded that these drugs inhibit the enzyme because of covalent interaction with the flavin in an analogous manner. The test for this hypothesis was to isolate the flavin-peptide-inhibitor adduct and measure its absorption spectrum and the amount of bound inhibitor. Clorgyline, deprenyl and pargyline form analogous flavocyanines following inactivation of MAO, the result being (a) formation of a new chromophore with intense absorption at 408 nm, and (b) bleaching of FAD absorption at 455 nm, as judged by the change in absorption spectrum of MAO inactivated by these drugs (18). Flavocyanines are readily recognized by a prominent absorption peak at 380-390 nm with a very high extinction coefficient (E_{380}=34,000) (24). The absorption spectra of cysteinyl flavin isolated from beef liver and rat liver (18) and human placenta (20) inactivated by pargyline, deprenyl and clorgyline respectively are typical of flavocyanines (24). More than 90% of each of the (^{14}C)-inhibitors stoichiometrically bound to the enzyme preparations was recovered in association with the enzyme cysteinyl-flavin prosthetic group as flavocyanine (18). Thus it can be envisaged that the adduct formed at the active centers of MAO type A and type B with these inactivators involves covalent linkage to the N-5 of the flavin (Fig. 1.) (18).

(b) Non-selective hydrazine inactivators

It has been shown that when purified MAO preparations are treated with (^{14}C)-phenylhydrazine (25) or (^{14}C)-phenylethylhydrazine (26) these inhibitors stoichiometrically (mole/mole) bind to inactivate the enzyme. Binding to the FAD occurs at the active center of the enzyme. Recently Singer (23) has provided evidence for the binding of arylhydrazines to the C(4a) of the reduced flavin and to protein groups on the enzyme. When (^{14}C)-phenylethylhydrazine treated rat liver MAO is submitted to SDS-polyacrylamide gel electrophoresis in gels containing 0.1 M 2-mercapto-

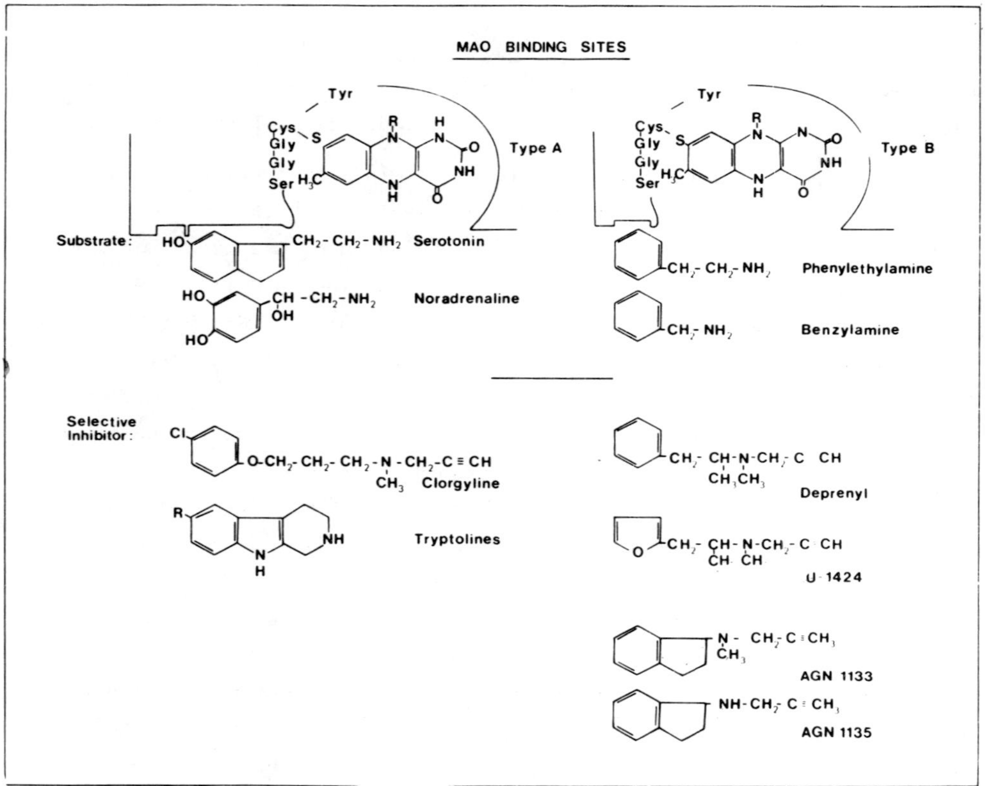

Figure 1. Schematic representation of the active sites of MAO types A and B, the binding sites of their substrates and selective inhibitors (18).

ethanol a single protein band having a molecular weight of 69,500 daltons migrates from cathode to anode, suggesting that each molecule of MAO consists of 2 subunits of equal molecular weight. On the basis of these results, the reported enzyme flavin content and the (^{14}C)-phenylethylhydrazine-binding capacity, it could be concluded that only one of the subunits should possess an active site and that MAO A and B types are not structurally different. However, if the (^{14}C)-phenylethylhydrazine inactivated MAO preparation was subjected to SDS-gel electrophoresis in the absence of 2-mercaptoethanol two bands of protein with molecular weights of 72,500 and 75,000 daltons could be separated and both bound approximately 1 mol of (^{14}C)-inhibitor per mole enzyme (mol wt. 150,000) (25). The suggestion has been made that the two bands represent isoenzymes of MAO. Callingham and Parkinson (27) have elegantly shown that the binding of ^{3}H-N-des-methylpargyline to each band can be selectively prevented if the enzyme preparations were preincubated with either clorgyline or deprenyl, thus supporting the above view that A and B MAO can be physically separated. Further it has recently been demonstrated by peptide mapping that the subunits of MAO A and B are different (28).

STRUCTURAL REQUIREMENTS FOR SELECTIVE INHIBITION

The results so far discussed indicate that the differences in the behaviour of MAO from rat and beef liver and human placenta are not artifacts, but reflect a genuine biological divergence. To summarize, it is clear that the differences in substrate specificity and inhibitor sensitivity of the enzyme forms do not reside in the mode of binding of (a) either substrate or inhibitor to the flavin prosthetic group or (b) the flavin prosthetic group to the MAO apoenzyme, since in both enzyme forms the flavin is covalently bound through its 8-α position to the thioether of cystein (Fig. 1). However, these differences may lie in the protein configuration in the vicinity of the active site. A closer look at the structure of MAO inhibitors show that these compounds resemble the substrates of MAO and in most cases are synthesized from an indole or phenylethylamine molecule (see Fig. 1). Structure-activity studies with derivatives of the acetylenic inhibitors, pargyline, clorgyline, deprenyl and AGN 1133 have shown that for the drug to act as an inhibitor of MAO A or B, the distance between the aromatic portion and N-group of the molecule is crucial. If the distance is equivalent to 3 or more carbon units the drug acts as a selective inhibitor of MAO A, as reflected in the structure of such inhibitors as clorgyline, M&B 9303 (15), Lilly 51461 (29), β-carbolines (Fig. 2) and α-methyltryptamine (14,15) (see Fig. 1). For the drug to be a selective MAO B inhibitor the distance should be 1 or 2 carbon units as in pargyline, N-desmethylpargyline, deprenyl, U-1424, AGN 1133 and AGN 1135 (15,16), so that in the B form of the enzyme the distance between the binding sites for the nitrogen and the aromatic portion of the substrate is shorter than in the A form. This may explain why the selectivity of MAO type B inhibitors for the B enzyme is not as pronounced as that of MAO A inhibitors for MAO type A (15). Access of MAO A inhibitors to the smaller MAO B active site may be more restricted than that of the MAO B inhibitors to the MAO A active site (15,16).

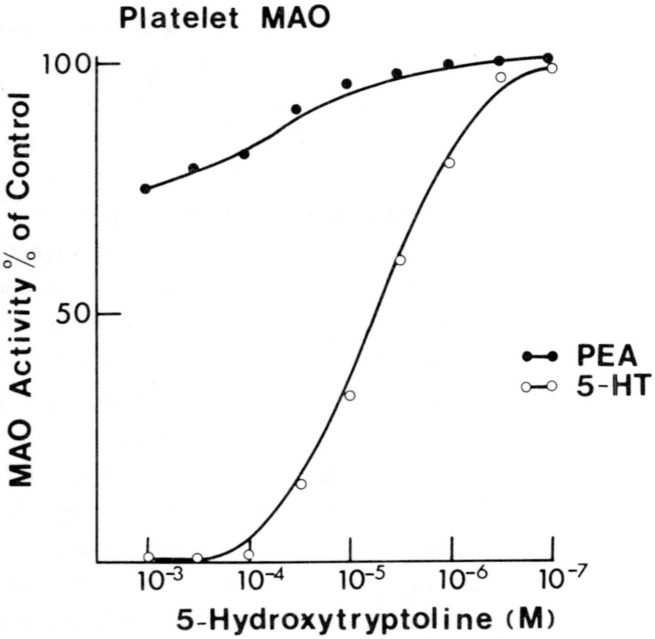

Figure 2. The selective inhibition of MAO type A by 5-hydroxytryptoline. Enzyme preparations were preincubated for 10 min. with 5-hydroxytryptoline prior to the addition of the substrates 5-hydroxytryptamine (5-HT) or phenylethylamine (PEA) (14). Six other derivatives of tryptolines tested were shown to be selective reversible inhibitors of MAO type A (14).

The biochemical studies so far discussed regarding the active site of the liver enzyme and its interaction with MAO inhibiting drugs are directly pertinent to the enzyme in the brain. Recently we have shown that purified brain MAO preparations contain covalently bound flavin, as cysteinyl-flavin, with the same turnover number as that in the oxidase from liver and kidney (22).

PHARMACOLOGICAL EFFECTS OF SOME IRREVERSIBLE INHIBITORS OF MAO TYPE B

Since most of the MAO activity in human brain is of type B (30,31), development of selective inhibitors of MAO B has led to the possibility of utilising the anti-depressant and anti-Parkinsonian properties of MAO inhibitors without reducing the ability of MAO type A in the gastrointestinal tract and liver to deaminate pressor amines such as tyramine (4). (-) Deprenyl, in contrast to clorgyline and other irreversible MAO inhibitors, has been shown not to potentiate the pressor effects of orally administered L-Dopa (10) or tyramine (32). In addition, (-) deprenyl inhibits the action of tyramine but not noradrenaline in a variety of isolated tissue preparations (9,33) as well as reducing tyramine pressor responses in the whole animal (34). This effect of (-) deprenyl has largely been attributed by Knoll (33) to inhibition of the high-affinity amine uptake system, thus limiting the entry of the indirectly-acting amines to the sympathetic nerve endings. The tyramine-antagonistic property, however, has been detected at doses of (-) deprenyl far in excess of those which selectively inhibit MAO B, as pointed out by Sandler et al. (35). Concentrations of (-) deprenyl in excess of 10^{-5}M inhibit tyramine responses, but these concentrations also inhibit non-selectively MAO types A and B (13). Similarly, tyramine pressor responses in the cat were reduced by a dose of 5 mg/kg deprenyl (34), although much lower doses are used clinically to produce selective inhibition of MAO type B (10). In order to explain the non-potentiation of tyramine responses by such low, selective doses of (-) deprenyl, it may be unnecessary to invoke a separate tyramine-antagonistic property for deprenyl. Selective inhibition of MAO type A by clorgyline, however, does potentiate the effects of amphetamine (36) and tyramine (35). The essential difference between the action of these inhibitors may result from the activity of intraneuronal MAO being composed largely of type A (37).

Work with another selective irreversible inhibitor of MAO B, AGN 1135, has shown that inhibition of the pharmacological effects of tyramine is not a unique property of (-) deprenyl (38). In the isolated rat vas deferens preparation, AGN 1135 inhibited contractile responses to tyramine at concentrations of 10^{-5}M to 10^{-4}M without altering responsiveness to norepinephrine (Fig. 3). Tyramine responses were potentiated, however, both in the case of AGN 1135 and (-) deprenyl, when the inhibitors were subsequently washed out of the organ bath.

These concentrations of AGN 1135 and (-) deprenyl caused complete irreversible inhibition of MAO type A and B activity, which presumably resulted in potentiation of the action of the indirectly-acting amine, whereas the specific tyramine-antagonistic effect of these drugs was a

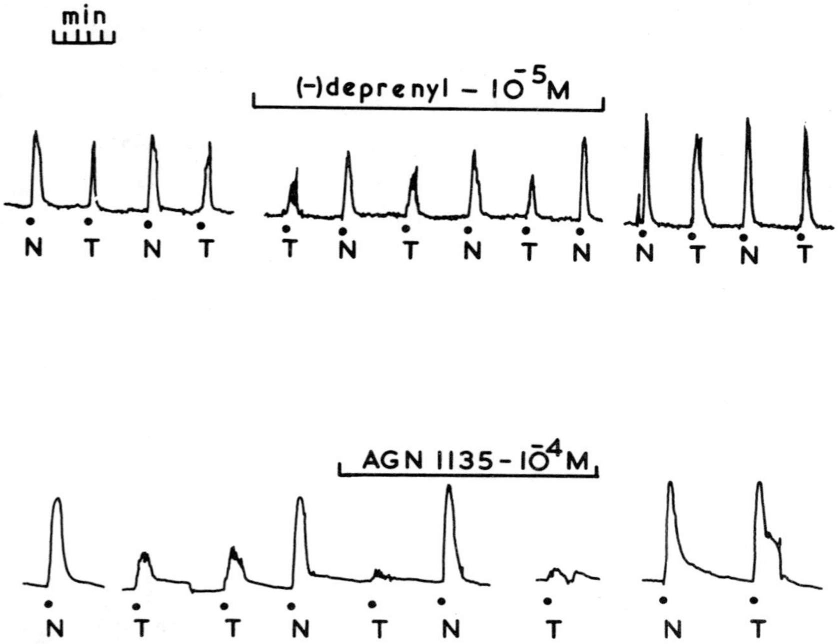

Figure 3. Isometric contractions of isolated rat vas deferens. Responses to noradrenaline (N, 0.5 μg/ml) and tyramine (T, 5 μg/ml). AGN 1135 or (-) deprenyl was present in the organ bath during the period shown by horizontal bar. Results of 2 separate experiments shown.

reversible phenomenon and dependent on presence of the drug in the system. By contrast, AGN 1133, which differs from AGN 1135 only in the presence of a N-methyl group, and is not as selective in its inhibition of MAO B, caused only potentiation of tyramine responses.

Uptake of ^{3}H-metaraminol and ^{3}H-tyramine by the isolated rat vas deferens was examined at the same concentrations of AGN 1135 and (-) deprenyl as those used in organ bath experiments. Only a 20% inhibition in ^{3}H-metaraminol uptake was prodûced by both drugs (Table 1) although desmethylimipramine (10^{-6}M) inhibited uptake by 70%. Similarly, ^{3}H-tyramine uptake was reduced only 15% by (-) deprenyl (10^{-5}M) and not at all by AGN 1135 (10^{-4}M)(33). This slight effect on amine uptake by AGN 1135 and (-) deprenyl would appear to be inadequate to explain the large inhibition of the contractile response to tyramine.

Table 1. Uptake of ^{3}H-metaraminol by isolated rat vas deferens.

	Control	$0^{o}C$	DMI $1x10^{-6}M$	AGN 1135 $1x10^{-4}M$	(-) Deprenyl $1x10^{-5}M$	$3x10^{-5}M$
Uptake dpm/mg per 5 min.	1394	232	370	1063	1138	1026
SEM	±27	±16	±52	±28	±93	±42
% control	100	17	28	79	81	73
P		<0.01	<0.01	<0.01	<0.01	<0.01

Whole vas deferens were incubated with inhibitors for 20 min. at $37^{o}C$ in Kreb's solution gassed with O_2/CO_2 (95%/5%). (^{3}H)-metaraminol (10^{-7}M) was added for a further 5 min. and uptake stopped by rapidly transferring organs to a large volume of Kreb's solution at room temperature. Vas deferens were then solubilised with Soluene 100 (Parkard Ltd.) and total radioactivity determined by liquid scintillation counting.

An alternative explanation for the selective antagonism of the tyramine effect may be offered by the possibility of an active efflux system mediating exit of noradrenaline from the sympathetic nerve ending following release of the neurotransmitter by a phenylethylamine (39). Des-methylimipramine has been shown to decrease the accelerated (^{3}H)-noradrenaline efflux produced by administration of β-phenylethylamine (40,41). (-) Deprenyl and AGN 1135, therefore, may inhibit active efflux to a greater extent than neuronal membrane uptake of amines.

The irreversible, propargyl derivative inhibitors of MAO possess a variety of actions on the sympathetic neurone which must be considered in assessing the central effects of these drugs. In carefully controlled, low doses, the major effect of AGN 1135 and (-) deprenyl may be selective inhibition of MAO type B. As the dose of (-) deprenyl is increased, two further effects become apparent; one is inhibition of noradrenaline release by indirectly-acting amines, and the other is an amphetamine-like sympathomimetic and animal behavioural effect. The latter actions were described by Simpson (42) in the cardiovascular system of the rat, Green and Youdim (3), on rat locomotor activity and has also been observed in the cardiovascular system of the dog (43). Increase in blood pressure and heart rat produced by (-) deprenyl in the rat were blocked by pre-treatment with 6-hydroxydopamine (42) showing that these effects were due to catecholamine release. In the case of AGN 1135, sympathomimetic effects were not observed (38) although the tyramine-antagonistic action was apparent in isolated preparations. (-) Deprenyl is metabolised to amphetamine and methamphetamine (44), but it is not known whether these metabolites contribute to the anti-depressant and anti-Parkinsonian properties of the drug. Indeed, since (-) deprenyl is the form used clinically, and since (-) isomers of amphetamines are less active than the (+) isomers, it has been suggested that significant pharmacological effect would not result from amphetamine produced metabolically (35). It remains to be seen whether AGN 1135 will also possess anti-depressant and anti-Parkinsonian properties in the human.

CONCLUSIONS

Existence of two distinct forms of MAO has permitted the development of selective inhibitors of the enzyme. Presently available inhibitors of MAO type B show relatively poor selectivity; however, further research could lead to the development of highly selective MAO B inhibitors, which have potential use as antidepressants and in the treatment of Parkinson's disease by inhibiting brain MAO without potentiating the peripheral effects of indirectly-acting sympathomimetic amines which are A-B substrates (e.g. tyramine). The effects of amines which are MAO B substrates (e.g. β-phenylethylamine) would be potentiated by such compounds, but no deleterious effects of such potentiation have as yet been reported. Such drugs could also be designed which do not possess the intrinsic amphetamine-like activity of L-deprenyl.

The structural requirements for inhibition of active efflux of noradrenaline from sympathetic neurones induced by phenylethylamines is at present unknown, however, the possibility exists, that this property could be incorporated in the structure of either MAO A or MAO B selective inhibitors. Thus inhibition of either form of the enzyme without potentiation of the actions of sympathomimetic amines is feasible. Such an inhibitor of MAO B would also block the actions of β-phenylethylamine, which may reduce its antidepressant property.

The clinical effectiveness of such specific drugs remains to be determined.

ACKNOWLEDGMENT

This work was supported by grants from the National Council for Research and Development, Prime Minister's Office, Jerusalem, and the Dr. Ronald Lawrence Neurophyschopharmacological Research Fund, Technion, Israel.

REFERENCES

1. Youdim, M.B.H. (1975). In: MTP International Review of Science. Ed. H. Blaschko. Butersworth, London, p.165.

2. Costa, E. and Sandler, M. (1972). Monoamine Oxidase - New Vistas. Raven Press, New York.

3. Green, A.R. and Youdim, M.B.H. (1975). Brit. J. Pharmacol., 55, 415.

4. Youdim, M.B.H. (1977). In: Neuroregulators and Psychiatric Disorders. Eds. E. Usdin, D. Hamburg and J. Barchas. Oxford University Press, New York, p. 57.

5. Bakhle, Y.S. and Youdim, M.B.H. (1979). Brit. J. Pharmacol., 65 147.

6. Zeller, E.A. (1963). Ann. N.Y. Acad. Sci., 107, 809.

7. Youdim, M.B.H., Collins, G.G.S. and Sandler, M. (1969). Nature, 223, 626.

8. Johnston, J.P. (1968). Biochem. Pharmacol., 17, 1285.

9. Knoll, J. and Magyar, K. (1972). Adv. Biochem. Psychopharmacol., 5, 393.

10. Birkmayer, W., Riederer, P., Ambrozi, L. and Youdim, M.B.H. (1977). Lancet, 1, 439.

11. Lees, A.J., Kohout, L.J., Shaw, K.M., Stern, G.M., Elsworth, J.D., Sandler, M. and Youdim, M.B.H. (1977). Lancet, 2, 791.

12. Mendlewicz, J. and Youdim, M.B.H. (1978). J. Neural Transmn., 43, 279.

13. Fowler, C.J., Callingham, B.A., Mantle, T.J. and Tipton, K.F. (1978). Biochem. Pharmacol., 27, 97.

14. Oppenheim, B., Youdim, M.B.H., Goldstein, S. and Hefetz, A. (1978). Israel J. Med. Sci., 14, 1096.

15. Kalir, A., Sabbagh, A. and Youdim, M.B.H. (1980). Brit. J. Pharmacol. (in press).

16. Knoll, J. (1979). Trends Neurosc., 2, 111.

17. Houslay, M.D. and Tipton, K.F. (1974). Biochem. J., 139, 645.

18. Salach, J.I., Detmer, K. and Youdim, M.B.H. (1979). Molec. Pharmacol., 16, 234.

19. Murphy, D.L. and Donnelly, C.H. (1974). Adv. Biochem. Psychopharmacol., 12, 71.

20. Salach, J.I. and Detmer, K. (1979). In: Monoamine Oxidase Strucutre, Function and Altered Function. Eds. T.P. Singer, R.W. Von Korff and D.L. Murphy. Academic Press, New York, p.121.

21. Youdim, M.B.H. and Sandler, M. (1968). In: Biochemical Aspects of Prenylamine. Ed. F. Cedrangolo. Biochimica Appl. 14. Hoechst, Italia, Milano. p. 175.

22. Salach, J.I., Singer, T.P., Yasunobu, K.T., Minamura, N. and Youdim, M.B.H. (1976). In: Monoamine Oxidase and Its Inhibition. Eds. G.E.W. Wolstenholme and J. Knight, Elsevier, Amsterdam, p.57.

23. Singer, T.P. (1979). In: Monoamine Oxidase, Structure, Function and Altered Function. Eds. T.P. Singer, R.W. Von Korff and D.L. Murphy. Academic Press, New York, p. 7.

24. Maycock, H.L., Abeles, R.H., Salach, J.I. and Singer, T.P. (1976). Biochemistry, 15, 114.

25. Patek, D.R. and Hellerman, L. (1974). J. Biol. Chem., 249, 2373.

26. Collins, G.G.S. and Youdim, M.B.H. (1975). Biochem. Pharmacol., 24, 703.

27. Callingham, B.A. and Parkinson, D. (1979). In: Monoamine Oxidase Structure Function and Altered Functions. Eds. T.P. Singer, R.W. Von Korff and D.L. Murphy. Academic Press, New York, p.81.

28. Pintar, J.E., Cawthon, R.M., Costa, M.R.C. and Breakefield, X.O. (1979). In: Monoamine Oxidase, Structure, Function and Altered Function. Eds. T.P. Singer, R.W. Von Korff and D.L. Murphy, Academic Press, New York, p. 185.

29. Fuller, R.W., Slater, I.H. and Mills, J. (1979). In: Monoamine Oxidase, Structure, Function and Altered Function. Eds. T.P. Singer, R.W. Von Korff and D.L. Murphy. Academic Press, New York, p. 317.

30. Riederer, P., Youdim, M.B.H., Rausch, W.D., Birkmayer, W., Jellinger, K. and Seemann, D. (1978). J. Neural Transmn., 43, 217.

31. Squires, R.F. (1972). Adv. Biochem. Psychopharmacol., 5, 355.

32. Elsworth, J.D., Glover, V., Reynolds, G.P., Sandler, M., Lees, A.J., Phuapradit, P., Shaw, K.M., Stern, G.M. and Kumar, P. (1978). Psychopharmacology, 57, 33.

33. Knoll, J. (1978). J. Neural Transmn., 43, 177.

34. Knoll, J., Vizi, E.S. and Magyar, K. (1972). In: Recent Developments of Neurobiology in Hungary III. Results in Neuroanatomy, Neurophysiology, Neuropathophysiology and Neuropharmacology. Ed. K. Lissak, Budapest: Publishing House of the Hungarian Academy of Sciences, p. 167.

35. Sandler, M., Glover, V., Ashford, A. & Stern, G.M. (1978). J. Neural Transmn., 43, 209.

36. Simpson, L.L. (1978). J. Pharmacol. exp. Ther., 205, 392.

37. Goridis, C. and Neff, N.H. (1971). Evidence for a specific monoamine oxidase associated with sympathetic nerves. Neuropharmacology, 10, 557.

38. Finberg, J.P.M., Sabbagh, A. and Youdim, M.B.H. (1979). In: Enzymes and Neurotransmitters in Mental Disease. Eds. E. Usdin and M.B.H. Youdim, Wiley, London (in press).

39. Trendelenburg, U. (1979). In: The Release of Catecholamines from Adrenergic Neurones. Ed. D.M.Paton, New York, Pergamon Press, p. 333.

40. Paton, D.M. (1973). Brit. J. Pharmacol., 49, 143P.

41. Raiteri, M., del Carmine, R. and Bertolini, A. (1977). Mol. Pharmacol., 13, 746.

42. Simpson, L.L. (1978). Biochem. Pharmacol., 27, 1591.

43. Goldberg, L.I. personal communication.

44. Reynolds, G.P., Elsworth, J.D., Blau, K., Sandler, M., Lees, A.J. and Stern, G.M. (1978). Br. J. Clin. Pharmacol., 6, 542.

Neurotransmitters and their Receptors
Edited by U.Z. Littauer, Y. Dudai, I. Silman,
V.I. Teichberg and Z. Vogel

The Serotinergic Receptor in Rat Hippocampus

Menahem Segal

Department of Isotope Research, The Weizmann Institute of Science, Rehovot, Israel

ABSTRACT

The effects of serotonin (5HT) on neuronal activity were studied in the in-vivo and in-vitro rat hippocampus. Electrical stimulation of the raphe nuclei or iontophoretic application of 5HT caused suppression of spontaneous activity of hippocampal neurons. Early components of evoked commissural responses were depressed but late components were augmented by priming stimulation of the raphe. 5HT caused hyperpolarization associated with a decrease in input resistance in hippocampal neurons recorded from the in-vitro slice preparation. Several experiments indicate that 5HT produces its effects by increasing conductance for K^+ ions. Indeed, topical application of 5HT causes a transient rise in extracellular K^+ concentration ($[K^+]_o$). A spatial distribution of 5HT induced changes in $[K^+]_o$ parallels a spatial distribution of $[^3H]$5HT binding sites in the hippocampus. It is suggested that 5HT activates K^+ conductance and that a differential effect of 5HT in various fields of the hippocampus can underly its complex action seen in the intact brain.

INTRODUCTION

Serotonin (5HT), one of the main monoamine neurotransmitters, has been the subject of numerous investigations in recent years. Its biochemistry and pharmacology (1-5), brain distribution (6-11) and functions (12-15) are well characterized. Compared with the wealth of information gathered in these disciplines, relatively little was known until recently about the postsynaptic mechanism of action of 5HT in the brain.

The hippocampus (HPC) constitutes a major target organ of the serotonergic nucleus raphe medianus (MR) (6,7,8,10,16). Studies employing various anatomical and biochemical techniques have characterized the efferents of the MR and their terminals in the HPC. These studies demonstrate an uneven distribution of serotonergic fibers and terminals in the HPC; a heavy concentration of fibers was found in the dentate gyrus, and fewer fibers in the CA3 and CA1 molecular and pyramidal layers (6,16). The monosynaptic MR-HPC connection was selected as a model system for a serotonergic synapse in the brain.

The in-vivo studies

Initial studies (17) have demonstrated that electrical stimulation of the MR produced a long lasting inhibition of spontaneous activity of hippocampal neurons. This inhibition was modulated by serotonergic drugs; methysergide antagonized the inhibitory responses and chlorimipramine, a reuptake blocker, potentiated them. The responses were nearly absent in rats treated with 5HT depleting drugs (i.e. PCPA). Iontophoretical application of 5HT inhibited spontaneous activity of most cells tested in the HPC (17,18), as well as elsewhere (1,3,19,20,21). Furthermore, some 5HT antagonists (e.g. methysergide) exhibited at least a partial antagonistic action on the depressant effects of 5HT in the HPC (Fig. 1).

The effects of MR stimulation on HPC activity may not be a result of a simple activation of an inhibitory monosynaptic connection. MR-originated fibers terminate also in regions afferent to the HPC and may thereby affect HPC activity indirectly. This possibility was demonstrated in a study on the MR-septal connection. Stimulation of the MR caused an inhibition of medial septal neurons (22) which are known to project an excitatory cholinergic input into the HPC. The multitude of response types found in the HPC to MR stimulation (17) may therefore reflect both mono and polysynaptic connections between the raphe nuclei and the HPC.

The awake freely moving rat preparation offers the advantages of studying effects of stimulation in the absence of anesthesia over prolonged periods of time. Furthermore, interactions with natural stimuli can be analyzed. Effects of raphe stimulation on commissural responses were measured in awake rat (23). Stimulation of the commissural path activated a characteristic short latency (5-15 msec) monosynaptic excitatory response in region CA1 of the HPC (24). When MR was stimulated prior to commissural stimulation, it produced a decrease in the short-latency-response to the commissural stimulation (Fig. 2). In addition, it facilitated the formation of a longer latency (20-35 ms) excitatory response to the same stimulation. The efficiency of the MR priming stimulation was reduced after depletion of 5HT by PCPA. It appears that in addition to its suppressive action of spontaneous and primary evoked potentials, MR stimulation can facilitate the formation of long-latency excitatory responses to commissural stimulation in the HPC.

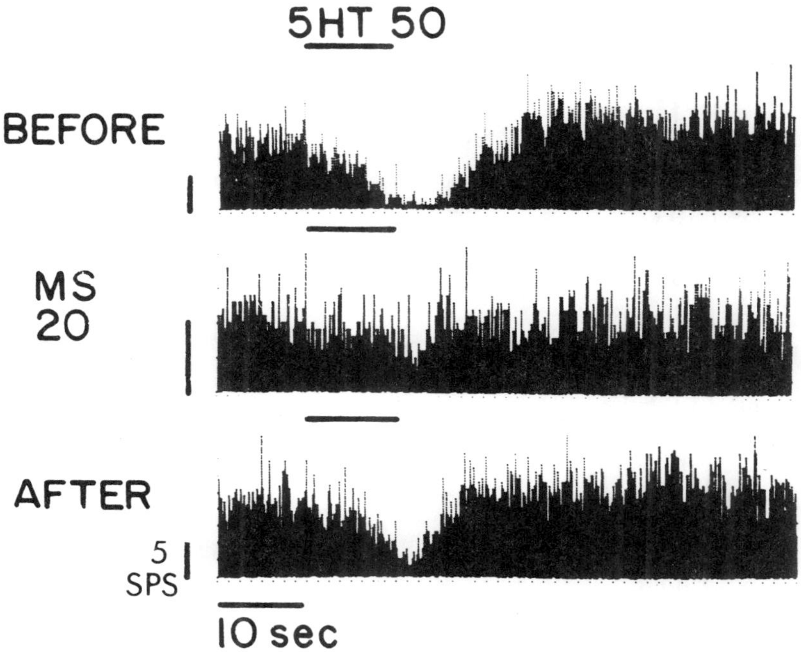

Fig. 1. Effects of methysergide (MS) on the suppression of hippocampal cellular activity by 5HT. Three successive peri-stimulus time histograms (PSTH), each consisting of 10 trials. Top histogram, before MS; 5HT, applied with a current of 50 nA for a duration indicated by the horizontal bar, cuased a reversible cessession of spontaneous extracellular activity. Middle, MS was administered continuously with a current of 20 nA. Bottom, after termination of MS current, a partial recovery from MS effects is seen. Ordinate, spikes per second. (From 17).

The pathways involved in this dual action as well as its mechanisms will be discusses later.

The in-vitro studies

Experiments aimed at elucidating the ionic mechanism of 5HT action in the HPC were conducted in the *in-vitro* hippocampal slice preparation (25). Hippocampi of decapitated rats were rapidly dissected, sliced into 300-400μm slices and superfused with controlled physiological solutions. Intracellular activity was recorded via glass micropipettes from neurons in the pyramidal layer of region CA1. Membrane potentials and responses of the neurons to hyperpolarizing and depolarizing current pulses as well as stimulation of local afferents were measured. 5HT was

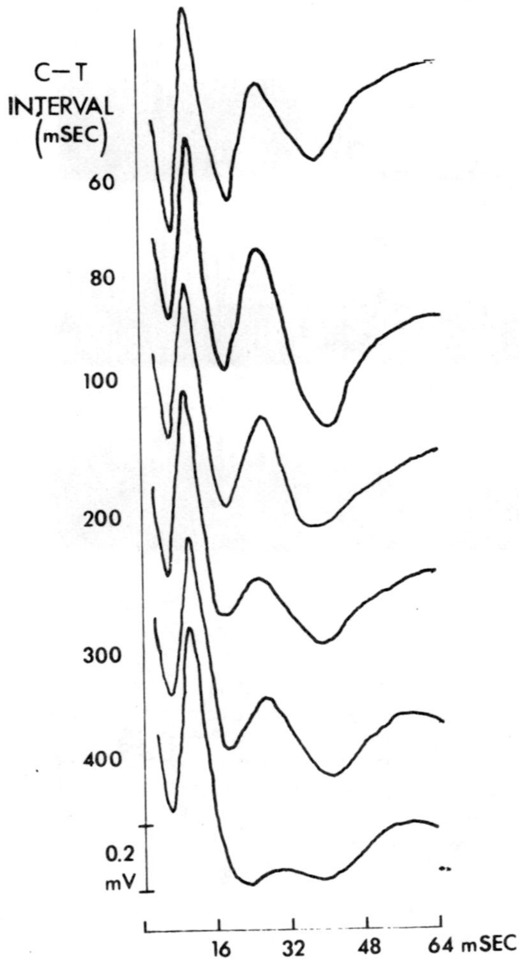

Fig. 2. Effects of MR conditioning stimulation on hippocampal responses to commissural stimulation. MR conditioning (C) stimulation (0.2 msec 5V, 3 pulses applied within 20 msec) was applied at indicated intervals before the test (T) stimulation of the contralateral hippocampus. Each trace consists of 16 successive responses recorded from stratum radiatum of area CA1, averaged with an Ortec signal averager (23). Note the presence of a secondary potential at short but not long C-T intervals. Negativity up.

applied in a droplet on the surface of the slice or via iontophoresis. Resting potentials of -55 to -80 mV could be recorded continuously for at least 1 hr. In most of the cells tested, applications of 5HT produced a hyperpolarization of 3-5 mV associated with a 20-30% decrease in input resistance as measured by responses to hyperpolarizing current pulses (Fig. 3). Whenever present, spontaneous spike discharges were reduced or even abolished by 5HT. These effects were observed when 5HT was applied on the pyramidal layer near the recording electrode but not when applied in the dendritic areas. The responses to 5HT were significantly reduced in the presence of methysergide in the superfusion medium. Although there

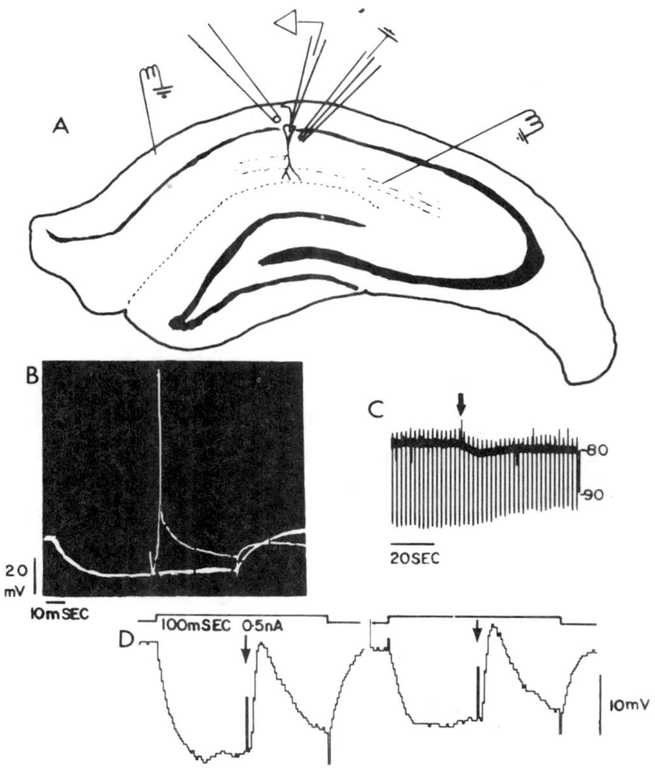

Fig. 3. 5HT effects in the hippocampal slice preparation. A. The arrangement of stimulating and recording electrodes. Intracellular recording was made from cells in the pyramidal layer of region CA1. A monopolar stimulating electrode was routinely placed in the stratum radiatum (right). Another stimulating electrode (optional) was placed in the alveus, to invade antidromically the recorded cells. A 5-barrel micropipette or a single wide-bored pipette were placed at various distances from the recording electrode. B. A typical oscillographic record of a cellular response to a hyperpolarizing current pulse and an action potential arising from an EPSP produced by stimulation of the stratum radiatum. C. A chart record of membrane potential and responses to hyperpolarizing current pulses applied at a rate of 0.5 Hz before and after application of 5HT (0.5 mM, arrowhead).

was a marked decrease in resistance in all measured neurons, the excitatory post synaptic potentials (EPSP's) were only slightly affected (Fig. 3).

An analysis of current-voltage plots before and after application of 5HT revealed that the reversal potenatial for 5HT actions is about -85 to -90 mV. This is in the range of the equilibrium potential of K^+-

ions. Several experiments excluded the involvement of Cl^-, another ion known to be associated with hippocampal inhibition, from mediating 5HT action; replacement of Cl^- in the medium by propionate ions did not affect 5HT action although the replacement caused significant changes in resting membrane potentials and in PSP's. Addition of ammonium ions to the medium did not change the sensitivity of 5HT either. The effects of 5HT were smaller in a medium containing 10 mM K^+ compared to those found in normal (5 mM K^+) medium. These and similar experiments have demonstrated for the first time in mammalian CNS, that 5HT acts by increasing conductance of K^+-ions (gK^+) across the neural membrane, and thereby hyperpolarizing the neurons. This rise in gK^+ was not Na^+ of Ca^{++} dependent. The hypothesis that 5HT acts by increasing gK^+ could be tested directly with the use of K^+ sensitive electrodes (26). In a recent series of experiments (27) it was indeed found that 5HT but not norepinephrine, caused a 0.5-2 mM rise in extracellular K^+ concentrations ($[K^+]_o$). This rise was partially antagonized by methysergide. A comparison of the effects of 5HT in the different regions of the hippocampal slice revealed that 5HT was about equally effective in regions CA1 and the dentate gyrus in elevating $[K^+]_o$ but was almost non effective in region CA3 (Fig. 4). This was not due to a physiologically inactive region since neurons in this region still reacted to afferent stimulation; and resting $[K^+]_o$ was similar to that in other regions of the slice.

5HT Receptors in the rat hippocampus

Results from several laboratories indicate that among all brain regions studied, the HPC contains the highest number of high affinity 5HT binding sites (4,5). This observation contrasts the low concentration of endogenous 5HT or raphe-originated 5HT-containing fibers. The present experiments were designed to varify the neuronal localization and to search for an intrahippocampal regional distribution of 5HT receptors. Initial experiments have confirmed the presence of a single high affinity (Kd=5 nM) binding site specific for ^{3}H-5HT (Fig. 5). Hippocampal injection of kainic acid (KA, 1μg/1μℓ) known to cause degeneration of neurons (28,29) caused a nearly complete disappearance of specific 5HT binding sites in the injected HPC. This experiment indicates that the serotonin binding sites are restricted to neuronal membranes and not to glial cells. The differential distribution of ^{3}H-5HT binding sites was measured in the following regions; the dentate gurus (DG), region CA3, the molecular and

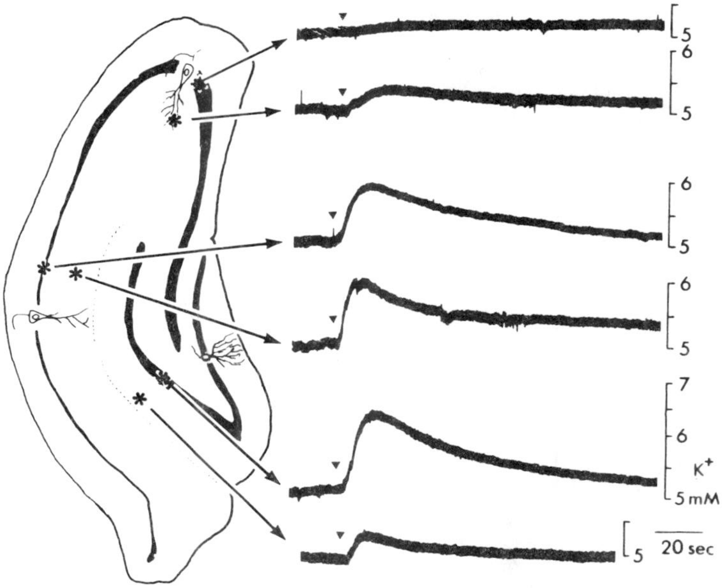

Fig. 4. Regional distribution of changes in $[K^+]_o$ produced by 5HT in the HPC. Recording electrodes were placed in the areas marked with asterisks and 5HT was applied near the recording electrodes. Note the large increases in $[K^+]_o$ recorded in CA1 and in the dentate granular layer and the relative absence of responses in area CA3 (top). (From 27).

radiatum layers of region CA1 (M-CA1), and the pyramidal, oriens and alveus of CA1 (P-CA1). It was found that DG, P-CA1 and M-CA1 bind specifically about the same amount of $[^3H]$-5HT but that region CA3 binding is only about 50% of that found in the other regions. This finding corroborates results of the physiological experiments and indicates that the 5HT receptors in CA1 region may be evenly distributed along the soma-dentritic axis and that region CA3 is relatively poor in 5HT receptors.

DISCUSSION

An attempt to present a coherent scheme of the action of 5HT in the HPC has to take into consideration several seemingly conflicting observations presented above and elsewhere (17,23). Stimulation of the MR causes inhibition of spontaneous hippocampal cellular activity (17). A similar effect is seen when 5HT is applied iontophoretically. On the other hand, priming stimulation of MR can facilitate formation of a late excitatory response in region CA1 to stimulation of the commissural path. Priming

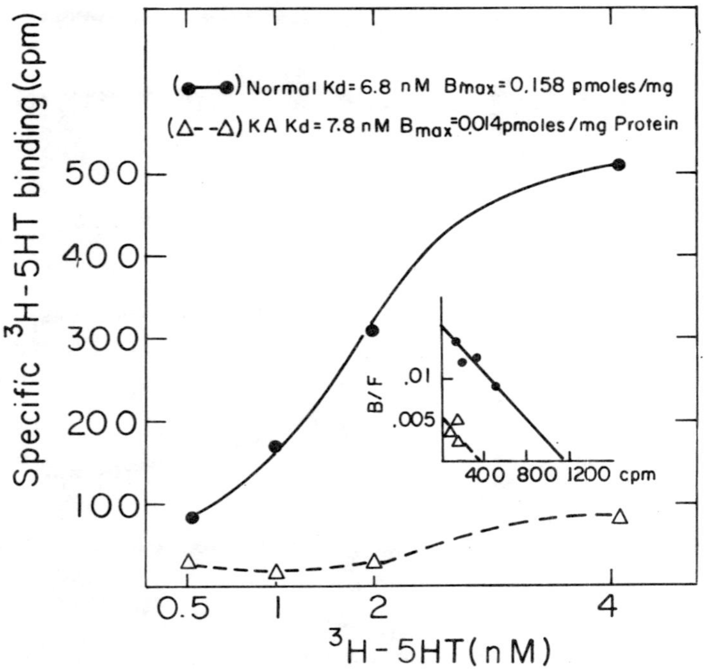

Fig. 5. Specific binding of ^{3}H-5HT to membranes of normal and KA treated hippocampus. Insert: a scatchard analysis of the binding data. The methods were adapted from Nelson et al. (5).

stimulation of MR was also reported to alter responses of the dentate gyrus to a test stimulus applied to the perforant path (30,32). It was suggested that the serotonergic input serves as a gating mechanism for incoming information in the dentate gyrus, but the exact nature of this gate was not clarified. The results of the intracellular study suggest one possible explanation for the opposite effects of 5HT on spontaneous and evoked activity in the HPC; 5HT caused a long lasting hyperpolarization associated with a decrease in input resistance and spontaneous firing although it did not affect EPSP's produced by stimulation of excitatory afferents. This can be expressed as an increase in signal (EPSP) to noise (spontaneous activity) ratio but it cannot explain the net increase in long latency excitatory response to commissural stimulation (Fig. 2). The long latency of the late excitatory response indicates that a polysynaptic pathway is being activated in the presence of 5HT. The action of 5HT in region CA1 contrasts the weak effects of 5HT in CA3, containing a rela-

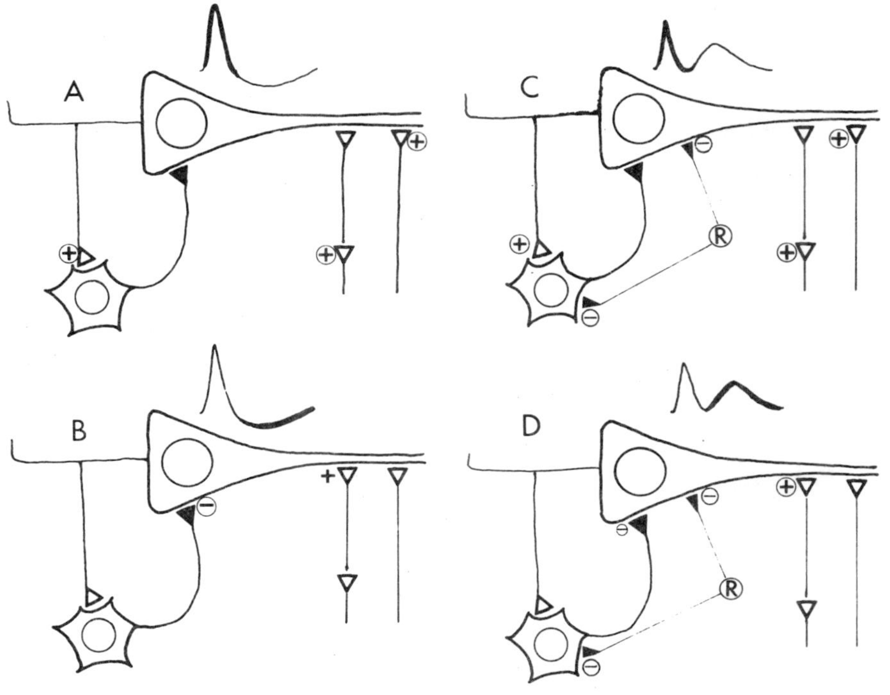

Fig. 6. A model of the effects of 5HT on responses of hippocampal cells to commissural stimulation. A. and B. Responses in the relative absence of inhibitory 5HT input. (A) Excitatory commissural synapses evoke a response of pyramidal neurons which excite the interneurons (B). These, in turn, inhibit the pyramidal neurons, such that the later phase of excitation, coming from the Schaffer collateral system is unable to trigger the neurons. Averaged evoked responses are derived from Figure 2. C. and D. Responses to commissural stimulation in the presence of 5HT input. (C) Excitatory responses to commissural stimulation are smaller than in (A) in the presence of raphe (R) originated inhibitory input. The interneurons, in turn, produce a weaker inhibition which is unable to mask the secondary excitatory input (D).

tively low number of ^{3}H-5HT binding sites. It is hypothesized that in the relative absence of 5HT activation, stimulation of the contralateral hippocampus excite neurons in both CA3 and CA1 regions. CA1 pyramidal neurons excite the local interneurons (33) which, in turn, inhibit the pyramidal cells by a potent GABA mediated feedback mechanism (Fig. 6). While inhibited by the local synapses, these pyramidal cells do not react to the secondary wave of excitation arriving from the Schaffer collaterals of CA3 neurons activated by the same commissural stimulation. When the serotonergic system is effective, the initial response of CA1 pyramids to commissural stimulation is slightly reduced (Fig. 6). The interneurons, also inhibited by 5HT, are not excited by the pyramids and in turn, do not inhibit the pyramids. CA3 neurons, not affected by the serotonergic input, send a relatively large secondary excitatory wave onto CA1 pyramids via the Schaffer collaterals. Since EPSP's in CA1 are not affected by 5HT, and in the relative absence of interneuron-originated GABA mediated inhibition, CA1 pyramids are now excited by this CA3 input and therefore produce a long latency excitatory response.

This mechanism can explain the presence of long latency responses observed in CA1 region. Similarly, the gating mechanism suggested for the action of 5HT in the dentate gyrus can actually act along the same principles; there is a known connection between CA3 and the dentate activity. A differential efficacy of 5HT in the dentate and CA3 can affect this modulatory action to produce the gating mechanism.

The present studies have contributed to the understanding of this unique control system in the brain and to the understanding of the post-synaptic action of 5HT. A major question of interest is now _when_ is this 5HT system activated in the normal brain. Studies along this line, using recording of activity of MR neurons in the awake freely moving rat will undoubtedly contribute to the building of a comprehensive picture of 5HT action of the brain.

REFERENCES

1. Bloom, F.E., Hoffer, B.J., Siggins, G.R., Barker, J.L., and Nicoll, R.A., 1972, Effects of serotonin on central neurons: microiontophoretic administration, _Fed. Proc._, 31:97.

2. Costa, E., Gessa, G.L. and Sandler, M., 1974, Serotonin - new vistas; biochemistry and behavioral and clinical studies, _in_: Adv. Biochem. Psychopharmacol. Vol. III, Raven Press, New York.

3. Weight, F.F. and Salmoiraghi, G.C., 1968, Serotonin effects on central neurons, _Advances Pharmacol._, 6:395.

4. Bennett, J.P. Jr. and Snyder, S.H., 1976, Serotonin and lysergic acid diethylamide binding in rat brain membranes: relationship to post-synaptic serotonin receptors, _Molec. Pharmacol._, 12:373.

5. Nelson, D.L., Herbet, A., Bourgoin, S., Glowinski, J. and Hamon, H., 1978, Characterization of central 5-HT receptors and their adaptive changes following intracerebral 5,7-dihydroxytryptamine administration in the rat, Mol. Pharmacol., 14:983.

6. Azmitia, E.D., 1978, The serotonin producing neurons of the midbrain median and dorsal raphe nuclei, in: "Handbook of Psychpharmacology", Vol. 9, LL. Iversen, S.D. Iversen and S.H. Snyder, eds., Plenum Press, New York.

7. Azmitia, E. and Segal, M., 1978, The efferent connections of the dorsal and median raphe nuclei in the rat brain, J. Comp. Neurol., 179:641.

8. Conrad, L.C.A., Leonard, C.M. and Pfaff, D.W., 1974, Connections of the median and dorsal raphe nuclei in the rat: an autoradiographic and degeneration study, J. Comp. Neurol., 156:179.

9. Bobillier, P., Seguin, S., Petitjean, F., Salvert, D., Touret, M., and Jouvet, M., 1976, The raphe nuclei of the cat brain stem: A topographical altas of their efferent projections as revealed by autoradiography, Brain Res., 113:449.

10. Moore, R.Y. and Halaris, A.E., 1975, Hippocampal innervation by serotonin neurons of the midbrain raphe in the rat, J. Comp. Neurol., 164:171.

11. Segal, M. and Landis, S., 1974, Afferents to the hippocampus of the rat studied with the method of retrograde transport of horseradish peroxidase, Brain Res., 78:1.

12. Akil, H. and Liebeskind, J.C., 1975, Monoaminergic mechanisms of stimulation produced analgesia, Brain Res., 94:279.

13. Jacobs, B.L., Wise, W.D. and Taylos, K.M., 1974, Differential behavioral and neurochemical effects following lesions of the dorsal or median raphe nuclei in rats, Brain Res., 79:353.

14. Jouvet, M., 1969, Biogenic amines and the states of sleep, Science, 163:32.

15. Lorens, S.A. and Yunger, L.M., 1974, Morphine analgesia two way avoidance, and consummatory behavior following lesions in the midbrain raphe nuclei of the rat, Pharmacol. Biochem. Behav., 2:215.

16. Gage, F.H., Thompson, R.G. and Valdes, S.J., 1978, Endogenous norepinephrine and serotonin within the hippocampal formation during the development and recovery from septal hyper-reactivity, Pharmacol. Biochem. Behav., 9:359.

17. Segal, M., 1975, Physiological and pharmacological evidence for a serotonergic projection to the hippocampus, Brain Res., 94:115.

18. Segal, M., 1976, 5HT antagonists in rat hippocampus, Brain Res., 103:161.

19. Phillis, J.W., Tebēcis, A.K. and York, D.H., 1967, The inhibitory action of monoamines on lateral geniculate neurons, J. Physiol. (Lond.)., 190:563.

20. Roberts, M.H.T. and Straughan, D.W., 1967, Excitation and depression of cortical neurones by 5-hydroxytryptamine, J. Physiol., 193:269.

21. Wang, R.Y. and Aghajanian, G.K., 1977, Inhibition of neurons in the amygdala by dorsal raphe stimulation: mediation through a direct serotonergic pathway, Brain Res., 120:85.

22. Segal, M., 1976b, Brainstem afferents to the rat medial septum, J. Physiol. (Lond.), 261:617.

23. Segal, M., 1977, Effects of brainstem priming stimulation on hippocampal response to interhemispheric stimulation in the awake rat, Exp. Brain Res., 28:529.

24. Andersen, P., 1960, Interhippocampal impulses II apical dendritic activation of CAl neurons, Acta Physiol. Scand., 48:178.

25. Segal, M., 1980, Effects of serotonin in the hippocampal slice preparation, J. Physiol., in press.

26. Heinemann, V., Lux, H.D. and Zander, K.J., 1977, Effects of norepinephrine and DB-c-AMP on active uptake of K^+ in the cerebral cortex of cats, in: "Iontophoresis and Transmitter mechanisms in the mammalian central nervous system", J.S. Kelly and R.W. Ryall, eds., Elsevier Biomedical Press, New York.

27. Segal, M. and Gutnick, M., 1980, Effects of serotonin on extracellular potassium concentration in the rat hippocampal slice, Brain Res., in press.

28. Olney, J.W., Rhee, V. and Ho, O.L., 1974, Kainic acid, a powerful neurotoxic analogue of glutamate, Brain Res., 77:507.

29. Coyle, J.T. and Schwarcz, R., 1976, Lesions of striatal neurons with kainic acid provides a model for Huntington's chorea, Nature, 263:244.

30. Winson, J., 1977, Effect of median raphe stimulation on neuronal transmission through the dentate gyrus in the freely moving and anesthetized rat, Neuroscience Society, p. 656.

31. Winson, J. and Abzug, C., 1977, Gating of neuronal transmission in the hippocampus: efficacy of transmission varies with behavioral state, Science, 196:1223.

32. Assaf, S.Y., and Miller, J.J., 1978, Heterosynaptic modification of neuronal transmission in the dentate gyrus of the rat, Society for Neuroscience Abstracts, 4:205.

33. Andersen, P., 1964, Pathway of postsynaptic inhibition in the hippocampus, J. Neurophysiol., 27:608.

34. Zimmer, J., 1971, Ipsilateral afferents to the commissural zone of the fascia dentata, demonstrated in decommissurated rats by silver impregnation, J. Comp. Neurol., 142:393.

Neurotransmitters and their Receptors
Edited by U.Z. Littauer, Y. Dudai, I. Silman,
V.I. Teichberg and Z. Vogel

Adaptive Changes in Central Serotonin Receptors After Long-Term Drug Treatment in Rats

T. Mennini, E. Poggesi, S. Caccia, C. Bendotti, F. Borsini and R. Samanin

Istituto di Ricerche Farmacologiche 'Mario Nigri', Via Eritrea, 62, 20157-Milan, Italy

ABSTRACT

Central serotonin receptors can change in number and sensitivity after repeated treatment with drugs acting on brain serotonin. Chronic treatment with d-fenfluramine, a serotonin releaser, caused a significant decrease in the number of 3H-serotonin binding sites. The effect was observed in the diencephalon after 14 days of treatment and in the cortex after 28 days. In the whole forebrain binding was significantly reduced after 28 days of treatment but not after 7 or 14 days, although the magnitude of the decrease was of the same order at all three times. Metachlorophenyl-piperazine (mCPP), a direct agonist at serotonin receptors, produced a reduction in the number of binding sites in the forebrain only after 28 days of treatment. Metergoline, a serotonin antagonist, significantly increased 3H-serotonin binding sites in the striatum, hippocampus and cortex after 28 days of treatment. Treatment for the same length of time with d-fenfluramine and metergoline changed the effect of mCPP on food intake in parallel with changes of 3H-serotonin binding.
The specificity of the changes of central serotonin receptors and sensitivity induced by d-fenfluramine and metergoline is discussed.

Several studies have shown that in brain tissue the sensitivity of target cells to catecholamines can be modified in opposite directions (1): hypersensitivity to catecholamine agonists (2,3) and an increase in the number of catecholamine receptor sites (4) are induced by various drugs which reduce the action of catecholamines on postsynaptic receptors. Functional hyposensitivity (5,6) and a decrease in the number of catecholamine receptor sites(7,8,9) have been found after prolonged overstimulation of these receptors.

Much less clear is whether similar mechanisms exist in the serotoninergic system. When the present study was started there was only one article in the literature, to our knowledge, reporting no changes of 3H-serotonin

(3H-5HT) binding in brain cortex of rats chronically treated with l-5-hydroxytryptophan (l-5HTP), chlorimipramine (Cl-IMI)or metergoline (10). Since the first two drugs are supposed to enhance serotonin transmission (11) and the third is a central serotonin antagonist (12),the data led the authors to question the existence of long-term adaptive mechanisms for 5HT similar to those found for catecholamines.

On the other hand, increases in the behavioral effects of serotonin agonists have been found by various authors in animals with selective lesions of central 5HT neurons or on withdrawal of long-term treatment with 5HT antagonists (13,14,15). Although no direct evidence of actual changes in receptors was presented, these findings were generally interpreted as indicative of postsynaptic supersensitivity in central 5HT receptors.

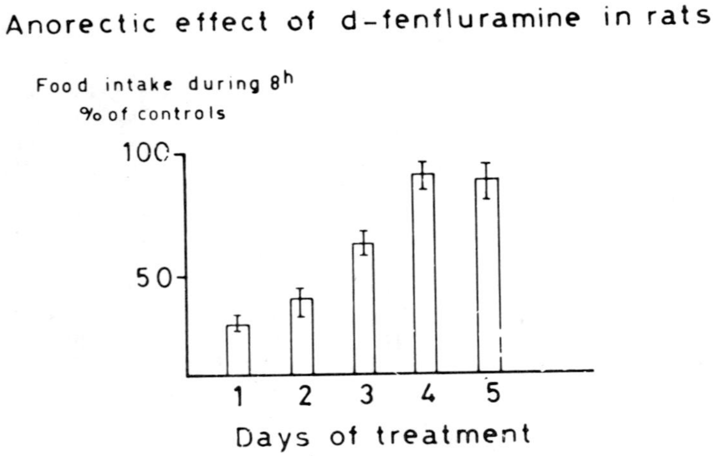

Fig. 1 - Data are mean values ± S.E. of 4 animals.
Food intake was measured using an eatometer according to the procedure described by Blundell et al. (45).
5 mg/kg i.p. of fenfluramine HCl were used.

Data from our laboratory (Fig.1) and others (16,17) show that tolerance rapidly develops in rats to the anorectic activity of fenfluramine, an effect shown to be due to the drug's ability to release 5HT from nerve terminals in the brain (18,19,20). This tolerance cannot be attributed to changes in drug kinetics, since drug levels were the same in the brain after a single or repeated fenfluramine doses (Table 1). Therefore, in analogy with what is known about drugs acting on catecholamines,a possible explanation is that the dynamics of 5HT receptors change after long-term treatment with fenfluramine.

TABLE 1 - Telencephalon levels (μg/g ± S.E.) of d and l fenfluramine(F) and d and l norfenfluramine (NF) after acute or chronic administration of racemic fenfluramine (3 mg/kg i.p.)to rats, 30 min after the last injection.

Treatment (mg/kg i.p.)x days	Telencephalon levels (μg/g± S.E.)			
	dF	dNF	lF	lNF
Fenfluramine (3)x 1	4.1±0.3	0.6±0.03	2.2±0.1	2.3±0.3
Fenfluramine (3)x 10	3.7±0.1	0.4±0.03	2.4±0.3	1.4±0.1

Fenfluramine was measured by gas chromatography, as described by Caccia *et al.* (46)

To check this hypothesis we decided to reconsider the possibility that changes in brain 5HT receptors after long-term treatment with 5HT agonists and antagonists can be revealed in appropriate experimental conditions.In selecting the conditions offering the best chances of finding adaptive 5HT receptor modifications and considering the possible factors leading to Wirz Justice's failure to reveal 3H-5HT binding changes,we reasoned that, apart from any system's intrinsic ability to develop adaptive changes or not, one important factor is the availability of pharmacological means to ensure a prolonged,intense effect on the system examined. The short-lasting effect of apomorphine (21), for instance, might account for the difficulties in detecting changes in dopamine receptor sensitivity when using pharmacologically active doses of this drug. Only recently has a clear-cut subsensitivity of dopamine target cells been found after treatment with apomorphine dipivaloyl ester (6), a long-acting apomorphine-like derivative (22),indicating the importance of persistent drug action for inducing significant receptor changes. The possibility must therefore be considered that a single daily injection of 5HTP or Cl-IMI, as used by Wirz Justice,may not have caused sufficient stimulation of 5HT receptors to induce significant reduction of 3H-5HT binding sites.

In order to select the most appropriate drug for 5HT receptor stimulation, we studied the ability of various agents to release 5HT and/or directly stimulate 5HT receptors in an *in vitro* model, assuming that drugs affecting these mechanisms offered the best chance of activating serotonin transmission *in vivo*. As shown in table 2, among the

TABLE 2 - Effect of drugs on 3H-5HT system *in vitro*

Drug	3H-5HT binding IC_{50}	3H-5HT uptake IC_{50}	3H-5HT release SC_{20}
d Fenfluramine	$>10^{-5}$	5.2×10^{-7}	1×10^{-6}
mCPP	6.2×10^{-7}	1.3×10^{-6}	7.1×10^{-6}
Quipazine	3.8×10^{-6}	3.7×10^{-7}	$>10^{-5}$
MK-212	$>10^{-5}$	5.0×10^{-6}	$>10^{-5}$
LM 5008	$>10^{-5}$	2.0×10^{-7}	$>10^{-5}$

Binding studies were done as described by Samanin *et al.* (25).
IC_{50} for displacement of 3H-5HT binding are the molar drug concentrations causing 50% displacement of specific 3H-5HT binding [7 nM] and were calculated from a log-dose effect plot based on 3 points at least.
Uptake and release studies in synaptosomal preparations were performed as described by Mennini et al. (47).
IC_{50} = [M] causing 50% inhibition of 3H-5HT uptake, calculated from a log-dose probit analysis based on four points.
SC_{20} = [M] producing 20% stimulation of release

$$\frac{\%\ \text{release with drug} - \%\ \text{release control}}{\%\ \text{release control}} \times 100$$

calculated from log-dose effect plot based on 3 points at least.
Data are mean values of 3-4 replications, ranging less than 25%.

various drugs purported to activate the 5HT system, fenfluramine was the strongest in releasing 5HT from nerve terminals, whereas mCPP showed the highest affinity for 5HT binding sites. As regards their effect *in vivo*, both drugs markedly reduce food intake in rats, mCPP being slighly more active than fenfluramine; their effect is significantly reduced by pretreatment with metergoline (19,23), confirming our previous findings that reduction of food intake in rats is a reliable index of drugs increasing central 5HT transmission (24,25,26).

Analysis of the pharmacokinetic patterns of mCPP and fenfluramine show up the considerable differences for the two drugs.

TABLE 3 - mCPP (μg/ g ± S.E.)in different brain areas after injection of 2.5 mg/kg i.p. to rats

hours after injection	Hippocampus	Hypothalamus	Telencephalon
0.5	4.38±0.12	3.81±0.22	5.18±0.41
1.0	4.02±0.24	2.77±0.09	3.35±0.18
2.0	1.76±0.10	1.71±0.12	1.40±0.15

Each value is the mean ± S.E. of 6 determinations.
See Samanin et al. (25) for methodological details .

TABLE 4 - d and l Fenfluramine and d and l norfenfluramine levels (μg/g) after injection of dl fenfluramine (5 mg/kg i.p.)to rats.

hs after injection	Hippocampus				Hypothalamus				Telencephalon			
	dF	dNF	lF	lNF	dF	dNF	lF	lNF	dF	dNF	lF	lNF
1	4.81 ±0.04	0.75 ±0.02	3.92 ±0.20	2.25 ±0.06	4.45 ±0.18	0.77 ±0.03	3.06 ±0.12	2.45 ±0.05	5.51 ±0.14	0.73 ±0.07	3.76 ±0.18	2.65 ±0.07
8	1.33 ±0.10	1.93 ±0.23	0.23 ±0.02	3.58 ±0.28	0.96 ±0.02	1.22 ±0.25	0.27 ±0.01	2.38 ±0.10	1.41 ±0.11	1.79 ±0.21	0.24 ±0.01	3.18 ±0.19

Each value is the mean ± S.E. of 6 rats.
Fenfluramine was measured gas chromatographically as described by Caccia et al. (46)

When equiactive doses of the two drugs are given there is only about 1 μg/g of mCPP in various areas of rat brain two hours after injection (Table 3), whereas the total amount of fenfluramine and active metabolites is still nearly 5 μg/g 8 h after drug treatment (Table 4). Since all metabolites and isomeric forms of fenfluramine enhance 5HT transmission (27) and reduce food intake (Table 5),this should obviously be taken into account when comparing the stimulant effects of mCPP and fenfluramine on 5HT receptors.

As regards the pharmacological means of reducing serotonin function, we chose metergoline because in our experience this is one of the most potent, long-lasting 5HT antagonists in the rat. This long-lasting action might in fact help explain the failure of Wirz Justice (10) to find 5HT

TABLE 5 - Anorectic activity in rats of the two optical isomers of fenfluramine and of norfenfluramine : test lasting 1 hour.

Drug	ED_{50} (mg/kg i.p.) for inhibiting food intake
d-Fenfluramine	1.29 (0.86-1.95)
l-Fenfluramine	2.96 (1.70-5.13)
d-Norfenfluramine	0.80 (0.50-1.15)
l-Norfenfluramine	1.93 (1.41-2.66)

Figures in parentheses are 95% confidence limits.
See Garattini *et al.* (27) for experimental details.

receptor changes after metergoline treatment,since these authors made their binding studies 15 hours after the last injection of metergoline,at which time functionally important amounts of metergoline or active metabolites were presumably still left,as indicated by the fact that a functional 5HT deficit has been observed 24 h after a single injection of metergoline (12). Therefore, the metergoline left could have interfered with 5HT binding analysis in their experiments. In order to minimize this risk for the drugs used in our experiments we discontinued treatment 4 days before binding assay.

Another important point to be considered in the Wirz-Justice study is that they measured 3H-5HT binding using only one concentration of the ligand,thus limiting analysis of relative changes in the affinity and number of binding sites. The importance of Scatchard plot analysis is illustrated,as we will see later,by the fact that if substantial amounts of endogenous 5HT are left in the membrane preparation,treatments changing brain 5HT levels may produce significant changes in the apparent K_D of 3H-5HT binding which can mask changes in receptor number if only one ligand concentration is used.

In our experiments , female CD-COBS rats,weighing 180-220 g,were treated for 14 or 28 days with two daily intraperitoneal injections(at 9 a.m. and 6 p.m.) of d-fenfluramine hydrochloride (2.5 mg/kg) or metergoline maleate (1 mg/kg),dissolved in 1% ascorbic acid. Controls received an equal volume of the vehicle. On day 5 after the last drug dose,rats were killed by decapitation and their brains were rapidly removed and dissected on ice, according to Glowinski and Iversen (28), into the following regions : cortex, hippocampus, striatum,diencephalon and brainstem (midbrain + pons + medulla oblongata). Membrane preparation and binding assay were as described by Bennett and Snyder (29) and Samanin et al. (25). Binding results were calculated by Scatchard plot analysis and B_{max} values were compared by a two-tailed Student's t test.

TABLE 6 - Effect of chronic treatment with metergoline or d-fenfluramine on 3H-serotonin binding sites in different rat brain regions.

Brain regions	3H-5HT binding - B_{max} (pmoles/g)				
	Vehicle	Metergoline 2 x 1 mg/kg i.p.		d- Fenfluramine 2 x 2.5 mg/kg i.p.	
		14 days	28 days	14 days	28 days
Brainstem	10.9±0.6	11.8±1.0	11.3±1.3	10.4±1.1	8.2±1.3
Diencephalon	14.1±0.6	12.0±0.9	17.5±0.6	9.5±0.4**	9.8±0.5**
Striatum	14.5±0.7	13.1±0.9	18.9±0.45*	14.1±0.2	12.1±0.8
Hippocampus	17.5±0.7	19.0±2.8	22.3±0.9*	15.5±0.5	13.8±1.3
Cortex	15.0±0.8	12.3±0.7	22.0±1.0*	14.5±1.5	11.2±0.3**

Data are mean values ± S.E. of 3 replications for drug treated animals, and 12 replications for vehicle treated rats /i.e. 3 vehicles for each of the four experiments,calculated together after checking that the variance of the four groups was not statistically different (Bartlett and Box, x^2 test)/

* $p<0.05$ } significantly different from vehicle - Student's t test
** $p<0.01$ }

Table 6 shows the effect of repeated treatment with fenfluramine or metergoline on 3H-5HT binding sites in the five rat brain regions examined. Metergoline did not alter 3H-5HT binding in any brain areas examined when given for 14 days,but after 28 days a significant increase was found in the striatum,hippocampus and telencephalon. The lack of effect in the diencephalon and brainstem may indicate different regional sensitivity of central 5HT receptors to antagonists,as shown by other authors using electrophysiological methods for studying central 5HT receptor responses (30,31,32). The fact that 14 days of treatment with metergoline caused no significant changes in 3H-5HT binding confirms the importance of the length of drug exposure for revealing changes of 5HT receptor sites.

After 14 days of treatment,fenfluramine caused a significant decrease in the number of 3H-5HT binding sites in the diencephalon, but no effect was observed in the other brain areas examined. After 28 days, a significant reduction of binding sites was also found in the telencephalon,but in the brainstem,striatum and hippocampus only a non-significant tendency was seen. The decrease of 3H-5HT binding after fenfluramine is the first direct evidence of development of subsensitivity in central 5HT receptors after repeated treatment with a drug which increases serotonin release from nerve terminals.

As for metergoline, the fenfluramine data underline the importance of the length of treatment for revealing regional adaptive mechanisms in the brain.Moreover, substances with different modes of action on brain 5HT such as 5HTP, Cl-IMI and fenfluramine can affect 5HT neurons differently in different brain areas,so regional development of receptor changes differs too. This could have contributed to Wirz-Justice's failure to find 5HT receptor changes, tested in only one brain area. For instance we found no changes of 3H-5HT binding in the brainstem with any drug or length of treatment,indicating a resistence of this area to develop changes in the number of 5HT receptors sites after prolonged drug administration. The drug dosage too can be important for revealing adaptive responses of receptors in central monoamine neurons. For instance, doses of fenfluramine larger than those used in the present study can cause such a marked depletion of brain 5HT (33,34) as to result in functional deficit, rather than activation, of central 5HT neurons. That some 5HT depletion had occurred even with a relatively low dose of fenfluramine is indicated by the fact that the apparent Kd was reduced by about 40% in the cortex of 28-day fenfluramine treated rats (Fig. 2), and the same result was seen in the diencephalon of rats receiving fenfluramine for 14 and 28 days. Actual examinations of 5HT levels in membrane preparations from fenfluramine treated animals showed a 5HT decrease of about 20% compared to control values. In order to minimize the influence of endogenous 5HT on Kd, in subsequent studies we incubated membrane preparations for 10 min at 37°C before assay. This eliminates most 5HT bound to the membrane fraction, as shown by Nelson _et al._ (35).

As a next step, we compared the effects of mCPP and fenfluramine treatment to see whether changes of 5HT receptors occur when postsynaptic receptors are directly activated by a 5HT-like chemical. In these experiments a 7-day treatment was included to reveal early receptor changes during

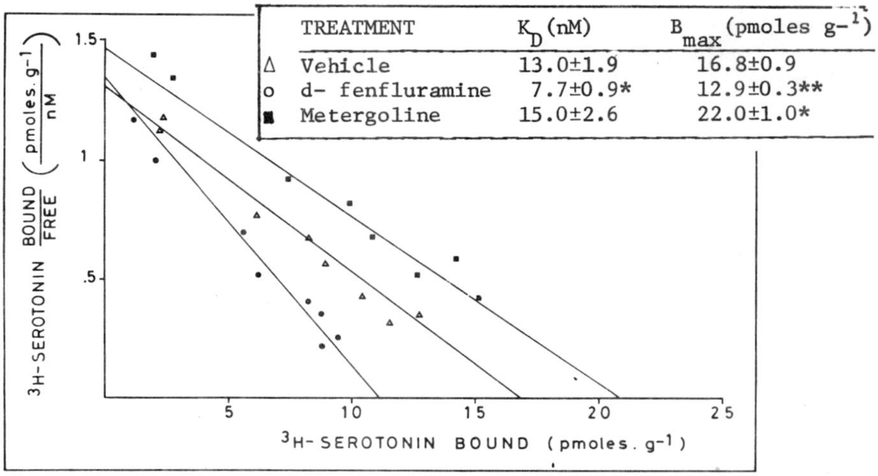

Fig. 2 - Scatchard plots of 3H-serotonin specifically bound to rat cortex membranes.
Specific binding of increasing concentrations of 3H-5HT to cortex membranes from control and treated rats was assayed using concentrations of 3H-5HT ranging from 1 nM to 40 nM , see (48) for methodological details.
Points on the Scatchard plots represent the mean values of 3 determinations,each made on two animals.
The K_D and B_{max} are the mean values ± S.E. of 3 Scatchard plots obtained from points other than those shown in the figure.
Statistical comparisons were made by a two-tailed Student's t test.
* $p < 0.05$ (
** $p < 0.01$) compared with vehicle treated animals

mCPP treatment. Rats were given two daily injections of fenfluramine or mCPP for 7,14 and 28 days, and we studied 3H-5HT receptor binding in forebrain and brainstem on the 5th day after stopping treatment.

Table 7 shows the effect of treatment on 3H-5HT binding sites in the forebrain. Fenfluramine caused a significant reduction of binding after 28 days,but no effect after 7 or 14 days,although the magnitude of the decrease was of the same order at all three times. Surprisingly, mCPP produced a reduction in the number of binding sites in the forebrain only after 28 days treatment. As discussed above, this can be explained by the different duration and intensity of receptor stimulation due to the different kinetics of the two drugs.

TABLE 7 - 3H-serotonin binding sites (pmoles/g tissue) in rat forebrain

Treatment	Days of treatment		
	7	14	28
Vehicle	27.2±2.6	25.8±0.7	28.6±0.8
d-fenfluramine 2x2.5 mg/kg i.p.	22.3±1.9	22.6±1.9	22.4±0.8**
mCPP 2x10 mg/kg i.p.	26.2±2.4	25.6±1.0	21.8±2.7**

Data are means ± S.E. of 6 animals. B_{max} are calculated by Scatchard plot analysis of single forebrains.

** $p < 0.01$ Dunnett' s test

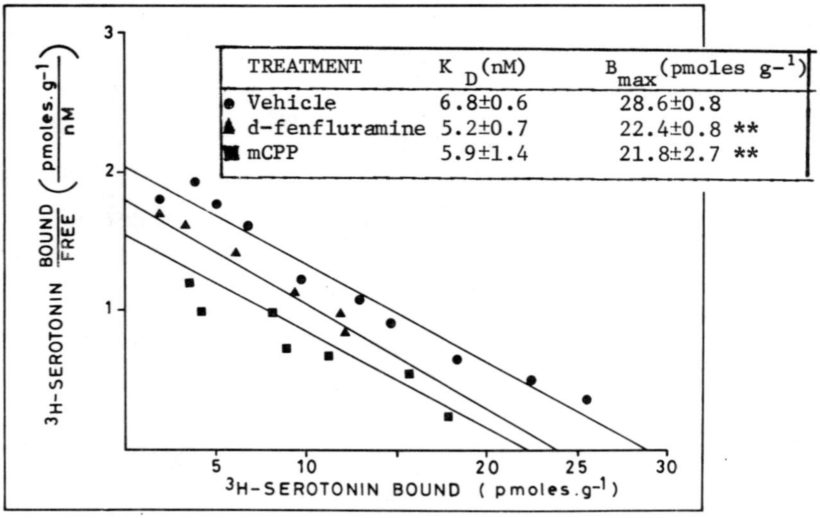

Fig. 3 - The same as for Fig.2 ,except that membrane preparations were incubated 10 min at 37°C before assay. Scatchard plots were obtained from single rat forebrain. The K_D and B_{max} are the means ± S.E. of 6 determinations.
Statistical comparisons between values were made by Dunnett's test.
** $p < 0.01$

The K_D values were not changed in either treatment (Fig. 3), as might have been expected after removal of endogenous serotonin during membrane preparation. No changes in K_D or B_{max} were obtained in the brainstem (Table 8) confirming the resistence of this area to develop changes of 5HT receptors.

TABLE 8 - 3H-serotonin binding sites(pmoles/g tissue)in rat brainstem.

Treatment	Days of treatment		
	7	14	28
Vehicle	15.7±2.3	16.4±1.4	15.0±1.0
d-Fenfluramine 2x2.5 mg/kg i.p.	17.1±3.1	15.7±2.2	15.0±0.8
mCPP 2x10 mg/kg i.p.	16.5±2.7	17.7±0.7	13.3±1.2

Data are means ± S.E. of 6 animals.
B_{max} are calculated by Scatchard plot analysis of single brainstems.

Although further studies are necessary to establish the exact time-course of brain regional changes after different treatments, the present studies clearly show that adaptive modification occurs in central serotonin receptors after repeated treatment with drugs acting on brain serotonin. Until now, conflicting results have been reported on the development of supersensitivity in 3H-5HT binding studies. Combined lesions of raphe nuclei, where most serotoninergic neurons innervating the forebrain originate (36), were found to cause an increase in the apparent affinity for 3H-5HT binding sites in the rat forebrain (29). Since drugs like reserpine and p-chlorophenylalanine, which markedly deplete brain 5HT, had the same effect, the enhanced binding was interpreted in terms of reduced competition for receptors by endogenous 5HT (29). Another study reported no development of 5HT receptor supersensitivity after lesions of central 5HT neurons (37). Subsequently, more refined studies (35) in which most endogenous 5HT bound to the P2 fraction from rat brain was eliminated showed that intraventricular administration of 5,7 dihydroxy-tryptamine resulted in a significant increase in the number of 3H-5HT binding sites in the hippocampus 18 days after injection. A significant increase in specific 3H-5HT binding to forebrain membranes was recently reported following repeated treatment of rats with parachlorophenylalanine

(38) while a decrease in number of binding sites was reported after long-term administration of tricyclic antidepressants, MAO inhibitors and D-LSD (39,40,41). The magnitude of the changes in maximal binding of 3H-5HT is similar in most conditions, and very close to that produced by chronic neurotransmitter depletion or receptor blockade in the dopamine system (42,43), indicating that long-term adaptive changes in receptor numbers are of limited entity.

One aspect of the functional significance of changes in central 5HT receptors is illustrated in the present study by the increase and decrease respectively in the anorectic effect of mCPP in animals treated with metergoline and fenfluramine. The anorectic effect of mCPP has been recently found to depend on its ability to act as 5HT agonist at central post-synaptic receptors (23), and we chose it as a tool for revealing behavioral changes depending on 5HT receptor sensitivity.

TABLE 9 - Effect of repeated treatment with fenfluramine or metergoline on anorectic activity of mCPP in rats

Treatment	Food intake % of control days of treatment		
	7	14	28
Vehicle	25	28	35
d-Fenfluramine 2x 2.5 mg/kg	90***	72**	56*
Metergoline 2x1 mg/kg	-	7*	0***

see Samanin _et al._ (48) for experimental details.

mCPP (2.5 mg/kg) was injected intraperitoneally 30 min before food intake was tested.

Each value is the mean of 6 determinations varying less than 20%.

* $p < 0.05$
** $p < 0.01$ F_i
*** $p < 0.005$

Table 9 shows that mCPP reduced food intake by 60-70% in vehicle treated animals. In rats treated with fenfluramine the same dose of mCPP caused less reduction of food intake, but animals which had received metergoline, when injected with mCPP, did not consume any food at all during the 1 h intake test.

The effect of fenfluramine is evident even after 7 days treatment, when the reduction in serotonin binding sites was not statistically significant, although the magnitude of the decrease was of the same order at all the three times of treatment. Assuming that tolerance to mCPP's effect is entirely dependent on receptor reduction, this indicates that non-significant changes in neurotransmitter binding sites may be sufficient to cause marked changes in behavioural or pharmacological effects. Although it cannot be excluded that changes in mCPP activity could result from different drug metabolism and/or distribution in animals pretreated with fenfluramine or metergoline, this likelihood is weakened by the fact that 4 days elapsed between drug discontinuation and mCPP experiments, and the changes of mCPP activity parallel the changes in the number of 5HT receptor sites in the direction postulated.

TABLE 10 - Effect of repeated treatment with d-fenfluramine or metergoline on Apomorphine stereotypy in rats.

Treatment	Total score ± S.E. Days of treatment	
	14	28
Vehicle	11.0±1.3	11.1±1.0
d-Fenfluramine 2x2.5 mg/kg i.p.	14.8±0.5	10.7±1.3
Metergoline 2x1 mg/kg i.p.	11.4±1.4	11.5±1.4

see Samanin et al. (48) for experimental details.
Apomorphine (2.5 mg/kg) was injected subcutaneously 30 minutes before stereotypy was assessed.
Each value is the mean ± S.E. of 6 determinations.

Moreover, the effect of apomorphine was not modified by either drug used (Table 10), indicating drug specificity, since repeated treatment with drugs acting on brain dopamine have been reported to cause marked changes in the pharmacological effects of apomorphine (3,6).
A further criterion for specificity is that either agonist or antagonist treatments fail to change α and β receptor binding in the rat forebrain (tables 11,12) with the exception of a small but significant reduction (12%) of 3H-DHA binding after 28 days' treatment with fenfluramine.

TABLE 11 - Effect of repeated treatment with d-fenfluramine, metergoline or mCPP on 3H-WB 4101 binding to rat forebrain membranes

Drug	pmoles/g ± S.E. Days of treatment		
	7	14	28
Fenfluramine 2x 2.5 mg/kg i.p.	2.1±0.2 (6)	2.8±0.1 (6)	2.6±0.2 (6)
Metergoline 2x1 mg/kg i.p.	2.2±0.1 (4)	3.1±0.1 (4)	2.8±0.1 (6)
mCPP 2x10 mg/kg i.p.	2.4±0.2 (6)	2.9±0.1 (6)	3.0±0.1 (6)
Vehicle	2.2±0.4 (5)	2.8±0.1 (6)	3.0±0.1 (6)

Binding of 3H-WB 4101 was determined as described by Greenberg et al. (49) using 0.22 nM H-WB 4101. Data are means ± S.E.

TABLE 12 -Effect of repeated treatment with d-fenfluramine, metergoline or mCPP on H-dihydroalprenolol binding to rat forebrain membranes

Drug	pmoles/g ± S.E. Days of treatment		
	7	14	28
Fenfluramine 2x2.5 mg/kg i.p.	3.8±0.1 (6)	3.1±0.2 (6)	2.8±0.2** (6)
Metergoline 2x1 mg/kg i.p.	3.8±0.1 (6)	3.7±0.1 (6)	3.2±0.1 (6)
mCPP 2x10 mg/kg i.p.	3.7±0.1 (6)	3.8±0.3 (5)	3.2±0.1 (6)
Vehicle	3.4±0.3 (6)	3.2±0.3 (6)	3.6±0.3 (6)

Binding of 3H-DHA was determined as described by Bylund and Snyder (50) using 1 nM 3H-DHA. Data are means ± S.E. of 6 animals.

** $p < 0.01$ Dunnett's test .

In conclusion the present data clearly indicate that it is possible to cause hyper- and hyposensitivity to central 5HT receptors after chronic exposure to drugs acting specifically at the serotoninergic neurons. These changes in central 5HT receptors could explain the increased behavioral effects of 5HT agonists in animals subjected to long term treatment with 5HT antagonists (13,14,15) and the rapid tolerance to the anorectic effect of fenfluramine in various animal species (16,17,44). Slow modifications at the receptors in response to long-term drug treatment may constitute therefore a common feature among the various neurotransmitters in the brain, and thus provide an interesting tool for studying the neurochemical basis of behavior.

ACKNOWLEDGEMENTS

This work was supported by a C.N.R. contract.

REFERENCES

1. Schwartz, J.C.,Costentin,J., Martres,M.P., Protais,P. and Baudry,M. Neuropharmacology 17: 665-685 (1978).

2. Gianutsos, G., Drawbaugh, R.B., Hynes, M.D. and Lal, H. Life Sci. 14: 887-898 (1974).

3. Tarsy, D. and Baldessarini,R.J. Neuropharmacology 13: 927-940 (1974).

4. Burt, D.R., Creese, I. and Snyder, S.H. Science 196: 326-328 (1977).

5. Chiel, H., Yehuda, S. and Wurtman, R.J. Life Sci. 14: 483-488 (1974).

6. Scatton, B. and Worms, P. Naunyn Schmiedeberg's Arch. Pharmacol. 303: 271-278 (1978).

7. Howlett, D.R. and Nahorski, S.R. Brain Res. 161: 173-178 (1979).

8. Wolfe, B.B., Harden, T.K., Sporn, J.R. and Molinoff, P.B. J.Pharmacol.Exp.Ther. 207: 446-457 (1978).

9. Sporn, J.R., Harden, T.K., Wolfe, B.B. and Molinoff, P.B. Science 194: 624-626 (1976).

10. Wirz-Justice, A., Krauchi, K., Lichtsteiner, M. and Feer, H. <u>Life Sci.</u> 23: 1249-1254 (1978).

11. Garattini, S. and Samanin, R. in: <u>Serotonin in Health and Disease</u>, W.B.Essman ed., Vol.2 pp.247-293, Spectrum Publ., New York (1978).

12. Mawson, C. and Whittington, H. <u>Br.J.Pharmacol.</u>, 39: 223P (1970).

13. Trulson, M.E., Eubanks, E.E. and Jacobs, B.L. <u>J.Pharmacol. Exp.Ther.</u> 198: 23-32 (1976).

14. Klawans, H.L., D'Amico, D.J. and Patel, B.C. <u>Psychopharmacologia</u> 44: 297-300 (1975).

15. Klawans, H.L., D'Amico, D.J., Nausieda, P.A. and Weiner W.J. <u>Psychopharmacology</u> 55: 49-52 (1977).

16. Le Douarec, J.C. and Neveu, C. In: <u>Amphetamines and Related Compounds</u>, E.Costa and S. Garattini eds., pp.75-105, Raven Press, New York (1970).

17. Ghosh, M.N. and Parvathy, S. <u>Br.J.Pharmacol.</u> 57: 479-485 (1976).

18. Garattini, S., Buczko, W., Jori, A. and Samanin, R. <u>Postgrad.Med.J.</u> 51: suppl.1, 27-35 (1975).

19. Jespersen, S. and Scheel-Krüger, J. <u>J.Pharm.Pharmacol.</u> 25: 49-54 (1973).

20. Samanin, R., Ghezzi, D., Valzelli, L. and Garattini S. <u>Eur.J.Pharmacol.</u> 19: 318-322 (1972).

21. Garattini, S., Fanelli, R., Jori, A., Consolo, S., Ladinsky, H. and Samanin, R. In: <u>International Symposium on Piribedil 1st.</u>Proceedings Monastir, Nov.27-Dec.1,1972, Servier Res.Institute, Paris, pp.240-244 (1975).

22. Baldessarini, R.J., Walton, K.G. and Borgman, R.J. <u>Neuropharmacology</u> 15: 471-478 (1976).

23. Samanin, R., Mennini, T., Ferraris, A., Bendotti, C., Borsini, F. and Garattini S. <u>Naunyn Schmiedeberg's Arch. Pharmacol.</u> 308: 159-163 (1979).

24. Samanin, R., Bendotti, C., Miranda, F. and Garattini, S. J.Pharm.Pharmacol. 29: 53-54 (1977).

25. Samanin, R., Caccia, S., Bendotti, C., Borsini, F., Borroni, E., Invernizzi, R., Pataccini, R. and Mennini, T. Psychopharmacology in press.

26. Samanin, R., Bendotti, C., Bernasconi, S. and Pataccini, R. In: Central Mechanisms of Anorectic Drugs, S. Garattini and R. Samanin, pp.233-242, Raven Press, New York (1978).

27. Garattini, S., Caccia, S., Mennini, T., Samanin, R., Consolo, S. and Ladinsky, H. Curr.Med.Res.Opinion 6: suppl.1, 15-27 (1979).

28. Glowinski, J. and Iversen, L.L. J.Neurochem. 13:655-669 (1966).

29. Bennett, J.P.Jr. and Snyder, S.H. Mol.Pharmacol., 12: 373-389 (1976).

30. Bradley, P.B. and Briggs, I. Br.J.Pharmacol. 50: 345-354 (1974).

31. Haigler, H.J. and Aghajanian, G.K. J.Neural Transmission 35: 257-273 (1974).

32. Segal, M. Brain Res. 103: 161-166 (1976).

33. Garattini, S., Bizzi, A., de Gaetano, G., Jori, A. and Samanin, R. In: Recent Advances in Obesity Research I, pp.354-367, Newman, London (1975).

34. Garattini, S., Bonaccorsi, A., Jori, A. and Samanin, R. In: Obesity: Causes, Consequences and Treatment, L.Lasagna ed. pp.70-80, Medcom Press, New York (1974).

35. Nelson, D.L., Herbet, A., Bourgoin, S., Glowinski, J. and Hamon, M. Mol.Pharmacol. 14: 983-995 (1978).

36. Dahlström, A. and Fuxe, K. Acta Physiol.Scand. 62: suppl. 232, 1-55 (1964).

37. Fillion, G.M.B., Rousselle, J.C., Fillion, M.P., Beaudoin, D.M., Goiny, M.R., Deniau, J.M. and Jacob, J.J. Mol.Pharmacol. 14: 50 -59 (1978).

38. Steigrad, P., Tobler, I., Waser, P.G. and Borbély, A.A. Naunyn-Schmiedeberg's Arch.Pharmacol. 305: 143-148 (1978).

39. Segawa, T., Mizuta, T. and Nomura, Y. Eur.J.Pharmacol. 58: 75-83 (1979).

40. Savage, P.D., Frazer, A. and Mendels, J. Eur.J.Pharmacol. 58: 87-88 (1979).

41. Trulson, M.E. and Jacobs, B.L. Life Sci. 24: 2053-2062 (1979).

42. Creese, I., Burt, D.R. and Snyder, S.H. Science 197:596-598 (1977).

43. Burt, D.R., Creese, I. and Snyder, S.H. Science 196: 326-328 (1977).

44. Pinder, R.M., Brogden, R.N., Sawyer, P.R., Speight, T.M. and Avery, G.S. Drugs 10: 241-323 (1975).

45. Blundell, J.E., Latham, C.J., and Leshem, M.B. J.Pharm. Pharmacol. 28: 471-477 (1976).

46. Caccia, S. and Jori, A. J.Chromatogr. 144: 127-131 (1977).

47. Mennini, T., Pataccini, R. and Samanin, R. Br.J.Pharmacol. 64: 75-82 (1978).

48. Samanin, R., Mennini, T., Ferraris, A., Beńdotti, C. and Borsini, F. Brain Res. in press

49. Greenberg, D.A., U'Prichard, D.C. and Snyder, S.H. Life Sci. 19: 69-76 (1976).

50. Bylund, D.B. and Snyder, S.H. Mol.Pharmacol. 12: 568-580 (1976).

Neurotransmitters and their Receptors
Edited by U.Z. Littauer, Y. Dudai, I. Silman,
V.I. Teichberg and Z. Vogel

Modulation of Serotonin Receptors by Steroid Sex Hormones in the Rat Brain

Anat Biegon and David Samuel

Department of Isotope Research, The Weizmann Institute of Science, Rehovot, Israel

Abstract

The binding of ^{3}H-5HT to crude membrane preparations from rat brain appears to be modulated by fluctuations in the endogenous levels of sex steroids. Thus, ^{3}H-5HT binding in basal forebrains (containing the hypothalamus, septum and preoptic area) of female rats in proestrous and estrous is 40% lower than in diestrous females or in male rats. Scatchard analysis indicates a reduction in the number of available binding sites (Bmax). ^{3}H-5HT binding to cortex, hoppocampus and caudate does not change across the estrous cycle.

50 µg estradiol benzoate (EB) in oil, given subcutaneously to ovariectomized female rats (3 weeks post operation) causes a 40% increase of the number of ^{3}H-5HT receptors 48 hours post injection, in the basal forebrain but not in the cortex. On the other hand, incubation of crude membranal preparations from whole rat forebrain with low concentrations of EB (10^{-10} - 10^{-8}M) for two hours, causes a reduction of 20-40% in the apparent number of ^{3}H-5HT receptors.

We conclude that estradiol reduces ^{3}H-5HT binding due to a fast (2h) effect on membranes, while increasing the number of ^{3}H-5HT receptors in a slow process (48h), probably estrogen receptor-mediated. These changes in 5HT-receptor binding may play a role in the control of sexual behavior and ovulation in the female rat.

The density of postsynaptic receptors is one of the factors determining the efficiency of neurotransmission in the nervous system. Both pharmacological and surfical manipulations were shown to affect receptor density (1,2,3). However, changes in receptor density in the brains of intact animals under physiological conditions have not been reported so far.

During the estrous cycle of the female rat, changes in hormonal secretion patterns are accompanied by changes in monoamines (4,5) and in behavior. We used the intact, freely cycling female rat as a model for investigating changes in serotonin receptor density and the involvement of the steroid sex hormone, estradiol. We have measured the binding of labeled serotonin (^{3}H-5HT, N.E.N., 30.2 Ci/mole) to several brain regions from freely cycling female rats. Males were included in the study in order to compare our binding data with those previously reported (3,6, 7)

Adult (12-14 week old) male and female Wistar rats from a local breeding colony were kept under controlled lighting (12 h. dark - 12 h. light) and temperature 24 $\pm$ 1°C), with food and water available ad lib.

Females underwent daily vaginal smears and only those exhibiting at least 3 consecutive regular 4 day cycles were included in the study. Animals were sacrificed by decapitation between 12 h and 14 h. The brains were quickly removed and dissected in the cold. Brain regions (basal forebrain, hippocampus, cortex, caudate) from 2-3 animals were pooled and homogenized in 50 mM Tris HCl buffer, pH 7.6, using a polytron. The homogenate was spun at 30,000xg for 19 min, washed and spun again. The pellet was then homogenized in 50 mM Tris HCl buffer, pH 7.4, containing 100 μM pargyline and 0.2% ascorbic acid, and incubated at 37°C for 10 min. 1 ml samples of this homogenate were added to test tubes containing the appropriate concentrations of label in 0.5 ml, and 0.5 ml of buffer with or without cold serotonin to a final concentration of 1 μM. After 10 min at 37°C, the tubes were transferred to an ice water bath and the contents filtered through GF/B glass fiber filters, followed by 2x5 ml washes with ice cold buffer. The filters were then transferred to vials and shaken overnight with 10 ml of toluene-triton scintillation fluid, and counted in a Packard Tri-Carb scintillation counter, at 30% efficiency.

The binding characteristics found in the males are in good agreement with those previously reported for the high affinity site of serotonin: a Kd of 1-3 nM and a Bmax of 0.16-0.20 pmoles/mg protein (measured according to the method of Lowry (8) (Fig. 1)). In the females, there is a clear and significant reduction in the number of serotonin binding sites in proestrous and estrous in comparison with diestrous (Fig. 1). The differences in Kd were statistically significant. The results from this series of experiments are summarized in Table 1.

TABLE 1

Binding characteristics of ^{3}H-5HT to basal forebrains from males and females at different stages of the estrous cycle. Results are the means ± S.E.M. of 2-6 experiments.

	♂	PE	E	D_1	D_2
Kd (nM)	2.8 ±0.07	1.9 ±1.0	1.9 ±0.5	1.7 ±0.6	2.5 ±0.3
B_{max} (pm/mg protein)	0.17±0.02	0.11±0.01*	0.12±0.01*	0.18±0.03	0.15±0.03

*Significantly lower ($P < 0.05$) than males, D_1 and D_2; as determined by Anova + Duncan's test.

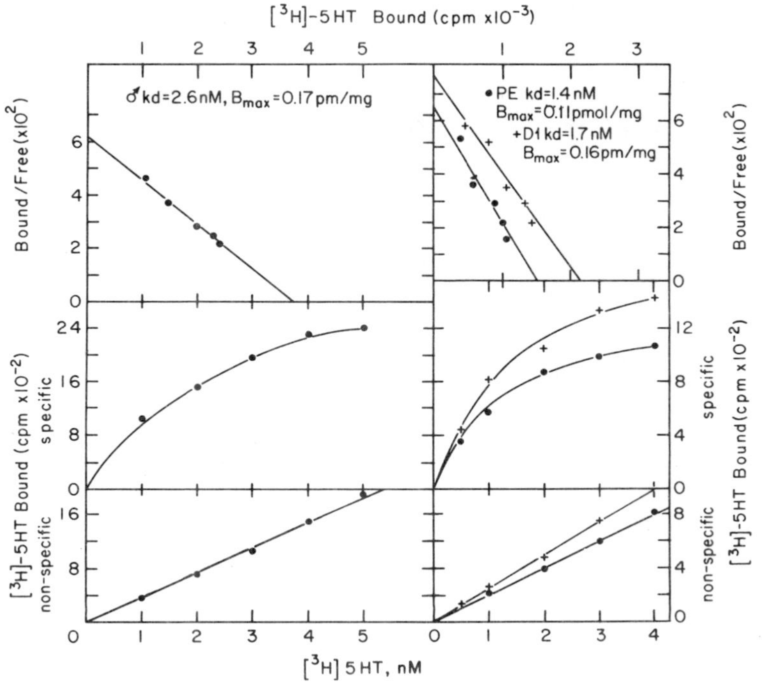

Fig. 1. Binding of ^{3}H-5HT to basal forebrains from male and female rats. The top drawings are the Scatchard plots of the binding data. ♂ = males, PE = Proestrous, D_1 = diestrous-1 females.

The binding of labeled serotonin (5nM) to other brain regions was also measured (Fig. 2). The specific binding to hippocampus in proestrous females was lower than in diestrous; a pattern similar to the one found in the basal forebrain. However, the differences were smaller, and the difference between estrous and diestrous females did not reach statistical significance. In the cortex and caudate, no effect of the cycle on serotonin binding was observed.

The possible involvement of estrogens was investigated. A subcutaneous injection of 50 µg estradiol benzoate in 0.1 ml peanut oil, at 11.00 am. produces, 48 hours later, a significant increase in the binding of ^{3}H-5HT to the basal forebrains of ovariectomized females, as compared to oil-injected, ovariectomized controls (Fig. 3). A Scatchard analysis of the binding data shows that this is the result of an increase in the concentration of binding sites amounting to approximately 25%.

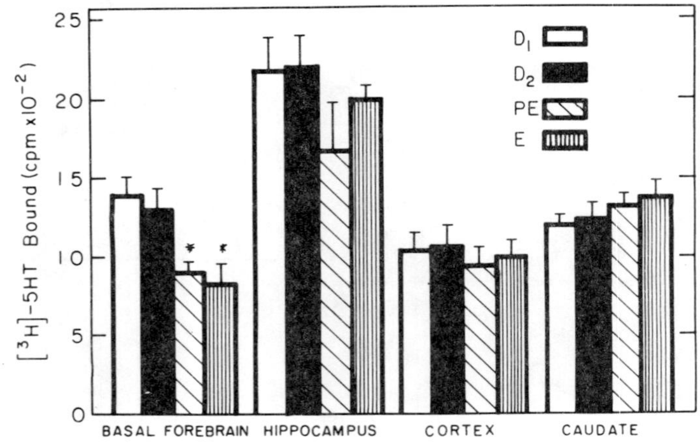

Fig. 2. Specific binding of ^{3}H-5HT (5nM) to several brain regions from female rats at different stages of the estrous cycle. D_1 = diestrous-1; D_2 = diestrous-2; PE = proestrous; E = estrous. The results are means $\pm$ S.E.M. of 2-6 determinations.

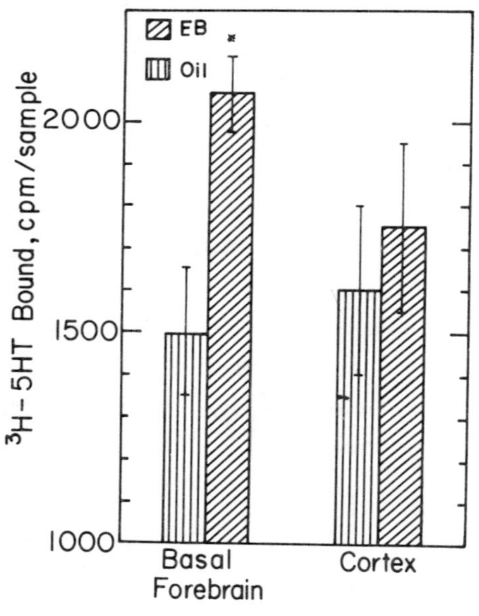

Fig 3. Effect of 50 μg estradiol benzoate (EB) on the binding of ^{3}H-5HT to forebrains of ovariectomized female rats. Animals were injected with EB or vehicle at 11 am and sacrificed 48 h later. N=9. *$p < 0.05$ compared to oil control. Student's t-test.

This finding can explain part of the increase in 5HT binding between proestrous and diestrous. However, an additional contribution could be the effect of a fast decrease in 5HT binding due to estrogen on the day of proestrous. This possibility was investigated *in vitro*. On 2 h incub-incubation of crude membrane preparations from whole forebrains with estradiol (10^{-10} - 10^{-4} M), we found a marked decrease in the specific binding of ^{3}H-5HT, 2.5 nM. Complete saturation experiments were then performed in the presence of 10^{-10}, 10^{-9} and 10^{-8} M estradiol. Scatchard plots of the data revealed a decrease in the density of binding sites. The results are summarized in Table 2.

TABLE 2

Effect of 2 h incubation with estradiol benzoate (EB) on the binding of ^{3}H-5HT to crude membrane preparation from rat brain.

Treatment	^{3}H-5HT bound cpm/mg protein	Kd (nM)	B_{max} (pm/mg P)
Tris Buffer control	390±40		
Tris-P.V.P. control	335±40	5.0	0.23
EB, 10^{-10}M	225±25	5.0	0.14
EB, 10^{-9}M	216±12	4.7	0.08
EB, 10^{-8}M	240±40	5.7	0.15
EB, 10^{-7}M	275±3		
EB, 10^{-6}M	250±50		
EB, 10^{-5}M	238±6		

EB was dissolved in hot glacial acetic acid and buffered with solid trisma base to pH 7.4, in 3.5% P.V.P. The control samples were incubated with tris-acetate buffer, pH 7.4, with 3.5% P.V.P.

CONCLUSIONS

5HT receptor density is modulated by naturally occuring changes in hormonal secretion. It is low on proestrous and estrous, when hormone levels are maximal, and high on diestrous. Since 5HT is known to inhibit sexual behavior (9,10) and ovulation (11), a reduction in 5HT transmission on proestrous and estrous (when sexual behavior and ovulation occur) is to be expected.

The proposed mechanism is a biphasic effect of estradiol: A fast reduction in 5HT binding due to the effect of the hormone on the post-synaptic membrane, and a slow increase in 5HT binding due to increased

5HT receptor synthesis mediated through the estragen receptor interacting with DNA expression (12). This is in keeping with the known modulatory effect of estrogen on progestin receptors in the brain (13) and α-adrenergic receptors in the periphery (14).

References

1. Burt, D.R., Creese, I. and Synder, S.H. Science 197, 596, 1977.

2. Dolphini, A., Adrieu, J., Hamon, M. and Bockaert, J. Mol. Pharmacol. 15, 1, 1979.

3. Nelson, D.L., Herbert A., Burgon, S., Glowinski, J. and Hamon, M. Mol. Pharmacol. 14, 983, 1978.

4. Greengrass, P.M. and Tonge, S.R. J. Pharm. Pharmac. 23, 897, 1971.

5. Kueng, W., Wirz-Justice, A., Menze, B. and Chapuis-Arndt, E. Neuro-endocrinol. 21, 289, 1976.

6. Fillion, G., Gillion, M.P. Spirakis, C., Bahers, J.M. and Jacob, J. Life Sci. 18, 65, 1976.

7. Whitaker, P.M. and Seeman, P. Psychopharmacology 59, 1, 1978.

8. Lowry, O.H., Rosebrough, N.J., Fair, A.L. and Randall, R.J. J.Biol. Chem. 193, 265, 1951.

9. Carter, S.C. and Davis, J.M. Behav. Rev. 1, 213, 1977.

10. Meyerson, B.J., Correr, H. and Eliasson, M. In: Advances in biochemical psychopharmacology, Vol.II, p.229, Raven Press, N.Y. 1974.

11. O'Steen, W.K. Endocrinology 74, 885, 1964.

12. Chan, L. and O'Malley, B.W. New Eng. J. Med. 294, 1322, 1976.

13. MacLusky, N.J. and McEwen, B.J. Nature 274, 276, 1978.

14. Roberts, J.M. Goldfien, R.D., Insel, P.A., Tsuchiya, A.M. and Goldfien, A. Clin. Res. 26, A494, 1978.

Neurotransmitters and their Receptors
Edited by U.Z. Littauer, Y. Dudai, I. Silman,
V.I. Teichberg and Z. Vogel

The Lipid Fluidity of Synaptic Membranes and the Binding of Serotonin and Opiate Ligands

David S. Heron[1], Moshe Hershkowitz[1], Meir Shinitzky[2] and David Samuel[1]
Departments of Isotope Research[1] and Membrane Research[2],
The Weizmann Institute of Science, Rehovot, Israel

ABSTRACT

The binding of [^{3}H]-serotonin, [^{3}H]-D-ala-enkephaline and [^{3}H]-naloxone to membrane preparations from rodent brains was investigated as a function of changes in membrane fluidity. The microviscosity ($\bar{\eta}$) of synaptic membranes can be increased by *in vitro* incubation with either cholesteryl hemisuccinate (CHS) or stearic acid, resulting in an up to five-fold increase in the specific binding of [^{3}H]-serotonin and up to two-fold increase in the binding [^{3}H]-D-ala-enkephaline and [^{3}H]-naloxone. The binding of serotonin increases progressively reaching a maximum at 1.75$\bar{\eta}$ units relative to control, while that of opiate ligands reaches a maximum at 1.35 relative $\bar{\eta}$ units. Further addition of CHS causes a sharp decline in the binding of those ligands. Fluidization of synaptic membranes, by treatment with lecithin or linolic acid, causes a decrease in the binding of all three ligands. The changes in binding could be reversed by first treating with CHS and then with lecithin or vice versa. These observations can be explained in terms of the vertical displacement of protein receptors in the synaptic membrane. In untreated brain tissue, the accesibility (Bmax) of serotonin receptor binding sites constitutes only about 20% and that of opiate receptor sites about 60% of the potential binding capacity stored in the membrane. These results are of interest owing to their possible implications in a number of physiological processes - such as aging of the CNS, or addiction, which may be associated with modulation of membrane lipid fluidity.

The accessibility of synaptic receptors to ligand binding can be modulated by changes in membrane lipid fluidity both *in vitro* and *in vivo*. The shift in the equilibrium position of membrane proteins (1-4) including enzymes and receptors, plays a key role in the modulation (5) or receptor function in many cellular processes, such as neurotransmisson. The accessibility of a receptor binding site, a prerequisite for its function, and the extent and direction of its displacement by changes in membrane fluidity are determined by the geometry of the receptor in its immediate lipid environment. When lipid microviscosity is decreased, the β-adrenergic receptor for instance, has been shown to be more exposed in liver cell membranes (6), less exposed in rabbit reticulocyte membranes (7) and unaffected in turkey erythrocytes (8).

We have therefore studied the changes in the accessibility and binding characteristics of both serotonin and opiate receptors in synaptic membranes, using cholesterol or its hemisuccinate ester for increasing viscosity and egg-lecithin for fluidization.

The media for modulating the lipids in membrane were prepared in the following manner: A hot solution of cholesteryl hemisuccinate (CHS) in glacial acetic acid (40 mg/ml) was diluted to 100 vols by 50 mM Tris-HCl buffer, pH 7.4, containing 3.5% polyvinyl pyrrolidone (PVP, M.W. 40,000). The pH was then readjusted to 7.4 with solid Tris free base and the resulting translucent suspension of CHS in 170 mM Tris-acetate buffer, used for modulating membrane fluidity (9). Solutions of egg lecithin (80 mg/ml) stearic acid (6 mg/ml) and linoleic acid (6 mg/ml) in glacial acetic acid were prepared and used in a similar manner.

Three different membrane preparations of increasing purity obtained from the forebrains of male Balb BL mice were used: (a) Crude membrane preparation (Crude homogenate); (b) Crude synaptosomal membrane preparation (P_2M) prepared as described by Hershkowitz (10) and (c) Synaptic plasma membranes (SPM) prepared as described by Morgan et al. (11). The pellets from each preparation were suspended in 10 vols of Tris-HCl buffer (100 mg tissue/ml) and incubated for two hours at room temperature with continuous shaking, with amounts between 1 and 30 ml of the lipid suspension described above per 1 ml of membrane suspension. The samples were then centrifuged at 42,000xg for 10 minutes, the pellets washed twice and resuspended in 50 mM Tris-HCl buffer (pH 7.4) for the assays described below.

The membrane lipid microviscosity, $\bar{\eta}$, of the various membrane preparations, before or after lipid treatment, was determined by fluorescence depolarization using 1,6-diphenyl-1,3,5-hexatriene (DPH) as a probe (12). A suspension of membranes (containing about 40 μg protein) was incubated with a DPH dispersion (2 ml) for 30 minutes at 25°C. The degree of fluorescence polarization, P, was then determined at 25°C, and the lipid microviscosity - the reciprocal of fluidity - determined by the empirical relation, $\bar{\eta} = 2P/(0.46-P)$.

Binding assays using [^{3}H]-serotonin were performed on either crude homogenates or the P_2M preparation according to the method of Bennet and Snyder (13) with minor modifications. In a standard experiment the assay mixture contained 1 ml of a tissue suspension (corresponding to 20 mg tissue or about 1.5 mg protein), 0.5 ml [^{3}H]-serotonin (final concentration between 0.5 and 8.0 mM) and either 0.5 ml Tris-HCl buffer, pH 7.4, containing 10^{-4}M pargyline and 0.2 mg/ml ascorbate, or the same buffer also containing 10 μM (final concentration) unlabeled serotonin. The mixtures were incubated for 10 minutes at 37°C, placed in ice-water, and finally filtered by suction through GF/B filter, followed by 2x5 ml washes with ice-cold buffer.

Opiate ligand binding was determined as described by Pasternak et al. (14) with minor modifications. The reaction mixture contained 1.95 ml of tissue suspension (20 nM [^{3}H]-naloxone or 1.0 nM D-ala-2-(tyrosyl-3,5-^{3}H) enkephaline, final concentration), with or without 20 μl of unlabeled morphine (10^{-5}M final concentration). The samples were incubated for 40 minutes at room temperature in the [^{3}H]-d-ala-enkephaline or [^{3}H]-naloxone binding assays in the absence of sodium. In the [^{3}H]-naloxone assay, in the presence of 100 mM sodium chloride the incubation was for 2 hours at 0°C. The samples were then processed as described for serotonin. Following filtration, all samples were incubated with toluene-triton scintillation liquid and counted in a Packard scintillation counter at 33% efficiency. All assays were done in triplicates, together with triplicates containing unlabeled ligands. Specific binding is defined as total minus non-specific binding, i.e. in the presence of unlabeled ligands. Non-specific binding constituted about 40% of the total in the serotonin binding assay and about 20% of the total in both opiate ligands assays.

Fig. 1 depicts Scatchard plots (15) of [^{3}H]-serotonin binding to a crude membrane preparation at different microviscosity values. The non-linear control curve indicates the existence of both high and low affinity binding sites. Table 1 summarizes the data from a number of binding experiments. The Kd values, obtained for untreated membranes are in agreement with published values (16,17). The capacity and Kd of both high- and low-affinity sites increase progressively with increasing microviscosity. At high values of $\bar{\eta}$, the differences between the slopes of high- and low-affinity sites appear to decrease, with a trend towards the expression of only low affinity sites. When the membranes are slightly fluidized with lecithin their binding capacity appears to increase, in addition to the increase in Kd of both high- and low-affinity sites. Further fluidization however, causes the expected decrease in biding capacity and only high-affinity sites can be detected. The slopes (Fig. 1) become steeper with increasing lipid fluidity, until at very low $\bar{\eta}$ values they become positive.

Binding data over a wide range of $\bar{\eta}$ values and ligand concentrations, obtained in a series of independent experiments, are summarized in Figure 2. The binding of [^{3}H]-serotonin first increases as $\bar{\eta}$ increases, reaching a five-fold maximum at $\bar{\eta}$ values of about 1.75, relative to control, and then declines sharply. On the other hand, slight fluidization of the membranes causes a small but significant increase in binding, but upon further increase in membrane fluidity, a significant decrease in binding is observed.

Table 2 summarizes a series of competition experiments which confirm the substrate specificity of the newly accessible serotonin receptors. Various drugs, known to compete for serotonin sites, displace bound [^{3}H]-serotonin to varying degrees. As $\bar{\eta}$ increases, the binding of the various drugs competing for serotonin sites is slightly reduced, although the profile of their potencies and substrate specificity is preserved. GABA and atropine do not compete for serotonin sites at any of the $\bar{\eta}$ values tested.

Fig. 3 summarizes opiate binding data from an extensive series of experiments carried out in a similar manner to those described for serotonin. Increasing the fluidity of P_2M membranes by incubation with increasing amounts of egg-lecithin (region A of Fig. 3) causes a decrease (up to 50%) in the binding of [^{3}H]-D-ala-enkephaline and of [^{3}H]-naloxone (both in the presence and absence of 100 mM sodium). Incubations of these membranes with increasing amounts of CHS (region B) causes a progressive increase in $\bar{\eta}$ with a concomitant increase in the binding of both ligands (in the absence of sodium). Ligand binding reaches a maximum of 65-90% above control when $\bar{\eta}$ is increased by 35%, and on further increase in microviscosity by means of CHS, decreases sharply (region C). When determining [^{3}H]-naloxone binding in the presence of sodium ions, the well known sodium shift (18) was observed i.e. an almost two fold increase of binding as compared to that in the absence of sodium. However, further increase of $\bar{\eta}$ with CHS fails to increase ligand binding, only regions A and C being observed.

In order to demonstrate the reversibility of the changes in receptor site accessibility, we have carried out the experiments summarized in Table 3. The membrane sample was first fluidized with egg lecithin, one half of this sample was then assayed for binding and the expected decrease found. On treating the other half of the sample with CHS, $\bar{\eta}$ increased with a concomitant increase in binding, thus demonstrating the reversibility in region A of Fig. 3. Analogous experiments were carried out in reverse, the results clearly showing reversibility of the changes in $\bar{\eta}$ and binding in region B as well. However when the samples were treated with large amounts of CHS, so as to reach $\bar{\eta}$ values beyond the critical point (between regions B and C of Fig. 3), and then fluidized, by treating with egg-lecithin no increase in binding after the second treatment was observed. Instead, further reduction in binding occurred, indicating that some irreversible change had taken place.

Table 4 presents $\bar{\eta}$ values of membranes obtained from different brain regions of Balb BL mice and in other rodent species. Although these measurements were made on crude preparations, these data indicate that a wide range of lipid microviscosity of membranes from different brain regions exists. The data also indicate that the microviscosity values, obtained after various lipid treatments, are within the range obtained for untreated preparations.

The data presented here can be summarized as follows: As the membranes become more viscous, the specific binding of serotonin increases steadily. The specific binding of [^{3}H]-serotonin, as a function of the microviscosities, $\bar{\eta}$, has a complex profile (Fig. 2). In the region where $\bar{\eta}$ increases, the binding appears to be biphasic and reaches a maximum at 1.75 relative $\bar{\eta}$ units. Above this level serotonin binding decreases sharply. This behavior may reflect a progressive, though unequal, exposure of different binding sites for serotonin. In the third phase, at $\bar{\eta} > 1.75$ relative units, the decrease in binding indicates an irreversible loss, or shedding of receptors.

The results on opiate binding are qualitatively similar, although it should be noted that the critical point of which the receptors are shed is quite different, ($\bar{\eta} = 1.35$ relative units) from that of serotonin receptors, (Fig. 3).

The Scatchard plots of the specific [^{3}H]-serotonin binding (Fig. 1) indicate a progressive response to changes in membrane microvisocity. As the number of both low- and high-affinity sites increases, their Kd values also increase (indicating lower affinity) with increasing $\bar{\eta}$. The dis-

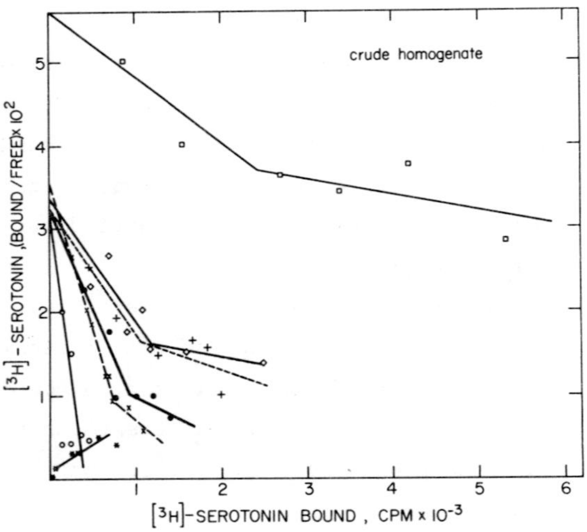

Fig. 1

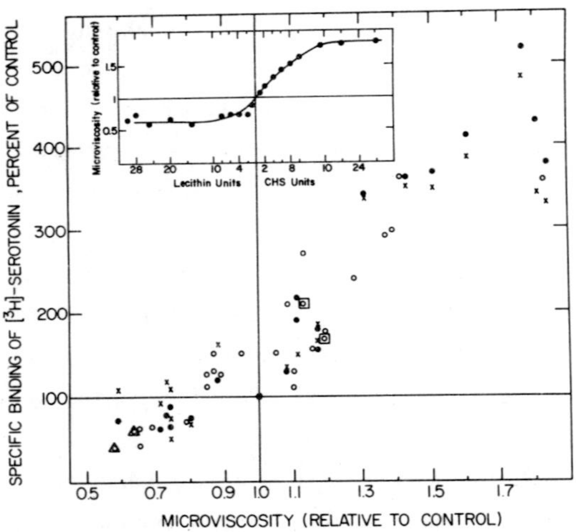

Fig. 2

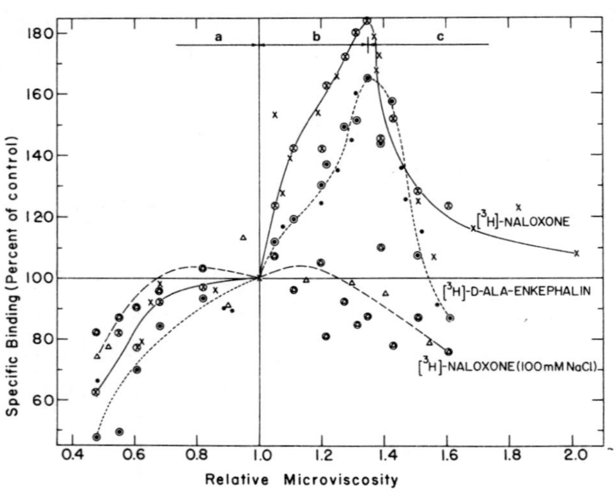

Fig. 3

FIGURE LEGENDS

Fig. 1. Scatchard plot of the binding of [^{3}H]-serotonin at 37°C as a function of concentration at different $\bar{\eta}$ values. Portions of crude homogenates (prepared from 10-20 pooled mouse brains) were incubated with varying amounts of CHS or lecithin. Control (untreated) samples were incubated with Tris-acetate buffer, pH 7.4 containing 3.5% PVP. The membrane microviscosity and binding were determined, each point being the mean of triplicate samples with a standard error of less than 5%. Each experiment was done at least twice with similar results. ◇ - ◇, $\bar{\eta}$=9.90; 0-0, $\bar{\eta}$=7.49; ●-●, $\bar{\eta}$=6.75 (control);□ -□, $\bar{\eta}$=5.80; x-x, $\bar{\eta}$=5.39.

Fig. 2. Specific binding of [^{3}H]-serotonin as a function of membrane microviscosity ($\bar{\eta}$). Portions from the same mouse brain suspension were incubated with varying amounts of lipids (see below). Control samples were incubated with 170 mM Tris-acetate buffer, pH 7.4. Each set of experimental points contains data from a single and separate experiment. Points to the left of the vertical line were obtained after treatment with lecithin. Points to the right of the vertical line were obtained after treatment with CHS. ●, P_2M fractions incubated with 6 nM [^{3}H]-serotonin; x, P_2M fractions incubated with 1 nM [^{3}H]-serotonin; o, crude homogenate incubated with 2 nM [^{3}H]-serotonin;⊡,△, same as above but after treatment with stearic acid and linoleic acid, respectively. Insert: Representative experiment showing membrane microviscosity of P_2M fraction as a function of lipid incubation volume. Each unit of CHS or lecithin represents one volume of lipid suspension (CHS - 0.4 mg/ml, lecithin - 0.8 mg/ml) per volume of membrane suspension (100 mg/ml). Values of $\bar{\eta}$ and [^{3}H]-serotonin binding capacity of the control samples are: $\bar{\eta}$ (crude homogenate) = 5.26; specific [^{3}H]-serotonin binding to crude homogenate = 2.0 pmoles/g tissue; $\bar{\eta}$ (P_2M) = 6.75; binding of [^{3}H]-serotonin to P_2M fraction at 1 nM ligand = 0.72 pmoles/g tissue; binding of [^{3}H]-serotonin to P_2M at 6 nM ligand = 2.98 pmoles/g tissue.

Fig. 3. Specific binding to P_2M fraction of [^{3}H]-naloxone (X), [^{3}H]-naloxone in the presence of 100 mM sodium chloride (Δ) and [^{3}H]-D-ala-enkephalin (●), as a function of membrane microviscosity ($\bar{\eta}$). The number of binding sites in untreated membranes were 2.80 fmol/mg original tissue weight for [3H]-D-ala-enkephalin, 3.78 fmol/mg for [^{3}H]-naloxone in the absence of sodium and 6.81 fmol/mg for [^{3}H]-naloxone assayed in the presence of 100 mM soidum ions. The microviscosity of control samples is 6.58 ± 2% poise.

Table 1. Summary of [^{3}H]-serotonin Binding Experiments at Different Microviscosity, $\bar{\eta}$, Values.

Preparation	$\bar{\eta}$, poise 25°C	Kd		Capacity	
		High-Affinity Site nM	Low-Affinity Site nM	High-Affinity Site pmoles/g tissue	Low-Affinity Site pmoles/g tissue
Crude Membranes	7.49	2.82	11.60	15.91	48.30
	6.75	1.55	11.60	5.19	20.10
	5.26 (untreated)	0.95	4.14	3.05	6.55
	5.02	1.49	5.27	4.85	12.64
	4.45	0.64	2.50	2.26	4.00
	4.35	0.29	-	0.90	-
P_2M	9.90	3.44	7.11	23.30	37.20
	7.49	1.99	5.10	7.40	12.75
	6.75 (untreated)	0.76	9.87	2.64	7.40
	5.80	2.68	-	3.27	-
	5.39	1.22	-	2.37	-

Table 2. Displacement of Bound [^{3}H]-Serotonin from Mouse Forebrain Homogenates at Different Microviscosity Values ($\bar{\eta}$)

Drug	BINDING (CPM)	
	Microviscosity ($\bar{\eta}$, poise, 25°C)	
	5.26 (untreated)	6.25
None	1508	4300
Serotonin (10^{-5}M)	940 (100%)	2208 (100%)
Serotonin (10^{-6}M)	1050 (81%)	2746 (74%)
Methysergide (10^{-6}M)	1228 (49%)	3463 (40%)
Metergoline (10^{-6}M)	1165 (60%)	3364 (45%)
Cinanserinė (10^{-6}M)	1356 (27%)	3884 (20%)
Mianserine (10^{-6}M)	1230 (49%)	3646 (31%)
Methiothepin (10^{-6}M)	1224 (50%)	3576 (35%)
Fluxethine (10^{-6}M)	1306 (21%)	4097 (10%)
Imipramine (10^{-6}M)	1390 (21%)	4272 (1.3%)
Haloperidol (10^{-6}M)	1214 (52%)	4177 (5.9%)
Atropine (10^{-6}M)	1612 (-)	5214 (-)
GABA (10^{-6}M)	1680 (-)	5179 (-)

Membranes were prepared and treated as described in Materials and Methods. Equal amounts of membranes were incubated with 4mM [^{3}H]-serotonin and with the various drugs listed above. The binding was assayed as described. Each value is the mean of triplicate samples which varied less than 15%. For each drug used, the percent of displacement occurring with 10^{-5}M unlabelled serotonin is given in parenthesis. The IC_{50} of serotonin and of methysergide were determined by incubation with 5 different concentrations of the unlabelled drugs and were found to be 10^{-8}M and 2.10^{-6}M respectively, in the untreated preparation ($\bar{\eta}$ = 5.26), and 8.10^{-7}M and 10^{-6}M when $\bar{\eta}$ = 6.25.

Table 3. Reversibility of Opiate and Serotonin Binding at Different Microviscosity Values.

	Control (untreated)	Lecithin (x14) →	CHS (x6)	CHS (x6) →	Lecithin (x15)	CHS (x18) →	Lecithin (x10)
Microviscosity ($\bar{\eta}$ poise 25°C)	6.58	4.05	7.11	8.35	5.80	10.85	9.62
[^{3}H]-D-ala-enkephaline (Specific binding, cpm)	664(100)	461(69)	554(83)	1095(165)	672(101)	737(111)	669(101)
[^{3}H]-naloxone Specific binding, cpm)	574(100)	447(77)	512(80)	881(153)	633(110)	677(118)	564(98)
[^{3}H]-serotonin (Specific binding, cpm)	1135(100)	784(69)	1548(136)	2324(205)	1225(108)	3726(108)	2950(260)

Samples were first treated with egg-lecithin (numbers in parenthesis at top indicate ratio of volumes of lipid suspension to membrane suspension) and then washed thoroughly. Half of the sample was assayed for microviscosity and ligand binding (as indicated) and the other half treated with CHS, washed thoroughly, and the microviscosity and binding re-determined. Experiments were done in both directions, as indicated. Numbers in parenthesis are percent of control.

Table 4. Membrane Microviscosity Values, $\bar{\eta}$, of Various Brain Regions and Different Species.

Species	Preparation	Brain Region	P	$\bar{\eta}$, 25°C poise
Balb BL male mice (6-8-week old)	P_2M	Cerebral Cortex	0.310	4.15
" " "	"	Hypothalamus	0.310	4.15
" " "	"	Thalamus	0.315	4.35
" " "	"	Hippocampus	0.315	4.35
" " "	"	N. Caudatus	0.322	4.67
" " "	"	Cerebellum	0.327	4.90
" " "	"	Midbrain	0.336	5.39
" " "	"	Brain Stem	0.355	6.75
" " "	"	Whole Brain	0.351	6.41
" " "	SPM	Whole Brain	0.301	3.78
" " "	Crude Homogenate	Forebrain	0.333	5.26
C_{57} BL/6J (lean male mice)	"	"	0.331	5.14
C_{57} BL/6J-ob/ob (obese male mice)	"	"	0.342	5.80
(C_3H/eb x C_{57} BL/6J)F_1 (7-week old male mice)	"	"	0.333	5.26
(C_3H/eb x C_{57} BL/6J)F_1 (2.5-year old mice)	"	"	0.344	5.95
Rats (male Wistar)	"	"	0.346	6.01

Membranes were prepared from the forebrains of 3-10 animals. Values are the mean of at least two experiments, which varied less than 10%.

placement of the receptor proteins may of course also affect their rotational and lateral movement, as well as cause critical changes to their tertiary and quaternary structure. Apparently, both high-affinity and low-affinity sites can markedly change their binding characteristics in response to the conditions imposed by the surrounding lipids and eventually reach a situation where the distinction between them is abolished. It could very well be that the serotonin binding sites all have the same basic chemical structure which, in different environments, have different binding characteristics. The observation, that at low lipid viscosities ($\bar{\eta} < 0.8$ relative units) the serotonin receptors detected are of high affinity, while at high lipid viscosities ($\bar{\eta} > 1.3$ relative units) the receptors are predominantly of the low affinity type (see Table 1), may have an alternative explanation. Low- and high-affinity sites may be located at different levels along the vertical axis of the receptor molecule. As the latter is displaced vertically to the plane of the membrane, the relative contribution of each of these sites is changed as indicated by the Scatchard plot parameters. In the case of the opiate receptor, when $\bar{\eta}$ increases the affinity for agonists decreases while that for antagonist increases (to be published).

A most interesting finding is that in the untreated preparations, the apparent binding capacity of serotonin receptors constitutes only about 20% (Fig. 2) and that of the opiate receptors about 60% (Fig. 3) of the potential binding capacity stored in the membrane. The binding of an agonist to a receptor is just the initial step in a sequence of events. The next step, the activation of adenylate cyclase, has been reported to be enhanced by increasing lipid fluidity (8,19). The final response of target cells of different membrane fluidity could therefore be the result of two opposing processes - the accessibility of receptors, which decreases with lipid fluidization, and the activation of adenylate cyclase, which increases with lipid fluidization. One may, therefore, expect an optimal lipid fluidity for the maximal response of each receptor. It should be mentioned that other processes involved in neuronal transmission, such as release and reuptake, may also change in response to changes in synaptic membrane lipid fluidity.

The three main parameters, which determine membrane lipid fluidity *in vivo*, are the cholesterol to phospholipid ration (C/PL), the sphingomyelin to lecithin ratio (S/L) and the degree of saturation of the phospholipid acyl chains (12,20). A change in any of these parameters will contribute to changes in lipid microviscosity, though to a different extent (12). In aging animals, these ratios have been reported to increase (21-23). The increase in the lipid viscosity of synaptic membranes, (see Table 4), could in fact initially increase receptor accessibility, and it has been reported (24) that the number of serotonin binding sites in brains from old men is about two-fold higher than in those from young adults, and consists of only low-affinity sites. With increasing synaptic membrane viscosity the exposed receptors can eventually overshoot the point of optimal activity, and become more vulnerable to degradation. Some of the behavioral aspects of aging, associated with the serotoninenergic system (e.g. loss of sleep, appetite, and libido), could be accounted for by this process.

Table 4 shows that membranes prepared from various brain regions differ in their microviscosities. This might be a partial explanation of the heterogeneity of receptor sites in the brain. Consistent with our findings that midbrain is composed of more viscous membranes as compared to cerebral cortex and hippocampus, Bennet and Synder (13) have shown that Kd of [^{3}H]-serotonin is lower (i.e. has higher affinity) in cortex and hippocampus as compared to midbrain, which is in agreement with our findings on fluidity.

The technical assistance of Mali Israeli and the help of Shoshana Newman in the preparation of this manuscript is gratefully acknowledged.

REFERENCES

1. Borochov, H. and Shinitzky, M. (1976) Proc. Natl. Acad. Sci. USA 73. 4526-4530.

2. Borochov, H., Abbott, R.E., Schachter, D. and Shinitzky, M. (1979) Biochemistry 18, 251-255.

3. Muller, C.P. and Shinitzky, M. (1979) Brit. J. Haem. 42, 355-362.

4. Shinitzky, M. and Souroujon, M. (1979) Proc. Natl. Acad. Sci. USA 76, 4438-4440.

5. Shinitzky, M. (1979) in Physical and Chemical Aspects of Cell Surface Events and Cellular Regulation, eds. Blumenthal, R. and deLisi, C. (Elsevier/North-Holland, Amsterdam), pp. 173-181.

6. Bakardijieva, A., Galla, H.J. and Helmreich, E.J.M. (1979) Biochemistry 18, 3016-3023.

7. Strittmatter, W.J., Hirata, F. and Axelrod, J. (1979) Science 204, 1205-1207.

8. Hanski, E., Rimon, G. and Levitzki, A. (1979) Biochemistry 18, 846-853.

9. Shinitzky, M., Skornick, Y. and Haran-Ghera, N. (1979) Proc. Natl. Acad. Sci. USA 76, 5313-5316.

10. Hershkowitz, M. (1978) Biochim. Biophys. Acta 542, 274-283.

11. Morgan, J.G., Wolfe, L.S., Mandel, P. and Gombos, G. (1971) Biochim. Biophys. Acta 241, 737-751.

12. Shinitzky, M. and Borenholz, Y. (1978) Biochim. Biophys. Acta 515, 367-394.

13. Bennet, J.P., Jr. and Snyder, S.H. (1976) Mol. Pharmacol. 12, 373-389.

14. Pasternak, G.W., Wilson, H.A. and Snyder, S.H. (1975) Mol. Pharmacol. 11, 478-484.

15. Scatchard, G. (1949) Ann. N.Y. Acad. Sci. 51, 660-672.

16. Fillion, G., Fillion, M.P., Spirokis, C., Bakers, J.M. and Jacob, J. (1976) Life Sci. 18, 65-74.

17. Nelson, D.L., Herbert, A., Bourgoin, S., Glowinski, J. and Hamon, M. (1978) Mol. Pharmacol. 14, 983-995.

18. Pert, C.B. and Snyder, S.H. (1974) Mol. Pharmacol. 10, 868.

19. Rimon, G., Hanski, E., Braun, S. and Levitzki, A. (1978) Nature 276, 394-396.

20. Shinitzky, M. and Inbar, M. (1976) Biochim. Biophys. Acta 433, 133-149.

21. Eisenberg, S., Stein, Y. and Stein, O. (1969) J. Clin. Invest. 48, 2320-2329.

22. Warner, M., Tolls, R.E., Hultin, J.V. and Mellecker, J. (1970) Z. Klin. Chem. Biochem. 8, 105-115.

23. Rouser, G. and Yamamoto, Y. (1968) Lipids 3, 284-287.

24. Shih, J.C. and Young, H. (1978) Life Sci. 23, 1441-1448.

Neurotransmitters and their Receptors
Edited by U.Z. Littauer, Y. Dudai, I. Silman,
V.I. Teichberg and Z. Vogel

The Adrenergic Receptor as the Locus of Antidepressant Therapy in Humans

R.H. Belmaker, B. Lerer, R.P. Ebstein and H. Dasberg

Jerusalem Mental Health Center – Ezrat Nashim, P.O.B. 140, Jerusalem, Israel

Abstract

B - adrenergic receptor subsensitivity has been proposed as a major effect of chronic treatment with antidepressant drugs in rats. A clinical trial of salbutamol, a B 2 adrenergic agonist, in depression provided human evidence for such receptor subsensitivity. Plasma cyclic AMP before treatment with salbutamol rose 267% in response to 0.25 mg salbutamol i. v. After one and three weeks of oral salbutamol treatment, depression scores declined in 11 depressed patients, while the plasma cyclic AMP response to i. v. salbutamol declined over 60%. The B-adrenergic adenylate cyclase remained subsensitive 4 days after cessation of salbutamol therapy. Lithium is another drug that markedly improves affective disorder. Data is presented that Li, too, reduces activity of B-adrenergic adenylate cyclase in humans.

Considerable research and theorizing in biological psychiatry over the past two decades has been based on the search for neurotransmitter abnormalities (1). Neurotransmitter metabolites in spinal fluid (CSF) and urine of mentally ill patients have been extensively studied (2). No clear etiologic correlate of schizophrenia, mania or depression has emerged, however. Drug treatment of mental illness has been found to be associated with some specific neurochemical changes, such as increased (3) homovanillic acid (HVA) accumulation in spinal fluid after neuroleptic treatment, or changes in urinary norepinephrine (NA) metabolite, MHPG, after treatment with certain tricyclic antidepressants (4). However, much other work has been unrevealing. For instance, high dose propranolol treatment of schizophrenia (5) was found to be devoid of effect on CSF amine metabolites (Table 1). It might have been expected that propranolol, by blocking NA receptors, would induce a compensatory pre-synaptic increase in NA and thus a rise in MHPG. The lack of MHPG change in human CSF might be due to a poor correlation between lumbar CSF MHPG and brain MHPG, or perhaps the NA system does not respond with pre-synaptic compensation to post-synaptic blockade, as does the DA system. In any case, CSF NA metabolites would seem to provide limited information about NA neurotransmission if a potent B-adrenergic antagonist did not affect MHPG.

The catecholamine hypothesis of depression had originally suggested that depression is associated with a reduction in functional NA levels at some central synapses (6). However, iprindole and other atypical but apparently effective antidepressants were found to have no effect on NA turnover (7). Moreover, tricyclic antidepressants of the classic vatiety that inhibit NA reuptake and thereby enhance synap-

Table 1. The effect of propranolol therapy on CSF amine metabolites and prolactin.

Patient No.	CSF propranolol ng/ml	HVA pmol/ml before	HVA pmol/ml after	5-HIAA pmol/ml before	5-HIAA pmol/ml after	MHPG pmol/ml before	MHPG pmol/ml after
1	29	282	467	199	224	74	74
2	78	241	176	106	67	44	37
3	55	419	267	157	84	51	41
4	20	214	165	138	94	82	29
5	42	163	140	87	80	45	47
6	11	130	122	89	83	34	34
7	16	175	325	124	157	41	48
8	1	98	167	104	113	33	40
9	35	141	202	84	112	50	65
10	70	90	121	49	46	30	31
$\bar{x} \pm$ SEM	40 ± 8	195 ± 31	215 ± 35	113 ± 13	106 ± 16	48 ± 5	44 ± 5

tic NA were found in pharmacokinetic studies to reach the brain quickly. Inhibition of reuptake could be expected to occur rapidly after onset of treatment, but therapeutic response to these agents in depression typically requires 2-4 weeks of continued treatment (8). These factors contributed to a disillusionment with concepts of neurotransmitter turnover as a key in understanding depression pathophysiology. Simultaneously, biochemical advances in cyclic AMP and receptor technology focussed attention on the receptor in depression. Receptor defects were hypothesized in the etiology of the illness (9). Sulser et al (10) studied the effects of chronic in vivo antidepressant treatment on the NA-sensitive adenylate cyclase in rat forebrain. They found that all antidepressant treatments, including electroshock (E.S.T.) and iprindole, induce subsensitivity of the NA-sensitive adenylate cyclase in rat forebrain. Moreover, induction of subsensitivity required continued in vivo treatment and its development paralleled the time course of human antidepressant effects. Sulser et al (10) suggested that a receptor sensitivity change and not a change in NA levels is the key factor in antidepressant therapy.

Human evidence for the concept of Vetulani and Sulser (10) seemed crucial, as animal experiments on sensitivity changes employ drug doses that are difficult to compare with those in human treatment. As part of a study on the antidepressant effects of salbutamol, we were able to evaluate the development of subsensitivity of B-adrenergic adenylate cyclase in humans.

Simon et al (11) had first reported antidepressant efficacy for salbutamol, a B-2 adrenergic agonist used routinely in the treatment of asthma. Schildkraut's original theory of depression as a deficiency of NA (6) had implied that a direct agonist may be effective in depression. However, available agonists either did not cross the blood-brain barrier or caused cardiac arythmias after more than brief use. The cardiac safety of salbutamol made clinical trial possible, and both uncontrolled (11) and controlled studies of Simon et al (12) suggested antidepressant effects.

Eleven depressed patients at the Jerusalem Mental Health Center were accepted for salbutamol treatment if other antidepressant treatments had not been successful. After a 14-day drug-free period, the patients received 0.25 mg salbutamol intravenously in a 10 minute infusion. Before the infusion and every 10 minutes thereafter for 70 minutes, blood was removed from an indwelling catheter into EDTA and placed on ice. The plasma was separated and stored at -70° until assay for cyclic AMP. After the first infusion the patients began oral salbutamol treatment at 2 mg four times daily, going up to 4 mg four times daily after 3 days. After 7-10 days the patients again received an intravenous infusion of salbutamol, at least 14 hours after the last oral dose. After 15-25 days of treatment a third intravenous infusion of salbutamol was given, again at least 14 hours after the last oral dose. After 3-4 weeks of salbutamol treatment, placebo was substituted, and a fourth infusion performed after 4 drug-free days.

Fig. 1 shows the plasma cyclic AMP response to i.v. salbutamol before, during and after chronic oral therapy. The plasma cyclic AMP response to the B-2 adrenergic agonist is over 267% of basal plasma cyclic AMP levels. Significant subsensitivity of the response is evident within 7 days of oral treatment. The statistical significance of the subsensitivity increases after 15-25 days of treatment, implying that subsensitivity has become more consistent among all the patients. The magnitude of the subsensitivity is over 60% of the salbutamol-induced rise in plasma cyclic AMP. Four days after cessation of treatment the subsensitivity has not diminished in magnitude, suggesting a relatively lasting change in receptor function. The half-life of salbutamol is short, and thus the subsensitivity 4 days after placebo substitution is clearly not dependent on residual salbutamol. Vetulani and Sulser (10) also reported that antidepressant-induced subsensitivity of rat forebrain NA-sensitive adenylate cyclase remains after cessation of antidepressant treatment. Such lasting effects are consistent with the lasting clinical effects of these treatments.

Fig. 2 shows the mean Hamilton Depression Scores (13) in the 11 patients. A significant improvement occurs within one week in this open clinical trial. Relapse occurs after cessation of salbutamol and the improvement is no longer significant when compared to baseline. There was no individual correlation between clinical response among the patients and induction of subsensitivity.

Fig. 3 shows the pulse response to salbutamol. Subsensitivity of the pulse response is clearly apparent and statistically significant. After 4 days of post-treatment placebo the pulse response returns closer to baseline than did the plasma cyclic AMP.

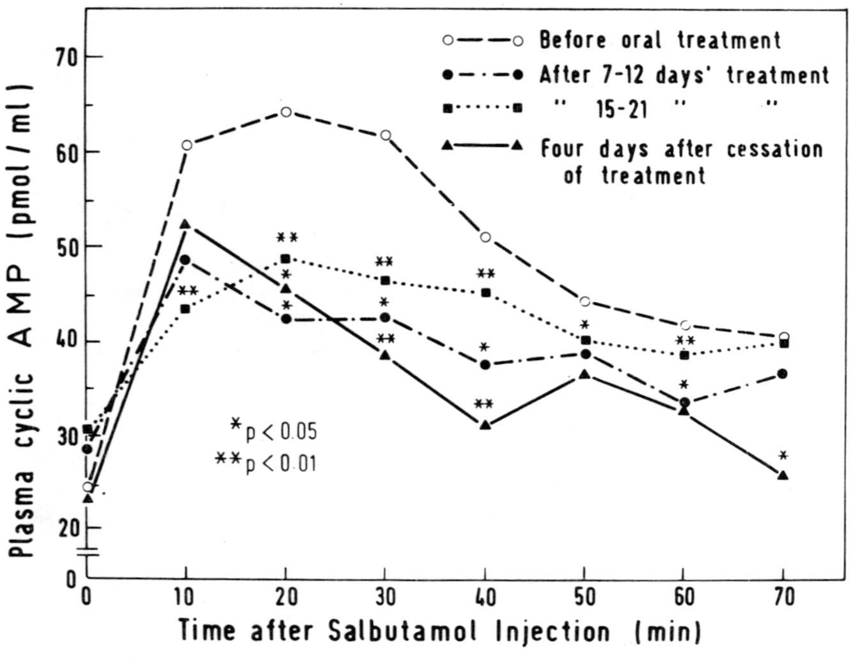

Fig. 1. The effect of chronic oral salbutamol treatment on the plasma cyclic AMP response to i.v. salbutamol.

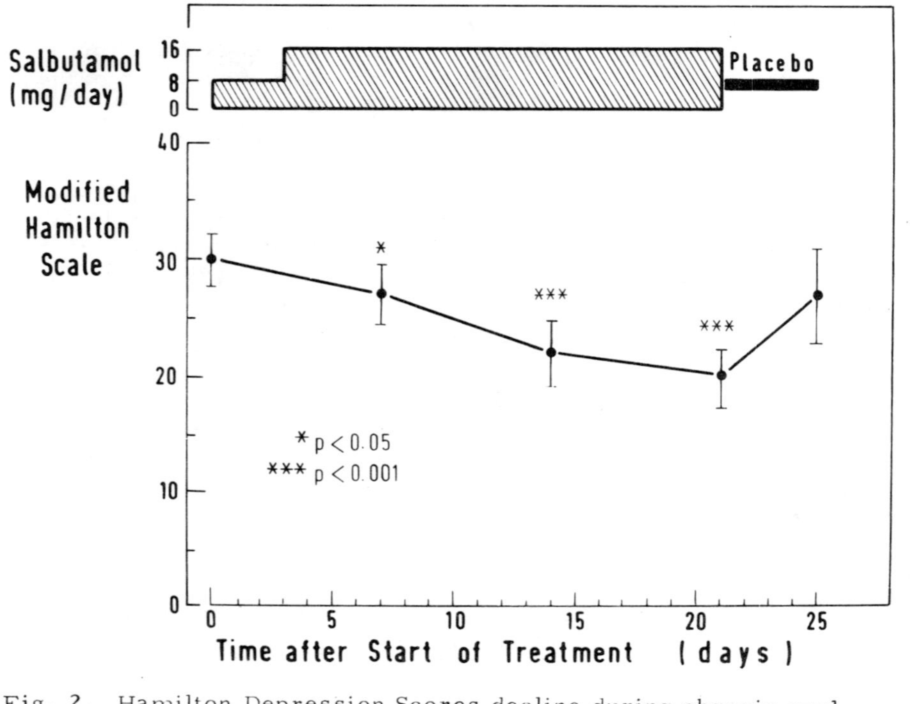

Fig. 2. Hamilton Depression Scores decline during chronic oral salbutamol therapy.

The above results support the concept that receptor sensitivity changes result from agonist availability changes in neurohormone systems (14). The role of receptor sensitivity changes after salbutamol treatment of depression demands further investigation of the function of B-2 adrenergic receptors in human brain. Molinoff (15) has suggested that these receptors are far less important than the B1 receptors. However the present results suggest that further research is necessary. An open trial such as ours is clearly not adequate proof of antidepressant efficacy for salbutamol, and controlled studies should be undertaken. The above study, however, can be seen as a prototype of receptor-oriented strategies in human depression research.

While Sulser et al (10) reported that E.C.T., MAO inhibitors, tricyclic antidepressants and other atypical antidepressants all induce subsensitivity of NA-sensitive adenylate cyclase, they did not report data on the effect of Li in this system. Li is a unique treatment in psychiatry with both antidepressant and antimanic properties (16). The antimanic properties of Li may be related to its ability to prevent receptor sensitivity increases in several systems (see Lerer, Ebstein and Belmaker, this volume). The antidepressant properties of Li could be related to Li effects on the NA-sensitive cyclic AMP accumulation that are similar to the effects reported by Sulser et al (10) for all other antidepressant treatments. Li inhibition of NA-sensitive adenylate cyclase has been reported from several laboratories (17, 18, 19). This inhibition can be demonstrated at Li concentrations within the therapeutic range (20). Unlike antidepressant-induced

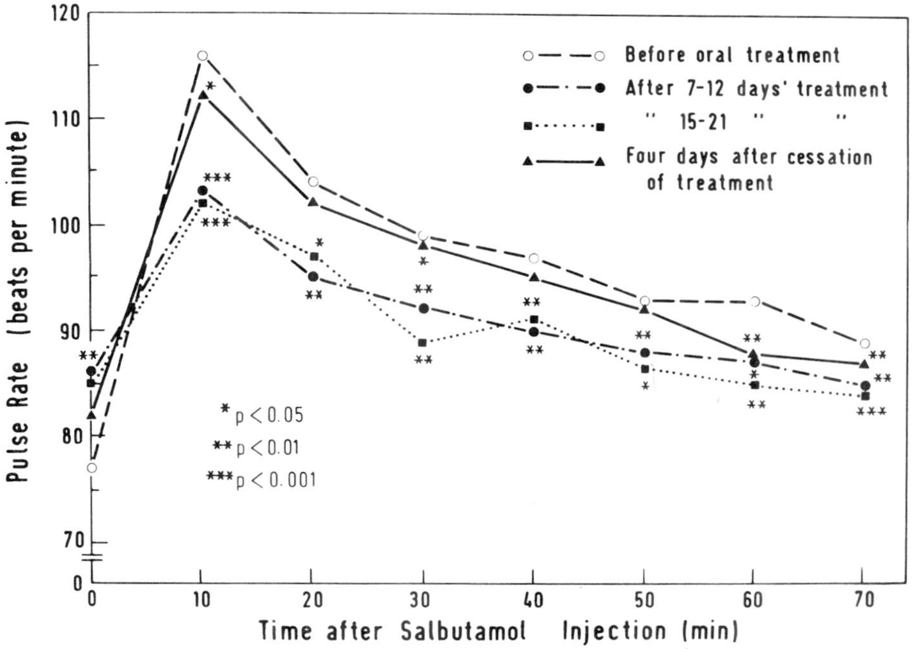

Fig. 3. The effect of chronic salbutamol on the pulse response to i.v. salbutamol

subsensitivity of the NA-sensitive adenylate cyclase, Li inhibition of NA-sensitive adenylate cyclase occurs in vitro as well as after chronic in vivo treatment. Thus the Li effect is more like that of a classic inhibitor of NA neurotransmission. However, chronic Li treatment does not lead to a compensatory supersensitivity of B-adrenergic receptors (22) or B-adrenergic adenylate cyclase (21), unlike propranolol or classic B-receptor antagonists (15). Moreover, Li does not affect B-adrenergic receptor binding to agonists or antagonists in vitro . Thus it has been suggested that Li inhibits the B-adrenergic receptor adenylate cyclase complex at a site distal to the receptor recognition site itself (21).

Fig. 4 shows the effect of chronic Li pre-treatment (oral 0.2% LiCl in food for 3 weeks) on the NA-sensitive adenylate cyclase in rat cortex ex vivo (21). Li plasma levels were determined in carotid blood obtained at sacrifice. The Li effect is marked, although the plasma Li levels are at the high end of the therapeutic range. It seemed important to evaluate this effect in humans receiving more clearly therapeutic doses of Li as a chronic treatment. Using the epinephrine-induced rise in plasma cyclic AMP in humans as a model, Ebstein et al showed that low plasma Li concentrations (0.71 mM) markedly inhibited peripheral B-adrenergic adenylate cyclase in humans. The epinephrine-induced rise in plasma cyclic AMP had previously been shown (16) to be due to stimulation of B-adrenergic adenylate cyclase. The protocol was similar to that described for salbutamol above,

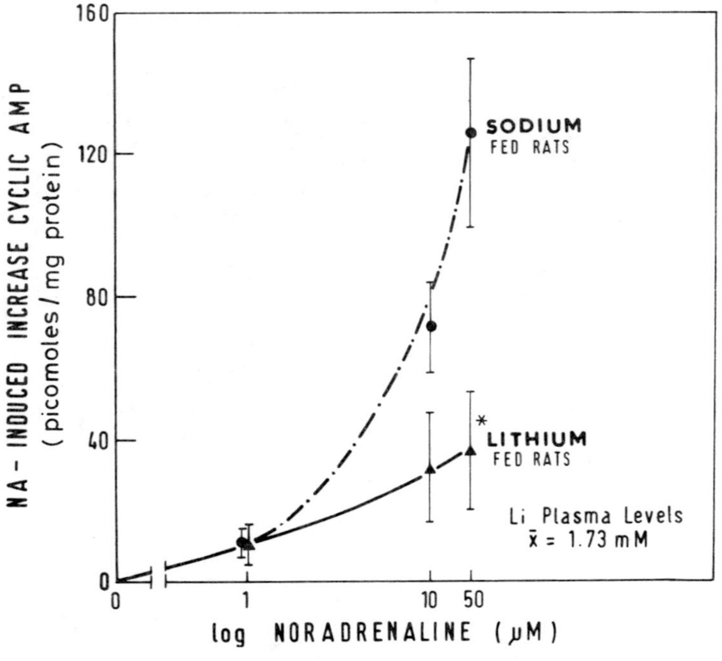

Fig. 4. The effect of chronic Li on the NA-induced increase in cyclic AMP in rat cortical slices.

using however 0.5 mg epinephrine subcutaneously as the stimulus. The Li inhibition in this system has been repeated by Friedman et al (23) using isoproterenol i.v. in human volunteers, and more recently again by our laboratory (24) in a new Li-treated and control group (Fig. 5). It should be noted that all the subjects in Fig. 5 receiving Li had been in chronic treatment, and thus the time course of the Li effect on human B-adrenergic adenylate cyclase is not clear as in the case of the salbutamol trial described above. However, the animal in vitro work would suggest that Li inhibition of the B-adrenergic adenylate cyclase is a direct dose-related drug effect. Inhibition in vivo in humans might be expected to occur when pharmacokinetic factors achieve adequate intracellular Li concentrations. Estimates for achievement of steady state Li brain levels after onset of Li therapy in humans are 6-10 days. Indeed, this time lag agrees well with the time lag required for clinical antimanic effects of Li in humans. Data on the time course of Li effects on depression or on the prevention of depression are more difficult to obtain, especially since clinicians tend to use lower doses and more conservative Li dosing schedules in depression than in mania. The above data raises the possibility that the antidepressant effects of Li are related to its ability to decrease B-adrenergic adenylate cyclase activity, as has been proposed for other antidepressant treatments by Sulser et al. The addition of human evidence for effects of both salbutamol and Li on B-adrenergic adenylate cyclase supports the concept that such effects can take place at normal therapeutic doses of psychoactive drugs.

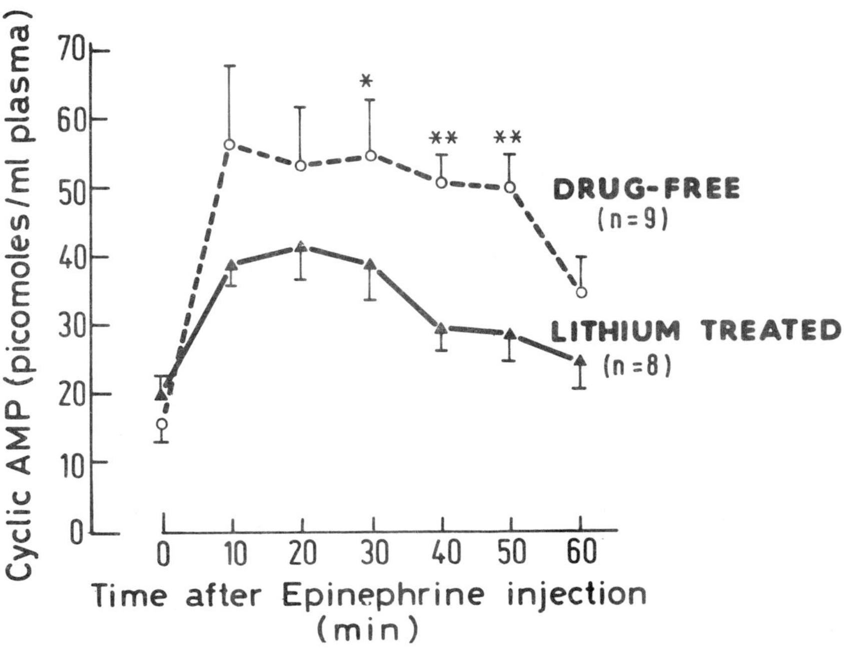

Fig. 5. The effect of chronic Li on the plasma cyclic AMP response to epinephrine.

References

(1) Van Praag, H.M. Depression and schizophrenia: A contribution on their chemical pathologies. Spectrum Public., New York, 1977.

(2) Mendels, J., Stinnet, J.L., Burns, D. and Frazer, A. Amine precursors and depression. Arch. Gen. Psychiatry, 32: 22-30, 1975.

(3) Post, R.M. and Goodwin, F.K. Time-dependent effects of phenothiazines on dopamine turnover in psychiatric patients. Science, 190: 488-489, 1975.

(4) Maas, J.W., Fawcett, J.A. and Dekirmenjian, H. 3-Methoxy-4-hydroxyphenylglycol (MHPG) excretion in depressive states: pilot study. Arch. Gen. Psychiatry, 19: 129-134 1968.

(5) Belmaker, R.H., Ebstein, R.P., Dasberg, H., Levy, A., Sedvall, C. and van Praag, H.M. The effect of propranolol treatment in schizophrenia on CSF amine metabolites and prolactin. Psychopharmacology, 63: 293-296, 1979.

(6) Schildkraut, J. J. The catecholamine hypothesis of affective disorders: a review of supporting evi dence. Am. J. of Psychiatry, 122:509-522.

(7) Zis, Athanasios P. and Goodwin, Frederick K. Novel antidepressants and the biogenic amine hypothesis of depression. Arch. Gen. Psychiatry, 36: Sept. 79.

(8) Baldessarini, R. J. The basis for amine hypotheses in affective disorders. Arch. Gen. Psychiatry, 32: 1087-1093.

(9) Bunney, W.E., Post, R.M., Andersen, A.E. and Kopanda, R.T. A neuronal receptor sensitivity mechanism in affective illness (a review of evidence). Communications in Psychopharmacology, 1: 393-405, 1977.

(10) Sulser, F., Vetulani, J. and Mobley, P.L. Commentary: mode of action of antidepressant drugs. Biochemical Pharmacology, 27: 257-261, 1978.

(11) Simon, P., Lecrubier, Y., Jouvent, R., Puech, A.J. Allilaire J. F. and Widlocher, D. (1978). Experimental and clinical evidence of the antidepressant effect of a beta adrenergic stimulant. Psychological Medicine, 8: 335-338.

(12) Lecrubier, Y., Puech, A. J., Jouvent, R., Simon, P. and Widlocher, D. A beta adrenergic stimulant salbutamol vs. clomipramine in depression: a controlled study. Bri. J. Psychiatry, in press.

(13) Hamilton, M. Devel opment of a rating scale for primary depressive illness. Brit. J. Soc. Clin. Psychol., 6:278-296, 1967.

(14) Baudry, M., Martres, M.P. and Schwartz, J.C.: Modulation in the sensitivity of noradrenergic receptors in the CNS studied by the responsiveness of the cyclic AMP system. Brain Res. 116: 111-124, 1976.

(15) Minneman, K.p., Dibner, M.D., Wolfe, B.B. and Molinoff, P.B. B_1-and-B_2-adrenergic receptors in rat cerebral cortex are independently regulated. Science, 204: 866-868, 1979.

(16) Ebstein, R.P., Belmaker, R.H., Grunhaus, L. and Rimon, R. Lithium inhibition of adrenaline-sensitive adenylate cyclase in humans. Nature, 259: 411-413, 1976.

(17) Forn, J. and Valdecasas, F.G. Effects of lithium on brain adenylate cyclase activity. Biochem. Pharmacol. 20: 2773-2779, 1971.

(18) Ebstein, R.P. and Belmaker, R.H. Lithium and brain adenylate cyclase. In: Lithium: Controversies and unresolved issues. T.B. Cooper, S. Gershon, N.S. Kline and M. Schou, eds. Excerpta Medica, Amsterdam, 1979.

(19) Reches, A., Ebstein, R.P. and Belmaker, R.H. Differential effect of lithium on noradrenaline-and-dopamine-sensitive accumulation of cyclic AMP in guinea pig brain. Psychopharmacology 58: 213-216, 1978.

(20) Belmaker, R.H. and Ebstein, R.P. Adenylate cyclase and the mechanism of lithium action. In: Neuropsychopharmacology, B. Saletu, ed. Pergamon Press, Oxford, 1979.

(21) Ebstein, R.P., Hermoni, M. and Belmaker, R.H. The effect of lithium on noradrenaline-induced cyclic AMP accumulation in rat brain: inhibition after chronic treatment and absence of supersensitivity. J. Pharmacol. and Experimental Therapeutics, in press.

(22) Rosenblatt, J.E., Pert, C.B., Tallman, J.F., Pert, A. and Bunney, W.E. Jr. The effect of impramine and lithium on α and B receptor binding in rat brain. Brain Res. 160: 186-191, 1979.

(23) Friedman, E., Oleshansky, M.A., Moy, P. and Gershon, S. Lithium and Catecholamine-induced plasma cyclic AMP elevation. In: Lithium: Controversies and unresolved issues. T. B. Cooper, S. Gershon, N.S. Kline and M. Schou, eds. Excerpta Medica, Amsterdam, 1979.

(24) Belmaker, R.H., Kon, M., Ebstein, R.P. and Dasberg, H. Partial inhibition by lithium of the epinephrine-stimulated rise in plasma cyclic GMP in humans. Biological Psychiatry, in press.

Neurotransmitters and their Receptors
Edited by U.Z. Littauer, Y. Dudai, I. Silman,
V.I. Teichberg and Z. Vogel

Receptor Mechanisms of Lithium Action in Affective Disorder

B. Lerer, R.P. Ebstein and R.H. Belmaker

Jerusalem Mental Health Center – Ezrat Nashim, P.O.B. 140, Jerusalem, Israel

Abstract

Lithium is an effective drug in the treatment of manic-depressive illness. It has no direct effects on receptor binding but prevents changes induced by other drugs in DA-receptor number, B-adrenergic receptor number, and B-adrenergic adenylate cyclase.

Lithium (Li) is an effective drug in the prevention of manic and depressive episodes (1). Numerous theories have been advanced to explain its mechanism of action, but none has been proven. Effects of Li on sodium and other electrolytes have been shown (2) as have effects of Li on enkephalins (3) and on serotonin metabolism (4). Very few of the Li effects noted in the literature have been demonstrated to occur at therapeutically equivalent Li concentrations, however. In addition, many of Li's biochemical effects are transient and disappear after chronic administration, and are thus unlikely to be related to Li's continuing therapeutic efficacy in patients.

Recently, receptor technology has made possible the study of Li effects on neurotransmitter receptors. Therapeutic Li concentrations do not affect receptor binding to agonists or antagonists in vitro in the dopamine, α-noradrenaline or B-noradrenaline receptor paradigms (5). Thus Li is not a classic receptor agonist or antagonist in these systems. Chronic in vivo treatment with Li leads to no change in DA receptors, a very small (17-27%) increase in α-NA receptors and a very small (10-13%) decrease in B-NA receptors (6). These small changes are difficult to relate to Li's marked clinical effects.

Bunney recently suggested that affective disorder, the recurrence of attacks of depression alternating with mania, may be related to cyclical changes in receptor sensitivity (6). Considerable interest then greeted the report of Pert et al (7) that chronic Li treatment in vivo could prevent the haloperidol-induced increase in DA-receptor number. Pert et al (7) fed animals haloperidol for 3 weeks, leading to a mean increase of 23% in (3H) spiroperidol binding. Simultaneous feeding of Li 0.2% in wet food, leading to therapeutically-equivalent Li plasma concentrations of 0.8 to 1.0 mEq/L completely prevented the haloperidol-induced increase in DA-receptors. Moreover, DA receptor supersensitivity after 3 weeks of haloperidol could be shown by Pert et al

(7) by behavioral techniques as well as biochemical ones. Apomorphine-induced stereotypies were significantly increased in animals pre-treated with haloperidol, but this increase could be completely blocked by administration of Li concurrent with the haloperidol. Pert et al (7) suggested that Li may act in manic-depressive illness by stabilizing receptor number and preventing changes hypothesized by Bunney et al (6) to be involved in the pathogenesis of affective disorder.

A major difficulty in connecting the finding of Pert et al (7) with Li's mechanism of action in affective disorder is the absence of clear support for a role of DA in the pathogenesis of affective disorder. Tricyclic antidepressants that are useful in the depressed phase of affective disorder do not, at clinically relevant dosages, affect reuptake of DA nearly as much as they affect reuptake of NA or serotonin (8). While DA-blocking neuroleptics are of some clinical value in mania, they are clearly less specific than Li and may not be truly normalizing in this disease (9). It may be that Li's ability to prevent receptor number changes may also occur in other neurotransmitter systems more relevant to affective disorder. The finding of Pert (7) et al relating to DA receptor changes may merely be the first glimpse at a more general property of Li. The true clinical utility of the finding of Pert et al (7) could well be in the area of tardive dyskinesia, which has been strongly connected to increases in DA-receptor number after chronic neuroleptic treatment. Clinical trials should be conducted to determine whether concurrent Li treatment with neuroleptics can neutralize the potential of neuroleptics to induce tardive dyskinesia.

In attempting to examine whether Li can prevent receptor sensitivity changes in other neurotransmitter systems, Friedman et al (10) examined the effect of Li on increased serotonergic receptor activity induced by reserpine in mice. Serotonergic receptor activity was investigated employing 5-methoxy-DMT-induced head twitches. Li pretreatment did not prevent the behavioral supersensitivity ascribed to serotonin in this paradigm. Treisser & Kellar (11) studied the effect of chronic Li on reserpine-induced increases in B-adrenergic receptor number in rat cortex. They fed rats Li 0.25% for two weeks and then administered a loading dose of reserpine (1.0 mg/kg i.p.) followed by daily injections of reserpine (0.1 mg/kg i.p.) for three weeks. They found that reserpine treatment alone increased mean B-receptor number from 8.9 pmol/gm of (3H) DHA binding to 12.4 pmol/gm of (3H) DHA binding. Concurrent Li treatment prevented the development of reserpine-induced supersensitivity, reducing the mean B-adrenergic receptor number to 9.4 pmol/gm of (3H) DHA binding. Li levels in plasma were 0.8 - 1.1 mM. They did not study NA-mediated behaviors, however. Interestingly, no study has yet reported whether chronic Li pretreatment can prevent the reserpine-induced behavioral depression in rats.

B-adrenergic receptor number is parallel to B-adrenergic adenylate cyclase activity in numerous systems (12). Li has been reported to directly inhibit adenylate cyclase activity (13). The NA-sensitive adenylate cyclase has been reported to be the most sensitive adenylate cyclase to Li inhibition (14). Li inhibition of NA-sensitive adenylate cyclase occurs at the high end of the therapeutic range in vitro and can also be demonstrated ex vivo after 3 weeks of continuous Li feeding to rats (15). As a bridge between the previous work on Li effects on B-adrenergic adenylate cyclase and the more recent work on Li effects on receptor number changes, we decided to evaluate the effect of Li on reserpine-induced increases in adenylate cyclase activity. Rats were fed Li 0.15% in food for 3-5 weeks leading to plasma levels of 0.4 mM in carotid blood obtained at sacrifice. Reserpine was administered by i.p. injection for 4 days (loading dose 5 mg/kg, then 2.5 mg/kg for 3 days). NA-stimulated adenylate cyclase activity was measured in cortical slices as previously described (15). The results are shown in Table 1.

Table 1. The effect of chronic Li pretreatment on the reserpine-induced increase in cyclic AMP accumulation.

	Control	Reserpine	Lithium	Reserpine + Li
basal	91±36 (s.e.m.)	108±20	72±16	66±19
10uM NA	154±27	452±109	181±30	378±65
50uM NA	207±71	615±97[a]	250±23	310 ±73[b]

a) $p < .01$ (one-tail) student's $t = 3.1$, reserpine vs. control
b) $p < .03$ (one-tail) student's $t = 2.23$, reserpine plus Li vs reserpine

Cyclic AMP values in p moles/mg protein represent the mean of 5 experiments on separate days, each experiment using four rat brains in each of the four groups.

It is clear from Table 1 that Li prevents reserpine-induced increases in adenylate cyclase activity. This is consistent with the data of Treiser & Kellar (11). Li at the low plasma concentrations in this study cannot be shown to inhibit NA-sensitive adenylate cyclase ex vivo (comparing the Li only column on table 1 with control). However, effects of Li to directly inhibit adenylate cyclase require continued presence of Li, unlike the changes in receptor number induced by reserpine and prevented by Li in the paradigm above. Since the rat cortical slices are pre-incubated in vitro after sacrifice of the Li-fed animal, Li may well equilibrate with the medium, and direct inhibition of adenylate cyclase may be difficult to demonstrate at low Li concentrations.

The theory that Li's clinical mode of action involves stabilizing receptor number is supported by the above study. A study showing Li prevention of behavioral supersensitivity in the NA system would seem to be a crucial missing leg of the triad of receptor, adenylate cyclase and behavior. Further research must also ask whether Li can prevent receptor changes in the other direction: subsensitivity. Rosenblat et al (5) noted that Li did not prevent the B-adrenergic receptor number decline induced by chronic imipramine treatment of rats. They did not, however, present data in detail, and the issue is a crucial one. Li in clinical practice prevents both depression and mania in bipolar manic-depressive patients. One is therefore tempted to demand a biphasic action for the drug biochemically. Further experimentaion should ask whether Li prevents desimipramine-induced subsensitivity of NA-sensitive adenylate cyclase (16), and whether Li prevents electroshock (E.C.S.) induced subsensitivity of NA-sensitive adenylate cyclase (16) or E.C.S.-induced reduction in rat cortical B-adrenergic receptor number. (17). In humans, salbutamol treatment of depression has recently been shown to induce subsensitivity of the plasma cyclic AMP response to i.v. salbutamol (see Belmaker et al, this volume). Would Li co-treatment prevent salbutamol-induced subsensitivity of the B-adrenergic adenylate cyclase in humans? If not, it would seem that Li can prevent receptor sensitivity changes in one direction only and a second mechanism must be discovered to explain Li's bidirectional action in the clinic.

References

(1) Baastrup, P.C. and Schou, M. Lithium as a prophylactic agent. Its effect against recurrent depressions and manic-depressive psychosis. Arch. Gen. Psychiatry, 16: 162-172, 1967.

(2) Baer, L., Kassir, S. and Fieve, R.R. Lithium-induced changes in electrolyte balance and tissue electrolyte concentration. Psychopharmacologia 17:216, 1970.

(3) Byck, R. Peptide transmitters: a unifying hypothesis for euphoria, respiration, sleep and the action of lithium. Lancet 11: 72-73, 1976.

(4) Mandell, A.J. Effects of lithium on serotonin synthesis. In: The Neurobiology of Lithium, W.E. Bunney and D.L. Murphy (eds.) Neurosciences Research Program Bulletin, v.14 no. 2, 169-173, 1976.

(5) Rosenblatt, J.E., Pert, C.B., Tallman, J.F., Pert, A. and Bunney, W.E. Jr. The effect of imipramine and lithium on α-and B-receptor binding in rat brain. Brain Research 160: 186-191, 1979.

(6) Bunney, W.E. Jr., Post, R.M., Andersen, A.E. and Kopanda, R.T. A neuronal receptor sensitivity mechanism in affective illness (a review of evidence). Psychopharmacol. Commun. 1: 393-405, 1977.

(7) Pert, A., Rosenblatt, J., Sivit, C., Pert, C.B. and Bunney, W.E. Jr. Long-term treatment with lithium prevents the development of dopamine receptor supersensitivity. Science, 201: 171-173, 1978.

(8) Van Praag, H.M. Depression and schizophrenia: a contribution on their chemical pathologies. Spectrum Publications, New York, pp. 33-37, 1977.

(9) Belmaker, R.H. and Van Praag, H.M. Mania: Disease entity or symptom cluster. In: Mania: an evolving concept. R.H. Belmaker and H.M. Van Praag (eds.) Spectrum Publications, New York (in press).

(10) Friedman, E., Dallob, A. and Levine, G. The effect of long-term lithium treatment on reserpine induced supersensitivity in dopaminergic and serotonergic transmission. Life Sci. 25: 1263-1266, 1979.

(11) Treiser, S. and Kellar, K.J. Lithium: effects on adrenergic receptor supersensitivity in rat brain. Europ. J. Pharmacol., 58: 85-86.

(12) Lefkowitz, R.J. and Williams, L.T. (1978). Molecular mechanisms of activation and desensitization of adenylate cyclase coupled beta-adrenergic receptors. In: Advances in Cyclic Nucleotide Research. W.J. George, W.J. and L.J. Ignarro (eds. 9: 1-17.

(13) Forn, J. and Valdecasas, F.G. Effects of lithium on brain adenylate cyclase activity. Biochem. Pharmacol. 20: 2773-2779, 1971.

(14) Belmaker, R.H. and Ebstein, R.P. Adenylate cyclase and the mechanism of lithium action. In: Neuropsychopharmacology, B. Saletu et al, eds., Pergamon Press, Oxford, 1979.

(15) Ebstein, R.P., Hermoni, M. and Belmaker, R.H. The effect of lithium on noradrenaline-induced cAMP accumulation: Inhibition after chronic treatment and absence of supersensitivity. J. Pharm. Exp. Ther. (in press).

(16) Vetulani, J. and Sulser, F. Action of various antidepressant treatments reduces reactivity of noradrenergic cyclic AMP-generating system in limbic forebrain. Nature (London) 257: 495-496, 1975.

(17) Bergstrom, D.A. and Kellar, K.J. Effect of electroconvulsive shock on monoaminergic receptor binding sites in rat brain. Nature, 278: 464-466.

Neurotransmitters and their Receptors
Edited by U.Z. Littauer, Y. Dudai, I. Silman,
V.I. Teichberg and Z. Vogel

Clinical Implications of the Molecular Model of Tardive Dyskinesia

J. Bannet, MD[1], R.H. Belmaker, MD[2] and R.P. Ebstein, PhD[2]

[1] *Department of Psychiatry, Hadassah University Hospital, Jerusalem, Israel*
[2] *Mental Health Center – Ezrath Nashim, Jerusalem, Israel*

ABSTRACT

Increases in 3H-spiroperidol binding in rat caudate after chronic haloperidol treatment is used as an animal model of tardive dyskinesia. Individual pharmacogenetic differences and the effects of interrupted treatment are studied in this system. DA receptor agonist treatment, based on work in the animal model, is presented for a patient with tardive dyskinesia.

Tardive dyskinesia (TD) is a persistent neurological disorder which develops after prolonged neuroleptic use in some schizophrenic patients(1). TD is characterized by repetitive, involuntary movement of the mouth, lips and tongue ("bucco linguo masticatory syndrome") and occasionally involves limbs and trunk as well(2). The reported incidence of TD varies greatly(3) but a reasonable estimate is that 20% of patients taking neuroleptic drugs exhibit symptoms of this disease(2). The most important factors contributing to the development of TD are age, length of hospitalization and exposure to high-dose drug therapy(4). Once developed, TD is usually resistant to treatment and often persists long after neuroleptic therapy is stopped(3). Appearance of TD frequently occurs only after cessation of neuroleptic treatment, and in such cases reintroduction of drug therapy is sometimes successful in controlling the dyskinesia. Similarly, the occurrence of TD when drug therapy is ongoing can often be effectively treated by raising the daily dose. This paradoxical use of a drug to control its own side effect is the main clinical evidence which supports current molecular concepts of TD.

Biochemical theories of TD are based on the common property of all neuroleptic drugs in blocking dopamine receptors(5) and the subsequent development of behavioral(6, 7) and biochemical(8, 9, 10) supersensitivity. Klawans et al(9) have suggested that "TD results from denervation hypersensitivity of striatal dopamine receptors". Supersensitivity enables the fraction of DA molecules which "slip by" neuroleptic blockade to activate a greatly sensitized DA receptor. Clinical evidence to support this model of TD is the paradoxical finding discussed above that neuroleptic therapy is the best immediate treatment of these dyskinesias. Higher doses of neuroleptic drugs reestablishes effective dopamine blockade which had been overcome by receptor sensitization. The appearance of TD which coincides with cessation of neuroleptic treatment is understandable as an "unmasking" of a supersensitive DA receptor when neuroleptic treatment is stopped.

Biochemical evidence to support the supersensitive DA receptor model of TD has been obtained with the development of new techniques to study DA receptors at the molecular level(8). Receptor binding assays have permitted quantitative measurement of changes in receptor number after neuroleptic treatment(7, 8, 10). These reports have demonstrated a compensatory increase in rat brain receptor number averaging 43% without a change in affinity after 3-4 weeks of neuroleptic treatment. Similarly, autopsy studies of schizophrenic patients demonstrate increased DA receptor number in specific brain regions from patients previously treated with neuroleptic drugs(11). Although most of the available evidence supports neuroleptic-induced DA supersensitivity as a useful model of TD, some clinical findings are not consistent with the animal model. Tarsy and Baldessarini(12) have criticized dopamine supersensitivity as a model of TD because of the apparent discrepancy between the rapid development by three weeks of elevated DA receptor number in animal studies and the slow onset of TD in patients. Moreover, it is clear that only a fraction of humans treated for years with neuroleptics develop TD, whereas individual differences have not been studied in the response of DA receptor number to haloperidol treatment.

We therefore evaluated DA receptor number in individual rat and mouse caudates after haloperidol or drug-free feeding. After 3 months of haloperidol treatment of rats there was a 78% increase in caudate DA receptor number, accompanied by a significantly increased variance in the number of DA receptors in haloperidol-treated compared with control rats[Fig.1]. Although 3 inbred mouse strains (C57Bl, C3H and CBA) also showed significant increases in DA receptor number after 3 months of haloperidol treatment, <u>no</u> increased variance was observed after haloperidol treatment. Wild type mice from a genetically heterogeneous population showed increases in DA receptor number after chronic haloperidol treatment accompanied by a significantly increased variance in receptor number of the drug-treated group.

Fig.1

The effect of 3 weeks and 3 months oral haloperidol treatment on striatal DA receptor number in individual rats. (The number of receptor sites and K_D was determined by scatchard plot for each individual rat striatum).
The variance of DA receptor number is significantly increased after haloperidol treatment (F ratio = 3.1, p<.01 at 3 weeks; F ratio = 5.7, p<.001 at 3 months).

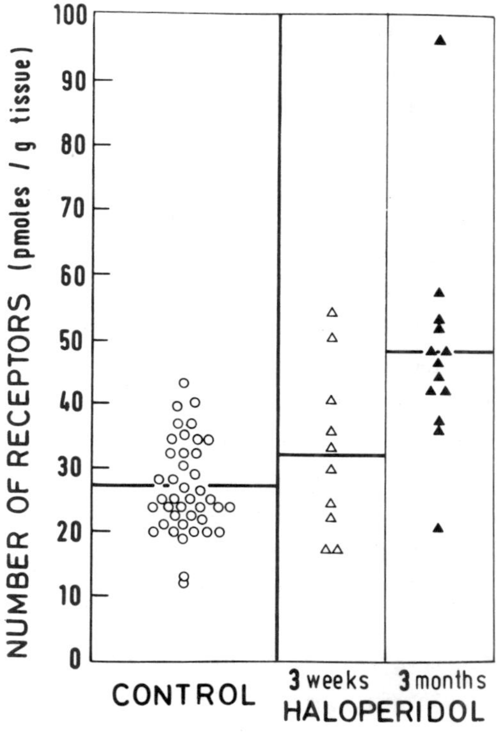

The heterogeneity in individual response to neuroleptic treatment in our animal experiments may be similar to the clinical situation in which TD develops in only a fraction of treated patients(3). Our results suggest a possible pharmaco-genetic susceptibility to haloperidol-induced increases in receptor number which manifests itself only after chronic exposure to drugs. The biochemical mechanism underlying DA receptor susceptibility to haloperidol treatment is unknown, although individual differences in brain neuroleptic levels might explain the observed increase in variance in response to neuroleptic treatment. However, the results of Muller and Seeman(15), showing a lack of correlation between daily drug dose and development of supersensitivity in the range of 0.5mg/kg to 10mg/kg haloperidol, suggest that pharmokinetic differences are not important factors in neuroleptic-induced increases in DA receptor number. Our results demonstrate the importance of measuring individual values after exposure to neuroleptics when using genetically heterogeneous populations. The common practice of pooling striata from several animals may mask genetic variability relevant to drug-induced changes in DA receptor number.

Increased variance of DA receptor number in animals treated with neuroleptics is parallel to the findings observed when striatal DA receptor number is measured in brains obtained from individual schizophrenic patients treated with neuroleptic drugs prior to death(16). Analysis of the published data of Owen et al(16) shows an increased variance in mean DA receptor number in striata obtained from neuroleptic-treated patients compared to control brains ($F=10.6$, $p<.001$). This suggests that genetic predisposition may also be important in determining the response of individual patients to neuroleptic treatment and may have important implications in drug treatment of schizophrenia. Perhaps genetic correlates of tardive dyskinesia, such as specific HLA types or red cell enzyme polymorphisms could be discovered and individuals at risk for tardive dyskinesia could avoid neuroleptic treatment.

As another approach to the prevention of TD, "drug holidays" for neuroleptic-treated patients have been advocated(2). Since prospective studies are extremely difficult in this area and could take years to yield a definitive answer, a study of drug holidays in an animal model of TD seems relevant. We therefore examined the influence of long term haloperidol administration versus intermittent administration[Fig.2] on Sabra wild mice. (3H)Spiroperidol binding is significantly increased after 5 ($p<.01$) or 10 ($p<.001$) weeks of haloperidol treatment, but 10 weeks of drug holiday treatment is no different from 5 or 10 weeks of continual treatment.

Animal models in psychiatry, as in all medicine, can be instructive but not definitive. Definitive evidence on the value of drug holidays for prevention of tardive dyskinesia can come only from a well-designed clinical study. However, the absence of a positive effect of drug holiday on the molecular model of tardive dyskinesia can serve to quell premature enthusiasm for drug holidays. There is no physiological reason why intermittent blockade of dopamine receptors by neuroleptic drugs may not enhance, rather than reduce, compensatory receptor number increases. The preliminary clinical study of Jeste and associates(17) points in the same direction.

Fig.2

The effect of chronic haloperidol on (3H)spiroperidol binding in mouse striatum. (concentration of (3H)spiroperidol was 1nM in reaction mixture)

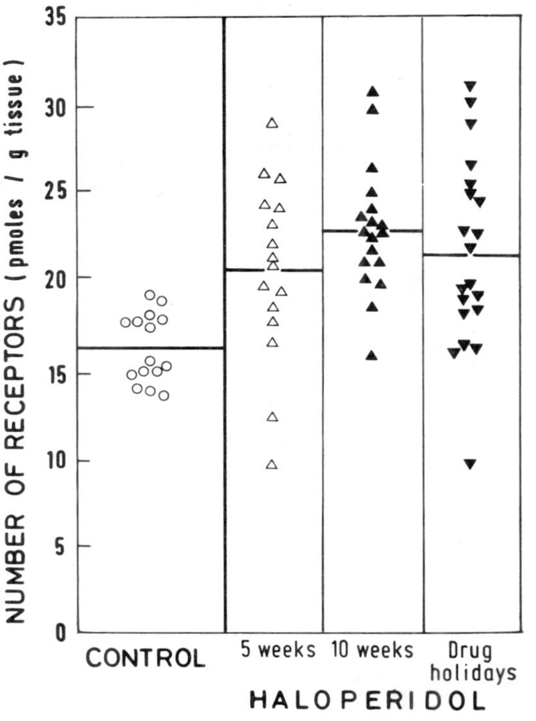

Novel methods of treating TD could also be profitably examined using a valid animal model of this disorder. For example L-dopa therapy worsens TD in humans by increasing dopamine neurotransmission onto already increased numbers of dopamine receptors. However Friedhoff(18) suggests that a period of L-dopa therapy may succeed in reducing the number of dopamine receptors to normal by a process opposite to that which led to their increase. That is, receptor agonist induced receptor hyposensitivity may be used to treat receptor antagonist induced receptor hypersensitivity. This suggestion has been studied and confirmed in tardive dyskinesia model in rats(18, 19). Using this idea in a clinical research protocol we treated a 61 year old chronic schizophrenic patient, suffering for over 5 years from TD. For the evaluation of treatment two rating scales were used, the Abnormal and Involuntary Movement Scale (AIMS) for TD(20) and the Brief Psychiatric Rating Scale (BPRS) for schizophrenic symptoms(21).

Fig.3

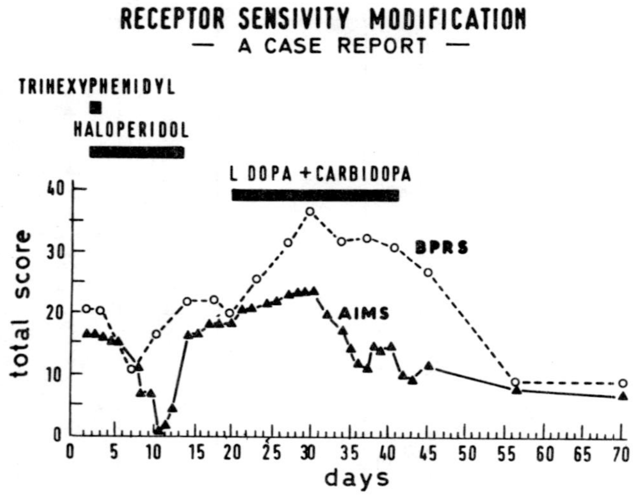

Fig. 3 illustrates the course of the patient whose TD improved markedly after initial withdrawal of the anticholinergic anti-Parkinson drug trihexyphenidyl. Total AIMS score declined from 16 to 0. Withdrawal of haloperidol (15mg/day) resulted in a return of TD (AIMS increases) as the hypothesized supersensitive DA receptors are unmasked. Onset of L-dopa (125mg/day) and carbidopa (12.5mg/day) led to further increase in AIMS scores along with an exacerbation of schizophrenic symptomatology (BPRS increases), as predicted by DA theories of schizophrenia and previous studies of acute L-dopa in schizophrenia(22). After cessation of L-dopa therapy AIMS scores and BPRS scores both drop markedly below baseline values. The results suggest successful induction of subsensitivity of DA receptors in the striatum possibly mediating TD and perhaps also, more speculatively, of DA receptors in the mesolimbic system whose overactivity contribute to schizophrenic symptomatology.

The above examples suggest the value of clinical-biochemical interactions in the understanding of a human illness, tardive dyskinesia. The molecular model of TD suggests the need for identifying pharmacogenetic risk factors, casts doubt on the value of drug holidays in preventing TD, and suggests that agonist induced subsensitivity may present a novel approach to treatment of TD. Further research on the molecular mechanism of supersensitivity is crucial in providing psychiatric clinicians with tools with which to regulate and restore receptor sensitivity in human illness.

REFERENCES

1) Kobayashi, R.M. Drug therapy of tardive dyskinesia. New Eng J Med 296, 257-260, 1977

2) Editorial. Tardive dyskinesia. Lancet 2, 447-448, 1979

3) Crane, G.E. Persistent dyskinesia. Brit J Psychiatry 122, 395-405, 1973

4) Chouinard, G., Annable, L. et al. Factors related to tardive dyskinesia. Am J Psych 136, 79-85, 1979

5) Snyder, S.H. The dopamine hypothesis of schizophrenia: focus on dopamine receptor. Am J Psychiatry 133, 197-202, 1976

6) Klawans, H.L., Rubovits, R. An experimental model of tardive dyskinesia. J Neural Trans 33, 235-246, 1972

7) Moore, K.E., Thornburg, J.E. Advances in Neurology. ed. I. Hanin and E. Usdin, Oxford, Pergamon Press, p.351, 1975

8) Burt, D.R., Creese, I. et al. Antischizophrenic drugs: chronic treatment elevates dopamine receptor binding in brain. Science 326-328, 1977

9) Klawans, H.L., Goetz, C. et al. Laevo dopa induced receptor hypersensitivity. Ann Neurol 2, 125-129, 1977.

10) Kobayashi, R.M., Fields, J.Z. et al. Brain transmitter receptors and chronic antipsychotic drug treatment: a model for tardive dyskinesia. In: Animal models in psychiatry. Ed. E. Usdin, New York, Pergamon, pp.405-409, 1978

11) Lee, T., Seeman, P. et al. Binding of H-neuroleptics and 3H-apomorphine in schizophrenic brains. Nature 274, 897-900, 1978

12) Tarsy, D., Baldessarini, R.J. The pathophysiological basis of tardive dyskinesia. Biol Psychiatry 12, 431-450, 1977

13) Ebstein, R.P., Pickholz, D. et al. Dopamine receptor changes after long term haloperidol treatment in rats. J Pharm Pharmacol 31, 558-559, 1979

14) Burt, D.R., Creese, I. et al. Properties of (3H)haloperidol and (3H)dopamine binding associated with dopamine receptors in calf brain membranes. Mol Pharmacol 12, 800-812, 1976

15) Muller, P., Seeman, P. Brain neurotransmitter receptors after long term haloperidol. Life Sci 21, 1751-1758, 1977

16) Owen, F., Crow, T.J. et al. Increased dopamine receptor sensitivity in schizophrenia. Lancet 2, 223-225, 1978

17) Jeste, D.V., Potkin, S.G. et al. Tardive dyskinesia reversible and persistent. Arch Gen Psychiatry 36, 585-590, 1979

18) Friedhoff, A.J. Receptor sensitivity modification:a new paradigm for the potential treatment of some hormonal and transmitter disturbances. Comp Psychiatry 18, 309-317, 1977

19) List, S.J., Seeman, P. Dopamine agonists reverse the elevated (3H)neuroleptic binding in neuroleptic pretreated rats. Life Sci 24, 1447-1452, 1979

20) ECDEU Assessment Manual. NIMH Psychopharmacology Research Branch. Rockville, Maryland, pp.534-535, 1976

21) ECDEU Assessment Manual. NIMH Psychopharmacology Research Branch. Rockville, Maryland, pp.157-169, 1976

22) Angrist, B.M., Sathananthan, G.S. et al. Behavioral effects of L-dopa in schizophrenic patients. Psychopharmacologia 31, 1-12, 1973

Neurotransmitters and their Receptors
Edited by U.Z. Littauer, Y. Dudai, I. Silman,
V.I. Teichberg and Z. Vogel

Neuronal Serotonin Receptors and Cyclic AMP: Biochemical, Pharmacological and Electrophysiological Analysis

Irwin B. Levitan and Alan H. Drummond*

Friedrich Miescher-Institut, P.O.Box 273, CH-4002 Basel, Switzerland

ABSTRACT

Application of micromolar concentrations of serotonin (5-hydroxytryptamine, 5HT) to an *Aplysia* abdominal ganglion causes identified neuron R15 to hyperpolarize. Voltage clamp analysis indicates that this results from activation of a K^+ conductance, allowing K^+ to move down its concentration gradient out of the cell. The response is mimicked by extracellular application or intracellular injection of cyclic AMP derivatives. It is also mimicked by intracellular injection of guanylylimidodiphosphate, which activates adenylate cyclase and causes cyclic AMP to accumulate in R15. The effects of low concentrations of 5HT are enhanced in the presence of the phosphodiesterase inhibitor Ro 20-1724. A number of analogs of 5HT (for example 6HT, tryptamine, bufotenine), at concentrations in the micromolar range, also cause R15 to hyperpolarize.

5HT applied to an abdominal ganglion causes cyclic AMP to accumulate within R15. 5HT also stimulates adenylate cyclase activity in membranes prepared from isolated R15 cell bodies. N-Methyl 5HT and bufotenine stimulate adenylate cyclase activity to the same extent as 5HT; that is, they are full agonists. Tryptamine, 6HT and d-LSD are partial agonists. A pharmacological analysis indicates that the 5HT receptor mediating neuron R15 hyperpolarization is very similar to that mediating adenylate cyclase stimulation.

All the criteria necessary to assign cyclic AMP a role in the response to a neurotransmitter have been satisfied in the present case. This is the first time all these criteria have been satisfied in a neuronal system. Accordingly, we conclude that the 5HT-induced hyperpolarization of *Aplysia* neuron R15 is mediated by cyclic AMP.

---

* Present address: Department of Pharmacology, University of Glasgow, Glasgow G12 8QQ, Scotland

INTRODUCTION

There is considerable evidence implicating serotonin (5-hydroxytryptamine; 5HT) as a neurotransmitter in vertebrate and invertebrate nervous systems. Its neurotransmitter function has been particularly thoroughly studied in the central ganglia of certain gastropod molluscs, where it is released upon pre-synaptic stimulation and produces different responses in different target cells (1-5). It has also been suggested that 5HT may act as a neuromodulator, that is as an agent which does not by itself change the membrane potential of a target cell, but rather changes the way in which the target cell responds to other inputs (6). There has been some indication that the neuromodulatory and neurotransmitter effects of 5HT might be mediated by cyclic AMP (4,5,7-9).

We have studied 5HT receptors in the marine snail *Aplysia californica* and the terrestrial snail *Helix pomatia*, using a combined pharmacological, biochemical and electrophysiological approach. The extraordinarily large, identifiable nerve cells present in these (and other) gastropods allow such multidisciplinary studies at the level of single, identified neurons. We have found that *Aplysia* and *Helix* 5HT (and dopamine) receptors can be measured by the binding of the radioactive ligand [^{3}H]-LSD (10-12), and have made use of this to define in detail the pharmacological profile of these receptors. Furthermore, we have shown that the 5HT receptors labelled by [^{3}H]-LSD are functionally coupled to the enzyme adenylate cyclase in neuronal membranes (11-13). Finally, we have demonstrated that 5HT causes identified *Aplysia* neuron R15 to hyperpolarize, and that the 5HT receptors involved in this response are also coupled to adenylate cyclase (14). In the present communication we summarize the evidence, accumulated during the past few years, that the 5HT-induced hyperpolarization of neuron R15 is mediated by cyclic AMP.

METHODS

The methodology used to carry out the biochemical and electrophysiological experiments described here is standard, and has been described in detail in other publications from our laboratory (10-18).

RESULTS

Electrical Activity in Neuron R15

Aplysia neuron R15 is an endogenous oscillator. It exhibits a pattern of activity consisting of "bursts" of action potentials, interrupted by interburst hyperpolarizations (Fig. 1A). This endogenous pattern can be altered by application of 5HT to the medium bathing the *Aplysia* abdominal ganglion (in which R15 is located). At low concentrations of 5HT there is am increase in the depth and duration of the interburst hyper-

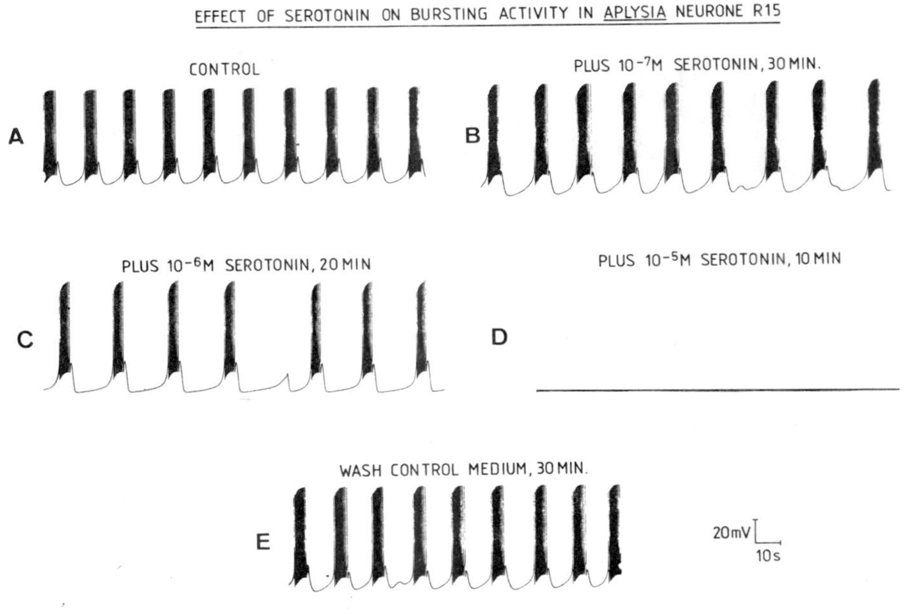

Fig. 1. Effects of bath application of different concentrations of 5HT on electrical activity in neuron R15. From ref. 14.

polarization phase (Fig. 1B). The effect is enhanced as the concentration of 5HT is raised (Fig. 1C), until eventually bursting is completely abolished and the membrane potential remains stable very close to the K^+ equilibrium potential (about -75 mV, Fig. 1D). The activity pattern returns to normal when the ganglion is washed with normal medium (Fig. 1E). The results shown in Fig. 1 are typical of over 30 separate experiments. Threshold effects of 5HT are usually seen at concentrations between 10^{-8}M and 10^{-7}M, and bursting is usually inhibited in the presence of 10^{-6}M to 10^{-5}M 5HT. At higher 5HT concentrations the net effect is often excitatory rather than inhibitory, apparently because 5HT can have several effects at high concentrations (see below).

Very similar effects on R15 bursting activity can be elicited by bath application of 8-parachlorophenylthio cyclic AMP, a cyclic AMP analog which is not susceptible to hydrolysis by phosphodiesterase. As shown in Fig. 2, increasing concentrations of this analog cause a progressive enhancement of the

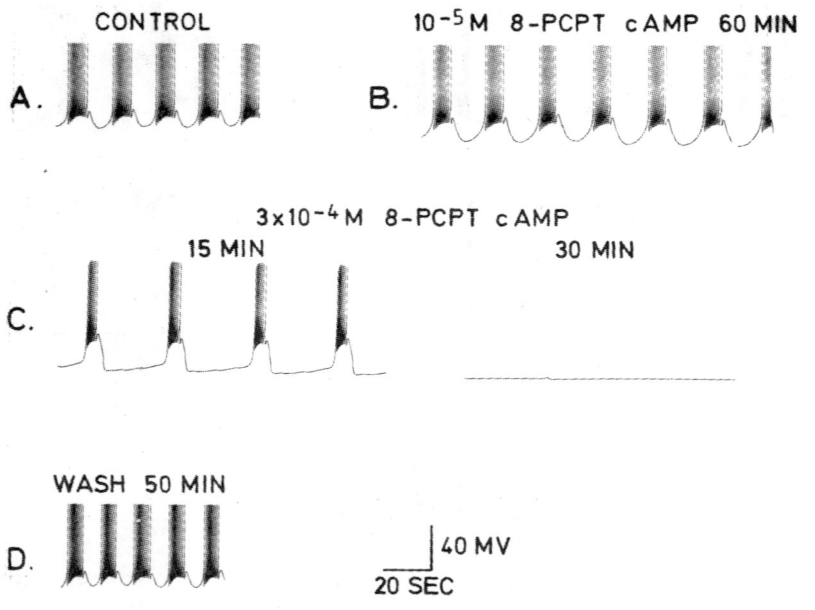

Fig. 2. Effects of bath application of different concentrations of 8-parachlorophenylthio cyclic AMP (8-PCPT cAMP) on electrical activity in neuron R15. From ref. 18.

interburst hyperpolarization, eventually with complete inhibition of bursting (Fig. 2C). The result is the same when the cyclic AMP analog is injected directly into R15 (ref. 16), indicating that its site of action is in this neuron and not on some pre-synaptic or non-neuronal element.

The mechanism of these effects of 5HT and cyclic AMP analogs has been investigated using voltage clamp techniques. Steady state current-voltage (I-V) curves of neuron R15 are shown in Fig. 3. Note that there is a characteristic region of negative slope between about -70 and -30 mV, which is thought to contribute to bursting behavior (19). In the presence of 5HT (Fig. 3A) or 8-benzylthio cyclic AMP (Fig. 3B - the effects of this analog are identical to those of 8-parachlorophenylthio cyclic AMP), the slope of the I-V curve at voltages more negative than -70 mV is increased, and the new curve intersects the control between -75 and -80 mV. This "reversal potential" for the response is close to the K^+ equilibrium potential (-75 mV, ref. 20), suggesting that the activation of a K^+ conductance may be responsible for the hyperpolarization seen in unclamped cells.

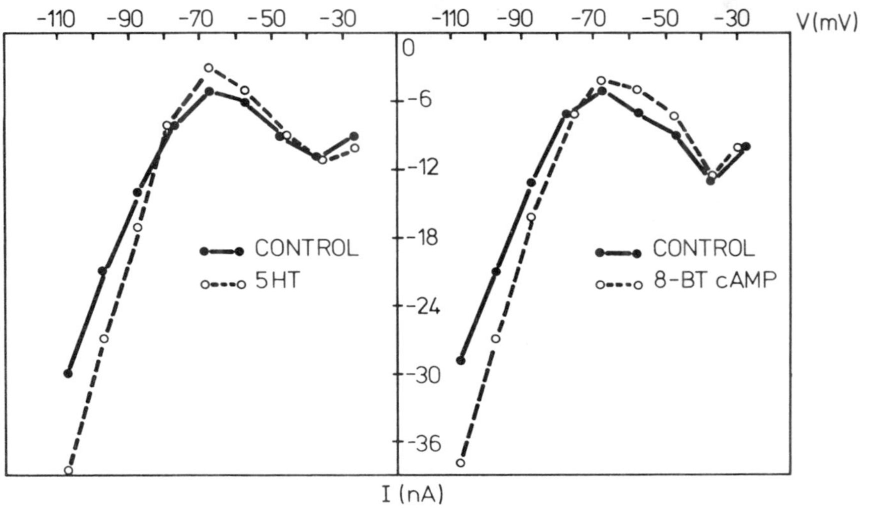

Fig. 3. Effects of 1 μM 5HT (left) or 0.3 mM 8-benzylthio cyclic AMP (8BT cAMP, right) on the current-voltage relationship in neuron R15. Modified from ref. 14.

This suggestion is confirmed by experiments in which the K^+ concentration in the bathing medium is changed, and the resulting I-V curves examined (14). Under these conditions the reversal potentials for the effects of 5HT and cyclic AMP analogs change as predicted by the Nernst equation for a K^+ conductance channel (14). In most experiments there is also an enhancement of the negative slope region of the I-V curve in the presence of 5HT or cyclic AMP analog (Fig. 3). This latter effect becomes more pronounced as the concentration of 5HT is increased, and it probably is responsible for the increased bursting seen in some unclamped cells at high 5HT concentrations. It may be due to an increase in a voltage-dependent Na^+ or Ca^{++} conductance, but its mechanism has not yet been investigated in detail. Treistman and Drake (21) have obtained similar voltage clamp data following intracellular injection of cyclic AMP analogs.

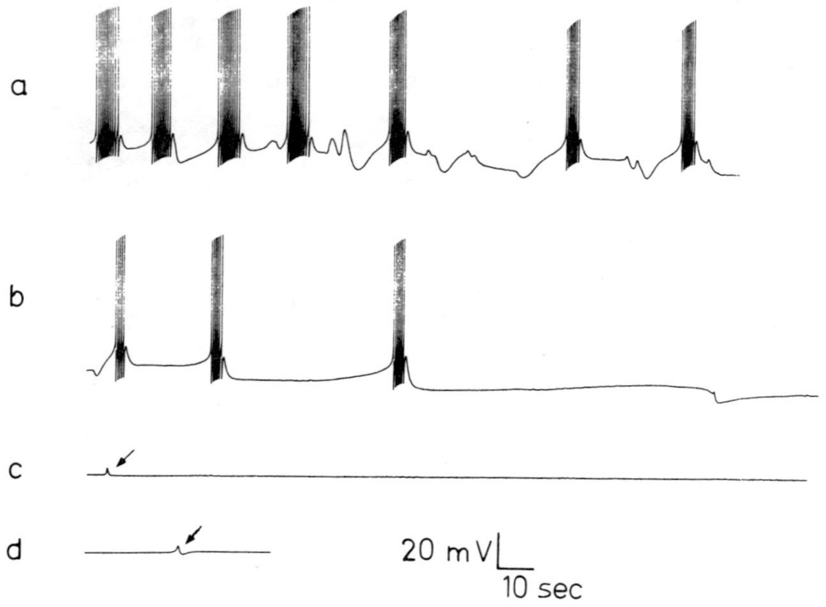

Fig. 4. Effects of intracellular injection of Gpp(NH)p on electrical activity in neuron R15. a) Normal pattern immediately before injection; b) 1-2 min; c) 2 hrs; d) 3.5 hrs after injection. From ref. 17.

Cyclic AMP levels can also be increased in R15 by intracellular injection of guanylylimidodiphosphate (Gpp(NH)p), a GTP derivative which activates adenylate cyclase in R15 (ref. 17) and in many other systems. Injection of Gpp(NH)p leads to abolition of bursting in R15 (Fig. 4); the membrane potential once again approaches the K^+ equilibrium potential. Treistman and Drake (21) have carried out a voltage clamp analysis of this response, and have found that Gpp(NH)p causes an apparent increase in K^+ conductance together with a change in the negative slope region of the I-V curve, very similar to that produced by 5HT or cyclic AMP analogs.

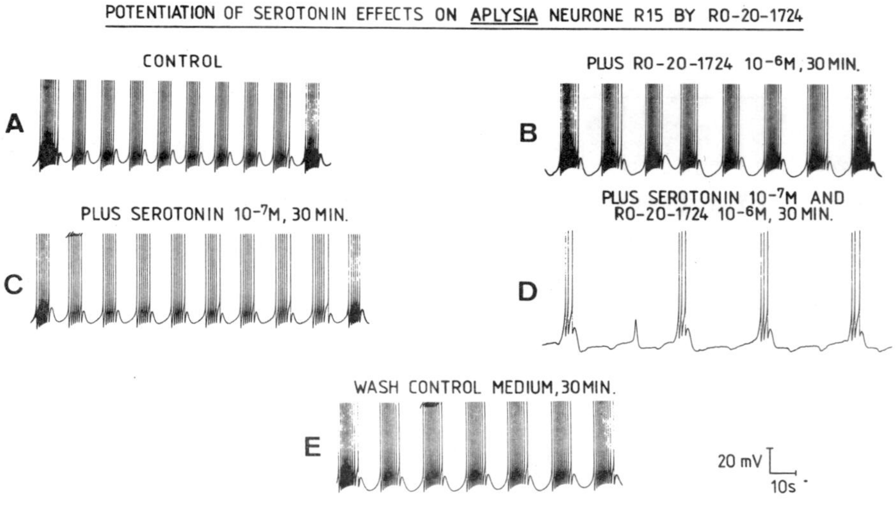

Fig. 5. Enhancement of the effects of low concentrations of 5HT on electrical activity in R15 by the phosphodiesterase inhibitor Ro 20-1724. Modified from ref. 14.

The effects of low concentrations of 5HT can be markedly enhanced by inhibition of phosphodiesterase, the enzyme responsible for hydrolysing cyclic AMP. As shown in Fig. 5, low concentrations of either 5HT or the phosphodiesterase inhibitor Ro 20-1724, added separately to the bath, have little or no effect on the activity of R15 in this experiment. However, when the two are added together, bursting is almost completely abolished (Fig. 5).

Serotonin Receptors and Cyclic AMP

When *Aplysia* ganglia are incubated together with 5HT, cyclic AMP accumulates in the whole ganglion (22), as well as in identified neuronal cell bodies isolated following the incubation (Table 1).

Table 1. 5HT causes cyclic AMP to accumulate in identified *Aplysia* neuronal cell bodies.

Cell	cyclic AMP (fmoles/cell)	
	Control	10^{-5}M 5HT
Left pleural giant neuron	230 ± 31	530 ± 93
R2	342 ± 60	615 ± 77
R15	29 ± 7	86 ± 21

Similar findings have been reported by Cedar and Schwartz (23). 5HT can also stimulate adenylate cyclase activity in membrane fractions prepared either from whole ganglion (Fig. 6) or

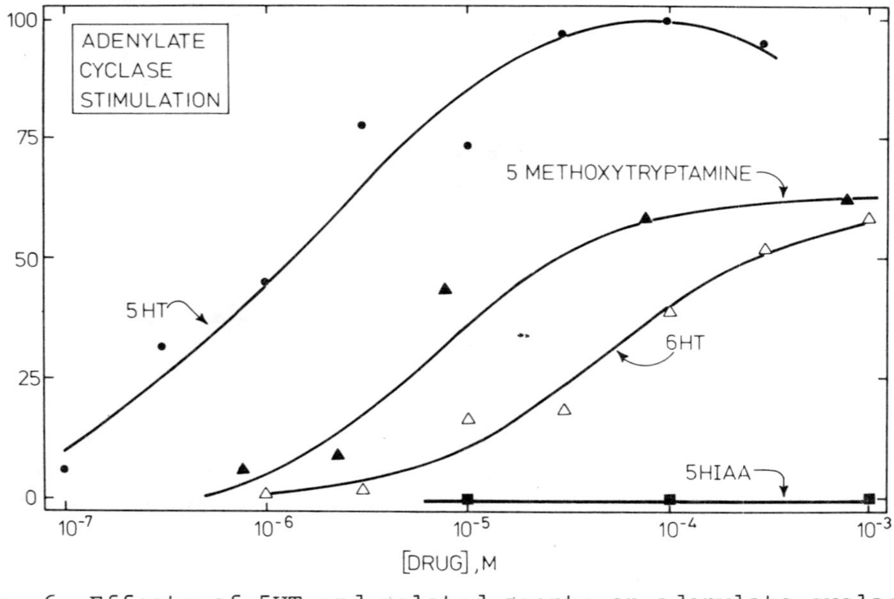

Fig. 6. Effects of 5HT and related agents on adenylate cyclase activity in a crude membrane preparation. The ordinate is the per cent stimulation of enzyme activity relative to the maximum stimulation by 5HT, which is arbitrarily set to 100%.From ref.12.

from isolated identified neuronal cell bodies (Table 2). The stimulation by 5HT ranges from 30 to 200%, and is observed at concentrations (Fig. 6) similar to those which alter bursting activity in R15 (Fig. 1).

Table 2. 5HT stimulates adenylate cyclase activity in membranes prepared from isolated identified *Aplysia* neuronal cell bodies. Modified from ref. 13.

Source of membranes	% Stimulation by 10^{-5}M 5HT
Left pleural giant neuron	57
R2	42
R15	33

Pharmacological Analysis of Serotonin Receptors

Aplysia 5HT receptors can be measured by binding of the radioactive ligand [^{3}H]LSD (10-12). Although [^{3}H]LSD also labels dopamine receptors, we have developed conditions which allow each of the receptors to be studied individually using this single ligand, and have defined the pharmacological profile of these receptors in considerable detail (10,12). In addition, we have examined the drug-sensitivity of the 5HT-sensitive adenylate cyclase; some examples of the effects of 5HT-related compounds on this enzyme activity are illustrated in Fig. 6. 5-Methoxytryptamine and 6HT are partial agonists in the adenylate cyclase system; that is they stimulate the activity of the enzyme, but the maximal response is lower than elicited by 5HT. Furthermore, 5HT is more potent (active at lower concentrations) than either of these partial agonists. 5-Hydroxyindoleacetic acid (5HIAA) is without detectable effect on adenylate cyclase activity (Fig. 6).

The effects of a wide range of drugs on [^{3}H]LSD binding to 5HT receptors, and on 5HT-sensitive adenylate cyclase activity, are summarized in Table 3. Note that the concentrations of drugs required for half-maximal inhibition of [^{3}H]LSD binding

Table 3. Pharmacological analysis of 5HT-sensitive [^{3}H]LSD binding, and 5HT-sensitive adenylate cyclase.
The concentrations of drugs required for half-maximal effects (EC_{50} or K_i values) in each assay are shown. Data taken from Tables II and IV in ref. 12.

Agent tested	EC_{50} or K_i value (μM)	
	[^{3}H]LSD binding	Adenylate cyclase
5HT and dopamine-like agents		
5HT	1.30	1.65
N-methyl-5HT	1.50	1.55
Bufotenine	2.10	1.25
Tryptamine	13	18
5-methoxytryptamine	2	6.2
6HT	75	26
5HIAA	--- a	--- a
Dopamine	>100	>100
Apomorphine	77	12
Ergot alkaloids and derivatives		
d-LSD	0.0012	0.010
l-LSD	12	>10
Ergotamine	0.002	0.047
Dihydroergocryptine	0.020	0.097
Neuroleptic drugs		
d-butaclamol	0.014	0.021
l-butaclamol	12	13
cis-flupenthixol	0.24	0.10
trans-flupenthixol	13	14
cis-chlorprothixene	0.13	0.11
trans-chlorprothixene	0.36	0.31
Spiroperidol	6.2	3.8
Pipamperone	17	9.5

[a] Too weakly active to measure accurately (EC_{50} or K_i > 300 μM).

correspond very closely to those required for half-maximal effects on adenylate cyclase (correlation coefficient r = 0.94 as calculated by regression analysis - see ref. 12). Furthermore, certain drugs exhibit a stereospecific interaction with 5HT receptors as measured in both assays; in particular, the d-isomers of LSD and butaclamol are several orders of magnitude more potent than the corresponding l-isomers (Table 3).

A similar pharmacological analysis has been carried out on the 5HT-induced hyperpolarization of neuron R15. This analysis has necessarily been more limited because of the difficulties involved in doing these experiments; nevertheless, the results fall into a consistent pattern, summarized in Table 4.

Table 4. Pharmacological analysis of 5HT-induced hyperpolarization of neuron R15; comparison with 5HT-sensitive adenylate cyclase. Modified from ref. 14.

Agent tested	Hyperpolarization in R15	Adenylate cyclase assay
	Threshold conc. (μM)	EC_{50} or K_i (μM)
Agonists		
5HT	0.02 - 0.10	1.65
N-methyl 5HT	0.05 - 0.10	1.55
Bufotenine	0.05 - 0.10	1.25
6HT	1 - 3	26
Tryptamine	0.50 - 2.00	18
5-methoxytryptamine	0.10 - 0.30	6.2
d-LSD	0.50 - 10	0.010
l-LSD	> 50	>10
Antagonists (measured in presence of 1 μM 5HT)		
d-butaclamol	2 - 10	0.021
l-butaclamol	>100	13

Compounds such as 5HT, N-methyl 5HT and bufotenine, which are full agonists in the adenylate cyclase assay, are agonists in producing hyperpolarization in R15. Tryptamine, 5-methoxytryptamine and 6HT are also agonists in both assays; the hyperpolarizing response cannot be quantitated sufficiently to determine whether they are full agonists, or partial agonists as they are on the cyclase. Furthermore, d-LSD (as an agonist or partial agonist) and d-butaclamol (as an antagonist) act stereospecifically in both assays. Finally, 5HIAA affects neither R15 electrical activity nor adenylate cyclase. Note also that, with the exception of d-butaclamol and d-LSD, the concentrations of these compounds required to produce their effects are similar in both assays (Table 4). These results make it likely that the same 5HT receptor mediates both cyclic AMP accumulation and hyperpolarization in R15. It is not clear why such high concentrations of d-LSD and d-butaclamol are required to affect electrical activity in R15; even at high concentrations, the effects of these drugs are often apparent only after 1-2 hours of bath application, and it is possible that the connective tissue sheath surrounding the abdominal ganglion acts as a selective diffusion barrier.

DISCUSSION

There have been suggestions that amine neurotransmitters, including 5HT, may act through cyclic AMP. It seems clear that at least some 5HT receptors are coupled to adenylate cyclase, since 5HT-sensitive adenylate cyclases have been described in vertebrate (24,25) and invertebrate (26) nervous systems. However, it is not clear what (if any) physiological responses are mediated by these 5HT receptors, and thus it has not been possible in these systems to assay whether cyclic AMP plays a physiological role.

Sutherland and his colleagues (27) suggested a number of criteria which must be satisfied before one may conclude that cyclic AMP mediates a physiological response, and Greengard (28) has modified these for application to neurotransmitter-evoked responses. Recent reports from several laboratories (4-9) have described 5HT-induced physiological changes in *Aplysia* nervous system and muscle which satisfy one or more of these criteria. All of the criteria have been fulfilled for the 5HT-induced hyperpolarization of neuron R15 described here: (1) the physiological response is mimicked by intracellular injection of cyclic AMP, or by activation of adenylate cyclase within R15; (2) the effects of 5HT are enhanced in the presence of a phosphodiesterase inhibitor; (3) 5HT causes cyclic AMP to accumulate in R15; (4) 5HT stimulates adenylate cyclase activity in membranes from R15 cell bodies; and (5) the 5HT receptor mediating adenylate cyclase stimulation is pharmacologically similar to that producing hyperpolarization. This is the first time that all the Sutherland-Greengard criteria have been satisfied in a neuronal system. Accordingly, we conclude that the 5HT-induced hyperpolarization of neuron R15, resulting from activation of a K^+ conductance, is mediated by cyclic AMP. Whether cyclic AMP acts by directly stimulating phosphorylation of some protein component of a K^+ channel, or whether its effect is indirect, for example by allowing entry of Ca^{++} which in turn activates a K^+ conductance (29), remains to be determined.

REFERENCES

1. Gerschenfeld, H., Science 171 (1971) 1252-1254.
2. Gerschenfeld, H. and Paupardin-Tritsch, D., J. Physiol. (Lond.) 243 (1974) 427-456.
3. Gerschenfeld, H. and Paupardin-Tritsch, D., J. Physiol. (Lond.) 243 (1974) 457-481.
4. Kaczmarek, L., Jennings, K. and Strumwasser, F., Proc. Natl. Acad. Sci. (USA) 75 (1978) 5200-5204.
5. Mandelbaum, D., Koester, J., Schonberg, M. and Weiss, K., Brain Res. 177 (1979) 388-394.
6. Kupfermann, I., Ann. Rev. Neurosci. 2 (1979) 447-465.
7. Weiss, K., Schonberg, M., Mandelbaum, D. and Kupfermann, I. Nature 272 (1978) 727-728.
8. Shimahara, T. and Tauc, L., Brain Res. 127 (1977) 168-172.
9. Klein, M. and Kandel, E., Proc. Natl. Acad. Sci. (USA) 75 (1978) 3512-3516.
10. Drummond, A., Bucher, F. and Levitan, I., Nature 272 (1978) 368-370.
11. Drummond, A., Bucher, F. and Levitan, I., Brain Res. 184 (1980) 163-177.
12. Drummond, A., Bucher, F. and Levitan, I., J. Biol. Chem. (1980) in press.
13. Levitan, I., Brain Res. 154 (1978) 404-408.
14. Drummond, A., Benson, J. and Levitan, I., in preparation.
15. Levitan, I., Bergström, E. and Simonet, M., J. Neurochem. 31 (1978) 1353-1359.
16. Treistman, S. and Levitan, I., Nature 261 (1976) 62-64.
17. Treistman, S. and Levitan, I. Proc. Natl. Acad. Sci.(USA) 73 (1976) 4689-4692.

18. Levitan, I. and Norman, J., Brain Res. 189 (1980) in press.

19. Barker, J. and Smith, T., in Abnormal Neuronal Discharges, edited by N. Chalazonitis and M. Boisson, Raven Press, New York (1978).

20. Kunze, D., Walker, J. and Brown, H., Fed. Proc. 30 (1971) 255.

21. Treistman, S. and Drake, P., in preparation.

22. Levitan, I., Madsen, C. and Barondes, S., J. Neurobiol., 5 (1974) 511-525.

23. Cedar, H. and Schwartz, J., J. Gen. Physiol. 60 (1972) 570-587.

24. von Hungen, K., Roberts, S. and Hill, D., Brain Res. 84 (1975) 257-267.

25. Enjalbert, A., Hamon, M., Bourgoin, S. and Bockaert, J., Mol. Pharmacol. 14 (1978) 11-23.

26. Nathanson, J. and Greengard, P., Proc. Natl. Acad. Sci. (USA) 71 (1974) 797-801.

27. Robison, A., Butcher, R. and Sutherland, E., Cyclic AMP, Academic Press, New York (1971).

28. Greengard, P., Nature 260 (1976) 101-108.

29. Heyer, C. and Lux, H.D., J. Physiol. (Lond.) 262 (1976) 349-382.

Neurotransmitters and their Receptors
Edited by U.Z. Littauer, Y. Dudai, I. Silman,
V.I. Teichberg and Z. Vogel

Pharmacology of Histamine Receptors in Mammalian Brain

J.C. Schwartz, G. Barbin, E.M. Duchemin, M. Garbarg, T.T. Quach, E. Rodergas and C. Rose
Unité 109 de Neurobiologie, Centre Paul Broca de l'I.N.S.E.R.M., 2ter, Rue d'Alésia, 75014 Paris, France

ABSTRACT

Cerebral H_1-receptors selectively mediate the histamine-induced glycogenolysis, a calcium-dependent process. H_1-receptors can be studied in the living animal with ^{3}H-mepyramine as ligand and their blockade seems to account for the sedative properties of a variety of psychotropic drugs.

In addition high-affinity binding sites for ^{3}H-histamine can be evidenced on cerebral membranes which could represent a class of postsynaptic receptors distinct from H_1- or H_2-receptors.

A variety of experimental approaches have, during the last years, fortified the conviction that histamine (HA) has to be considered as a neurotransmitter in mammalian brain (for recent reviews see 1, 2, 3). Thus this amine is synthesized at high rate, is held in discrete neuronal tracts evidenced by lesion studies, can be released upon depolarisation, affects the activity of target neurons and is efficiently inactivated by transmethylation and oxidative deamination. In addition another fraction of the amine seems to be held in mast-cells or closely related cells and might be involved in vascular control or immune responses.

In both cases, the messenger role of HA implies that it is recognized by specific receptors mediating its actions on target-cells. As for other putative neurotransmitters the conditions required to characterize these receptors i.e. selective pharmacological tools (agonists and antagonists) and suitable biological models have been recently met. They have allowed to demonstrate that HA receptors are indeed present in cerebral tissues, that they belong to various pharmacological classes and that they might represent targets for various types of psychoactive drugs.

AGENTS		ACTIVITY ON BIOLOGICAL SYSTEMS: Ileum contraction (H_1-receptors)	Atrium rate (H_2-receptors)
① **AGONISTS**		**Relative Agonist Potency**	
Histamine	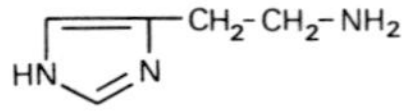	100	100
2 - Methylhistamine	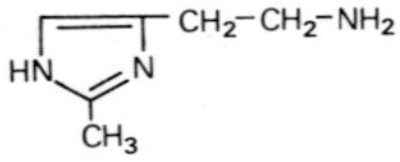	17	5
2 - Thiazolyl-ethlylamine	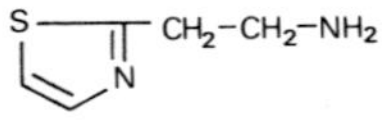	26	0.3
4 - Methylhistamine	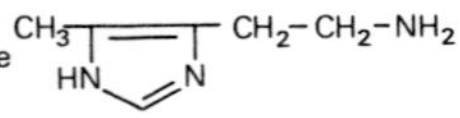	0.2	43
Dimaprit	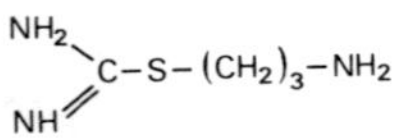	0.0001	70
Impromidine	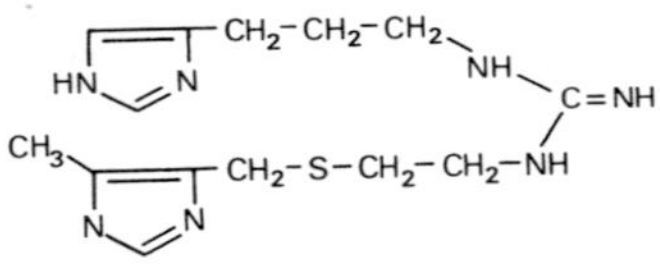	< 0.001	4,800
② **ANTAGONISTS**		**Antagonist activity (KB,M)**	
Mepyramine	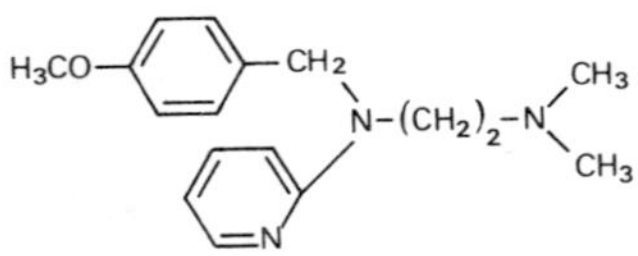	0.5×10^{-9}	—
Burimamide	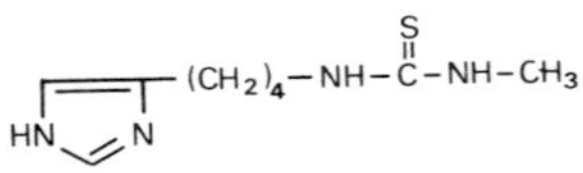	3×10^{-3}	7.8×10^{-6}
Metiamide	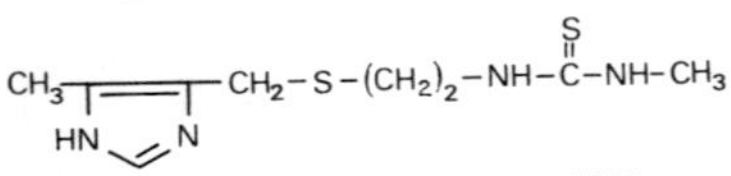	$>10^{-3}$	0.9×10^{-6}
Cimetidine	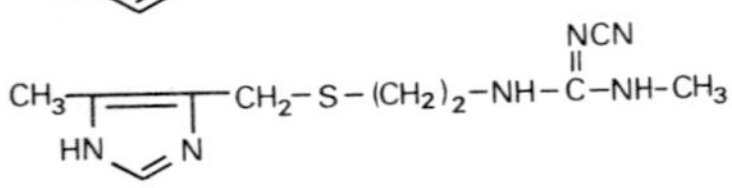	45×10^{-3}	0.8×10^{-6}

Fig. 1

ACTIVITY OF HISTAMINE AGONISTS AND ANTAGONISTS ON REFERENCE BIOLOGICAL SYSTEMS

I. PHARMACOLOGICAL TOOLS FOR THE CHARACTERIZATION OF HISTAMINE RECEPTORS

Starting from the forties, a large number of "classical antihistamines" (now termed H_1-antihistamines) have been synthetized. These agents, the prototype of which is mepyramine (Table 1) antagonise competitively and generally with high potency some typical actions of histamine: for instance the apparent dissociation constant (K_B) of mepyramine is around 10^{-9}M regarding blockade of HA-induced contractions of guinea-pig ileum.

However these agents are generally unable to antagonise several actions of HA (stimulation of gastric acid secretion, increase in heart rate) and the notion that the latters were mediated by distinct receptors has emerged. The existence of two separate populations of HA receptors termed H_1 and H_2 respectively has been largely confirmed by the availability of pharmacological agents able to mimic or conversely to block in a selective manner these various actions : in Table 1 are depicted the structure of these agents and their selectivity is shown by comparison of their relative agonist potencies (agonists) or apparent dissociation constants (antagonists) on typical biological systems.

From a practical point of view it must be stressed that whereas potent and highly selective H_2-receptor agonists like dimaprit and impromidine are available, this is not yet the case for H_1-receptor agonists. In addition the H_2-receptor antagonists available are still characterized by a rather low affinity and an inability to cross easily the blood-brain barrier : these features limit their experimental usefulness and render more likely the occurence of non-specific effects.

II. H_1-RECEPTORS AND GLYCOGENOLYSIS

There are few experimental models to study H_1-receptors in brain. Indeed their participation in the HA-induced accumulation of cyclic AMP has been clearly shown in slices from guinea-pig brain (4, 5, 6). But this model is a rather complex one because, in contrast to H_2-receptors, which appear to be directly associated withthecatalytic site of the enzyme adenylate cyclase, (7) H_1-receptors mediate indirect effects of HA on the synthesis of the nucleotide (6). The latter effects can only be evidenced when H_2-receptors linked with the cyclase are stimulated and they probably involve translocation of calcium ions.

Also, it has been recently shown that H_1-receptors mediate the HA-induced stimulation of cyclic GMP formation in a clone of neuroblastoma cells (8) as well as in bovine sympathetic ganglion (9) but clear evidence for a similar effect on the levels of this nucleotide in mammalian brain is still lacking.

We have recently devised a simple technique to evaluate the glycogenolytic action of various agents on brain tissues (10). When brain slices are incubated in the presence of ^{3}H-glucose, the ^{3}H-glycogen levels in tissues can be conveniently determined by counting the ethanol-insoluble radioactivity on pieces of filter paper. In addition to noradrenaline, whose glycogenolytic action mediated by β-receptors is well established, we have recently observed

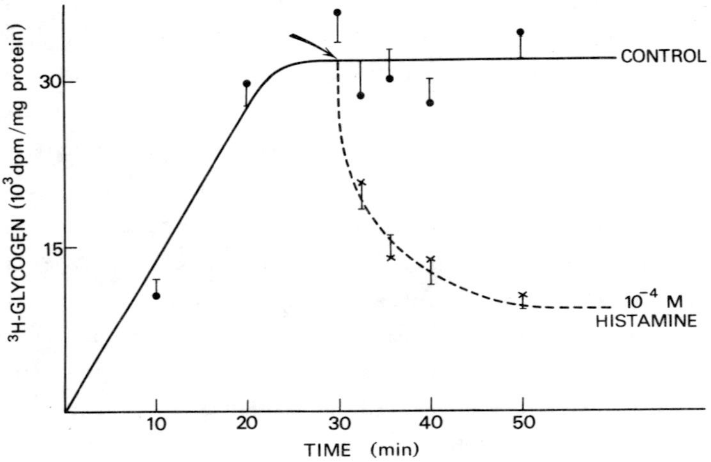

Fig. 2

TIME-COURSE OF ^{3}H-GLYCOGEN SYNTHESIS AND HA-INDUCED HYDROLYSIS IN SLICES FROM MOUSE CORTEX

Slices incubated in the presence of ^{3}H-glucose (33μCi.ml^{-1}). Addition of 100μM HA (arrow) at a time when a steady state level of ^{3}H-glycogen was reached, resulted in a rapid fall of the level of the ^{3}H-polymer. ^{3}H-glycogen was isolated by ethanol precipitation, using a filter paper technique (10).

that HA promotes in a few minutes the hydrolysis of approximately 70-80% of the ^{3}H-glycogen content of slices from mouse cortex (Fig. 2). This response to HA is concentration-dependent and occurs with an EC_{50} of 3μM, i.e. in the same range as the stimulation of cAMP accumulation in slices from guinea-pig brain. The potent glycogenolytic action of HA is mimicked by H_1-agonists like 2-thiazolylethylamine but dimaprit, a pure H_2-agonist, is totally ineffective. Whereas adrenergic, serotoninergic and H_2-receptor antagonists do not block the HA-induced glycogenolysis, H_1-antihistamines prevent, in a competitive manner, the breakdown of the polysaccharide. That typical H_1-receptors are selectively involved is confirmed by the estimation of the relative potencies of agonists and the apparent dissociation constants of various antihistamines, both sets of values being entirely consistent with interaction of HA with a pure population of H_1-receptors (Table 1). The recent development of a H_1-receptor radioassay using ^{3}H-mepyramine as a ligand (11,12) allows comparison of parameters of binding and of glycogenolytic responses. Thus the Kd value of ^{3}H-mepyramine binding in membranes from mouse cortex (3nM) is close to its apparent K_B evaluated from the parallel shift of the concentration-response curve to HA regarding ^{3}H-glycogen hydrolysis in slices from the same brain region, an observation which further supports the idea that identical sites are involved in the recognition of ^{3}H-mepyramine and in HA-induced glycogenolysis. However it appears that HA is significantly less potent in inhibiting ^{3}H-mepyramine binding (K_i = 45μM) than in initiating the glycogenolytic response (EC_{50} = 3μM), suggesting the existence of "spare receptors". This explanation is consistent with the high sensitivity of the glycogenolytic system to the action of various effectors : for instance the glycogenolytic action of noradrenaline occurs for much lower concentrations than those required to maximally stimulate cAMP accumulation in the same preparation (10).

TABLE I

EFFECTS OF HISTAMINE AGONISTS AND ANTAGONISTS ON ^{3}H-GLYCOGEN HYDROLYSIS IN CORTICAL SLICES

1. Agonists	"Relative potencies"
Histamine	100
Dimaprit	0.0001
4-Methylhistamine	1
2-Methylhistamine	12
2-Thiazolylethylamine	30
2. Antagonists	**K_i values (nM)**
Mepyramine	4.7
(+) Chlorpheniramine	2.0
Promethazine	5.0
Triprolidine	5.6

Slices were pre-incubated for 30 min. in the presence of ^{3}H-glucose, then incubated for 20 min. in the presence of histamine or histamine agonists in increasing concentrations. "Relative potencies" were calculated according to the equation

$$RP = \frac{EC_{50}\ \text{histamine}}{EC_{50}\ \text{agonist}} \times 100$$

To determine inhibition constants of different H_1-antagonists, histamine (50μM) alone or in the presence of these compounds in increasing concentrations were added simultaneously in the incubation tube. K_i values were calculated using the equation

$$K_i = \frac{IC_{50}}{1 + \frac{S}{K_a}}$$

That the process of "tachyphylaxis" or desensitisation i.e. decreased responsiveness upon prolonged exposures of tissues to agonists concerns biological responses to HA mediated by H_1-receptors is known for a long time : it was described on the contractions of guinea-pig ileum by Barsoum and Gaddum (13). More recently Richelson (14) showed desensitisation to occur regarding the stimulation of cGMP formation in neuroblastoma cells.

As shown in Fig. 3 desensitisation can also be observed on the glycogenolytic response to HA : the concentration-response curve is, in this case, shifted to the right without modification of the maximal response. The effect is specific for HA (or H_1-receptor agonists) and is reversible. The mechanism underlying this change is not yet entirely clear but seems to involve, at least in part, changes occuring at the receptor level since glycogenolytic responses to other agents are not modified and, furthermore, it is accompanied by a limited but significant decrease in the number of H_1-receptors as evaluated by ^{3}H-mepyramine binding (Quach et al., in preparation).

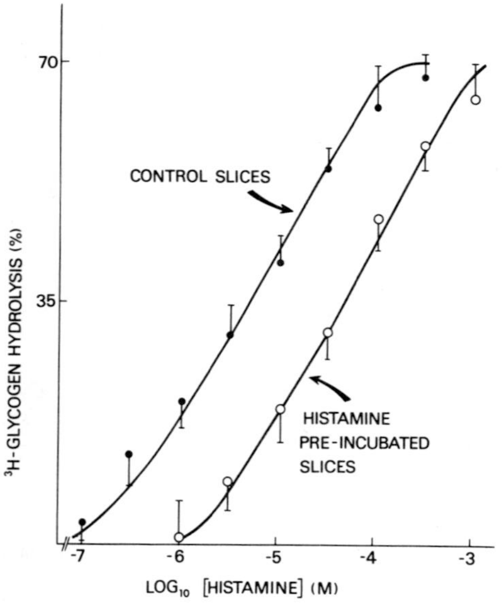

Fig. 3

THE EFFECT OF HA-PREINCUBATION ON HA-INDUCED HYDROLYSIS OF ^{3}H-GLYCOGEN IN SLICES FROM MOUSE CORTEX

Slices were preincubated without HA (controls) or with 50μM HA for 20 min., washed three times. Then ^{3}H-glycogen hydrolysis induced by HA at indicated concentrations, was determined. Results are expressed as percentage of basal level : 20.2 $\pm$ 1.0 dpm.10^3.mg protein^{-1} for controls and 20.9 $\pm$ 1.0 dpm.10^3. mg protein^{-1} for HA-preincubated slices.

III. CEREBRAL H_1-RECEPTOR OCCUPATION *IN VIVO* AND SEDATIVE PROPERTIES OF PSYCHOTROPIC DRUGS

In addition to classical *in vitro* binding studies which reveal many features of the recognition site of neurotransmitter receptors, *in vivo* studies of these receptors using ^{3}H-ligands administered systemically to the living animal provide complementary and often useful data (15, 16, 17, 18, 19).

Since ^{3}H-mepyramine has been recently proposed as a selective ligand of H_1-receptors from peripheral (20) as well as cerebral tissues (11, 12), we have explored the possible use of this ^{3}H-ligand in the living mouse.

Three criteria must be met to consider that the *in vivo* localisation of a given ligand selectively reflects the interaction with a class of receptors : i) the process should have a saturable character ii) the distribution of the ligand between brain regions should parallel that of the receptors as established by *in vitro* binding or other studies iii) the process should exhibit the pharmacological specificity expected for this class of receptors.

Following systemic administration of ligands like ^{3}H-pimozide (17) or ^{3}H-LSD (19) in low dosage the evaluation of the total radioactivity accumulated in brain regions allows the estimation of binding to dopamine and serotonin receptors, respectively. However, in the case of intravenously administered ^{3}H-mepyramine the criteria were not met, suggesting that receptor binding was obscured by non-selective distribution of the ligand. In contrast, when this non-specific component was eliminated by preparing cerebral homogenates from which the particulate fraction was isolated and rapidly washed on a filter, the retention of ^{3}H-mepyramine appeared to reflect binding to H_1-receptors.

Three minutes following i.v. administration, the *in vivo* binding of ^{3}H-mepyramine is maximal and represents approximately 10% of total ^{3}H-mepyramine level in tissue. It exhibits a regional heterogeneity paralleling ($r = 0.95$) that observed in *in vitro* binding studies (Table II).

The saturable character of ^{3}H-mepyramine binding *in vivo* is clearly shown in the cortex and data (Fig. 4) allow the estimation of binding parameters : Hill plot analysis leads to a n_H value non-significantly different from unity, presumably reflecting a non-cooperative interaction of the ^{3}H-ligand with the binding sites *in vivo* ; the ED_{50}, i.e. the mepyramine dosage ensuring, 3 min. after its administration, a half maximal occupation of binding sites in mouse cortex is extremely low (20μg.kg^{-1}) but this value cannot be directly compared with the Kd of ^{3}H-mepyramine for H_1-receptor binding *in vitro* (2.8nM) (21) ; finally the capacity of ^{3}H-mepyramine binding sites in

TABLE II

REGIONAL DISTRIBUTION OF IN VIVO AND IN VITRO ^{3}H-MEPYRAMINE BINDING IN MOUSE BRAIN

REGIONS	^{3}H-MEPYRAMINE BINDING	
	IN VIVO (pCi.mg protein^{-1})	IN VITRO (fmoles.mg protein^{-1})
Hypothalamus	52 ± 2	109 ± 6
Midbrain	45 ± 2	90 ± 12
Cortex	45 ± 1	75 ± 12
Brainstem	40 ± 3	70 ± 10
Cerebellum	32 ± 2	44 ± 8
Striatum	29 ± 1	49 ± 8
Hippocampus	25 ± 1	47 ± 5

For *in vivo* binding, mice were injected with 1μCi ^{3}H-mepyramine in the tail vein and were killed 3 min. later. Various brain areas were dissected out, homogenized in 0.05M phosphate buffer pH 7,5 and 1ml of the homogenate immediately filtered under vacuum. Filters were rinsed with 2 x 20ml cold buffer and radioactivity counted. Non-specific binding, i.e. ^{3}H-mepyramine remaining bound when 1mg.kg^{-1} mepyramine was simultaneously injected, represents less than 5% of the total. Values are the mean ± S.E.M. of 8 determinations.

In vitro binding of ^{3}H-mepyramine was measured on a particulate fraction obtained by homogenization of various brain areas into 30 volumes of phosphate buffer followed by two successive centrifugations (1850g.min. and 200,000g.min respectively). Membrane fractions were incubated for 30 minutes at 30°C in the presence of 5nM ^{3}H-mepyramine. Non-specific binding was evaluated in the presence of 2μM triprolidine. Values are the mean ± S.E.M. of 5-10 determinations.

mouse cortex is 57fmoles.mg protein^{-1}. Comparison of the latter value with the capacity of ^{3}H-mepyramine binding sites in a P_2 pellet from the same brain region (Bmax = 113fmoles.mg protein^{-1}) indicates a reasonably good agreement, if one considers the relative enrichment of this P_2 fraction which does not contain soluble proteins. Preliminary studies had shown that the binding evaluated under such conditions does not result from *in vitro* binding of the ^{3}H-ligand which might have occured artefactually following homogenization. Thus the level of ^{3}H-mepyramine bound was not significantly modified when brain tissue from mice injected with the ^{3}H-ligand 3 min. before sacrifice was homogenized together with brain tissue from animals injected with unlabeled mepyramine (200μg.kg^{-1}). These data indicate that the binding observed under our experimental conditions had occured *in vivo*. The pharmacological specificity of ^{3}H-mepyramine binding *in vivo* is shown by the large differences in inhibitory potency of agents : whereas most H_1-antihistamines are potent

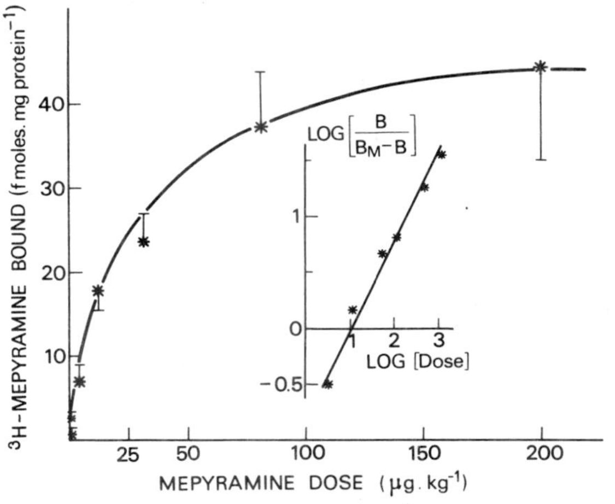

Fig. 4

IN VIVO ^{3}H-MEPYRAMINE BINDING IN THE CORTEX OF MICE AS A FUNCTION OF DOSAGE

Groups of 4 mice received 1µCi of ^{3}H-mepyramine i.v. together with non-radioactive mepyramine in increasing dosage. The non-saturable binding which was substracted represented approximatively 50% of the total at the highest dosage. Results expressed in fmoles.mg protein^{-1}, based on the specific activity of injected material. Hill plot of the same data (inset) gives a straight line with a slope not different from unity (nH = 0.96).

inhibitors, a variety of compounds devoid of H_1-receptor antagonist properties are ineffective (Table III). In addition, the much lower inhibitory potency of the levo-isomer of chlorpheniramine as compared to the dextro-isomer, the latter being also approximatively 200-fold more potent as a H_1-antihistamine (11) indicates that the *in vivo* binding is stereospecific. Finally, the lack of effect of scopolamine and atropine rules out a participation of muscarinic receptors, for which H_1-antihistamines have often affinity and reinforces the conviction that ^{3}H-mepyramine binding sites *in vivo* are, indeed, the H_1-receptors.

The important feature in our finding is that the ID_{50} of most H_1-antihistamine i.e. the dose resulting in the occupation of 50% of cerebral H_1-receptors, 1h after administration, is in the same range or even lower for several compounds than the mean therapeutic dosage, indicating that a substantial fraction of cerebral H_1-receptors are likely to be occupied during their clinical use. This strongly suggests that the central effects that most

TABLE III

INHIBITION OF ^{3}H-MEPYRAMINE BINDING IN MOUSE CORTEX IN VIVO BY VARIOUS PSYCHOTROPIC DRUGS IN THERAPEUTIC DOSAGE AND CORRELATION WITH CLINICAL SEDATIVE PROPERTIES

Drugs	Inhibition of ^{3}H-mepyramine binding (%)	Sedative effects
(1) H_1-Antihistamines		
Mequitazine (0.2)	1 ± 7^{NS}	+
(—)-Chlorpheniramine (0.1)	16 ± 3^{NS}	
Brompheniramine (0.2)	$51 \pm 3^{**}$	+++
Cinnarizine (1.2)	$60 \pm 6^{*}$	+++
(+)-Chlorpheniramine (0.1)	$69 \pm 4^{**}$	+++
Triprolidine (0.4)	$70 \pm 3^{**}$	+++
Cyproheptadine (0.2)	$75 \pm 1^{**}$	+++
Promethazine (1.0)	$77 \pm 6^{**}$	+++
(2) Antidepressants		
Iprindole (0.7)	19 ± 3^{NS}	+
Viloxazine (1.0)	20 ± 6^{NS}	+
Desipramine (1.0)	30 ± 8^{NS}	+
Imipramine (1.5)	$39 \pm 6^{*}$	++
Maprotiline (1.0)	$58 \pm 11^{**}$	++
Clomipramine (0.5)	$62 \pm 2^{**}$	++
Amitriptyline (1.0)	$85 \pm 6^{**}$	+++
Doxepine (2.0)	$86 \pm 7^{**}$	+++
(3) Neuroleptics		
Trifluoperazine (0.2)	9 ± 1^{NS}	+
Trifluperidol (0.1)	19 ± 6^{NS}	+
Haloperidol (0.2)	21 ± 7^{NS}	+
Pimozide (0.1)	25 ± 7^{NS}	+
Fluphenazine (0.2)	$32 \pm 2^{*}$	+
Droperidol (3.0)	$56 \pm 3^{**}$	+++
Thioridazine (1.0)	$66 \pm 2^{**}$	+++
Chlorpromazine (4.0)	$73 \pm 4^{**}$	+++
Levomepromazine (4.0)	$75 \pm 3^{**}$	+++
(4) Miscellaneous		
No significant inhibition observed after administration of the following drug: Diazepam (0.1) Meprobamate (6.0) Phenobarbital (2.0) Propranolol (1.6) Alprenolol (2.0) Salbutamol (0.04) Clonidine (0.006) Apomorphine (0.25) Cinanserine (1.2) Scopolamine (2.5) Atropine (2.5).		

Groups of 4-8 mice received the various drugs i.p. at the indicated dosage (mg.kg^{-1}) which represents the mean therapeutic dosage. One hour later 1μCi ^{3}H-mepyramine was given i.v. and mice killed 3 min. later. Results are express as percent ($\pm$ S.E.M.) of saline-treated mice (46.3 ± 3.9 pCi.mg protein^{-1}). * $p < 0.05$, ** $p < 0.001$. The qualitative sedation index was adapted from Van Praag (30) and Byck (31) for antidepressant drugs and neuroleptics, respec tively, and completed by data from Van Rossum (32), Brion (33) and Rickels (3

H_1-antihistamines share are due to occupation of these receptors. Prominent sedation is associated with the clinical use of most H_1-antihistamines, with an incidence ranging from 20 to 60% (22). Although these sedative properties cannot be easily demonstrated in behavioural studies in rodents, in humans

H_1-antihistamines elicit subjective symptoms like decreased attention or "mental clouding" as well as objective effects like increased sleep duration and changes in EEG patterns resembling those observed upon administration of barbiturates. That these effects are likely to result from blockade of post-synaptic receptors of histaminergic neurons in brain is consistent with the involvement of these neurons in the control of states of wakefulness, as suggested by i) the occurence of arousal reactions observed on EEG following intracerebral administration of histamine (23) ii) the anatomical disposition of the ascending histaminergic pathway projecting diffusely to telencephalic regions (24) and which seems to emanate from the mesencephalic reticular formation (25) iii) the circadian variation in histamine turnover in brain with a maximum during periods of arousal (26). Interestingly, mequitazine is a H_1-antihistamine characterized by a relatively good affinity for H_1-receptors _in vitro_, contrasting with a low potency in inhibiting the cerebral binding of ^3H-mepyramine _in vivo_. This suggests that the lack of significant sedative properties of this compound demonstrated by a double-blind clinical study (27) is related to a poor access of the drug to cerebral H_1-receptors when systemically administered. Thus the ratio of ID_{50}/Ki, much higher for mequitazine than other H_1-antihistamines, might predict clinical sedative actions of drugs of this class.

In addition to typical H_1-antihistamines, several tricyclic antidepressants (maprotiline, clomipramine, amitriptyline, doxepine) or neuroleptics (droperidol, thioridazine, chlorpromazine, levomepromazine) administered at therapeutic dosage inhibit by more than 50% ^3H-mepyramine binding _in vivo_, suggesting that extensive blockade of cerebral H_1-receptors is likely to occur during clinical utilisation. The H_1-antihistaminic activity of these drugs was generally noticed in traditional pharmacological testing during their development (in fact both the antidepressants and the neuroleptics were discovered per chance during the search of H_1-antihistamines) and has been recently confirmed regarding cyclic GMP formation in neuroblastoma cells (28) and ^3H-mepyramine binding in vitro (29, 12). The sedative effects of all these compounds is well established (30,31, 32, 33, 34) and contrasts with the lack of such effects in compounds from the same class (like viloxazine and desipramine among antidepressants or trifluoperazine and trifluperidol among neuroleptics) which all fail to substantially occupy H_1-receptors in the brain of the living mouse. Thus the good correlation between H_1-receptors occupation at therapeutic dosage and sedative side-effects (Table III) together with the observation that such side-effects occur with most typical H_1-antihistamines, strongly indicates that the sedative component in the spectrum of activity of a variety of psychotropic drugs might often be ascribed to blockade of cerebral H_1-receptors.

Indeed, sedation might also be produced via mechanisms other than blockade of H_1-receptors in brain. It has been shown that sedative properties of tricyclic antidepressants (35) and neuroleptics (36) are well correlated with their affinities for α-noradrenergic receptor binding sites evaluated in cerebral membranes *in vitro*. While our observations do not rule out that blockade of cerebral α-adreno-receptors also participate in the sedative side-effects of these compounds, it might be noticed that i) such blockade has not yet be proven to occur *in vivo* following systemic administration of therapeutic doses, ii) sedation does not appear to be a side-effect shared by all typical α-adreno-receptor antagonists (37) as it is by H_1-antihistamines, iii) the most sedative tricyclic antidepressants like doxepin present substantially more affinity for H_1-receptors than for α-adreno-receptors (28).

In any case ^{3}H-mepyramine binding *in vivo* might represent a useful test to predict sedative properties of new psychotropic agents and also, therefore, to develop agents devoid of this property , when it is considered as an unwanted side-effect.

IV. ROLE OF CALCIUM IN HISTAMINE ACTIONS MEDIATED BY H_1-RECEPTORS

Two main "second messengers" seem to be responsible for the intracellular events triggered by neurotransmitters and hormones on target cells : cyclic nucleotides and calcium ions. Histaminergic transmission seems to obey this rule as the imidazoleamine has been shown to elicit increases in cAMP or cGMP on various tissues and it is well known that it contracts smooth muscles, an effect generally mediated by H_1-receptors and presumably involving calcium ions.

An HA-sensitive adenylate cyclase has been characterised in cell-free preparations from guinea-pig cerebral cortex and hippocampus and seems selectively coupled with H_2-receptors (7, 38). However the cAMP response in brain slices is more complex as it involves both H_1- and H_2-receptors as demonstrated by analysis of the complex antagonism of the responses to HA by antihistamines belonging to each class (4,6). This view is strengthened by the additive response to dimaprit, a selective H_2-receptor agonist in supramaximal concentration and to 2-thiazolylethylamine, a predominantly H_1-agonist. Because H_1-receptors have never been shown to be associated with an adenylate cyclase and because in slices from guinea-pig hippocampus their stimulation elicits cAMP accumulation only when H_2-receptors are simultaneously stimulated we had speculated that the effect they mediate is probably indirect (6).

TABLE IV

INFLUENCE OF CALCIUM ON cAMP ACCUMULATION IN SLICES FROM GUINEA-PIG HIPPOCAMPUS

	cAMP (pmoles.mg protein-1)	
	2.6mM Ca^{++}	Ca^{++}-free
Control	6.7 ± 0.8	6.0 ± 0.8
Dimaprit (0.1mM)	24.6 ± 1.7	28.7 ± 1.5
Dimaprit (0.1mM) + TEA (1mM)	75.7 ± 6.4	54.2 ± 3.7*
Difference	51.1	25.5

The pooled slices were incubated for 30 min. in complete Krebs-Ringer bicarbonate medium under a constant stream of $O_2:CO_2$ (95:5). Then the slices were washed four times and resuspended either with complete medium (Ca^{++} 2.6mM) or with the same medium in which Ca^{++} was omitted.

* $p < 0.05$ when comparing with the cyclic AMP accumulation induced by the combination of dimaprit and 2-thiazolylethylamine (TEA) in normal medium (Ca^{++} 2.6mM).

Recently we have checked a possible involvement of calcium ions in this indirect effect. As summarized in Table IV it appears that in the absence of calcium ions in the incubation medium, the effect of the H_2-agonist is not significantly modified whereas that of 2-thiazolylethylamine is strongly reduced. In the same line the effect of dimaprit is enhanced in the presence of the ionophore A 23187, a compound which is inactive when added alone (not shown). Taken together, these data suggest that translocation of calcium ions is involved in the additive effects mediated by H_2- and H_1-receptors, respectively. It is not yet clear whether the effect mediated by H_1-receptors and calcium ions occurs at the level of the synthesis or the breakdown of the nucleotide because each process could account for the observed change.

In addition a similar action can be observed regarding the glycogenolytic effect of histamine which seems to depend on the availability of calcium ions in the incubation medium (Fig. 5). Because ^3H-glycogen hydrolysis elicited by HA, in contrast to that mediated by β-adrenergic receptors, is not markedly facilitated in the presence of phosphodiesterase inhibitors, it is likely that phosphorylase activation by HA involves the calcium system and not the cAMP one. Interestingly the HA-induced increase in cGMP in neuroblastoma cells (8), and cervical ganglion (9) is also mediated by H_1-receptors and similarly involves calcium. Hence it is tempting to speculate that in a large number of biologica systems, H_1-receptors might be associated with a translocation system for calcium ions.

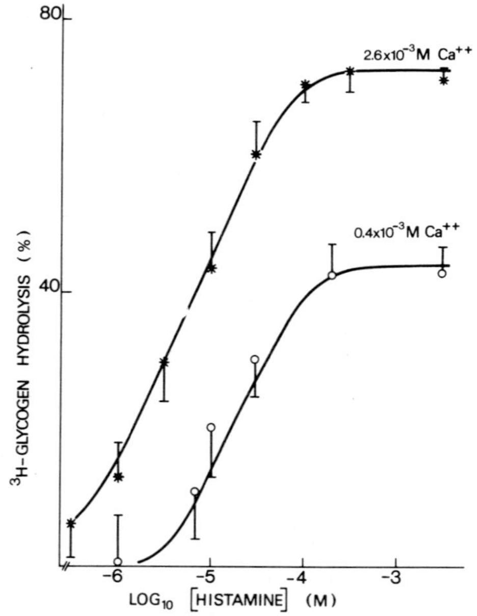

Fig. 5

^{3}H-GLYCOGEN HYDROLYSIS INDUCED BY HA IN SLICES FROM MOUSE CORTEX IN NORMAL KREBS-RINGER (2.6mM Ca^{++}) AND IN LOW-CALCIUM MEDIUM (0.4mM Ca^{++})

Slices were incubated for 30 min. in the presence of ^{3}H-glucose, then for 20 min. after the addition of increasing concentrations of HA, either in the normal or in the low-calcium medium. Results are expressed as percentage of basal ^{3}H-glycogen level = 38.5 $\pm$ 1.0dpm.10^3.mg protein^{-1} in normal medium and 43.2 $\pm$ 2.3dpm.10^3.mg protein^{-1} in low-calcium medium.

V. CHARACTERIZATION OF HIGH-AFFINITY BINDING SITES OF ^{3}H-HISTAMINE

Whereas ^{3}H-mepyramine represents a suitable ligand for H_1-receptors in brain, satisfactory ligands for other classes of HA-receptors are still to be developed. For instance, whereas H_2-receptors are indeed present in bra as evidenced by the stimulation of cAMP formation, ^{3}H-cimetidine, a H_2-anti-histamine, labels high-affinity sites presenting a pharmacological specificit clearly differing from that of H_2-receptors (39).

We have recently tried another approach, using ^{3}H-histamine as a ligand which has allowed us to evidence high-affinity binding sites in cerebra membranes. The kinetics of association and dissociation depicted in Fig. 6 lea to a value of 6nM for the Kd, obtained as the ratio of the two rate constants This value is in good agreement with the Kd value obtained by analysing the saturation kinetics on a Scatchard plot (Fig. 7). The same data indicate a

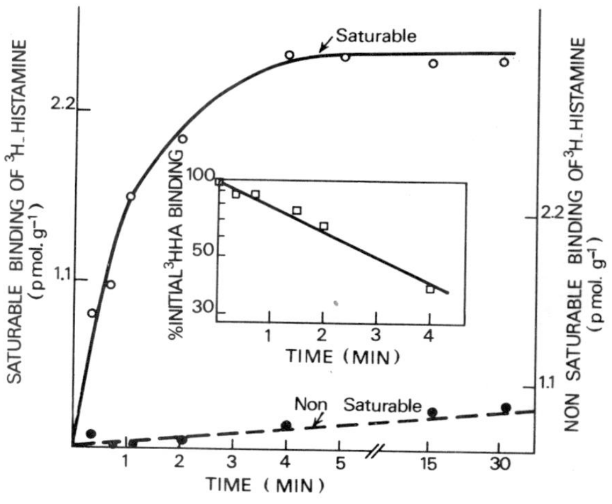

Fig. 6

KINETICS OF ^{3}H-HISTAMINE BINDING TO RAT CEREBRAL CORTEX

The time-course of binding of 10nM ^{3}H-HA (6.1Ci/mmol) to the particulate fraction (500μg protein per incubation) was determined at 30°C in the presence ("non-saturable" binding) or in the absence (total binding) of 5μM unlabeled HA. The second order rate constant for association (K_1) calculated from the initial slope of the association curve (up to 1.5 min.) and the known concentrations of the ligand (11nM) and binding sites (0.06nM) was $0.038\text{nM}^{-1}.\text{min.}^{-1}$. The inset represents the time-course of the dissociation of ^{3}H-HA binding ; after a 15-min. incubation at 30°C in the presence of 10nM ^{3}H-HA, 5μM unlabeled HA was added and the remaining binding measured at various time-intervals and a dissociation constant (k_2) of 0.23 min.^{-1} was obtained. The dissociation constant (K_D) obtained as the ratio of k_2/k_1 is 6.0nM.

maximal binding capacity of 7.8pmoles per g of original tissue and the absence of cooperative interaction as shown by the Hill coefficient close to unit (Fig. 7). The localisation and the developmental pattern of ^{3}H-HA binding sites in rat brain are consistent with the view that they represent post-synaptic HA-receptors. They are distributed in a markedly heterogenous fashion between brain regions, being abundant in regions containing high levels of L-histidine decarboxylase, a marker for putative HA nerve-terminals (40). There is, however, no strict correlation between the distribution of these sites and of the presynaptic marker, as also shown for other putative neuro-transmitters.

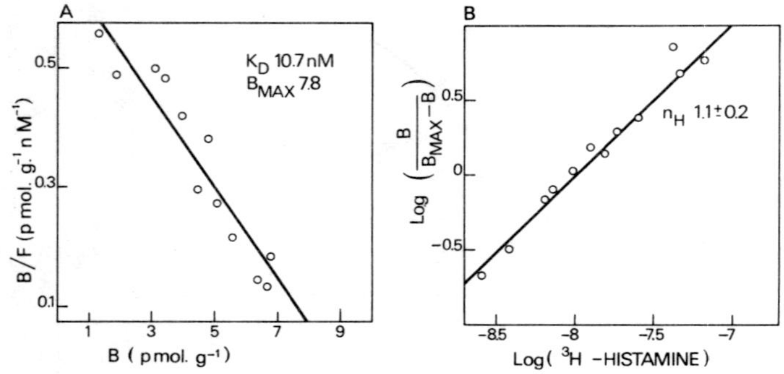

Fig. 7

SCATCHARD (A) AND HILL (B) REPRESENTATIONS OF THE SATURABLE BINDING OF ^{3}H-HISTAMINE TO A PARTICULATE FRACTION OF RAT CEREBRAL CORTEX

Tissue was homogenized in 100 volumes (w/v) of Tris-HCl buffer 50mM, pH 7.4 using a Teflon-glass Potter homogenizer. After centrifugation at 1000g.min. the supernatant was spun down at 3 x 10^5g.min. The resulting pellet was resuspended with a Dounce homogenizer in 70 volumes (w original tissue/ v) of Tris-HCl buffer containing 50mM NaCl and aliquots (about 10mg original tissue) were preincubated for 15 min. at 30°C. Fifteen min. incubations were done with increasing concentrations of ^{3}H-HA (6Ci/mmole) either alone or in the presence of 5μM unlabeled HA in order to determine total and "non-saturable" binding respectively ; then the reaction was stopped by rapid filtratio B represents the saturable binding of ^{3}H-HA (in pmoles.g tissue^{-1}) defined as ^{3}H-HA binding inhibited by 5μM HA, whereas F represents the concentration of free ^{3}H-HA (nM).

That ^{3}H-HA binding sites represent post-synaptic receptors is also consistent with the subcellular localization of these sites highly restricted to fractions containing synaptic membranes (Fig. 8). This view is further supported by the lesion data : there is an important loss of ^{3}H-HA binding sites in the striatum following local infusion of kainic acid, a neurotoxin ablating selectively neuronal perikarya which strongly suggests that these binding sites are localized upon neurons intrinsic to or emanating from this region. On the other hand following the lesion of the Medial Forebrain Bundle, which interrupts HA-synthesizing afferents to the striatum (41) no decrease in high-affinity binding sites of ^{3}H-HA occurs, ruling out their possible pre-synaptic localization. Interestingly there is even a small (+ 24%) but

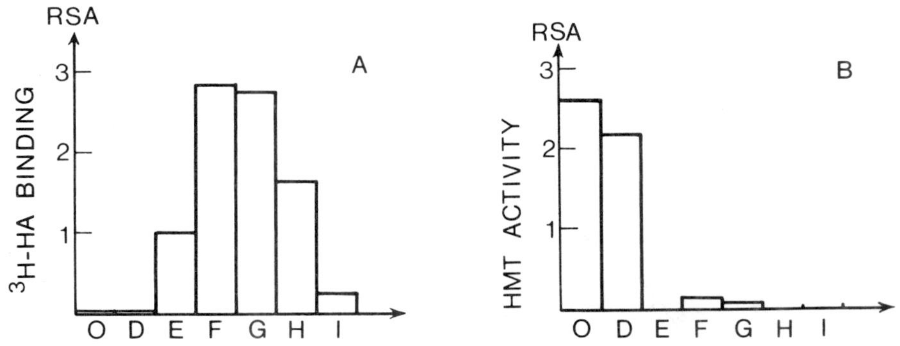

Fig. 8

DISTRIBUTION OF ^{3}H-HISTAMINE BINDING AND HISTAMINE-N-METHYLTRANSFERASE ACTIVITY IN SUBCELLULAR FRACTIONS FROM LYSED CRUDE MITOCHONDRIAL PELLET OF RAT CEREBRAL CORTEX

The cerebral cortex was homogenized in 10 volumes of 0.32M sucrose (w/v). After differential centrifugation of the homogenate, saturable ^{3}H-HA binding was measured in the crude nuclear pellet, the crude mitochondrial pellet and the microsomal fraction. Most of the ^{3}H-HA binding sites of the homogenate were recovered from the crude mitochondrial pellet (P_2). The P_2 fraction was lysed in distilled water and submitted to subfractionation on a sucrose gradient, according to Whittaker procedure. ^{3}H-HA binding as described in the legend of figure 7. HMT activity was measured according to the radioenzymatic method of Taylor et al. RSA (relative specific activity) refers to the ratio of the percentage of ^{3}H-HA binding or HMT activity to the percentage of protein in the same fraction. Values represent the means of data from three experiments on pooled tissues from three rats.

significant increase 10-12 days after the lesion. This recalls the situation observed for beta-adrenergic and dopamine receptors following interruption of catecholaminergic afferents and thought to correspond to denervation hypersensitivity (42). A clear denervation hypersensitivity to iontophoretically applied HA has been recently demonstrated in the guinea-pig hippocampus (43). In addition, the post-natal developmental pattern of ^{3}H-HA binding sites closely surimposes to the increase in HD activity, a reliable marker of histaminergic neurons (44).

Guanylnucleotides have been recently reported to alter the steady-state binding of agonists to a variety of receptors, reducing either their affinity or Bmax. The latter situation has been found for ^{3}H-HA binding in the presence of GTP and Gpp(NH)p in concentrations analogous to those required to affect other receptor bindings (Fig. 9). Although the significance of this effect remains to be clarified, this observation, in view of the general role of the guanylnucleotides in receptor function, reinforces the conviction that true receptors are labeled by ^{3}H-HA.

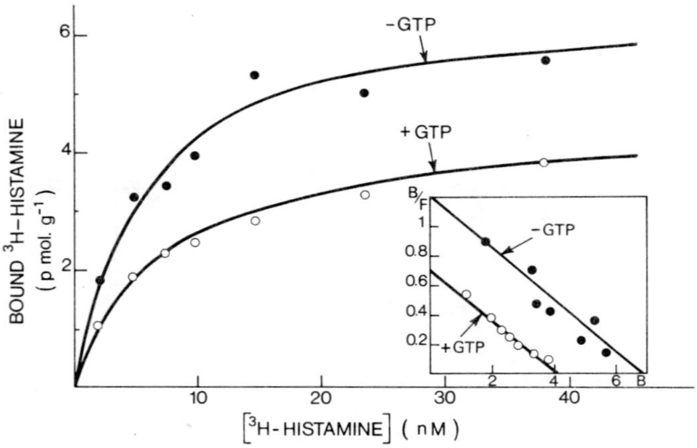

Fig . 9

EFFECT OF GTP ON ^{3}H-HISTAMINE BINDING TO RAT CEREBRAL CORTEX

The particulate fractions (600μg of protein) from the cerebral cortex of 3 rats were incubated with increasing concentrations of ^{3}H-histamine (60Ci/mmole) and the high-affinity binding determined as described in the legend of figure 7. GTP (100μM) was added (o) or omitted (•) in the buffer containing the ^{3}H-ligand. In the presence of GTP and ^{3}H-HA in increasing concentrations, the "non-saturable" binding was unchanged whereas the high-affinity binding was significantly reduced at every concentration of the ligand. Scatchard plot of the data (represented in the inset) indicated a 37% reduction of the maximal binding capacity in the presence of GTP whereas the dissociation constant (K_D = 5.9nM) was not significantly modified. The Hill coefficient was not different from unit in the presence of the nucleotide. ^{3}H-HA binding was decreased to the same extent in the presence of 100μM Gpp(NH)p. Other nucleotides did not inhibit significantly the high-affinity ^{3}H-HA binding.

Finally the pharmacological specificity of ^{3}H-HA binding sites has to be compared to that of receptors mediating the various biological actions of HA in the CNS in order to assess whether they involve identical recognition sites.

The histaminergic specificity of ^{3}H-HA binding sites is well shown by the lack of inhibitory potency of a large variety of putative neurotransmitters, contrasting with the significant potency of HA agonists like Nα-methylhistamine, Nα-Nα-dimethylhistamine, impromidine or dimaprit (Fig. 10). In the same way, it can also be noted that HA metabolites devoid of biological activity, like 3-methylhistamine or imidazoleacetic acid, are also inactive regarding inhibition of ^{3}H-HA binding.

Nevertheless it clearly appears that the ^{3}H-HA binding sites do not represent the recognition moiety of either H_1- or H_2-receptors. Thus the K_D of HA binding is approximately 1,000 times lower than the EC_{50} of the amine (in the micromolar range) regarding the various biochemical responses mediated by either H_1- or H_2-receptors as well as regarding inhibition of ^{3}H-mepyramine binding in brain. In the same way the inhibitory potency of various H_1- or H_2-agonists regarding ^{3}H-HA binding does not parallel their biological potency : this is well illustrated in the case of impromidine, a specific agonist of H_2-receptors which is 10-50 fold more potent than HA on various biological systems but approximately 30-fold less potent regarding inhibition of ^{3}H-HA binding. The difference is even more striking for H_1-agonists, like 2-methylhistamine or 2-thiazolylethylamine, which are approximately 4-time less potent than HA regarding biological responses mediated by H_1-receptors but 1000-time less regarding inhibition of ^{3}H-HA binding. Finally the apparent affinity of H_1-antihistamines (K_i values in the micromolar range) is not consistent with an interaction with H_1-receptors, for which their apparent dissociation constant is in the nanomolar range. The K_i of cimetidine and metiamide are grossly the same as their apparent dissociation constants regarding the inhibition of HA responses mediated by H_2-receptors but, as discussed above, the relative potency of H_2-agonists renders unlikely the idea that ^{3}H-HA binding reflects an interaction with typical H_2-receptors.

If ^{3}H-HA binding sites in brain are neither H_1- nor H_2-receptors what do they represent ?

Several hypotheses can be forwarded. One possibility is that these sites represent either H_1- or H_2-receptors in a modified state.

They might represent H_1- or H_2-receptors in one of their conformational states from which the transition into a lower affinity state might not occur easily in isolated membranes under our standard incubation conditions. This possibility is suggested by the selective action of guanylnucleotides. Interestingly, high-affinity binding sites for catecholamines and serotonin exhibiting a pharmacological specificity distinct from that of the corresponding adenylate cyclase or of the binding sites labeled with ^{3}H-antagonists have also been evidenced in brain tissues (45, 46).

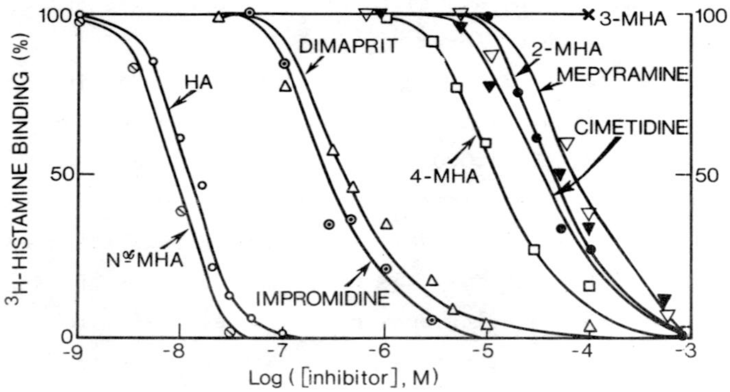

Fig. 10

INHIBITION OF ^{3}H-HISTAMINE BINDING BY VARIOUS HISTAMINERGIC AGENTS

A particulate fraction from cerebral cortex was incubated in the presence of various concentrations of the various agents together with 10nM ^{3}H-HA. Hundred percent represents the saturable binding of ^{3}H-HA (measured by the difference between values obtained in the absence and presence of 5μM unlabeled HA). The Hill plot of the inhibitions elicited by the various agents indicated a n_H value never different from unity. Besides the inactive HA metabolites, 3-methylhistamine and imidazole acetic acid, a series of putative neurotransmitters or related agents did not inhibit ^{3}H-HA binding even at concentrations higher than 50μM.

Another possibility is that ^{3}H-HA labels a class of HA receptors distinct from either H_1- or H_2-receptors. This is suggested by the recent identification of at least two classes of receptors mediating hyperpolarizing responses to HA of neurons in the cerebral ganglion of Aplysia Californica (47) : whereas H_1- or H_2-antagonists, particularly cimetidine, were in some cases effective, neither of the two types of receptors could be classified as strictly H_1- or H_2. In mammalian brain, the receptors mediating a large number of electrophysiological, neuroendocrinological or behavioral responses to HA have not yet been strictly identified. These responses were often shown to be blocked by H_1 and/or H_2-antihistamines administered locally in high dosage (or even in unknown concentration when iontophoretically-applied) but the relative lack of selectivity of these agents, (for instance most H_1-antihistamines have local anesthetic properties) and the technical limitations inherent to most of these physiological studies do not exclude that receptors other than H_1- or H_2-receptors were involved. Thus the possibility remains that ^{3}H-HA labels a class of post-synaptic receptors as yet non-identified by means of available pharmacological tools.

REFERENCES

1. SCHWARTZ J.C. (1977) Ann. Rev. Pharmacol. Toxicol. 17 : 325-339.
2. GREEN J.P., JOHNSON C.L. and WEINSTEIN H. In Psychopharmacology : A Generation of Progress, M.A. Lipton, A. DiMascio and K.F. Killam ed., Raven Press, New York, 1978, 319-332.
3. SCHWARTZ J.C., BARBIN G., BAUDRY M., GARBARG M., MARTRES M.P., POLLARD H. and VERDIERE M. In Current Developments in Psychopharmacology vol. 5, W.B. Essman and L. Valzelli ed., Spectrum Publication, Inc., New York, 1979, 173-261.
4. BAUDRY M., MARTRES M.P. and SCHWARTZ J.C. (1975) Nature 253 : 362-363.
5. DISMUKES K.R., ROGERS M. and DALY J.W. (1976) J. Neurochem. 26 : 785-790.
6. PALACIOS J.M., GARBARG M., BARBIN G. and SCHWARTZ J.C. (1978) Mol. Pharmacol. 14 : 971-982.
7. HEGSTRAND L.R., KANOF P.D. and GREENGARD P. (1976) Nature 260 : 163-165.
8. RICHELSON E. (1978) Science 201 : 69-71.
9. STUDY R.E. and GREENGARD P. (1978) J. Pharmacol. Exp. Ther. 207 : 767-778.
10. QUACH T.T., ROSE C. and SCHWARTZ J.C. (1978) J. Neurochem. 30 : 1335-1341.
11. HILL S.J., EMSON P.C. and YOUNG J.M. (1978) J. Neurochem. 31 : 997-1004.
12. TRAN V.T., CHANG R.S.L. and SNYDER S.H. (1978) Proc. Natl. Acad. Sci., U.S.A. 75 : 6290-6294.
13. BARSOUM G.S. and GADDUM J.H. (1935) J. Physiol., London 85 : 1-14.
14. TAYLOR J.D. and RICHELSON E. (1979) Mol. Pharmacol. 15 : 462-471.
15. YAMAMURA H.E., KUHAR M.J. and SNYDER S.H. (1974) Brain Res. 80 : 170-176.
16. PERT C.B. and SNYDER S.H. (1975) Life Sci. 16 : 1623-1634.
17. BAUDRY M., MARTRES M.P. and SCHWARTZ J.C. (1977) Life Sci. 21 : 1163-1170.
18. BYLUND D.B., CHARNESS M.E. and SNYDER S.H. (1977) J. Pharmacol. Expetl. Therap. 201 : 644-654.
19. DUCHEMIN A.M., QUACH T.T., ROSE C. and SCHWARTZ J.C. (1979) Life Sci. 24 : 401-410.
20. HILL S.J., YOUNG J.M. and MARRIAN D.H. (1977) Nature 270 : 361-363.
21. SCHWARTZ J.C., BARBIN G., DUCHEMIN A.M., GARBARG M., PALACIOS J.M., QUACH T.T. and ROSE C. In G.C. Pepeu, M. Kuhar and S.J. Enna eds., Receptors, Neurotransmitters and Peptide Hormones, Pergamon Press, Oxford, in press.
22. FAINGOLD C.L. In O. Eichler and Farah eds., Handbook of Experimental Pharmacology, vol. XVII, Part 2, Springer-Verlag, Berlin, 1978, 567-573.
23. WOLF P. and MONNIER M. (1973) Agents and Actions 3 : 196.

24. GARBARG M., BARBIN G., BISCHOFF S., POLLARD H. and SCHWARTZ (1976) Brain Res. 106 : 333-348.

25. SCHWARTZ J.C., BARBIN G., GARBARG M., LLORENS C., PALACIOS J.M. and POLLARD H. In P. Simon ed. Advances in Pharmacology and Therapeutics, vol. 2, Pergamon Press, Oxford, 1978, pp 171-180.

26. SCHWARTZ J.C., BARBIN G., GARBARG M., POLLARD H., ROSE C. and VERDIERE M. In E. Costa, E. Giacobini and R. Paoletti eds. First and Second Messengers in Nervous Tissues, Advances in Biochemical Psychopharmacology, vol. 15, Raven Press, New York, 1976, pp 111-126.

27. GERVAIS P., GERVAIS A., DE BEULE R. and VAN DER BIJL W. (1975) Acta Aller. 30 : 286.

28. RICHELSON E. (1978) Nature 274 : 176-177.

29. HILL S.J. and YOUNG M. (1978) Eur. J. Pharmacol. 52 : 397-399.

30. VAN PRAAG H.M. Van Gorcum, Assen, Amsterdam, The Netherlands, 1978.

31. BYCK R. In the Pharmacological basis of Therapeutics (eds. Godman L.S., and Gilman A.) 152-200 (Mac Millan Publishing Co, Inc., New York, 1975).

32. VAN ROSSUM J.M., JANSSEN P.A.J., BOISSIER J.R., JULOU L., LOEW D.M., MØLLER NIELSEN I., MUNKWAD I., RANDRUP A., STILLE G. and TEDESCHI D.H. In The Neuroleptics, Mod. Probl. Pharmaco-Psychiat., 5 : 23-70 (eds. Bobon D.P., Janssen R.A.J. and Bobon J., liege) (Karger, Basel/Münche/Paris, New York, 1970).

33. BRION S. (1975) J. Int. Med. Res. 3 : 87-91.

34. RICKELS K., CHUNG H., CSANALOSI L., SABLOSKY W. and SIMON J. (1973) Brit. J. Psychiat. 123 : 329-339.

35. U'PRICHARD D.C., GREENBERG D.A., SHEEHAN P.P. and SNYDER S.H. (1978) Science 199 : 197-198.

36. PEROUTKA S.J., U'PRICHARD, D.C., GREENBERG D.A. and SNYDER S.H. (1977) Neuropharmacology 16 : 549-556.

37. NICKERSON M. and COLLIER B. In The Pharmacological Basis of Therapeutics (eds. Goodman L.S. and Gilman A.) 533-547 (Mac Millan Publishing Co., Inc., New York, 1975).

38. GREEN J.P., JOHNSON C.L., WEINSTEIN H. and MAAYANI S. (1977) Proc. Natl. Acad. Sci., U.S.A. 74 5697-5701.

39. BURKARD W.P. (1978) Eur. J. Pharmacol. 50 : 449-450.

40. PALACIOS J.M., SCHWARTZ J.C. and GARBARB M. (1978) Eur. J. Pharmacol. 50 : 443-444.

41. GARBARG M., BARBIN G., FEGER J. and SCHWARTZ J.C. (1974) Science 186 : 833-835.

42. SCHWARTZ J.C., COSTENTIN J., MARTRES M.P., PROTAIS P. and BAUDRY M. (1978) Neuropharmacology 17 : 665-685.

43. HAAS H.L., WOLF P., PALACIOS J.M., GARBARG M., BARBIN G. and SCHWARTZ J.C. (1978) Brain Res. 156 : 275-291.

44. MARTRES M.P., BAUDRY M., SCHWARTZ J.C. (1975) Brain Res. 83 : 261-275.

45. BENNET J.P. and SNYDER S.H. Mol. Pharmacol. (1976) 12 : 373-389.

46. U'PRICHARD D.C., GREENBERG D.A. and SNYDER S.H. (1977) Mol. Pharmacol. 13 : 454-473.

47. GRUOL D.L. and WEINREICH D. (1979) Brain Res. 162 : 281-301.

C H O L I N E R G I C   S Y S T E M S

Neurotransmitters and their Receptors
Edited by U.Z. Littauer, Y. Dudai, I. Silman,
V.I. Teichberg and Z. Vogel

Studies of Postnatal Changes of Muscarinic Receptors in Mouse Brain

Yaacov Egozi, Yoel Kloog and Mordechai Sokolovsky

Department of Biochemistry, George S. Wise Faculty of Life Sciences, Tel-Aviv University, Tel-Aviv, Israel

Muscarinic receptor development in the various regions of the ICR mouse brain was studied by means of direct binding using the muscarinic antagonist N-methyl-4-piperidyl benzilate and by competition experiments using the muscarinic agonist oxotremorine. The quantity and density of receptors, the properties of antagonist and agonist binding were evaluated as a function of age in five regions. The most rapid development takes place in the medulla-pons and cerebellum with considerably slower maturation in the cortex, caudate-putamen and hippocampus. No change was seen in binding properties of the antagonist in any of the regions studied. On the other hand, in the medulla-pons, cerebellum and cortex, the agonist binding properties vary during development. Binding of oxotremorine can be accommodated by a 2-site model, i.e., variation in the binding reflects an increase in the proportion of high affinity sites and not a change in affinity constants at the two sites.

INTRODUCTION

Recent studies on the development of muscarinic receptors in mammalian brains (1-4) have been directed mainly towards the determination of the muscarinic binding capacities. Previous *in vitro* experiments indicated that the binding of both antagonists and agonists is complicated: binding of antagonists is followed by isomerization of the antagonist-receptor complex (5-7). The binding of agonists, deviates from a law of mass action and can be accommodated to a model which specifies binding to two or three sites with different affinities for agonists (8-10). The binding of muscarinic ligands is further complicated by the regional heterogeneity of binding found in mouse (7)(11) and in rat (9)(10) brains. We therefore investigated and report here the muscarinic receptor capacities and ligand binding properties in the developing ICR mouse brain using the specific tritrated muscarinic antagonist (^{3}H)-4NMPB and the agonist oxotremorine. While this work was in progress, developmental studies dealing with the binding of agonists to brain muscarinic receptors in rat (13) and inbred mice strains (14) were published.

MATERIALS AND METHODS

Materials:

Labeled and unlabeled compounds are the same as described previously (6)(7).

Methods:

Male ICR mice of different ages post partum were decapitated, brains were rapidly removed and the brain areas were dissected in a cold room. After dissection, brain regions (from 15-25 mice for the caudate-putamen, 10-15 mice for the hippocampus, and 5-10 mice for other regions) were homogenized in ice-cold 0.32 M sucrose using a motor-driven teflon pestle (950 rpm) in a glass homogenizer to yield a 2-10% homogenate (w/v). In order to achieve a constant receptor density the preparations were further diluted whenever necessary with 0.32 M sucrose to obtain the desired protein content. Direct binding studies using 50 μl aliquots of tissue preparations were carried out as previously described (7).

Specific binding is defined as the total minus the nonspecific, i.e. binding in the presence of 5×10^{-5}M of unlabeled 4NMPB or atropine. Protein was determined by the Lowry method using bovine serum albumin as a standard.

Competition experiments with (^{3}H)-4NMPB (2.0 nM) and the muscarinic agonist oxotremorine were performed with 0.05-0.1 nM (^{3}H)-4NMPB binding site concentrations (7). The competition curves were analyzed according to the two-site model described by Birdsall et al. (8)(9), as follows:

$$\frac{(RL)}{(RL)^o} = \frac{\alpha}{1 + K_{Happ}(A)} + \frac{(1 - \alpha)}{1 + K_{Lapp}(A)} \qquad \text{(Eq. 1)}$$

Where (RL) and $(RL)^o$ are the specific binding of (^{3}H)-4NMPB measured in the presence of agonist (A) and in its absence, respectively. α and $(1 - \alpha)$ are the proportions of the high and low affinity binding sites to which the agonist binds with affinity constants K_H and K_L respectively, where

$$K_H = K_{Happ} \quad (1 + K(L))$$

$$\text{and } K_L = K_{Lapp} \quad (1 + K(L)).$$

K is the affinity constant of (^{3}H)-4NMPB (L) meausred by direct binding. Curve fitting was carried out with a CDC6600 computer using a non linear least-squares regression computer program BMDPAR, revision date November 1978. (The program was developed at the Health Science Computing Facility of the University of California, Los Angeles. The Facility is sponsored by NIH Special Research Resources Grant RR-3).

The parameters of eq. 1 were allowed to vary continuously over a predetermined range, the criterion for best fit being the minimum deviation (F) defined in eq. 2.

$$F = \sum_{i=1}^{n} \left(\frac{(RL_i)}{RL^o} - \frac{\alpha}{1 + K_{Happ}(A_i)} - \frac{1 - \alpha}{1 + K_{Lapp}\ (A_i)}\right)^2 \qquad \text{(Eq. 2.)}$$

RESULTS

The development of muscarinic binding sites and their characteristics was followed in homogenates of the cerebellum, medulla-pons, cortex, hippocampus and caudate-putamen of newborn mice using the specific muscarinic antagonist (^{3}H)-4NMPB. The dissociation constants evaluated from Scatchard plots are given in Table I.

Table I: Dissociation constants (nM)[a] for (^{3}H)-4NMPB determined during ontogeny.

Age (day post-partum)	Cerebellum	Medulla-pons	Hippocampus	Caudate-putamen
1	0.55	0.56	0.19	0.21
5	0.47	0.50	0.31	0.3
10	0.65	0.70	0.19	0.18
16	0.75	0.55	0.24	0.28
20	1.05	0.62	0.38	0.35
30	0.74	0.76	0.25	0.25
105	0.72	0.72	0.29	0.29

[a]Values given are the means of 2-3 spearate experiments, each performed in triplicate, whose results varied by less than 30%.

As shown, the apparent dissociation constants of (^{3}H)-4NMPB from the muscarinic receptors remain unchanges for all brain regions studied during the course of maturation, i.e., from the first day after birth until adulthood. The small differences previously detected in adult mice between cerebellum or medulla-pons preparations and the other brain regions (7) is already manifested in newborn mice.

The kinetic approach to the study of antagonist-receptor interaction seems more adequate for detection of small variations in the binding characteristics between different brain regions, since small differences in the dissociation constants might reflect marked differences in the rates of association and dissociation of the muscarinic ligand to and from its receptors (7). We therefore studied the kinetics of dissociation of (^{3}H)-4NMPB in tissue preparations from 5-day old mice, using the radiosotope dilution technique (7). As Fig. 1 clearly demonstrates, the dissociation rates measured in preparations from 5-day old mice were similar to those obtained with adult mice for the medulla-pons and the hippocampus.

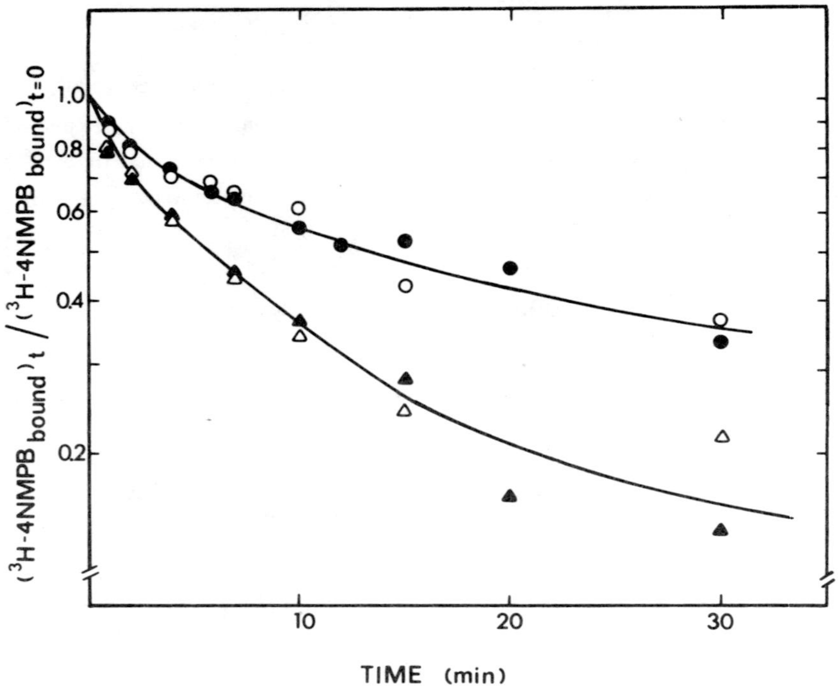

Fig. 1. Dissociation of (^{3}H)-4NMPB-receptor complexes. Samples (0.05 ml) were incubated for 30 min with 5.0 nM (^{3}H)-4NMPB in 2 ml modified Krebs buffer at 25°. Atropine (5×10^{-5}M) was then added, and the samples were filtered immediately (zero time) and at the times indicated. Specific (^{3}H)-4NMPB binding was determined as described in Methods. Each point in the figure is the mean of at least 6 samples whose standard error was less than 15%. Dissociation was determined with homogenates of cortex (o) and medulla-pons (Δ) prepared from mice 5 days after birth (open symbols) and from adult mice (closed symbols).

Moreover, the biphasic first order character of the dissociation plots observed previously in preparations from adult mice (7) is also seen in preparations from 5-day old mice. The biphasic character of the curves is probably due to the isomerization of (^{3}H)-4NMPB receptor complexes, as discussed in detail elsewhere (7)(11). The half time ($t_{1/2}$) values obtained for dissociation of these complexes in 5-day old adult mice are 14 min and 18 min for cortical preparation respectively, and 5 min and 6 min for the medulla-pons preparations respectively. Similar phenomena were observed in other brain regions.

The density of the muscarinic receptors in the various brain regions at different ages was evaluated from Scatchard plots of (^{3}H)-4NMPB binding and from protein determinations of the tissue preparations. The developmental pattern of muscarinic receptor density, expressed either as specific binding per mg protein or as receptor quantity (binding sites per whole tissue) are **shown** in Figs. 2 and 3 respectively.

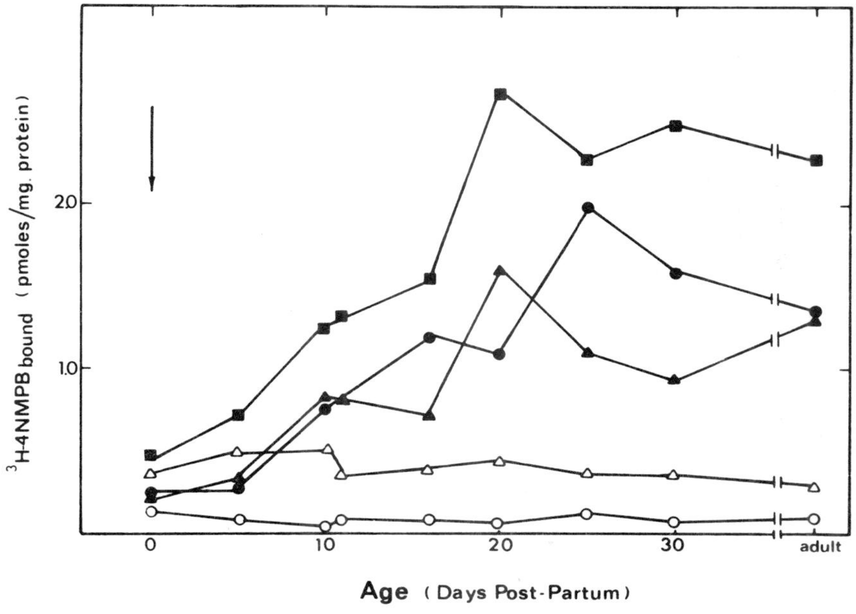

Fig. 2. Development of the density of (^{3}H)-4NMPB specific binding per mg protein in different mouse brain regions.
Values represent the means of 2-3 separate experiments whose results varied by less than 20%. o——o Cerebellum, Δ——Δ medulla-pons, ●——● hippocampus, ▲——▲ cortex, ■——■ caudate-putamen.

Tissue weight gain in the different regions is shown in Fig. 4. In the first two weeks after birth a rapid increase in tissue weight was observed in all regions, followed by a slower weight gain in the following two weeks. These increases do not parallel the developmental pattern of muscarinic receptor quantity (Fig. 3.), thus accounting for the difference in developmental pattern between receptor density and receptor quantity.

The ratio of protein concentration in the homogenates to original tissue weight was consistent for all regions and ages investigated (about 10%). Hence the pattern of receptor density development is the same regardless of the index used for tissue quantity, i.e., tissue weight or protein concentration.

The development of the characteristics of agonist binding to muscarinic receptor was studied by means of competition experiments, in which the potent muscarinic agonist oxotremorine was used to inhibit the binding of (^{3}H)-4NMPB, using preparations of the different brain regions from the day of birth until adulthood. In all experiments the concentrations of (^{3}H)-4NMPB binding sites was much lower (0.05-0.1 nM) than that of the labeled antagonist (2.0 nM) and of the apparent dissociation constant of the competing drug. Therefore the

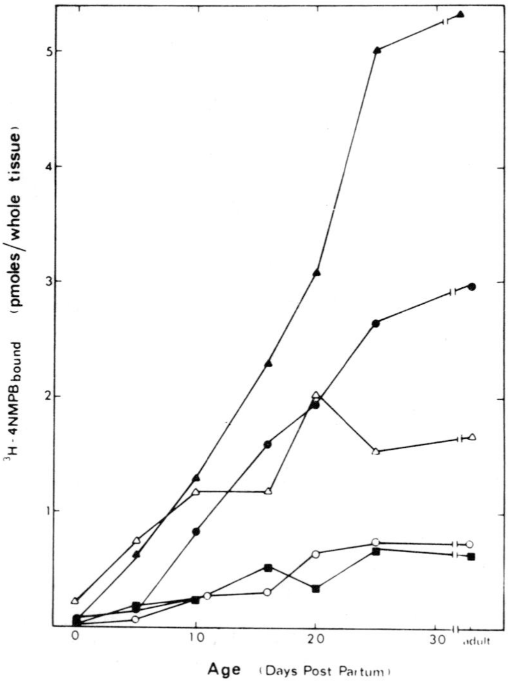

Fig. 3. Development of the total specific (^{3}H)-4NMPB binding per brain region.
o——o Cerebellum, △——△ medulla-pons, ●——● hippocampus, ▲——▲ cortex and ■——■ caudate-putamen.

concentrations of (^{3}H)-4NMPB and oxotremorine were virtually unchanged during the incubation period (free ligand ∿ total ligand).

The results of competition experiments on homogenates prepared from mouse brain at 5, 11 and 16 days after birth and from adult mouse brain are shown in Fig. 5 for the medulla-pons and the hippocampus and in Fig. 6 for the caudate-putamen, the cortex and the cerebellum.

At all ages and in all brain regions studied, oxotremorine (10^{-8}-10^{-4} M) inhibited the binding of 2.0 nM (^{3}H)-4NMPB. This wide range in effective oxotremorine concentration was most pronounced in adult medulla-pons and cerebellum, but was also observed in these brain regions with younger animals and to some extent in the other brain regions as well. In the medulla-pons and cerebellum homogenates the apparent affinities of oxotremorine at all ages were higher than those observed in the other regions, as revealed by I_{50} value (the concentration which inhibits 50% of specific (^{3}H)-4NMPB binding) measured in these regions (Table II). However, these inter-regional differences in I_{50} values are smaller (3 to 8 fold) at days 1 and 5 than in adults (20 to 30 fold).

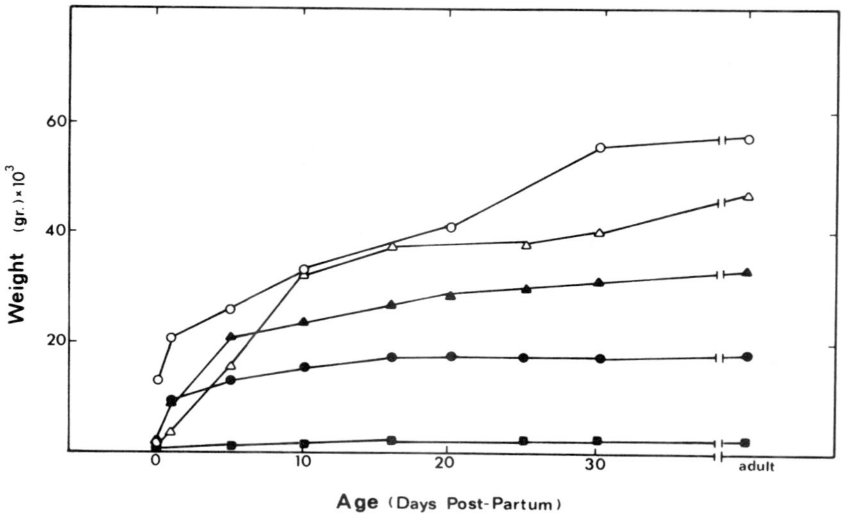

Fig. 4. Development of tissue weight of different mouse brain regions. Values presented are the means of at least 6 separate determinations. o——o Cerebellum, Δ——Δ medulla pons, ●——● hippocampus, ▲——▲ cortex and ■——■ caudate-putamen.

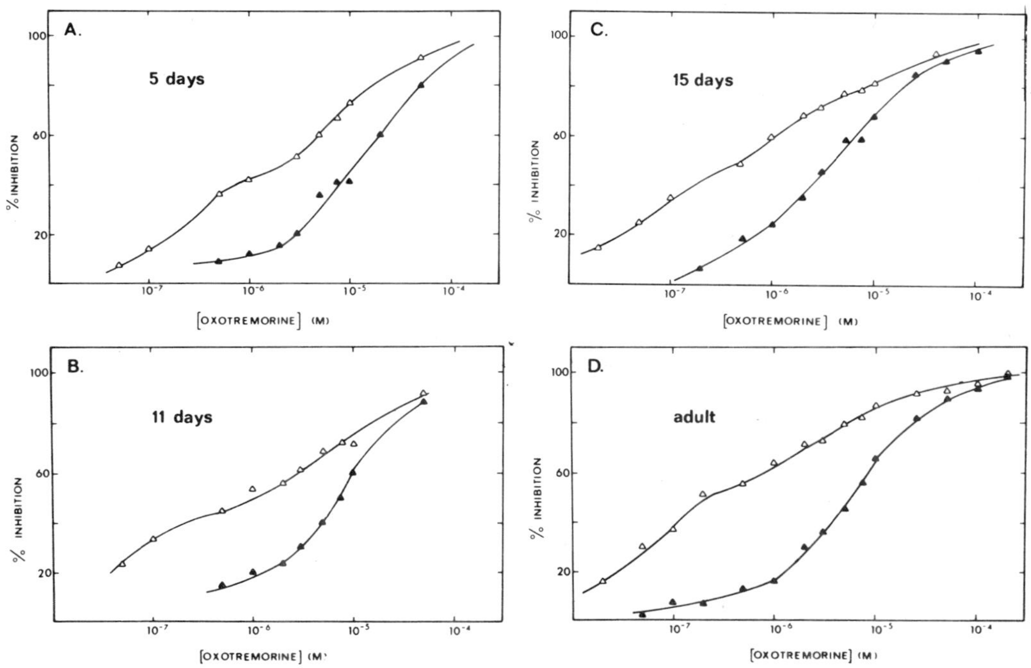

Fig. 5. Inhibition of (^{3}H)-4NMPB binding by oxotremorine during the development of the medulla-pons (Δ) and hippocampus (▲). Binding was determined in homogenates prepared from mice at the following post-partum ages: A - 5 days; B - 11 days; C - 15 days; D - adult (105 days).

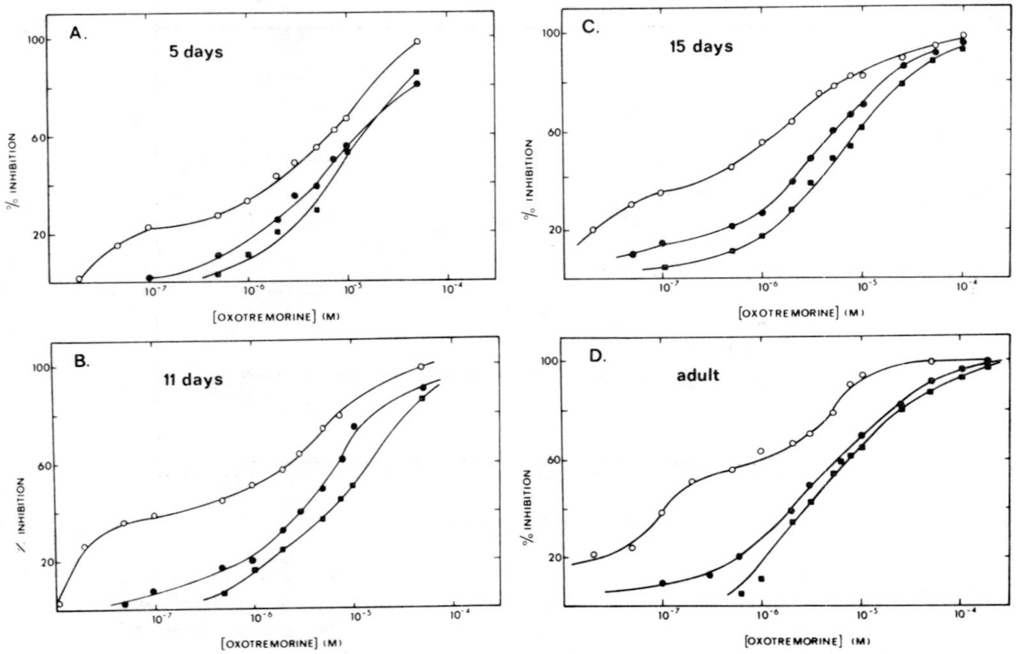

Fig. 6. Inhibition of (^{3}H)-4NMPB binding by oxotremorine during the development of the cortex (●), caudate-putamen (■) and cerebellum (o).
Binding was determined in homogenates prepared from mice at the following post-partum ages: A - 5 days; B - 11 days; C - 15 days; D - adult (105 days).

Table II: I_{50} values (μM) for oxotremorine determined by competition with 2 nM (^{3}H)-4NMPB during ontogeny.

Age (days post-partum)	Cerebellum	Medulla-pons	Cortex	Hippo-campus	Caudate-putamen
1	3.0 - 4.0	1.0 - 2.0	5.0 - 8.0	-	-
5-6	3.0 - 5.0	2.7	7.5	8.0 - 14.0	6.0 - 9.5
11	0.9 - 2.0	0.6 - 1.0	5.0 - 6.0	7.0 - 7.5	8.0 - 10.0
15-16	0.5 - 1.0	0.5 - 0.6	2.5 - 5.6	5.0 - 8.0	7.0 - 10.0
30	0.2 - 0.3	0.2 - 0.5	7.5	5.0 - 7.5	6.0 - 10.0
105	0.2 - 0.4	0.2 - 0.4	4.0 - 7.0	5.0 - 6.0	6.0 - 7.0

DISCUSSION

Postnatal development of muscarinic binding sites

The developmental pattern of the muscarinic binding sites in the different brain regions of ICR mice can be summarized as follows: 1. From day 1 up to day 5 post-partum, there is only a small increase in the total quantity of binding sites per whole tissue in the hippocampus, the caudate-putamen and the cerebellum, whereas in the medulla-pons and the cortex a considerable increase occurs. 2. The total quantity of muscarinic binding sites increased gradually from 5-6 days post-partum until it reaches adult values at about 20-25 days in all regions studied except for the medulla-pons, where adult values are reached earlier. At 10 days the quantity in the medulla-pons is about 75% of the adult value, while in the other brain regions it reaches 25-39% of the adult values. 3. The increase in the total quantity of binding sites per whole tissue between day 5 and the adult stage is greatest for the cortex and the hippocampus (about 25-fold) and least for the medulla-pons (less than 30 fold). In the caudate-putamen and the cerebellum the increase is about 6-10 fold.

The potent antagonist (^{3}H)-4NMPB has been shown to label muscarinic receptors both _in vitro_ (7)(11)(15)(16)(17) and _in vivo_((18) and the accompanying manuscript). It can therefore be concluded that the binding data summarized above relate to the development of the putative muscarinic receptors. This conclusion is further supported by the fact that (^{3}H)-4NMPB binding was inhibited by the muscarinic agonist oxotremorine in all regions and at all ages investigated.

There is a marked difference in the postnatal developmental pattern of muscarinic receptor density (i.e. binding sites per mg tissue or per mg protein) between the cortex, hippocampus and caudate-putamen, in which it increases, and the medulla-pons and cerebellum, in which it shows a slight decrease or remains unchanged (Fig. 2). Taken together with the data concerning total receptor quantity, these patterns can be understood in terms of the following scheme: In the hippocampus, caudate-putamen and cerebellum, the increase in tissue growth during the first 5 days after birth exceeds that of muscarinic binding sites (Fig. 3, 4). This early lag phase in muscarinic receptor development is absent in the medulla-pons and the cortex, where new receptors do accumulate (Fig. 3). In the next stage (5-6 days up to 20-25 days post-partum) new binding sites appear concomitantly with tissue growth. But while receptor formation in the cortex, the hippocampus and the caudate-putamen exceeds tissue growth, thus leading to increased density, the opposite is true for the medulla-pons and the cerebellum, so that an overall decrease in receptor density is observed. A decrease in binding site density is also seen in the cortex and the caudate-putamen between 20 and 25 days post-partum. This is clearly due to tissue weight gain and not to decrease in total receptor quantity (Figs. 3,4). The apparent discrepany in developmental pattern between muscarinic receptor quantity and its density emphasizes the need for caution in interpreting the developmental binding data.

The developmental pattern of muscarinic receptors has been shown to parallel that of other cholinergic markers, e.g., cholineacetyltransferase, acetylcholinesterase and high affinity choline uptake in the developing rat brain (1)(8). It therefore seems reasonable to use muscarinic binding as an index for the development of cholinergic mechanisms. The development of central muscarinic receptors in ICR mice presented in this study exhibits some significant parallels and differences when compared with data obtained for other rodents. Muscarinic binding site development reported for Wistar rats (1)(13) and Sprague-Dawley rats (3) clearly resemble that reported here for the hippocampus, the caudate-putamen and the cerebellum, i.e., a lag phase of about one weeks duration was observed after birth, followed by a marked increase in receptor density during the next 2-3 weeks. The reports also agree with regard to the rate of development in these regions in the different strains and species mentioned. There is a clear distinction, however, between mice and rats with regard to the medulla-pons,where muscarinic receptor density increases in rats (3)(13) but appears constant or decreases in mice as reported here and elsewhere (14).

Characteristics of (^{3}H)-4NMPB and oxotremorine binding during the post-natal perio

The binding data obtained for the muscarinic antagonist (^{3}H)-4NMPB indicate that neither its affinity for receptors nor the dissociation rates of (^{3}H)-4NMPB complexes change during the postnatal development. Similar observations regarding the affinity for receptors, have been noted in rat (1)(13), mouse (14) and rabbit brains (2) using the muscarinic antagonists (^{3}H)-QNB and (^{3}H)-N-methyl scopolamine. The data suggest that the nature of the muscarinic binding sites for antagonists does not change during the postnatal period. It is interesting to note that the small differences between dissociation constants for (^{3}H)-4NMPB measured in the cerebellum or medulla-pons and those measured in the other brain regions (7)(18) as well as the marked difference in the dissociation rates of (^{3}H)-4NMPB-receptor complexes between these regions, are observed at all ages investigated. These results support our previous conclusions on regional heterogeneity of antagonist binding (7)(11)(18).

The apparent dissociation constant measured for the agonist oxotremorine (I_{50}), like those for muscarinic antagonists, show little change during receptor development in the hippocampus, caudate-putamen and cortex of ICR mice.

In contrast, the competition curves for the cerebellum and the medulla-pons (Figs. 5,6) are flattened and both the I_{50} values and the shape of the curves changes as a function of age.

Flattened agonist/antagonist inhibition curves are well documented in the literature. A possible explanation was proposed by Birdsall et al. (8)(9), who suggested that agonists bind with differing affinities to two or three distinct binding site populations to which antagonists bind with the same affinity. The data obtained from inhibition of (^{3}H)-4NMPB binding by oxotremorine in the cerebellum and medulla-pons can be fitted by the two-site model, for all ages investigated with the exception of the cerebellum preparations from 1-day old mice, in which only one population of binding sites was observed (Table III). The binding parameters for oxotremorine were evaluated from the competition experiments (Fig. 5,6) by the best fit procedure using the nonlinear least squares program and eq. 1 (for details see Methods), and are summarized in Tables III and IV.

Table III: Affinity constants of oxotremorine to the high- and low-affinity binding sites (according to the two-site model) in the cerebellum during ontogeny

Age (days post-partum)	α	$K_H x10^{-6}$ (M^{-1})	$K_L x10^{-6}$ (M^{-1})	Residual sum of squares $x10^3$ A	B
5	0.26 ± 0.05	41.7 ± 18.5	0.28 ± 0.001	11.7	87
11	0.47 ± 0.06	29.8 ± 7.0	0.40 ± 0.015	21	198
16	0.60 ± 0.06	74.9 ± 24.1	0.32 ± 0.21	21.2	49
30	0.64 ± 0.08	42.4 ± 12.4	1.01 ± 0.58	7.1	78
105	0.64 ± 0.06	60.9 ± 23	0.83 ± 0.35	29.5	203

The binding parameters ± S.D. were calculated by the nonlinear least squares regression procedure for a two-site model as described in Methods. K_H and K_L are the affinity constants of oxotremorine to the high- and low-affinity binding sites respectively, and α denotes the proportion of the high affinity binding sites (eq. 1). In each case the residual sum of squares (A) is significantly lower than that obtained by fitting the data of the nonlinear regression method according to a one-site model (B). In each case the minimizing procedure showed convergence. The parameter values were all positive with real asymptotic standard deviation values.

Table IV: Affinity constants of oxotremorine to the high-and low-affinity binding sites (according to the two-site model) in medulla-pons during development.

Age (days post-partum)	α	$K_H x 10^{-6}$ (M^{-1})	$K_L x 10^{-6}$ (M^{-1})	Residual sum of squares x 10^3 A	B
5	0.43 ± 0.05	23.7 ± 7.1	0.49 ± 0.1	4.67	24
11	0.53 ± 0.03	70.4 ± 14.7	0.36 ± 0.07	7.2	10
16	0.61 ± 0.03	81.7 ± 11.7	0.53 ± 0.1	2.6	113
30	0.66 ± 0.026	98.7 ± 12	1.12 ± 0.26	1.45	37
105	0.61 ± 0.02	73.1 ± 8.1	0.73 ± 0.09	3.6	24

The data obtained suggest that the decrease in I_{50} values with age (Table II) in the cerebellum and medulla-pons stems mainly from the increase in proportion of high affinity binding sites in these regions (Tables III and IV). This increase occurs very rapidly in the first 11 days after birth and is completed at day 16. On the other hand, no significant changes were seen in the affinity of oxotremorine towards the high (K_H) or low (K_L) affinity binding sites (Tables III and IV).

Binding parameters for oxotremorine were similarly obtained for cortical preparations at different ages. Oxotremorine affinity constants K_H and K_L in the cortex were similar to those found in the medulla-pons and cerebellum, and likewise showed no change over the developmental period studied. At day-5 only one population of binding sites was observed. By day 11 two sites were observed and the proportions of high to low affinity binding sites later (at day 16) achieved adult values. In the caudate-putamen and hippocampus the proportion of high affinity binding sites at all ages investigated was very low (about 10%), and the best fit procedure for a two-site model could not therefore be used. However, both the I_{50} values and the shape of the inhibition curves as a function of postnatal age show very little change in these regions.

The developmental pattern of oxotremorine binding in the various regions of ICR mouse brain resembles that reported for rats for carbachol binding i.e. the main difference between the neonatal and adult cortical preparations is not in the I_{50} values for carbachol inhibition of (^3H)-antagonist binding but in the proportion of their high affinity binding sites (13).

In our previous reports on regional heterogeneity (7)(11), we observed marked differences in the Hill slope obtained with different agonists in a given brain region: in both the hippocampus and the caudate-putamen the value for oxotremorine is ca. 1.0, while for acetylcholine the value is ca. 0.5; on the other hand, in the medulla-pons the Hill slope value for both agonists was ∿ 0.5. Analysis of the antagonist/agonist inhibition curves according to the two-site model indicate (Table V) that these differences stem not only differences in the proportion of high and low affinity binding sites recorded for oxotremorine and carbamylcholine or acetylcholine. In the cortex, hippocampus and caudate-putamen the proportion of high affinity binding sites for oxotremorine is less than 15%, whereas it is 40-50% for carbamylcholine or acetylcholine. On the other hand, in the cerebellum and medulla-pons the values recorded for these three agonists approximated much more closely to each other (Table V). When comparing these results to those observed in other mammalian brains, it is again evident that by the same analysis of the inhibition data for agonists according to the two site model the proportion of high affinity binding sites for oxotremorine in rat cortex and frog cortex (6) is lower (∿ 18%) than that for carbamylcholine (40-50%) (9)(10)(19).

Table V: Proportion of high affinity binding sites for muscarinic agonists in adult mice.

	Cerebellum	Medulla-pons	Cortex	Hippocampus	Caudate-putamen
Acetylcholine	0.72 - 0.74	0.57 - 0.60	0.48 - 0.53	0.49 - 0.49	0.58 - 0.48
Carbamylcholine	0.65 - 0.58	0.59 - 0.61	0.23 - 0.23	0.30 - 0.42	0.46 - 0.49
Oxotremorine	0.64 - 0.66	0.65 - 0.66	0.19 - 0.18	∿ 0.1	∿ 0.1

The proportion of high affinity binding sites was evaluated from inhibition curves of binding of 2 nM (^{3}H)-4NMPB by agonists using the non linear least square regression procedure. Values given are those obtained from two separate experiments. In the hippocampus and caudate-putamen, estimated values are given for oxotremorine.

According to these observations we conclude that in the cortex, hippocampus and caudate-putamen agonist binding cannot be described solely in terms of the binding of agonist to fixed receptor sites of high and low affinities. On the other hand, in the cerebellum and medulla-pons this explanation seems to fit well. We therefore suggest that agonist binding may be explained by at least two mechanisms: (i) induced interconversion of the muscarinic receptors by agonists, reflected in differences in the ratio of high to low affinity binding sites for different agonists (e.g. in the cortex). In this respect it is important to note that interconversion between agonist sites has been inferred from agonist binding studies in mammalian brain (20)(21)(22) and in *Torpedo* presynaptic membranes (17)(23)(24). (ii) Different pre-existing states of muscarinic receptors result in marked regional differences in agonist binding (e.g., oxotremorine and carbamylcholine in the medulla-pons versus cortex). Either mechanisms may be a consequence of different mediators coupled with muscarinic activation, such as a pre- and postsynaptic process mediated by the muscarinic receptor((17) and the accompanying manuscript and references therein).

We have found marked differences in the affinity of agonists towards the presynaptic muscainic receptor of Torpedo electric organ and the postsynaptic receptor. The agonist binding pattern in Torpedo more closely resembles that found in the cerebellum or medulla-pons than in the cortex, and led us to suggest that these brain regions may be enriched in populations of presynaptic autoreceptors (17). If cholinesterase and cholineacetyl-transferase (11) are cholinergic markers for presynaptic membranes, then their high levels in the medulla-pons (3)(11) would support this suggestion. According to this hypothesis, the appearance of high affinity binding sites in the cerebellum and medulla-pons would indicate the appearance of presynaptic terminals on which muscarinic receptors are located, while the appearance of low affinity sites would indicate the appearance of postsynaptic receptors. Therefore, further understanding of agonist binding, and especially of the characteristics of pre- and postsynaptic muscarinic receptors, may serve as a tool for synaptogenic studies of the cholinergic synapses. However, recent experiments in our laboratory have indicated that interconversion between high and low affinity sites can be induced by a variety of factors such as guanine nucleotides (25), temperature, pH, sugars (26) etc. Hence, conclusions about the nature of these receptors and their "region-specificity" should await further and more detailed experimentation.

Acknowledgements

We are indebted to Drs. N.J.M. Birdsall and T. Bartfai for letting us read yet unpublished papers.

Mrs. Ronit Galron provided excellent technical assistance.

REFERENCES

1. Ben-Barak, J. and Dudai, Y. Brain Res. (1979) 166, 245-257.
2. Yavin, E. and Harel, S. FEBS Lett. (1979) 97, 151-154.
3. Coyle, J.T. and Yamamura, H.I. Brain Res. (1976) 118, 429-440.

4. Hiley, C.R. Brit. J. Pharmacol. (1976) 53, 427p-428p.

5. Kloog, Y. and Sokolovsky, M. Brain Res. (1977) 134, 167-172.

6. Kloog, Y. and Sokolovsky, M. Brain Res. (1978) 144, 31-48.

7. Kloog, Y., Egozi, Y. and Sokolovsky, M. Mol. Pharmacol. (1979) 15, 545-558.

8. Birdsall, N.J.M. and Hulme, E.C. J. Neurochem. (1976) 27, 7-16.

9. Birdsall, N.J.M., Burgen, A.S.V. and Hulme, E.C. Mol. Pharmacol. (1978) 14, 723-736.

10. Birdsall, N.J.M., Burgen, A.S.V. and Hulme, E.C. In: Recent Advances in Receptor Chemistry. Gualtieri, Giannella, Melchiorre Eds. (Elsevier/North Holland Biomedical Press) (1979) pp. 71-95.

11. Kloog, Y., Egozi, Y. and Sokolovsky, M. FEBS Lett. (1978) 95, 265-268.

12. Birdsall, N.J.M., Hulme, E.C. and Burgen, A.S.V. Proc. Roy. Soc. London, In press.

13. Kuhar, M.J., Birdsall, N.J.M. and Burgen, A.S.V. Brain Res. (1980) In press.

14. Aronstram, R.S., Kellogg, C. and Abood, L.G. Brain Res. (1979) 162, 231-241.

15. Kloog, Y., Heron, D.S., Korczyn, A.D., Sachs, D.I. and Sokolovsky, M. Mol. Pharmacol. (1979) 15, 581-587.

16. Kloog, Y., Sach, D.I., Korczyn, A.D., Heron, D.S. and Sokolovsky, M. Biochem. Pharmacol. (1979) 28, 1505-1511.

17. Kloog, Y., Michaelson, D.M. and Sokolovsky, M. Brain Res. (1980) In press.

18. Sokolovsky, M., Egozi, Y. and Kloog, Y. In Progress in Neural Sci. Vol. 7 (1980) In press.

19. Birdsall, N.J.M., Burgen, A.S.V. and Hulme, E.C. Brain Res. (1980) In press.

20. Aronstram, R.S., Hoss, W. and Abood, L.G. Eur. J. Pharmac. (1977) 46, 279-283.

21. Aronstram, R.S. and Eldefrawi, M.E. Biochem. Pharmacol. (1979) 28, 701-703.

22. Hedlund, B. and Bartfai, T. Mol. Pharmacol., (1979) 15, 538-544.

23. Kloog, Y., Michaelson, D.M. and Sokolovsky, M. FEBS Lett. (1978) 95, 331-334.

24. Michaelson, D.M., Avissar, S., Kloog, Y. and Sokolovsky, M. Proc. Natl. Acad. Sci. USA (1979) 76, 6336-6340.

25. Sokolovsky, M., Gurwitz, D. and Galron, R., Biochem. Biophys. Res. Comm. (1980) In press.

26. Gurwitz, D. and Sokolovsky, M., Biochem. Biophys. Res. Comm. (1980) In press.

Neurotransmitters and their Receptors
Edited by U.Z. Littauer, Y. Dudai, I. Silman,
V.I. Teichberg and Z. Vogel

Ontogenesis and Modulation of Cholinergic Receptors in Rat Brain

Yadin Dudai, Jacob Ben-Barak, Israel Silman and Herbert Gazit

Department of Neurobiology, The Weizmann Institute of Science, Rehovot, Israel

ABSTRACT

The majority of cholinergic receptors in the rat hippocampal formation are muscarinic and bind [^{3}H]quinuclidinyl benzilate ([^{3}H]QNB) with high affinity. The rate of development of these receptors under normal conditions resembles that of the hippocampal presynaptic marker, acetylcholinesterase, and both processes may reflect the functional maturation of cholinergic synapses. However, deafferentation studies performed during development and at maturity indicate that the development and the level of hippocampal muscarinic receptors do not depend upon normal establishment and maintenance of presynaptic contacts. Despite this lack of sensitivity to deafferentation, the level of muscarinic receptors in several brain regions, including the hippocampus, was found to be affected by pharmacological manipulations. Thus administration of the muscarinic agonist oxotremorine led to a small but significant decrease in the level of [^{3}H]QNB-binding sites in several brain regions during development and at maturity. In contrast, administration of the muscarinic antagonist scopolamine led to a small but significant increase in the level of [^{3}H]QNB-binding sites. In addition, chronic administration of organophosphates, which are potent cholinesterase inhibitors, led to a marked decrease in the number of muscarinic binding sites in various brain regions. Deafferentation, or concomitant administration of a muscarinic antagonist, prevented the organophosphate-induced decrease in receptor level. The above results could be explained by assuming that a high level of a muscarinic agonist (e.g. injected oxotremorine or excess of non-hydrolyzed acetylcholine) down regulates the receptor. Experiments in rat brain cell culture support this hypothesis. The apparent insensitivity of receptor levels to denervation, in contrast to the sensitivity to pharmacological manipulations, is discussed.

INTRODUCTION

Receptors for neurotransmitters may play a role in modulating the development and maintenance of synaptic connections (1). It is, therefore, of interest to study what factors determine the ontogenesis and sensitivity of such receptors in the brain. We have set out to investigate this question by a combination of anatomical, biochemical and pharmacological methods, employing the cholinergic muscarinic system in rat brain as a model, with special emphasis on the hippocampal formation.

In the following, we report the results of five sets of experiments which were aimed at characterizing the development of muscarinic receptors in rat brain and their regulation. First, the ontogenesis of muscarinic binding sites in the hippocampal formation is described and compared to that of other components of the cholinergic system in the region, i.e. acetylcholinesterase (AChE) and α-bungarotoxin-binding nicotinic sites. Second, the effect of cholinergic deafferentation on the development and maintenance of cholinergic receptors in the hippocampus is described. Third, the effect of exposure to a cholinergic agonist and to a cholinergic antagonist on receptor sensitivity *in vivo* is presented. Fourth, the effect on receptor sensitivity of a chronic inhibition of AChE, the enzyme that hydrolyzes acetylcholine, is described. Finally, results of experiments on the modulation of muscarinic receptor levels of rat brain cells in culture are presented. Taken together, our studies suggest that the development and the level of muscarinic binding sites in the hippocampus do not depend upon normal establishment of presynaptic contacts; however, conditions exist under which cholinergic ligands can regulate the level of muscarinic receptors in brain.

MATERIALS AND METHODS

Animals. Wistar male rats (from the Weizmann Institute Animal Breeding Center) were used for all experiments. At the appropriate age the rats were sacrificed, the brain immediately removed and the appropriate regions dissected on ice. When the hippocampal formation was dissected, it included the hippocampus, the dentate gyrus and the subiculum. Tissue was homogenized (100 mg/ml) in ice cold 0.32 M sucrose in a glass-Teflon homogenizer driven by a Heidolph motor at half-maximal speed.

Septal and fornix lesions were performed as previously described (2,3).

Drug injections. The organophosphate Tetram (O,O-diethyl-S-(β-diethylamino) ethyl phosphorothiolate) was dissolved in 0.2 ml propylene glycol and injected s.c. at doses of 0.04-0.16 mg/kg at a schedule described under Results. The muscarinic agonist oxotremorine and the muscarinic antagonist scopolamine were dissolved in saline and injected s.c.

at doses of 0.5 mg/kg and 10 mg/kg, respectively, according to the schedule described under Results. Controls were injected in parallel with the vehicle only.

Assays. Binding of α-[^{125}I]bungarotoxin (α-[^{125}I]Btx; 30-60 Ci/mmol) to homogenates was assayed by filtration over Millipore EGWP 02500 filters, as described in Ref. 4. Binding of [^{3}H]quinuclidinyl benzilate ([^{3}H]QNB, 29.4 Ci/mmol, New England Nuclear) to homogenates was assayed by filtration over glass-fiber filters (GF/C) as described in Ref. 4. Acetylcholinesterase (AChE) activity was determined as described by Johnson and Russell (5), employing [^{3}H]acetylcholine (100-500 Ci/mmole, Radiochemical Centre, Amersham) as substrate. Choline acetyltransferase (CAT) activity was determined as described by Fonnum (6), employing [^{3}H]acetyl CoA (2.67 Ci/mmol, New England Nuclear) as substrate. Protein was determined according to Lowry et al. (7), using BSA as a standard. Results of assays are presented as values of representative determinations or as mean ± SEM. Statistical significance was determined by a two-tailed t-test.

RESULTS

A. Properties and ontogenesis of cholinergic binding sites in rat hippocampus

The hippocampus may serve as a suitable model for studying the development of cholinergic receptors in brain and the possible role of these receptors in developmental processes such as axonal invasion and synaptogenesis. The region is one of the richest cholinergic structures in the brain (8). Detailed information is available on its anatomy and development (9-14). Only one extrinsic cholinergic afferent, the septo-hippocampal tract, which provides about 85% of the cholinergic innervation to the region, has been identified (8,15,16). A massive cholinergic deafferentation is thus feasible.

Rat hippocampus contains two types of membrane-bound cholinergic binding sites: one is of a muscarinic nature and binds the muscarinic antagonist QNB with high affinity; the other is of a nicotinic nature and binds the nicotinic antagonist α-Btx with high affinity. QNB-binding sites are considered cholinergic muscarinic receptors (17). The physiological function of hippocampal α-Btx-binding sites is not yet clear (18).

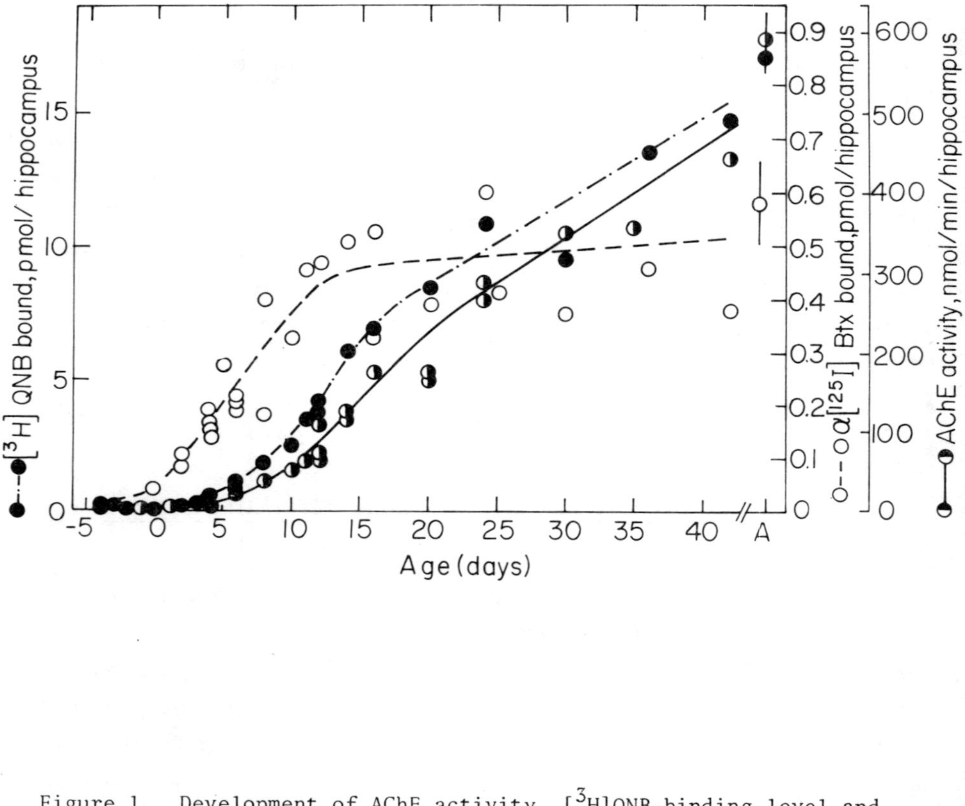

Figure 1. Development of AChE activity, $[^3H]$QNB-binding level and α-$[^{125}I]$Btx-binding level in the rat hippocampus as a function of age.

TABLE I: Binding properties of muscarinic and nicotinic sites in rat hippocampal homogenates

Ligand	K, [^{3}H]QNB-binding sites (M)	K, α-[^{125}I]Btx-binding sites (M)
[^{3}H]QNB	3×10^{-10}	-
α-[^{125}I]Btx	$>10^{-6}$**	2×10^{-9}
Atropine	1×10^{-9}	$>3 \times 10^{-4}$*
Scopolamine	5×10^{-10}	$>3 \times 10^{-4}$*
Dexetimide	4×10^{-10}	1×10^{-5}
DL-Muscarine	2×10^{-5}	$>3 \times 10^{-4}$*
Oxotremorine	1×10^{-6}	$>3 \times 10^{-4}$*
Acetylcholine***	1×10^{-5}	1×10^{-5}
Gallamine	6×10^{-6}	3×10^{-5}
Eserine	5×10^{-5}	2×10^{-4}
Nicotine	$>10^{-4}$*	1×10^{-6}
D-Tubocurarine	4×10^{-5}	2×10^{-6}
Dihydro-β-erythroidine	$>10^{-4}$*	1×10^{-5}
Decamethonium	6×10^{-5}	2×10^{-4}
Procaine	1×10^{-5}	3×10^{-4}*
DEFP	$>10^{-5}$*	$>10^{-5}$*
Concentration of sites	1.2 pmol/mg protein	0.04 pmol/mg protein

---

Aliquots of homogenate were preincubated for 30 min with the appropriate concentrations of ligands. Reaction was started by addition of either [^{3}H]QNB (final concentration 5 nM) or α-[^{125}I]Btx (final concentration 15 nM) and was carried out for 60 min (QNB binding) or 120 min (Btx binding) at 25°C. IC_{50} values were determined from plots of relative specific binding vs. ligand concentration and apparent affinities (K values) were estimated from the relation $K = IC_{50}/(1 + \frac{[L]}{Kd})$, were [L] is the labeled ligand concentration and Kd is its apparent dissociation constant. It should be noted that the Hill coefficient of some agonists for the binding sites is less than 1.0 and thus the affinities obtained by this calculation are only an approximation.

DEFP, diethylfluorosphophate, a potent AChE inhibitor.

---

* Little or no effect at this concentration

** Determined with non-labeled Btx

*** Determined in the presence of 10^{-5}M DEFP.

QNB-binding sites comprise the majority of cholinergic binding-sites in the rat hippocampus (about 17 pmol per adult hippocampus, or about 1.2 pmol per mg protein). Binding of [^{3}H]QNB (K_d = 0.3 x 10^{-9}M) to hippocampal homogenates is displaced by low concentrations of muscarinic ligands but not of nicotinic ligands (Table I). The binding properties of hippocampal α-Btx-binding sites are also presented in Table I, for comparison.

It has been shown by other groups that muscarinic binding sites are concentrated mainly in the hippocampal stratum radiatum and stratum oriens and in the dentate stratum moleculare (19,20). We have demonstrated that α-Btx-binding sites are concentrated in the outer third of stratum oriens and in the dentate polymorphic layer (21).

The muscarinic and nicotinic binding sites in the rat hippocampus differ not only in their concentration, binding properties and localization, but also in their ontogenesis. We found that [^{3}H]QNB-binding sites develop at a rate which resembles that of the development of AChE (the latter enzyme is considered to be of a presynaptic origin in the hippocampus) (Fig. 1). Both processes seem to proceed essentially in parallel with the maturation of most synapses in the region (12-14). In contrast, the level of α-Btx-binding sites attains mature values much earlier, before the majority of synaptogenetic events in the area are completed.

The studies described below are concerned only with [^{3}H]QNB-binding sites. Some additional properties of rat brain α-Btx-binding sites are described by us elsewhere (2,4,21).

B. Effect of cholinergic deafferentation on the development and the level of muscarinic binding-sites in rat hippocampus

As described above the rate of development of muscarinic receptors, as revealed by specific binding of [^{3}H]QNB, is similar to the rate of development of the hippocampal presynaptic marker, AChE. It is thus pertinent to ask whether the presynaptic terminals are essential for normal development of the postsynaptic receptors. Septohippocampal axons start to invade the hippocampus at about 4 days postnatal, and proceed toward the temporal end of the region until, about a week later, all parts of the hippocampal formation are innervated by cholinergic afferents (13). Major synaptogenetic events take place in the region between 11 and 25 days after birth (14). Lesions of the septum during the first postnatal days are thus expected to prevent the formation of most of the cholinergic synapses in the hippocampus. We set out, therefore, to investigate the effect of such lesions on the subsequent development of muscarinic receptors.

Septal lesion at an age of 2-4 days postnatal led to a permanent loss of the fimbria and to a significant (ca. 20%) reduction in size and weight of the adult hippocampus, apparently due mainly to reduction in dendritic layers (3). The weight reduction was evident only when the lesion was placed in newborn rats but not after adult lesions. A marked decrease was observed in the levels of AChE and CAT. The effect of this early lesion on AChE activity was already detected 2 days after the operation (Fig. 2). A small increase in AChE level was detected in lesioned animals until the third week after birth, but enzyme activity increased very little, if at all, subsequently (Fig. 2). In contrast, a sharp increase in AChE levels took place in non-lesioned animals during the third week after birth and total activity continued to increase gradually until an age of about 7 weeks. The residual AChE activity in the adult was dependent upon the age at which the lesion was performed: it was (28 ± 2)% of normal (expressed as total activity per hippocampus) after a lesion in 2-4 day old rats, (20 ± 2)% after a lesion in 13 day old rats, and (13 ± 1)% following adult lesion.

In contrast, [^{3}H]QNB-binding levels increased in a similar developmental pattern both in control and in early-lesioned animals (Fig. 2). Specific activity at maturity was essentially the same in lesioned and non-lesioned rats. Total binding per hippocampus was smaller in operated animals, but this reduction could be accounted for by the significant weight reduction and the slight decrease in protein content observed following early lesions. No significant difference was detected in the apparent K_d for [^{3}H]QNB and in the affinity of the muscarinic agonist oxotremorine, as estimated by displacement of [^{3}H]QNB binding, in homogenates of lesioned and control animals. No alterations were detected in the level or affinity of [^{3}H]QNB-binding sites after an adult lesion. Thus our results indicate that the development and the level of receptor sites, as revealed by [^{3}H]QNB-binding, does not seem to depend upon normal establishment of presynaptic contacts.

C. Effect of exposure to cholinergic ligands *in vivo*

The observation that massive denervation does not significantly affect the number of [^{3}H]QNB-binding sites suggests that muscarinic

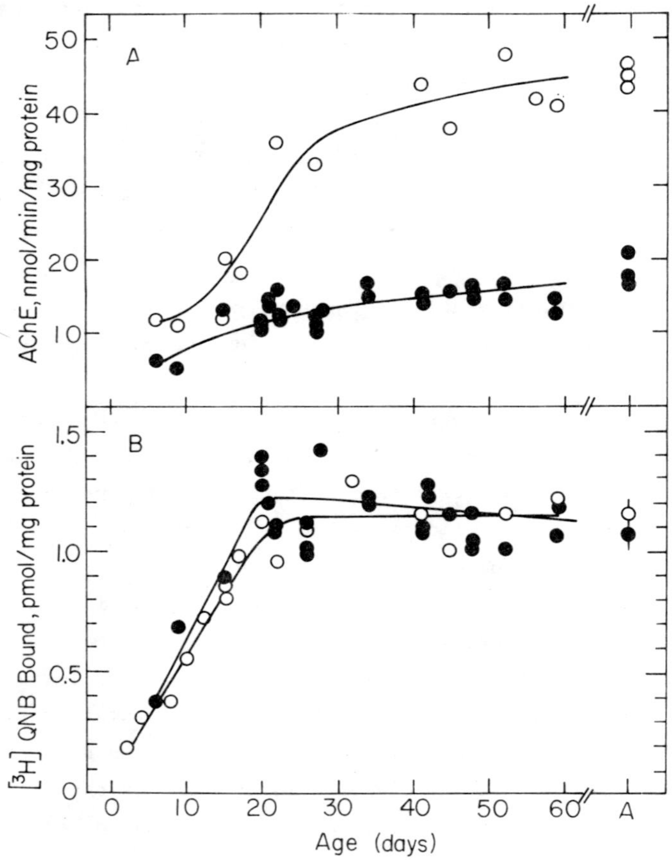

Figure 2. Development of AChE activity (A) and of [^{3}H]QNB-binding sites (B) in the hippocampus of early-septal-lesioned (●——●) and of control (o——o) rats as a function of age. The septal lesion was performed at day 4 postnatal.

TABLE II: Effect of in vivo administration of oxotremorine and scopolamine on [^{3}H]QNB-binding levels in various areas of rat brain

Region	Brain Stem		Hippocampus		Striatum		Cortex	
Age	Oxo	Scop	Oxo	Scop	Oxo	Scop	Oxo	Scop
11 days	78 ± 2**	111 ± 1	87 ± 4**	155 ± 3***	87 ± 4*	106 ± 5	83 ± 3***	129 ± 2***
21 days	92 ± 2*	117 ± 2***	94 ± 2	123 ± 3***	84 ± 2***	89 ± 3	95 ± 2	130 ± 4***
adult	85 ± 4**	106 ± 4	84 ± 3*	116 ± 1**	90 ± 2*	110 ± 1	94 ± 5	119 ± 4**

Rats were injected s.c. with oxotremorine (0.5 mg/kg, twice a day) or with scopolamine (10 mg/kg, once a day) in saline. Control animals were injected with saline only. Newborn rats were injected from birth until 24 hr before sacrifice at the indicated age. Adult rats were injected for 7 days with oxotremorine and for 30 days with scopolamine until 24 hr before sacrifice; the results for scopolamine effects on brain stem are given for a 7 day injection period only. Data are presented as mean ± SEM of percentage of control values, for 5-10 imals each.

* $P < 0.05$ (two tailed t-test).
** $P < 0.01$
*** $P < 0.001$

receptors in brain, in contrast to several other types of receptors (22,23), are not regulated by the availability of their ligands. However, several lines of evidence indicate that this is not the case and that conditions exist under which the level of muscarinic binding sites is modulated by their ligands.

The first piece of suggestive evidence comes from pharmacological experiments. Some muscarinic ligands can penetrate the blood brain barrier. Among them are the agonist oxotremorine and the antagonist scopolamine. We have investigated the effect of administration of these ligands, injected systematically, on the level of [^{3}H]QNB-binding sites in various brain regions. We were aware of the possibility that effects on the muscarinic sites *in vivo* may not necessarily be ascribed solely to a direct interaction of the injected ligand with the receptor; but such an effect, if revealed, may indicate a ligand-induced regulation and deserves further investigation.

Results of the *in vivo* ligand administration experiments are presented in Table II. It is seen that, in general, administration of the agonist oxotremorine induced a small but, in most cases, significant decrease in the level of [^{3}H]QNB-binding sites in various brain regions, both during development and at maturity. In contrast, administration of the antagonist scopolamine induced a significant increase in the level of [^{3}H]QNB-binding sites. The effect of oxotremorine was apparent after 24 hr and did not markedly increased upon further injections; the effect of scopolamine was apparent only after chronic injection for ca. one week. In both cases the alteration in [^{3}H]QNB-binding levels was apparently due to a change in the number of binding sites but not in affinity (Figs. 3,4).

D. Effect of exposure to organophosphates

If the presence of agonist leads to down regulation of the muscarinic receptor, as the results of oxotremorine administration may suggest, one should expect pharmacological manipulations which increase acetylcholine levels *in vivo* to induce a decrease in receptor levels. Inhibition of AChE may lead to accumulation of excess non-hydrolyzed acetylcholine in the vicinity of the receptor. Such inhibition may be obtained by administration of organophosphates, which are potent irreversible blockers of the enzyme and penetrate the blood-brain barrier. We have set out to investigate the effect of chronic administration of one such organophosphate,

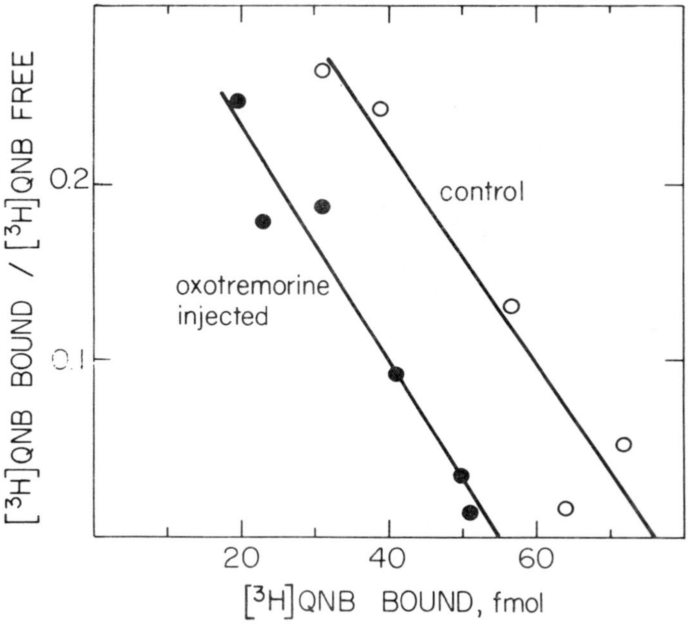

Figure 3. Binding of [^{3}H]QNB to a particulate brain-stem preparation from adult rats chronically injected with the muscarinic agonist oxotremorine (0.5 mg/kg, twice a day for 6 days) or with saline. Aliquots of homogenate were centrifuged at 20,000 xg for 30 min and the binding was assayed in the resuspended pellet. Data are presented as Scatchard plots. Each point is a mean of 3 animals. The figure is adapted from Ref. 40.

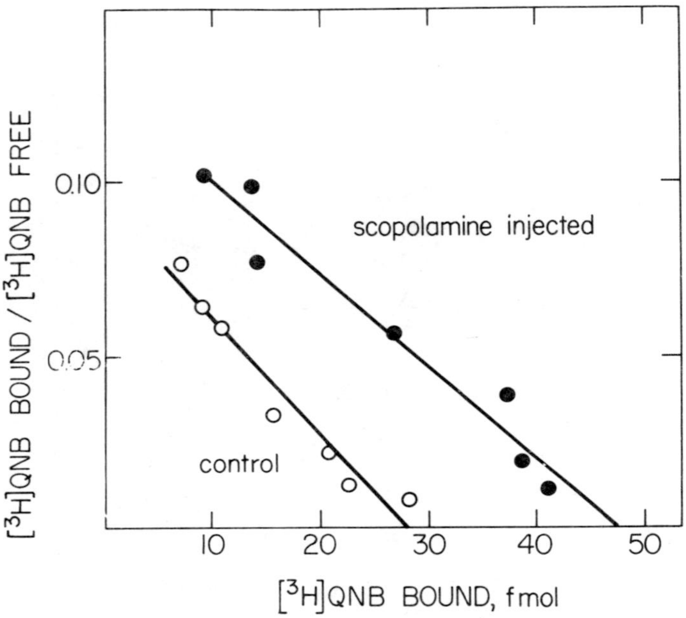

Figure 4. Binding of $[^3H]$QNB to a particulate hippocampal preparation from adult rats chronically injected with the muscarinic antagonist scopolamine (10 mg/kg once a day for 6 days) or with saline. Aliquots were prepared as in Fig. 3. Data are presented as Scatchard plots. Each point is a mean of 3 animals. The figure is adapted from Ref. 40.

TABLE III: AChE activity and $[^3H]$QNB-binding levels in rat brain following chronic administration of Tetram

Region	AChE activity, nmol/min/mg/protein				$[^3H]$QNB-binding level, pmol/mg protein			
	Control		Tetram		Control		Tetram	
Cortex	50 ± 4	100%	11 ± 1	22%	1.07 ± 0.05	100%	0.77 ± 0.10	72%
Hippocampus	35 ± 3	100%	9 ± 1	26%	0.70 ± 0.10	100%	0.38 ± 0.07	54%
Hypothalamus	24 ± 1	100%	10 ± 1	42%	0.35 ± 0.02	100%	0.31 ± 0.03	89%
Thalamus	44 ± 3	100%	9 ± 1	20%	0.63 ± 0.04	100%	0.42 ± 0.02	67%
Caudate	236 ± 16	100%	38 ± 2	16%	1.39 ± 0.06	100%	0.63 ± 0.05	45%
Brain stem	71 ± 4	100%	19 ± 2	27%	0.19 ± 0.04	100%	0.10 ± 0.01	53%

Male adult rats were injected s.c. 3 times weekly for 2 months with 0.16 mg/kg of Tetram in 0.2 ml propylene glycol. Control animals were injected with the vehicle only. AChE activity and QNB-binding levels were then determined in homogenates of the various brain regions. Values are mean ± SEM for 5-8 animals each.

TABLE IV: [^{3}H]QNB-binding levels in hippocampus and cortex of control and fornix-lesioned rats following chronic administration of Tetram

Treatment	Hippocampus		Cortex	
	pmol/mg	%	pmol/mg	%
Control	1.16±0.03	100	1.28±0.02	100
Tetram	0.89±0.03	77**	0.96±0.03	75**
Bilateral F.L. +Tetram	1.21±0.04	104	0.88±0.03	69**
Unilateral F.L. +Tetram, lesioned side	1.02±0.05	88*	0.86±0.03	67**
Unilateral F.L. +Tetram non-lesioned side	0.81±0.03	70***	0.88±0.04	69**

Bilateral or unilateral fornix lesions (=F.L.) were performed in adult male rats as previously described (2). Tetram was chronically administered as described in Ref. 39. AChE activity was reduced in both areas by the chronic exposure of Tetram to 13-15% of control and the lesion further decreased it in the hippocampus (but not in the frontal cortex) to 4-5% of control. Values are presented as mean ± SEM for 8 animals each and as percentage of control.

* $P<0.05$ (two tailed t-test)

** $P<0.001$

*** $P<0.001$, $P<0.01$ for the difference from the lesioned side.

Tetram, on [^{3}H]QNB-binding levels in various brain regions.

The chronic administration of Tetram at 0.16 mg/kg (i.e., 0.4 LD_{50}) led to a decrease of over 50% in AChE levels in all brain regions tested (Table III). The decrease observed ranged from over 60% in the hypothalamus to over 80% in the striatum. Values close to these were observed with doses of 0.08 mg/kg and above.

[^{3}H]QNB-binding levels were also reduced in most of the brain regions studied (Table III). The decrease observed for chronic treatment with 0.16 mg/kg Tetram ranged from 10% in the hypothalamus to over 50% in the striatum. Again decreases close to the maximum were obtained already at 0.08 mg/kg Tetram. A good correlation was obtained between the decreases in AChE activity as a function of Tetram dosage and the decreases in [^{3}H]QNB-binding levels in all areas except the hypothalamus. Scatchard plots revealed that the reduction in [^{3}H]QNB-binding was due to a decrease in the number of binding sites and not to a change in affinity. Tetram itself reversibly inhibited [^{3}H]QNB-binding <u>in vitro</u> only at relatively high concentrations and aliquots of homogenates from brain of treated animals, when mixed with homogenates from untreated animals, did not affect the [^{3}H]QNB-binding capacity or the AChE activity of the latter. It is thus unlikely that the effect of chronic administration of Tetram on the muscarinic binding sites <u>in vivo</u> was due to direct interaction of the organophosphate with the receptor. In addition, no significant decrease in [^{3}H]QNB-binding levels was detected in cortex, hippocampus or striatum from animals sacrified 24 hr after a single injection of 0.12 mg/kg Tetram, although a marked decrease was observed under such conditions in AChE levels.

We have also observed effects similar to those obtained with Tetram with another organophosphate, Paraoxon.

As stated above, the effect of organophosphates on the receptor may be explained by assuming that an increase in the level of acetylcholine, due to inhibition of the enzyme that hydrolyzes it, down-regulates the level of receptor. If this explanation is correct, then cholinergic denervation should prevent the effect of organophosphates on receptor levels. We decided, therefore, to test the effect of fornix lesion on the Tetram-induced decrease in [^{3}H]QNB-binding levels in the hippocampus. The results of such experiments are presented in Table IV. It is seen that the lesion clearly prevented the organophosphate-induced effect on receptor levels in the hippocampus but not in the frontal cortex, the

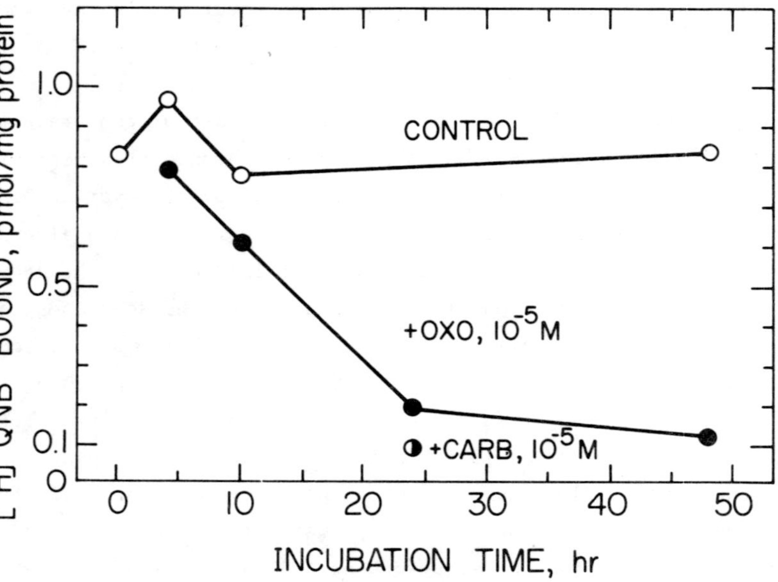

Figure 5. [^{3}H]QNB binding levels in rat cerebral cells in culture incubated in the presence and in the absence of muscarinic agonists. Dissociated brain cell cultures were prepared from fetal rat brain as described in Ref. 24. Aliquots of agonists were added at day 14 *in vitro*. The cells were rinsed at the indicated time, homogenized and centrifuged at 27,000 xg for 30 min. The pellet was resuspended and assayed for specific [^{3}H]QNB-binding as described in Ref. 24. OXO, oxotremorine, CARB, carbamylcholine.

AChE level in which is not significantly affected by destruction of the fornix. The data thus demonstrate that the presynaptic terminals are required for the organophosphate to exert its effect on muscarinic receptor levels in the rat hippocampus. Fornix lesion also depletes the hippocampus of non-cholinergic inputs; other possible mechanisms, e.g. involving heterosynaptic pathways, cannot therefore be utterly excluded as yet. Nevertheless, the observations are again compatible with the hypothesis that the decrease in the level of muscarinic binding-sites in brain, observed following administration of sublethal closes of organophosphates, is due to down-regulation of muscarinic receptors by the excess of non-hydrolyzed acetylcholine.

E. Effect of exposure to cholinergic ligands in culture

The *in vivo* studies described above provide evidence that conditions exist under which cholinergic ligands may modulate the level of muscarinic receptors, but an *in vitro* system may prove advantageous in elucidating the molecular mechanisms involved. We set out, therefore, to study the effects of exposure to cholinergic ligands on the level of muscarinic binding sites in rat cerebral cells in culture. Such cultures contain [^{3}H]QNB-binding sites with properties similar to those reported for mature brain (24).

We found that exposure to low concentrations of the muscarinic agonists oxotremorine and carbamylcholine markedly reduces the number of [^{3}H]QNB-binding sites in the cultures. In a typical experiment, about 75% reduction in receptor levels was detected after 24 hr incubation with 10^{-5}M oxotremorine (Fig. 5). In contrast, incubation with 10^{-6}M atropine for 24 hr led to an increase of 25% in [^{3}H]QNB-binding levels.

The *in vitro* experiments thus provide more direct evidence for the regulation of [^{3}H]QNB-binding sites by muscarinic ligands. Experiments to elucidate the molecular mechanisms underlying this regulation are now in progress.

DISCUSSION

Our studies demonstrate that the development of normal levels of [^{3}H]QNB-binding sites in rat hippocampus may proceed normally even in the absence of cholinergic presynaptic signals, one of which is the transmitter itself. Deafferentation in an adult brain also does not significantly affect [^{3}H]QNB-binding levels in the hippocampus. The latter observation is in accord with the lack of receptor-mediated muscarinic supersensitivity in several other systems studied to date (25-27).

Taken alone, these results suggest that the level of muscarinic receptors is not sensitive to the presence of acetylcholine. However, our pharmacological experiments suggest that this is not necessarily the case. Thus administration of a muscarinic agonist leads to a small but significant decrease in the number of [^{3}H]QNB-binding sites in several brain regions; administration of a muscarinic antagonist leads to a small but significant increase in the number of [^{3}H]QNB-binding sites in several brain regions, and administration of an organophosphate, which causes marked inhibition of AChE, leads also to a marked decrease in the level of [^{3}H]QNB-binding sites in several brain regions. In addition, the *in vitro* studies demonstrate marked ligand-induced alterations in muscarinic receptor level.

Supersensitivity induced by antagonists may be ascribed to the blocking of the agonist binding-site and hence to the prevention of a putative agonist-induced decrease in the number of binding-sites (e.g., Ref. 28). If prevention of receptor occupancy by an agonist is sufficient to induce supersensitivity one should expect to detect muscarinic supersentivity following denervation, but this is not the case. So why do hippocampal muscarinic receptors respond by supersensitivity to exposure to an antagonist but not to denervation? Several hypotheses may be suggested. One possibility is that a residual acetylcholine level, of non-septal origin, may be adequate to maintain normal receptor levels, since denervation depletes the hippocampus of most of its AChE activity. Another possibility is that the cell responds by supersensitivity to an antagonist-induced conformational change in the muscarinic receptor molecule and the presence of an agonist need not be invoked. A third possibility is that the presence of presynaptic terminals is required for supersensitivity to occur in this system. The observation that the effect is already observed at day 4 postnatal, before cholinergic septal afferents are detected in the hippocampus, does not seem to favor such an hypothesis. Finally it is possible that muscarinic receptors may be heterogeneous not only with respect to their ligand binding properties (29), but also with respect to their long-term regulation by ligands. Thus, for example, one might postulate the presence of postsynaptic receptors which do not display denervation supersensitivity, and of distinct putative extrasynaptic receptors which are modulated by pharmacological manipulations.

The ligand-induced modulations in muscarinic receptor level observed *in vitro* (see above and Refs. 30-32) seem to be analogous to those obtained *in vivo* after injections of muscarinic drugs. The *in vivo* effects of the agonist are smaller than those observed *in vitro*. This may be due to several possibilities:

a. Only a small fraction of the ligands injected *in vivo* reach the receptors and occupy them only for short periods.

b. Desensitization processes, leading to altered agonist binding properties, may differ *in vivo* and *in vitro*.

c. The cholinergic ligands, in addition to their direct occupancy-induced effect on postsynaptic receptor levels, may activate indirectly additional mechanisms which can counteract the direct effect of the ligand on the receptor level. For example, oxotremorine may bind to putative muscarinic presynaptic receptors which regulate acetylcholine release, leading to inhibition of release and hence to a decreased level of total agonists in the cleft (33).

d. As mentioned above, it is possible that muscarinic receptors *in vivo* are heterogenous with regard to regulation by ligands and that only part of them respond by altered level to occupancy by agonists or antagonists. The proportion of the latter type may be higher in culture.

Further studies on the regulation of muscarinic binding sites in rat brain cell cultures may shed light on some of the molecular mechanisms underlying modulations in the sensitivity of muscarinic receptors *in vitro*. It is plausible to assume that such ligand-induced modulations play a role in the etiology of some pathological conditions. Thus, for example, a decrease in cholinergic activity is implicated in tardive dyskinesia (34) and it was suggested that this may be due to chronic desensitization of muscarinic receptors resulting from prolonged exposure to acetylcholine (31). A ligand-induced decrease in the number of muscarinic receptors may be involved in some of the neurological and affective disorders observed in humans after exposure to sublethal doses of organophosphates (35-38). Further studies on the modulation of muscarinic receptors may lead not only to better understanding of factors that determine the efficacy of transmission in brain but may also elucidate

ACKNOWLEDGMENTS

This work was supported by grants from the United-States-Israel Binational Science Foundation, Jerusalem, and from the Israel Center for Psychobiology-Charles Smith Family Foundation, Jerusalem (to Y.D.). Y.D. is incumbent of the Barecha Foundation Career Development Chair.

REFERENCES

1. Changeux, J.P. and Danchin, A., Selective stabilization of developing synapses as a mechanism for the specification of neural networks, Nature 264 (1976) 705-712.

2. Dudai, Y. and Segal, M., α-Bungarotoxin binding sites in rat hippocampus: Localization in postsynaptic cells, Brain Res. 154 (1978) 167-171.

3. Ben-Barak, J. and Dudai, Y., Early septal lesion: Effect on the development of the cholinergic system in rat hippocampus, Brain Res. 185 (1980) 323-324.

4. Ben-Barak, J. and Dudai, Y., Cholinergic binding sites in rat hippocampal formation: Properties and ontogenesis, Brain Res. 166 (1979) 245-257.

5. Johnson, C.D. and Russell, R.L., A rapid simple radiometric assay for cholinesterase suitable for multiple determinations, Analyt. Biochem. 64 (1975) 229-238.

6. Fonnum, F., A rapid radiochemical method for the determination of choline acetyltransferase, J. Neurochem. 24 (1975) 407-409.

7. Lowry, O.H., Rosebrough, N.J., Farr, A.L. and Randall, R.J., Protein measurement with the Folin phenol reagent, J. Biol. Chem. 193 (1951) 265-275.

8. Lewis, P.K. and Shute, C.C.D., The cholinergic limbic system: Projection of hippocampal formation, medial cortex nuclei of the ascending cholinergic reticular system and the subfornical organ and supraoptic crest, Brain 90 (1967) 521-539.

9. Altman, J. and Das, G.D., Autoradiographic and histological evidence of postnatal hippocampal neurogenesis in rats, J. Comp. Neurol. 124 (1965) 319-335.

10. Angevine, J.B., Time of neuron origin in the hippocampal region, Exp. Neurol. 2 Suppl. (1965) 1-70.

11. Bayer, S.A. and Altman, J., Hippocampal development in the rat. Cytogenesis and morphogenesis examined with autoradiography and low-level X-irradiation, J. Comp. Neurol. 158 (1974) 55-80.

12. Cotman, C., Taylor, D. and Lynch, G., Ultrastructural changes in synapses in the dentate gyrus of the rat during development, Brain Res. 63 (1973) 205-213.

13. Matthews, D.A., Nadler, J.V., Lynch, G.S. and Cotman, C.W., Development of cholinergic innervation in the hippocampal formation of the rat. I. Histochemical demonstration of acetylcholinesterase activity, Develop. Biol. 36 (1974) 130-141.

14. Nadler, J.V., Matthews, D.A., Cotman, C.W. and Lynch, G.S., Development of cholinergic innervation in the hippocampal formation of the rat. II. Quantitative changes in choline acetyltransferase

and acetylcholinesterase activities, Develop. Biol. 36 (1974) 142-154.

15. Lewis, P.K., Shute, C.C.D. and Silver, A., Confirmation from choline acetylase analysis of a massive cholinergic innervation to the rat hippocampus, J. Physiol. 191 (1967) 215-224.

16. Storm-Mathisen, J., Quantitative histochemistry of acetylcholinesterase in rat hippocampal region correlated to histochemical staining, J. Neurochem. 17 (1970) 739-750.

17. Yamamura, H.I. and Snyder, S.H., Muscarinic cholinergic binding in rat brain, Proc. Nat. Acad. Sci. 71 (1974) 1725-1729.

18. Hunt, S. and Schmidt, J., The relationship of α-bungarotoxin binding activity and cholinergic termination within the rat hippocampus, Neurosci. 4 (1979) 585-592.

19. Kuhar, M.J. and Yamamura, H.I., Localization of cholinergic muscarinic receptors in rat brain by light microscopic radioautography, Brain Res. 110 (1976) 229-243.

20. Rotter, A., Birdsall, N.J.M., Field, P.M. and Raisman, G., Muscarinic receptors in the central nervous system of the rat. II. Distribution of binding of [^{3}H]propylbenzilylcholine mustard in the midbrain and hindbrain, Brain Res. Rev. 1 (1979) 167-183.

21. Segal, M., Dudai, Y. and Amsterdam, A., Distribution of an α-bungarotoxin-binding cholinergic nicotinic receptor in rat brain, Brain Res. 148 (1978) 105-119.

22. Raff, M., Self regulation of membrane receptors, Nature 259 (1976) 265-266.

23. Thesleff, S. and Sellin, L.C., Denervation supersensitivity, Trends in Neurosci. 3, (1980) 122-126.

24. Dudai, Y. and Yavin, E., Ontogenesis of muscarinic receptors and acetylcholinesterase in differentiating rat cerebral cells in culture, Brain Res. 155 (1978) 368-373.

25. Burt, D.R., Muscarinic receptor binding in rat sympathetic ganglia is unaffected by denervation, Brain Res. 143 (1978) 573-579.

26. Sachs, D.I., Kloog, Y., Korczyn, A.D., Heron, D.S. and Sokolovsky, M., Denervation, supersensitivity and muscarinic receptor in cat iris, Biochem. Pharmacol. 28 (1979) 1513-1518.

27. Rotter, A., Birdsall, N.J.M., Burgen, A.S.V., Field, P.M., Smolen, A. and Raisman, G., Muscarinic receptors in the central nervous system of the rat. IV. A comparison of the effects of axotomy and deafferentation on the binding of [^{3}H]propylbenzilylcholine mustard and associated synaptic changes in the hyppoglossal and pontine nuclei, Brain Res. Rev. 1 (1979) 207-224.

28. Siman, R.G. and Klein, W.L., Cholinergic activity regulates muscarinic receptors in central nervous system cultures, Proc. Nat. Acad. Sci. USA 76 (1979) 4141-4145.

29. Birdsall, N.J.M., Burgen, A.S.V. and Hulme, E.C., The binding of agonists to brain muscarinic receptors, Mol. Pharmacol. 14 (1978) 723-736.

30. Galper, J.B. and Smith, T.W., Properties of muscarinic acetylcholine receptors in heart cell cultures, Proc. Nat. Acad. Sci. USA 75 (1978) 5831-5835.

31. Taylor, J.E., El-Fakanany, E. and Richelson, E., Long term regulation of muscarinic acetylcholine receptors on cultured nerve cells, Life Sci. 25 (1979) 2181-2187.

32. Shifrin, G.S. and Klein, W.L., Regulation of muscarinic acetylcholine receptor concentration in cloned neuroblastoma cells, J. Neurochem. 34 (1980) 993-999.

33. Szerb, J.C., Hadhazy, P. and Dudar, J.D., Release of [^{3}H]acetylcholine from rat hippocampal slices: Effect of septal lesion and of graded concentrations of muscarinic agonists and antagonists, Brain Res. 128 (1977) 285-291.

34. Van Woert, M.H., Parkinson's disease, Tardive dyskinesia and Huntington's Chorea, in Biology of Cholinergic Function (A.M. Goldberg and I. Hanin, eds.), Raven Press, N.Y. (1976), pp. 583-601.

35. Gershon, S. and Shaw, F.M., Psychiatric sequelae of chronic exposure to organophosphorus insecticides, Lancet 1 (1961) 1371-1374.

36. Biskind, M. and Mobbs, R.F., Psychiatric manifestations from insecticide exposure, J. Am. Med. Ass. 220 (1972) 1248.

37. Levin, H.S., Rodnitzky, R.L. and Mick, D.L., Anxiety associated with exposure to organophosphate compounds, Arch. Gen. Psychiat. 33 (1976) 225-228.

38. Korsak, R.J. and Safo, M.M., Effect of chronic organophosphate pesticide exposure on the central nervous system, Clin. Toxicol. 11 (1977) 83-95.

39. Gazit, H., Silman, I. and Dudai, Y., Administration of an organophosphate causes a decrease in muscarinic receptor levels in rat brain, Brain Res. 174 (1979) 351-356.

40. Ben-Barak, J., Gazit, H., Silman, I. and Dudai, Y., *In vivo* modulation of muscarinic receptor levels in rat brain by cholinergic ligands, Submitted for publication.

Neurotransmitters and their Receptors
Edited by U.Z. Littauer, Y. Dudai, I. Silman,
V.I. Teichberg and Z. Vogel

Muscarinic Receptor Binding: Modulation by Nucleotides and Ions

E.C. Hulme, N.J.M. Birdsall, C.P. Berrie and A.S.V. Burgen
National Institute for Medical Research, Mill Hill, London N.W.7 1AA, U.K.

SUMMARY

GTP analogues strongly inhibit the binding of agonists and enhance the binding of antagonists to muscarinic acetylcholine receptors in rat heart, but only exert small effects in rat brain. In the heart, low ionic strength conditions generate heterogeneity in the binding curve for the classical antagonist N-methylscopolamine; this heterogeneity is abolished by micromolar concentrations of guanine nucleotides, which also appear to convert high affinity agonist binding sites to low affinity sites. Inorganic ions potentiate the effects of nucleotides on agonist binding, but inhibit their effects on antagonist binding.

INTRODUCTION

Guanine nucleotides strongly inhibit the binding of potent agonists to muscarinic receptors in heart homogenates (1-3). Under near physiological conditions of ionic strength, effects on the binding of antagonists are limited to a small enhancement of the affinity constant (1-2). Under such conditions, binding curves for muscarinic agonists in both brain and heart preparations are flattened in appearance, and best described by the superposition of several Langmuir isotherms, corresponding to discrete populations of agonist binding sites (1-8), while the binding of classical antagonists is adequately described by the simple Langmuir isotherm, indicating the presence of apparently homogeneous populations of antagonist binding sites (7-8). We have now made the novel observation that in the heart, alteration of ionic conditions can lead to the appearance of heterogeneity in antagonist binding profiles, and to the emergence of a strong nucleotide effect on the antagonist-receptor interaction.

MATERIALS AND METHODS

Binding measurements were made using a microcentrifugation assay as described previously (8). Whole rat hearts were homogenised (1) in a buffer containing 20 mM hepes, buffered to pH 7.5 with tris base (tris/hepes), filtered through cheesecloth, pelleted, and the pellet resuspended in tris/hepes buffer. Homogenates were diluted to a final tissue concentration of 20 mg wet weight/ml, supplemented with inorganic salts as appropriate, preincubated for 10 min at 30°C and then pipetted in 1 ml aliquots into microcentrifuge tubes containing ^{3}H-N-methyl-scopolamine (^{3}H-NMS)* and unlabelled competing drugs and nucleotides as indicated. Incubations were carried out for 20 min at 30°C (10 min with hydrolysable nucleotides) and terminated by centrifugation for 5 min at 14,000 g. Some incubations were performed in a buffer containing 100 mM NaCl/10 mM $MgCl_2$/20 mM hepes, adjusted to pH 7.5 with NaOH (Na/Mg/hepes) as described previously (1).

Non specific binding was measured by the inclusion of 10^{-6} M unlabelled 3-quinuclidinylbenzilate in the incubation medium, and subtracted from total binding to obtain receptor-specific binding.

Binding curves were fitted to a multiple site model of binding described by the equation

$$P\ (\text{occupancy}) = \sum_i \frac{\alpha_i K_i C}{1 + K_i C}$$

where α_i is the proportion of the ith binding site, whose affinity constant for the ligand C is denoted K_i. Both the fitting procedure and other aspects of data analysis were as described previously (4,8).

RESULTS

Nucleotide effects in the presence of sodium and magnesium ions

Figure 1 shows binding curves for (a) the potent muscarinic agonist carbachol, and (b) the antagonist ^{3}H-N-methylscopolamine measured in Na/Mg/hepes buffer in the absence and presence of 10^{-3} M GTP. In the absence of GTP, the binding curve for the agonist was very flattened; analysis by least-squares curve fitting to a multiple sites model of binding revealed the presence of two major populations of binding sites, with affinity constants of 2 x 10^7 M^{-1} (superhigh affinity sites; SH) and 5 x 10^5 M^{-1} (high affinity sites; H) comprising 33% and 56% of the total, and a minor population of low affinity sites (L) with an affinity of 10^4 M^{-1} making up the remainder. In the presence of the nucleotide, the curve shifted to much higher carbachol concentrations,

* Abbreviations used: NMS - N-methylscopolamine; GTP - guanosine triphosphate; GMPPNP - 5'- guanylylimidodiphosphate; GMPPCP - guanylyl (β,γ-methylene-diphosphonate; GTPγS - guanosine 5'-O(3-thiotriphosphate).

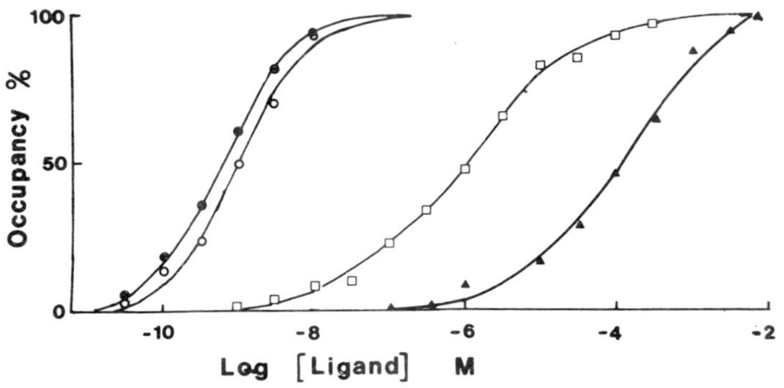

Figure 1. Binding of ^{3}H-NMS (●,O) and carbachol inhibition of binding of ^{3}H-NMS (3×10^{-10} M;□,▲) to rat heart muscarinic receptors in Na/Mg/hepes buffer in the absence (O,□) and presence (●,▲) of 10^{-3} M GTP.

and steepened. Curve fitting showed an apparent conversion of almost all the SH and H sites to L sites (SH:H:L = 0:15:85), with an accompanying increase in the I_{50} for carbachol from 6×10^{-7} to 5×10^{-5}M.

In contrast, the binding curve for NMS underwent a small shift towards higher affinity but remained well described by a simple Langmuir isotherm with affinity constant 1.1×10^{9} M^{-1} in the absence and 1.8×10^{9} M^{-1} in the presence of GTP.
The size of the GTP-induced shift was related to the pharmacological efficacy of the ligand, being large for potent agonists, small for partial agonists, and small or negative for antagonists. Only guanine nucleotides were active in eliciting these effects; adenine nucleotides were essentially inactive.

Nucleotide modulation of brain muscarinic receptors

In contrast to the heart, nucleotide effects on brain muscarinic receptor binding were small. Figure 2 shows the effect of 10^{-3} M GTP on the binding of carbachol to a broken cell preparation from the rat medulla pons, in Na/Mg/hepes buffer. The I_{50} for carbachol decreased from 3×10^{-7} M to 10^{-6} M in the presence of nucleotide; the ratio of SH:H:L determined by curve fitting altered from 49:37:14 to 20:41:39.

The effect of the nucleotide in the rat cerebral cortex was yet smaller. Despite the small absolute magnitude of the effects, the nucleotide specificity was similar to that seen in the heart, and GTP and the nonhydrolysable analogue GMPPNP were active at sub-micromolar concentrations. These effects, although small, thus appear to be genuine.

Nucleotide effects in the absence of inorganic ions

In tris-hepes buffer, in the absence of inorganic ions, a rather surprising phenomenon came to light; the binding of NMS to muscarinic receptors in the heart no longer conformed to the simple Langmuir isotherm, but, as illustrated in figure 3, the Scatchard plot became very non-linear. Curve fitting indicated the presence of two populations of sites, a minor population (19%) having an affinity constant of 7×10^{9} M^{-1}, and a major population having an anomalously low affinity constant, 2.5×10^{8} M^{-1}. Addition of GMPPNP caused an increase in the low affinity binding constant and apparent conversion of low to high affinity sites (Figure 3, Table 1). The effect was readily perceptible at 10^{-8} M GMPPNP, and almost complete at 10^{-6} M nucleotide; at 10^{-4} M GMPPNP the Scatchard plot for NMS binding was completely linear, defining an affinity constant of 5.5×10^{9} M^{-1}, a value of 2.5 times that measured in Na/Mg/hepes buffer in the presence of nucleotides. The NMS affinity constant measured in the cerebral cortex shows a similar enhancement in low ionic strength media (15) even in the absence of nucleotides.

It was possible to compute the carbachol binding to each class of NMS binding sites separately, from measurements of inhibition of the binding of a low concentration of ^{3}H-NMS (2×10^{-10} M) which predominantly occupies the high affinity antagonist binding sites, and of a high concentration of the ^{3}H-ligand (10^{-8} M) which occupies both high and low affinity sites.

Table 1. Effect of GMPPNP on binding constants for ^{3}H-NMS

GMPPN P(M)	K1 (M^{-1})	K2 (M^{-1})	α2	Bmax (pmoles)
0	6.9×10^{9}	2.5×10^{8}	0.81	0.21
10^{-8}	3.6×10^{9}	3.0×10^{8}	0.50	0.20
10^{-6}	2.8×10^{9}*		-	0.21
10^{-4}	5.9×10^{9}*		-	0.21

* deviation from simple Langmuir isotherm too small to allow unconstrained 2-site fit.

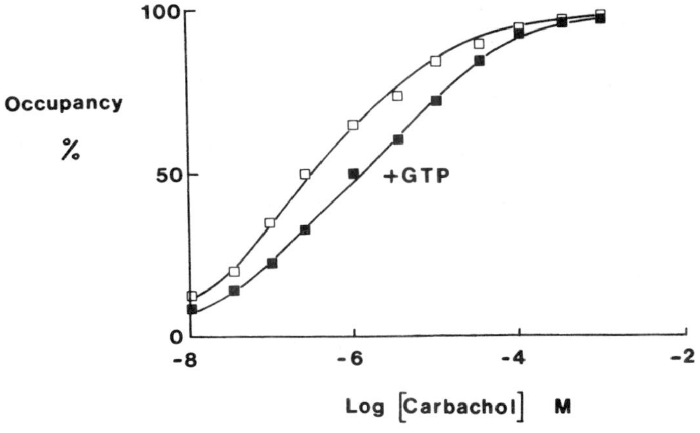

Figure 2. Binding of carbachol to muscarinic receptors in a homogenate of rat medulla pons in Na/Mg/hepes buffer in the absence (■) and presence (□) of 10^{-3} M GTP.

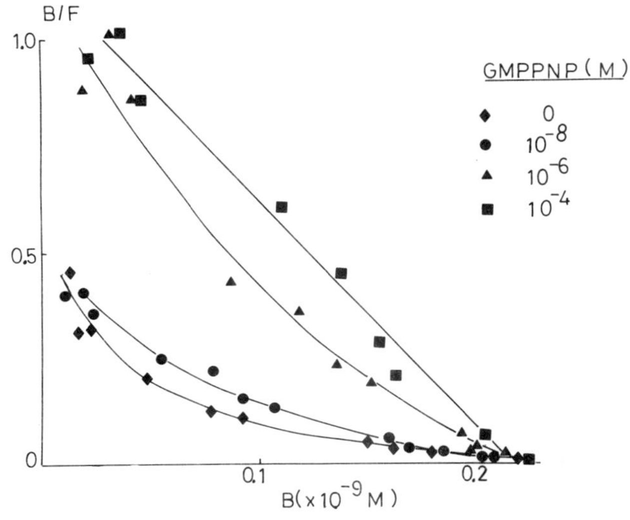

Figure 3. Scatchard plots of binding of ^{3}H-NMS to rat heart homogenate in tris/hepes buffer; effect of increasing concentrations of GMPPNP.

Figure 4 shows the results of such a set of measurements. The differences between the two carbachol binding curves are rather small, and each curve is flatter than the simple Langmuir isotherm, indicating that both high and low affinity NMS binding sites are associated with a heterogeneous population of agonist binding sites.

By taking a weighted average of curves such as those shown in figure 4 (the weights corresponding to the fractional abundance of the binding sites), it is possible to compute the intrinsic binding curve for carbachol to the population of binding sites actually present in the homogenate. In Figure 5 such a curve has been compared with a carbachol inhibition curve measured in the presence of 10^{-4} M GMPPNP, the latter curve having been corrected for the parallel shift induced by occupancy of the receptor by ^{3}H-NMS. Under these low ionic strength conditions, the reduction of the I_{50} for carbachol was only 5-fold; curve fitting showed an apparent conversion of SH to H sites, the ratio changing from 6:1 in the absence to 1:3 in the presence of the nucleotide. There seemed to be little alteration in the low affinity region of the binding curve, although small effects could easily be concealed within the cumulative errors of the measurements and calculations.

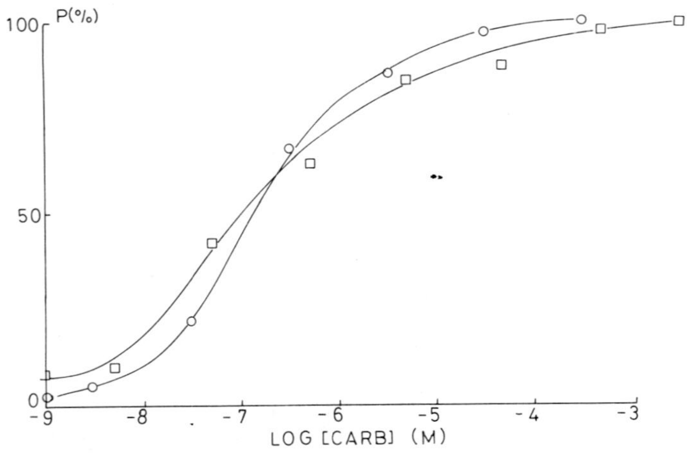

Figure 4. Binding of carbachol to high (□) and low (O) affinity NMS sites in rat heart homogenate in tris/hepes buffer.

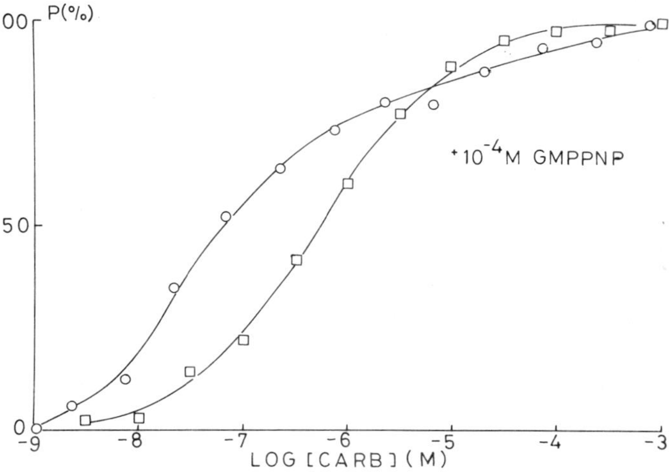

Figure 5. Intrinsic binding curves for carbachol to muscarinic receptors in rat heart homogenate in tris/hepes buffer in the absence (O) and presence (□) of 10^{-4} M GMPPNP.

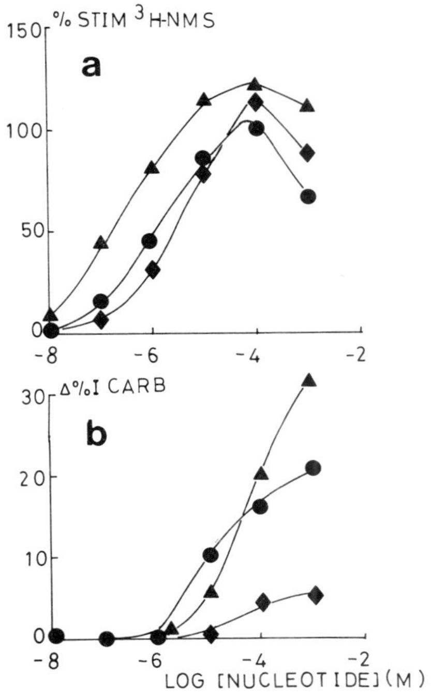

Figure 6. Effects of GTPγS (▲), GMPPNP (●) and GMPPCP (◆) on binding of (a) ^{3}H-NMS (expressed as % stimulation of binding over control) and (b) carbachol (expressed as change in % inhibition of binding of 2 x 10^{-10} M ^{3}H-NMS by 3 x 10^{-6} M carbachol) to rat heart homogenate in tris/hepes buffer.

Figure 6a shows the effect of 3 nonhydrolysable analogues of GTP, namely GTPγS, GMPPNP and GMPPCP on the binding of a low fixed concentration of ^{3}H-NMS. All three nucleotides strongly potentiated NMS binding at concentrations in the range 10^{-7} - 10^{-5} M, the most potent being GTPγS (EC_{50} = 2×10^{-7} M) GMPPNP having intermediate potency (EC_{50} = 5×10^{-7} M; mean of 3 experiments) and the least potent being GMPPCP (EC_{50} = 3×10^{-6} M). All three nucleotides gave similar maximum enhancements, and all began to inhibit at the highest concentrations tested (10^{-3} M); the reason for the latter appears to be related to the significant enhancement of the ionic strength of the incubation medium given by this concentration of the nucleotide, and its counterions. Unlike the guanine nucleotides, the adenine nucleotides failed to potentiate NMS binding at 10^{-4} M.

Figure 6b shows the effects of these nucleotide analogues on inhibition of the binding of 2×10^{-10} M ^{3}H-NMS by 3×10^{-6} M carbachol which gave ca 75% inhibition in the absence of nucleotides. All three analogues opposed the inhibitory actions of carbachol, but at much higher concentrations than those active on ^{3}H-NMS binding. The difference between the dose response curves was greatest for GTPγS; here the EC_{50} for enhancement of antagonist binding was 2×10^{-7} M while that for inhibition of carbachol binding was greater than 10^{-5} M. However, the discrepancy became smaller at lower carbachol concentrations, indicating that the binding of nucleotides and carbachol is in some respects competitive. Again, adenine nucleotides were without effect on agonist binding.

The effects of near saturating concentrations of the nucleotide analogues on the binding of 3×10^{-6} M carbachol were markedly different. The rank order of inhibition of carbachol binding at 10^{-3} M nucleotide was GTPγS > GMPPNP > GMPPCP. GMPPCP in particular had only small inhibitory actions on agonist binding. Preliminary experiments have shown that GTP and GDP produce maximum effects approximately equivalent to those given by GTPγS and GMPPNP respectively.

DISCUSSION

Our studies have shown that the binding properties of rat heart muscarinic receptors are strongly modulated by guanine nucleotides. Large effects of guanine nucleotides are also apparent in some other peripheral tissues (Hulme et al., in preparation). In contrast, muscarinic receptors in the brain are much less subject to nucleotide perturbation, at least in the areas so far examined.

As in other such systems, this nucleotide modulated population of muscarinic receptors is linked to the enzyme adenylate cyclase (9-12). Although there is no direct evidence, it seems likely that as in the case of the β-receptor, the linkage is mediated by a guanine nucleotide binding protein (13), present in the cell membrane, whose state of association with the receptor is governed by conformational changes induced by nucleotides and by changes in the receptor governed by the binding of agonists and antagonists.

Under near physiological conditions of ionic strength, the inhibitory effects of guanine nucleotides on muscarinic agonist binding far outweigh the enhancement of antagonist binding. Under such conditions, the nucleotide effects thus present the now classical appearance of a shift in the binding profiles of potent agonists with little effect on antagonist binding (14).

In contrast, in heart homogenates in the absence of inorganic ions, there is a strong effect of guanine nucleotides on antagonist binding. Under these conditions, only a small proportion of the total receptors (ca 20%) bind NMS with high affinity, while the remainder relax into a conformational state which displays low affinity for the antagonist, differing in this respect from brain muscarinic receptors, whose affinity for NMS is enhanced under such conditions (15).

Low concentrations of guanine nucleotides such as GMPPNP restore these sites to high affinity. Much higher concentrations of the nucleotides are needed to elicit inhibition of agonist binding. Preliminary experiments have suggested that the binding of guanine nucleotides and agonists can behave in a pseudo competitive manner. One plausible interpretation of these findings is that the binding of GTP or its analogues induces a conformational transition in the receptor which opposes or excludes the agonist-induced conformational change, but which may under certain conditions, favour the binding of antagonists.

REFERENCES

1. Berrie, C.P., Birdsall, N.J.M., Burgen, A.S.V. and Hulme, E.C. (1979) Biochem. Biophys. Res. Commun. 87, 1000-1005.

2. Wei, J-W., and Sulakhe, P.V. (1979) Eur. J. Pharmac. 58, 91-92.

3. Rosenberger, L.B., Roeske, W.R. and Yamamura, H.I. (1979) Eur. J. Pharmac. 56, 179-180.

4. Birdsall, N.J.M., Burgen, A.S.V., and Hulme, E.C. (1978) Mol. Pharmacol. 14, 723-736.

5. Birdsall, N.J.M., Hulme, E.C. and Burgen, A.S.V. (1980) Proc. Roy. Soc., in press.

6. Galper, J.B., Klein, W. and Caterall, W.A. (1977) J. Biol. Chem. 252, 8692-8699.

7. Fields, J-Z., Roeske, W.R., Morkin, E. and Yamamura, H.I. (1978) J. Biol. Chem. 253, 3251-3258.

8. Hulme, E.C., Birdsall, N.J.M., Burgen, A.S.V. and Mehta, P. (1978) Mol. Pharmacol. 14, 737-750.

9. Murad, F., Chi, Y-M., Rall, J.W. and Sutherland, E.W. (1962) J. Biol. Chem. 237, 1233-1238.

10. Watanabe, A.M., McConnaughey, M.M., Strawbridge, R.A., Fleming, J.W., Jones, L.R. and Besch, H.R. (1978) J. Biol. Chem. 253, 4833-4836.

11. Jacobs, K.H., Aktories, K., and Schultz, G. (1979) N-S Arch. Pharmac. 310, 113-120.

12. Birdsall, N.J.M., Berrie, C.P., Burgen, A.S.V. and Hulme, E.C. (1980) in Receptors for neurotransmitters and peptide hormones (eds. Pepeu, Kuhar, Enna) in press.

13. Pfeuffer, T. (1977) J. Biol. Chem. 252, 7224-7234.

14. Maguire, M.E., van Arsdale, P.M. and Gilman, A.G. (1976) Mol. Pharmacol. 12, 335-339.

15. Birdsall, N.J.M., Burgen, A.S.V., Hulme, E.C. and Wells, J.W.W. (1977) Brit. J. Pharmacol. 59, 503p.

Neurotransmitters and their Receptors
Edited by U.Z. Littauer, Y. Dudai, I. Silman,
V.I. Teichberg and Z. Vogel

Muscarinic Receptors: Solubilization Criteria and Binding Assay Optimization

H. Gorissen, G. Aerts and P. Laduron

Department of Biochemical Pharmacology, Janssen Pharmaceutical Research Laboratories, B-2340 Beerse, Belgium

Two different solubilization methods, namely the salt and digitonin extraction, of the muscarinic receptor from mammalian brain were compared in four species. On the ground of their hydrodynamic properties, it is clear that, contrary to digitonin extracts, muscarinic salt extracts do not display the characteristics of molecularly dispersed systems. Moreover the muscarinic solubilized receptors appear as a homogeneous system in the various species under our experimental conditions. The charcoal adsorption technique, was selected as the most convenient procedure for the determination of this soluble macromolecular complex.

Muscarinic receptors from bovine (1-3) and rat (4) brains may be successfully solubilized by treating microsomal membranes with the natural detergent digitonin. This extraction procedure seems to indicate that these receptor proteins are endo-membrane macromolecular components. Alternatively high salt concentration (NaCl 2N) has been presented as effective for the solubilization of muscarinic receptors from rat (5, 6) and bovine (7) brains, suggesting an exo-membrane localization of those biomacromolecules (5, 6). This ambiguity may be resolved by simultaneously submitting both extracts, to the same analytical solubilization criteria, namely the gel-filtration on Sepharose CL-4B and the sedimentation through sucrose gradients.

Microsomal fractions (P) from the striata of rat, calf, dog and cat, as from rat forebrain were prepared (8) and kept in 2 vol. water at -16° C. Extraction was carried out by treating these fractions at 0° C in 4 vol., either by 1 % suspended digitonin (with or without 0.25 M sucrose) for 15 min (4, 9), or by NaCl 2N for at least 4 h (5). Both extraction media were buffered with 10 mM sodium phosphate supplemented by 0.01 % NaN_3. After centrifugation at 117,000 x g for 1 h, the first supernatant (S_1) may be recentrifuged at 182,000 x g for 1 h to give a second supernatant called S_2. Salt extracts were additionaly dialysed at 0°C between the two centrifugation steps. Aliquots of the different preparations were incubated for 15 min at 30°C with [^{3}H]-dexetimide (2×10^{-9} M). Blank values were determined in the presence of a hundred-fold higher concentration of unlabelled dexetimide.

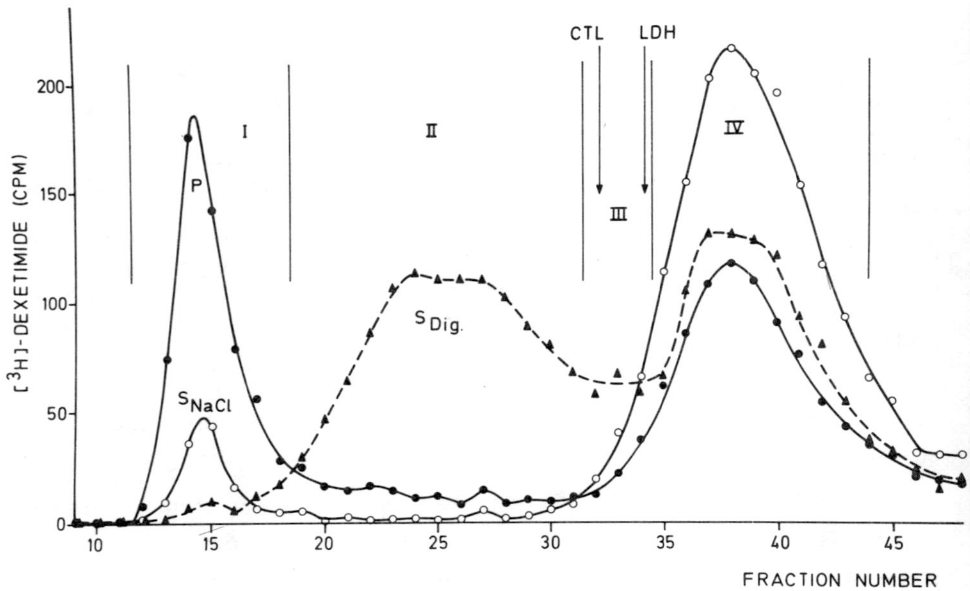

Fig. 1 - Gel-filtration on Sepharose CL-4B. Elution profiles of microsomal (—●—●—●—), digitonin (▲-▲-▲) and salt (—o—o—o—) preparations labelled by [^{3}H]-dexetimide (4×10^{-9} M). Aliquots of 0.1 ml of incubation mixture were layered on the top of the column (22 x 0.5 cm) and eluted at 2°C with 10 mM sodium phosphate buffer (pH 7.2) containing 0.03 % digitonin and 0.01 % NaN_3. Five-drop fractions (rate ~10 drops/min) were collected in counting vials. Arrows indicate the elution of the marker enzymes, catalase (CTL) and lactate dehydrogenase (LDH). Controls: when the different preparations were incubated in the presence of a hundred-fold concentration (4×10^{-7} M) of unlabelled dexetimide, the radioactivity was totally recovered in region IV.

As shown in Fig. 1, digitonin (S_{Dig}) and salt (S_{NaCl}) muscarinic extracts labelled by [^{3}H]-dexetimide present totally different elution patterns on Sepharose CL-4B columns. Indeed, compared to microsomal membranes (P), digitonin extracts were retarded on the gel (Fig. 1, II), while the corresponding salt preparations were excluded in the void volume as their original membranes (Fig. 1, I). Both extracts from the striata of four mammalian species showed, using this analytical approach, quite identical results. The second analytical procedure was based on the different centrifugation properties of both extraction media. The sedimentation patterns (Fig. 2 A) of the labelled digitonin extracts,

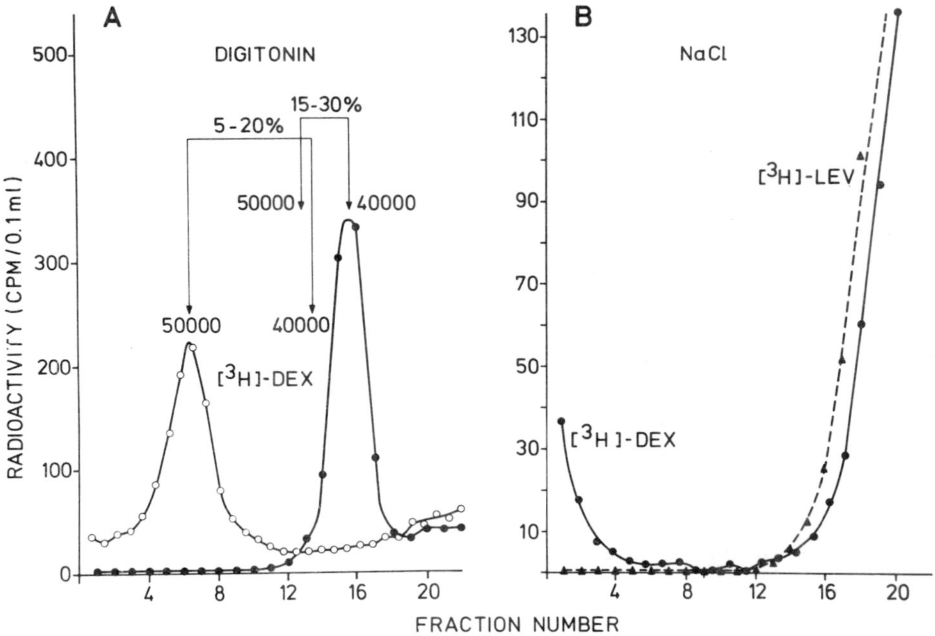

Fig. 2 - Gradient sedimentation radioactivity profiles. (A) Digitonin extracts (0.2 ml) from rat forebrain labelled by [^{3}H] dexetimide (2 x 10^{-9} M) were centrifuged for 16 h at 40,000 rev/min (SW 65 Ti rotor) through 15-30 % sucrose (●—●—●) and at 50,000 rev/min through 5-20 % sucrose (o—o—o). Arrows indicate the position of the peak after 16 h centrifugation in different conditions. (B) Salt extracts (0.2 ml) from rat forebrain labelled by 2 x 10^{-9} M [^{3}H]-dexetimide (●—●—●) and [^{3}H]-levetimide (-▲--▲-) were centrifuged for 16 h at 50,000 rev/min through 5-20 % sucrose. The gradients were buffered by 10 mM sodium phosphate (pH 7.2) and supplemented by 0.01 % NaN_3 and 0.03 % digitonin.

from the brain of the various species, were the same using different sucrose concentrations (5-20 and 15-30 %) and different speed conditions (40,000 and 50,000 rev/min). The peak of specific binding was shifted further to the bottom of the tube, either by using a higher speed, or a longer centrifugation time. However, with all the salt extracts, under comparable centrifugation conditions, a sedimentable specifically labelled material, was always recovered in the bottom of the tube (Fig. 2 B, fractions 1-3). Further, when dialysed salt extracts (S_1) are recentrifuged, the supernatant of the second centrifugation (S_2) is devoid of any specific binding. This is not the case for digitonin extracts where most of the binding measured in the first supernatant (S_1) was recovered in the S_2 fraction (88 to 104 %).

Various assay methods suited for the determination of the digitonin solubilized muscarinic receptor were checked. The different assay methods, namely the gel-filtration on Sephadex G-50 (4), the ammonium sulfate aggregation (2), the charcoal adsorption (10) and the ion-exchanger DEAE-cellulose (2) gave, using a dog striatal extract, similar IC_{50}-values for two enantiomeric drugs, i.e. dexetimide ($3.2-4.0 \times 10^{-9}$ M) and levetimide ($1.0-3.2 \times 10^{-6}$ M), with a comparable stereospecific effect. However, the specific binding obtained using the different methods varied from 3.9 to 6.6 pmol/ml. These differences were not related to dissociation phenomena, because [^{3}H]-dexetimide labelled very firmly the muscarinic receptor and there was almost no dissociation at 0°C (4). The two assay methods used by Hurko (2), namely the ammonium sulfate and DEAE-cellulose techniques, appeared equally effective, but yielded only 60 % of the binding detected by the gel-filtration. Moreover, the most sensitive, but also the most time consuming assay, the Sephadex gel-filtration, may be safely replaced by the charcoal technique which displays 90 % of the binding obtained by the gel-filtration. This was confirmed in four different species.

In conclusion, the salt extracted muscarinic receptors were not present as molecula-ly dispersed systems. Furthermore, the differences in binding characteristics described for the salt preparations of rat (6) and bovine (7) brains appeared not to be related to species specificity but more obviously to variations in the experimental procedures used for the enrichment and the determination of the muscarinic system after salt extraction. On the contrary the digitonin extracts from the brain of four species, showed that the muscarinic system has identical hydrodynamic (2, 4, 9) and binding (2-4) properties. Finally, comparison of various assay methods with different animal preparations indicated clearly that charcoal adsorption may be considered as the most suitable assay method for the determination of the muscarinic receptor in its soluble form.

ACKNOWLEDGEMENTS

Part of this work was supported by a grant from the I. W. O. N. L. We thank D. Ashton for his help in preparing the manuscript.

REFERENCES

1. Beld, A. J. and Ariëns, E. J. (1974) Eur. J. Pharmacol. 25, 203-209.
2. Hurko, O. (1978) Arch. Biochem. Biophys. 190, 434-445.
3. Aronstam, R. S., Schuessler, D. C. and Eldefrawi, M. E. (1978) Life Sci. 23, 1377-1382.
4. Gorissen, H., Aerts, G. and Laduron, P. (1978) FEBS Lett. 96, 64-68.
5. Bartfai, T., Anner, J., Schultzberg, M. and Montelius, J. (1974) Biochem. Biophys. Res. Commun. 59, 725-733.
6. Alberts, P. and Bartfai, T. (1976) J. Biol. Chem. 251, 1543-1547.
7. Carson, S., Godwin, S., Massoulié, J. and Kato, G. (1977) Nature 266, 176-178.
8. Laduron, P. (1977) Int. Rev. Neurobiol. 20, 251-281.
9. Gorissen, H., Aerts, G. and Laduron, P. (1979) FEBS Lett. 100, 281-285.
10. Gavish, M., Chang, R. S. L. and Snyder, S. H. (1979) Life Sci. 25, 783-790.

Neurotransmitters and their Receptors
Edited by U.Z. Littauer, Y. Dudai, I. Silman,
V.I. Teichberg and Z. Vogel

Agonist and Antagonist Interaction with Muscarinic Pre- and Postsynaptic Receptors: Biochemical Characterization

M. Sokolovsky, S. Avissar, Y. Egozi, D. Gurwitz, Y. Kloog and D.M. Michaelson

Department of Biochemistry, George S. Wise Faculty of Life Sciences, Tel-Aviv University, Tel-Aviv, Israel

The ligand binding properties of muscarinic receptors present in purified synaptosomal fraction isolated from the *Torpedo* electric organ and in several regions of the ICR mouse brain were studied using the tritiated antagonist N-methyl-4-piperidylbenzilate. Kinetic and equilibrium analysis of antagonist binding as well as competition experiments with several agonists were used to probe the nature of the binding sites and possible differences between specific muscarinic sites in the various preparations. In addition, the binding properties of discrete mouse brain regions following intracisternal 6-hydroxydopamine lesion were investigated. The localization of pre- and postsynaptic muscarinic receptors in view of their different binding properties is discussed.

INTRODUCTION

High affinity binding of tritium-labeled N-methyl-4-piperidylbenzilate (4NMPB) and atropine to homogenate from various regions of mouse brain was recently used to characterize the mechanism of binding to specific muscarinic sites (1-3). The binding assay with these antagonists using the filtration technique,enabled us to investigate the ligand specificity directly and in conjunction with detailed kinetic studies. The results of these experiments suggest that within the set of conditions created by our methodology for the definition and characterization of receptors by labeled ligands, mouse brain homogenates exhibit _functional heterogeneity_ (2)(4)(5) of muscarinic receptors. Regional heterogeneity was also inferred in the interaction of muscarinic receptors with agonists (6-8). One possible explanation for the _functional_ heterogeneity is the existence of pre- and postsynaptic receptors. The present work describes (i) the use of intracisternal 6-hydroxydopamine (6-OHDA) lesion for central presynaptic muscarinic receptor studies; (ii) the ligand binding properties of presynaptic muscarinic receptors of Torpedo (9 - 11) and compares them with those of the postsynaptic muscarinic receptors (5)(12); (iii) the possible relationship between ligand binding properties and functional heterogeneity.

MATERIALS AND METHODS

Labeled and unlabeled compounds are the same as described previously (5)(11).

Torpedo electric organs were homogenized and fractionated as described previously (13)(14). Fractions a_2 and a_3, which are the most enriched in synaptosomes and muscarinic receptors (9)(10), were pooled, diluted with 4 volumes of the homogenization buffer (0.8 M glycine, 1mM EGTA, pH 6.6) and centrifuged at 17500 g for 20 min. The pellet was resuspended so that each ml contained 1.2-2.4 mg protein. This preparation, which we shall refer to as the synaptosomal fraction, was used for the binding assays.

Adult male mice (ICR, 20-25 g) were injected intracisternally with 70 μg 6-OHDA (hydrobromide salt, Sigma, calculated as the free base) in 10 of saline containing 0.5% L-ascorbate. The mice were injected under light ether anesthesia and the wound closed with surgical clips. This proved to a satisfactory procedure since trial injections of a pigment revealed complete staining of the ventricles within seconds. A second group of mice received vehicle alone, using the same procedure. The injections were repeated after a 72 h interval. A third group of mice received daily i.p. injections of 0.5 mg/kg reserpine in 0.2 ml saline. Untreated mice were included in all experiments as controls.

Animals were killed by decapitation at various intervals after treatment, the brains removed, and discrete regions dissected out separately from each specimen (5). In all subsequent procedures each tissue was treated separately. Tissues were weighed and homogenized in 3 ml 0.32 M sucrose in a glass homogenizer using a motor-driven Teflon pestle (950 rpm). Homogenates were placed on ice and analyzed within 4 h. Norepinephrine uptake was determined with ^{3}H-NE (27.8 Ci/mmole, NEN) according to the method of White (15) with minor modifications, as follows: 0.1 ml aliquots of each tissue homogenate were added to 0.4 ml Krebs-bicarbonate buffer, pH = 7.4, final concentration 0.1 μM ^{3}H-NE. The buffer contained 10 μM EGTA and 0.02% L-ascorbate. Samples of each tissue homogenate were prepared in triplicate and incubated for 10 min at 37°C. Incubation was terminated by rapid filtration using cellulose-acetate filters (Millipore, 0.45 μ), followed by three washes with 3 ml saline. Filters were counted in a Packard Scintillation Counter (Prias P-L). Nonspecific NE uptake was determined at 0°C and subtracted from total counts. Direct binding studies, competition experiments and the analysis of binding kinetics were carried out as described in detail in previous reports (5)(11).

RESULTS AND DISCUSSION

When tissues treated with 6-OHDA were assayed 3 days after the second injection, a considerable decrease in NE uptake was observed in all brain regions studies (Fig. 1). Two doses of the neurotoxin were necessary to bring about a drastic reduction of NE uptake in the cortex; a higher dose in one injection was inappropriate due to high mortality.

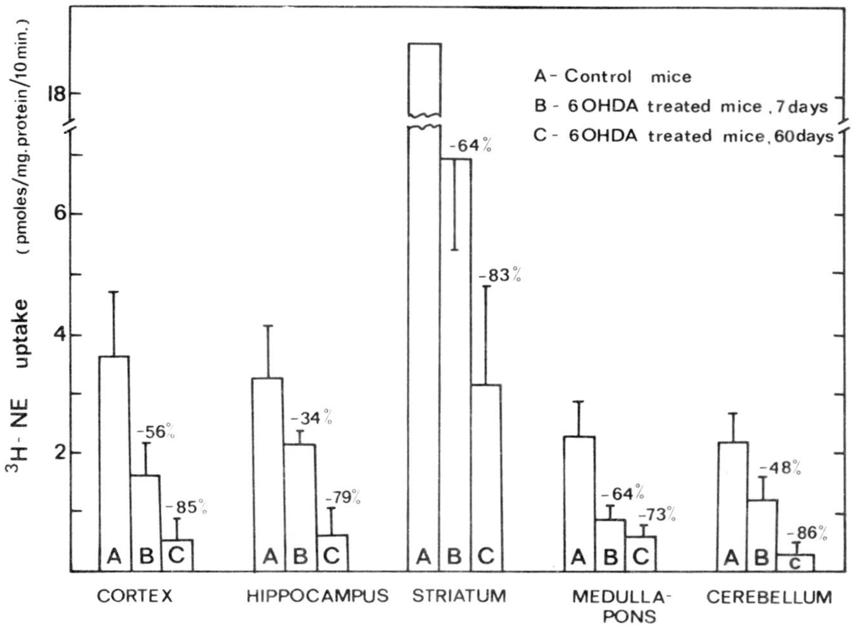

Fig. 1. (^{3}H)-NE uptake in different regions of control and 6-OHDA lesioned mice.
Data (12 experiments) are given as pmoles (^{3}H)-NE taken up by homogenate equivalent to 1 mg protein in 10 min at 37°. (^{3}H)-NE concentration was 0.1 μM. Decreases are statistically significant $p<0.01$.

In the striatum, medulla-pons and cerebellum,decreases in NE uptake showed a positive correlation with decreases in muscarinic receptor density (Fig. 2). Although NE uptake was decreased to the same extent in the cortex and hippocampus as in the other regions, no change was apparent in the muscarinic receptor density of these regions.

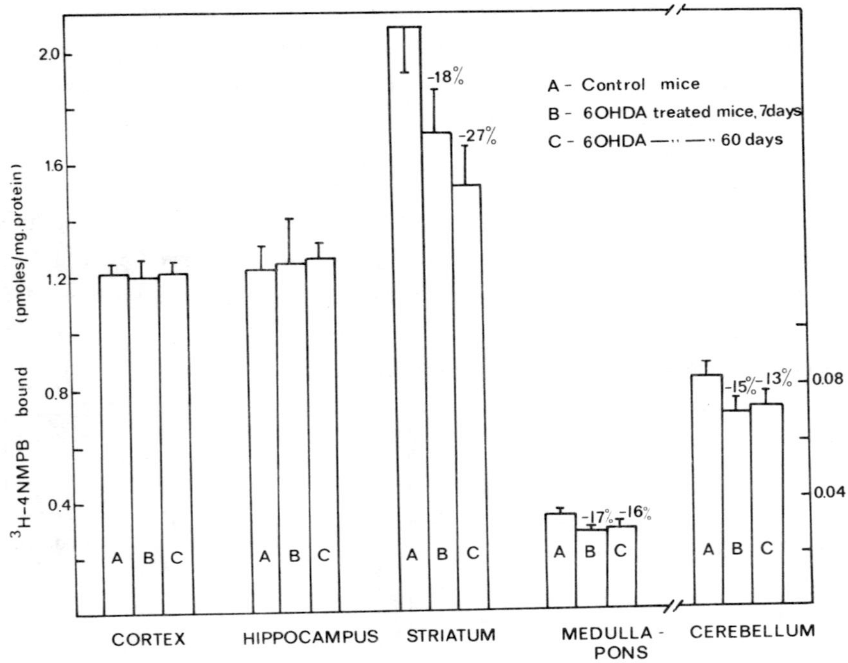

Fig. 2. (^{3}H)-4NMPB specific binding in different regions of mouse brain (12 experiments).
Numbers (%) indicate post-lesion differences in specific binding as compared with untreated group A. All differences indicated are statistically significant, $p<.01$. Differences between values for groups B and C are not significant, except in the striatum where $p<.05$.

When brain homogenates were prepared and assayed 60 days after lesion, values for NE uptake were decreased even further (Fig. 1.). However, muscarinic receptor density values were unchanged compared to those determi 3 days after the second injection, except in the case of the striatum, in which muscarinic receptor density decreased by a further 9% compared to the controls (Fig. 2.). In mice treated with saline vehicle or reserpine, muscarinic receptor density in all brain regions was unchanged.

The decrease in muscarinic binding after 6-OHDA lesion could not be accounted for by a reduction of affinity in any of the brain regions investigated, since no change in receptor affinity towards antagonists (NMPB and atropine) or agonists (oxotremorine, carbamylcholine and acetylcholine) could be detected.

In the light of current knowledge regarding 6-OHDA toxicity (16) several explanations for these findings may be considered: (a) Non-specific damage by the neurotoxin treatment. This can be reasonably ruled out, since degeneration of muscarinic receptors did not occur in the cortex and hippocampus although damage to catecholaminergic neurons, as manifested by decreases in NE uptake, took place to the same extent here as in the other regions studied. (b) Involvement of post-synaptic mechanisms, as proposed by Kato _et al_. (17). This is unlikely to explain our results, since reserpine treatment for one week had no effect on muscarinic receptor density. However, it should be noted that in the earlier study the technique used was unilateral nigral lesion. (c) Degeneration of catecholaminergic cell bodies and dendrites which had received cholinergic innervation. (d) Degeneration of catecholaminergic terminals which have presynaptic muscarinic receptors located on them.

It is difficult to distinguish between the two latter interpretations, due to lack of information regarding the exact time course of 6-OHDA toxicity in the CNS. A histochemical study by Descarries _et al_. (18) has demonstrated that degeneration of the adrenergic cell bodies of the locus ceruleus after intraventricular 6-OHDA injection is a slow process, completed only after 30 days. If this finding may be projected to all brain regions, our results would appear to reflect terminal degeneration which is completed within about a week (16), since no further decreases in muscarinic receptor density were apparent after 60 days (except in the striatum) beyond those already seen after 7 days. In the striatum the small further decrease in muscarinic receptor density probably reflects a later process of cell body degeneration. We therefore conclude that our data are best interpreted as a degeneration of presynaptic muscarinic receptors located on CA terminals in the medulla-pons and cerebellum.

Although the labeling of the muscarinic receptors with 4NMPB _in vitro_ enables one to evaluate many characteristics of the receptor binding site, it is possible that important functional characteristics may be obscured. Thus, changes in the number of muscarinic receptor sites under varying physiological and pharmacological conditions may be affected during the time in which one sacrifices the animal and prepares brain homogenates for receptor assay. For this reason, and because 4NMPB has a high affinity for the muscarinic receptor, we examined _in vivo_ its accumulation by various regions after s.c. injections of (^{3}H)-4NMPB (Fig. 3). At the time intervals indicated, the mouse brains were dissected and the regions under investigation were analyzed for accumulated radioactivity. As shown in Fig. 3, pretreatment of animals with (-)QNB inhibits (^{3}H)-4NMPB accumulation in all regions; the _in vivo_ specific binding is defined as the total radioactivity minus (^{3}H)-4NMPB accumulation after pretreatment with (-)QNB. As evident from the comparison shown in Table I, the regional distribution of the (^{3}H)-4NMPB after in vivo administration is essentially the same as the regional variation and binding capacities of 4NMPB assayed _in vitro_.

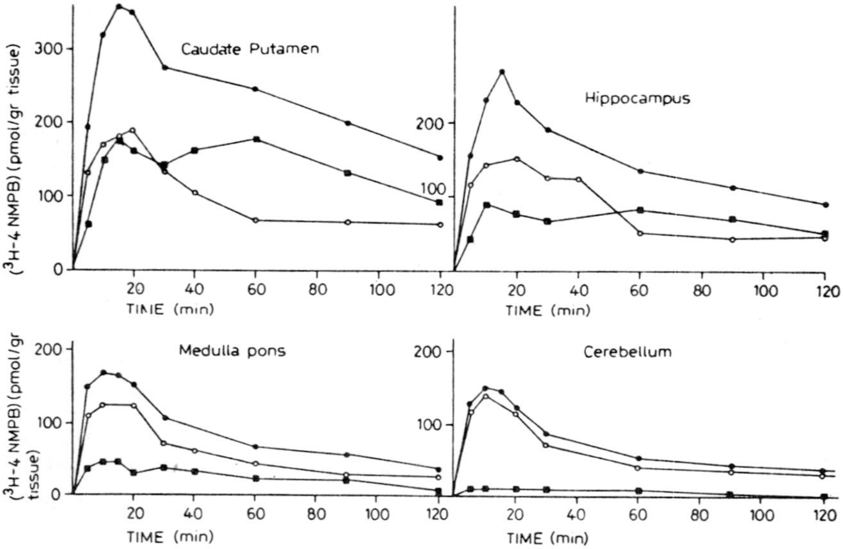

Fig. 3. Time course of (^{3}H)-4NMPB accumulation into various regions of mouse brain (●——●).
Mice were given 0.5 μCi of (^{3}H)-4NMPB (0.1 mg/kg) s.c. in 0.2 ml of saline and sacrificed after various time intervals. o——o Mice were pretreated with 3.3 mg/kg of (-)QNB for 10 min, followed by 0.5 μCi of (^{3}H)-4NMPB. ■——■ "specific binding" i.e. total accumulation of (^{3}H)-4NMPB minus its accumulation after pretreatment with (-)QNB. Each point represents the mean of at least three animals, which did not vary more than 10%.

The contention that muscarinic receptors in _Torpedo_ electric organ are presynaptic is based on the following observations: (i) Muscarinic binding sites copurify with intact _Torpedo_ synaptosomes (9)(14). (ii) _Torpedo_ synaptosomes contain only trace amounts of postsynaptic receptors (9)(10)(14). (iii) Activation of the synaptosomal muscarinic receptors results in inhibition of Ca^{2+} dependent AcCh release. This inhibition is revealed by muscarinic antagonists (10).

Table I: Regional distribution (*in vitro*) and accumulation (*in vivo*) of specific (^{3}H)-4NMPB binding in mouse brain *

Region	Binding capacity (pmoles/mg protein)		K_d(nM)
	In vivo	*In vitro*	
Cerebellum	0.1 ± 0.05	0.12 ± 0.01	1.15 ± 0.2
Medulla-pons	0.4 ± 0.06	0.29 ± 0.05	0.82 ± 0.02
Hippocampus	0.9 ± 0.1	1.05 ± 0.05	0.47 ± 0.03
Caudate putamen	1.8 ± 0.1	1.54 ± 0.38	0.38 ± 0.01
Cortex	0.9 ± C.1	0.91 ± 0.06	0.41 ± 0.03
Thalamus	-	0.61 ± 0.1	0.5 ± 0.06
Hypothalamus	0.3 ± 0.05	0.25 ± 0.04	0.8 ± 0.05

* The values given are the mean of at least 6 separate binding curves ± S.E.M. K_d values obtained from Scatchard plots.

Our study revealed the following properties of ligand binding to the *Torpedo* muscarinic receptor: Labeled antagonists bind with high affinity to the presynaptic receptor (∿190 fmol/mg protein), with saturability occurring at very low ligand concentrations (K_d = 0.3 ± 0.1 nM and K_d = 1.0 ± 0.2 nM for (^{3}H)-QNB and (^{3}H)-4NMPB respectively). As shown in Fig. 4, the potent muscarinic antagonists (-)QNB, (+)QNB and atropine inhibited the binding of (^{3}H)-4NMPB in a competitive manner. Equally significant for the characterization of the binding sites is the fact that the affinity ratio of the enantiomers of QNB, as measured by the ratio of their K_d values, holds both for binding experiments and for the bioassay in the intact organ. The identical stereoselectivity strongly indicates that the structural integrity of the membrane preparation is preserved in the binding experiments. Since in many preparations (1-3) (5)(19-22) it has been shown that the binding of muscarinic antagonists involves an isomerization step, we examined the possibility that this is also true for the presynaptic *Torpedo* muscarinic receptor.

As predicted from this sequential model, under slow isomerization conditions the dissociation rate of (^{3}H)-4NMPB-receptor complexes should be a function of the time of preincubation of the ligand with the receptors; this means that the rate of dissociation should be faster when the system has not reached equilibrium (i.e. the isomerization step is not yet completed) than at equilibrium. To test this possibility, the synaptosomal samples were incubated with a high concentration of (^{3}H)-4NMPB (20 nM), so that most of the binding sites were occupied within a few seconds, and the dissociation was measured after 20 sec or 3 min. The dissociation rate of (^{3}H)-4NMPB receptor complex measured 20 sec after formation of the ligand-receptor complex was so rapid that it could not be accurately analyzed by the filtration assay. However, the data clearly indicated that $t_{1/2} < 5$ sec. Dissociation rates measured after preincubation of 3 min and 30 min became progressively slower ($t_{1/2}$ = 1.5 and 6.5 min respectively).

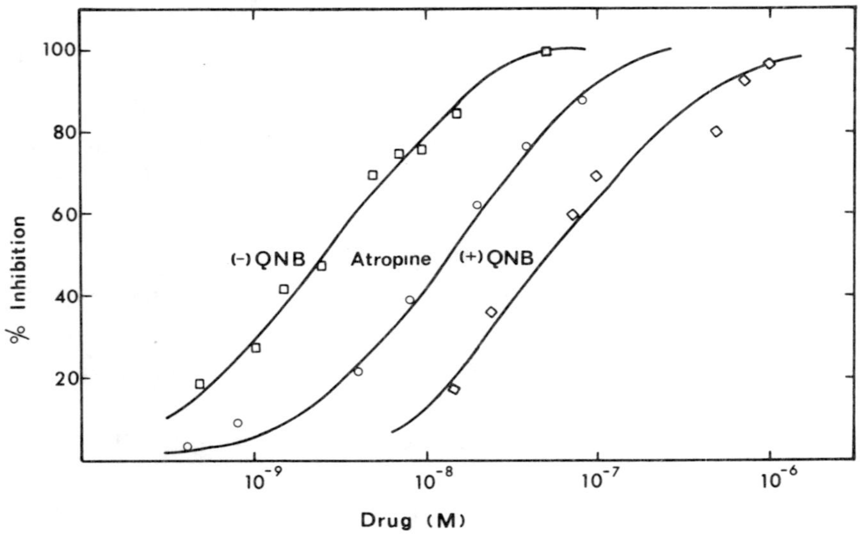

Fig. 4. Inhibition of (^{3}H)-4NMPB binding to the synaptosomal fraction by muscarinic antagonists.
Samples (0.1 ml) were incubated at 25° for 30 min in 2 ml buffer containing 2.0 nM (^{3}H)-4NMPB, and the concentration of unlabeled ligands indicated. Specific binding was determined as described in the text. Each point represents the average of triplicate determinations. (^{3}H)-4NMPB binding site concentration was 0.01-0.02 nM.

Thus the kinetic results obtained in this study could best be fitted by a two-step sequential isomerization model (5)(19): first the antagonist binds to the receptor, and then the receptor ligand complex undergoes isomerization (i.e. a conformational change). Exact values for the four kinetic parameters of this model are not yet known. However, the data yield the following conclusions: 1) isomerization occurs more slowly than the bimolecular receptor ligand reaction; 2) the dissociation rate of the ligand from the newly formed complexes ($k_{off} \simeq k_{-1} > 8.15\ min^{-1}$) is faster than the dissociation rate ($k_{off} = k_{-2} = 0.11\ min^{-1}$) from the equilibrated receptor antagonist complexes.

The muscarinic agonists oxotremorine, carbamylcholine, arecoline and AcCh inhibited binding of (^{3}H)-4NMPB (Fig. 5). Inhibition curves for these agonists were flattened, and were characterized by a Hill slope smaller than 1.0.

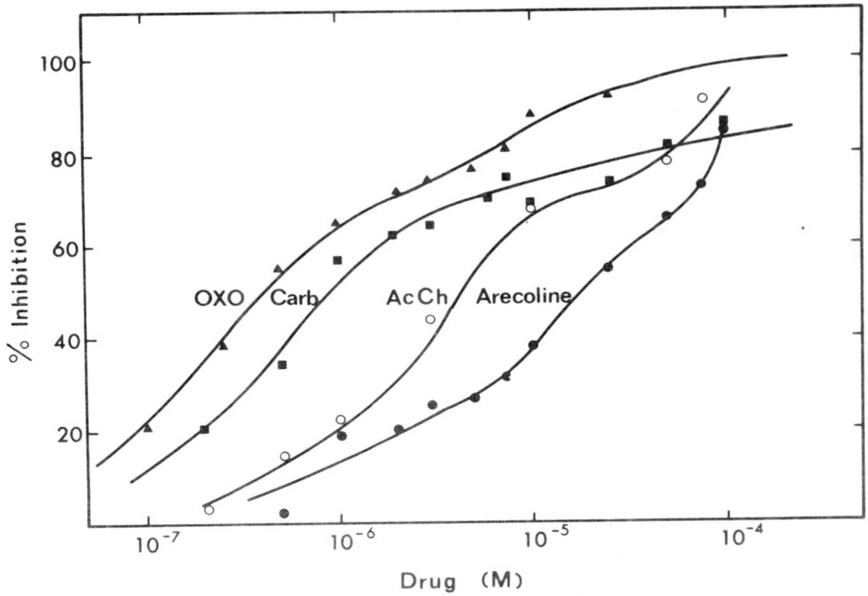

Fig. 5. Inhibition of (^{3}H)-4NMPB binding to the synaptosomal fraction by muscarinic agonists.
Each point represents the average of triplicate determinations.

As suggested by Birdsall *et al.* (6)(7), a possible explanation for the low Hill slopes of the agonist inhibition curves is that the agonists bind with different affinities to two or three distinct populations of binding sites to which the antagonists bind with the same affinity. In the *Torpedo* presynaptic preparation, the data obtained for inhibition of (^{3}H)-4NMPB binding by agonists can also be fitted by the two-site model specifying a high and a low affinity site. The solid lines in Fig. 5 for oxotremorine and carbamylcholine are the best fit lines obtained by a nonlinear least-squares program. The parameters thus obtained indicate that the affinity constants for high and low affinity binding sites are $K_H = 11.07 \pm 2.2 \times 10^{-6}M^{-1}$ and $K_L = 0.027 \pm 0.012 \times 10^{-6}M^{-1}$ for oxotremorine and $K_H = 6.7 \pm 2.1 \times 10^{-6}M^{-1}$

in the medulla-pons versus cortex). Either mechanism may be a consequence of different mediators coupled with muscarinic activation, such as pre- and postsynaptic process mediated by the muscarinic receptor ((11) and references therein). Guanine nucleotides have been shown to modify the binding of agonists to several neurotransmitters and hormonal receptors ((24) and references therein). In all these cases the affinity for agonists is decreased with no change in the affinity for antagonists. We have recently found (M. Sokolovsky and D. Gurwitz, unpublished results) that the binding properties of muscarinic receptors in homogenates of mouse medulla-pons and cerebellum are altered in the presence of guanine nucleotides. There is almost no change in affinity constant for antagonists, while there is an effect in agonist binding which is characterized by the conversion of high affinity sites to low affinity sites. Similar results could be seen using Gpp(NH)p and GDP. Minimal effects were found in homogenates of cortex, hippocampus and caudate-putamen. A similar effect has also been observed in the muscarinic receptors in rat mycocardium (25).

Table III summarizes some of the characteristics of muscarinic ligand binding to receptors in the medulla-pons and cortex as compared with those of the presynaptic Torpedo receptors.

Table III: Characteristics of ligand binding to muscarinic receptors

	Antagonist ((^{3}H)-4NMPB)		Agonist (oxotremorine)		Effect of	
	K_d(nM)	$t_{1/2}$(diss)	I_{50}(μM)	α	6-OHDA	GTP
Cortex	0.41	20 min	9.8	0.19	-	-
Medulla-pons	0.82	5 min	0.39	0.65	+	+
Torpedo synaptosomes	1.0	6.5 min	0.25	0.78		+

α = proportion of high affinity binding sites.

It can be seen that the binding pattern in Torpedo more closely resembles that found in the medulla-pons (and cerebellum, not shown) than in the cortex. This, together with the evidence presented in this report for the presence of presynaptic muscarinic receptors located on catecholamine terminals, suggests that the medulla-pons and cerebellum are enriched in populations of presynaptic receptors. If cholinesterase and cholineacetyl-

and $K_L = 0.012 \pm 0.006\ M^{-1}$ for carbamylcholine. The proportions of high affinity sites for these two agonists are 84% and 78% respectively.

In our previous reports on regional heterogeneity (5), we observed marked differences in the Hill slopes obtained with different agonists in a given brain region: in both the hippocampus and the caudate-putamen the value for oxotremorine is ca. 1.0, while for acetylcholine the value is ca. 0.5; on the other hand, in the medulla-pons the Hill slope value for both agonists was ∿ 0.5. Analysis of the antagonist/agonist inhibition curves (eg. Fig.6) according to the two-site model shows (Table II) that these stem not only from differences in the proportion of high and low affinity binding sites recorded for oxotremorine and carbamylcholine or acetylcholine.

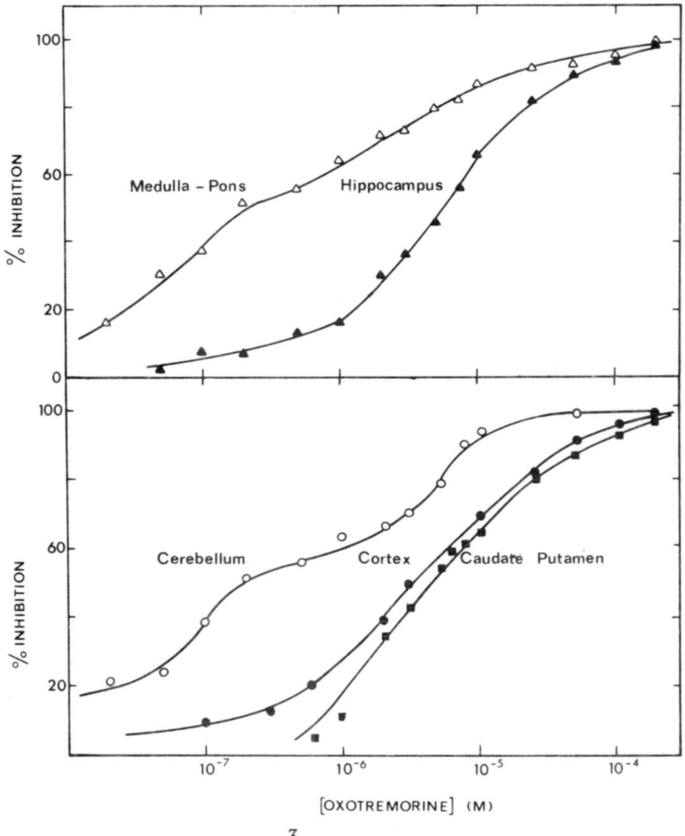

Fig. 6. Inhibition of (^{3}H)-4NMPB binding by oxotremorine. Samples were incubated at 25° for 30 min in 2 ml Krebs-Hensleit solution containing 2.0 nM (^{3}H)-4NMPB and oxotremorine in the concentrations indicated. Concentration of binding sites were in all cases < 0.1 nM.

In the cortex, hippocampus and caudate-putamen the proportion of high affinity binding sites for oxotremorine is less than 15%, whereas it is 40-50% for carbamylcholine or acetylcholine. On the other hand, in the cerebellum and medulla-pons the values recorded for these three agonists approximated much more closely to each other (Table II). When comparing these results to those observed in other mammalian brains, it is again evident that by the same analysis of the inhibition data for agonists according to the two-site model, the proportion of high affinity binding sites for oxotremorine in rat cortex and frog cortex (7)(8) is lower (∿ 18%) than that for carbamylcholine (40-50%).

Table II: Proportion of high affinity binding sites for muscarinic agonists in mice

Agonists	Cerebellum	Medulla-pons	Cortex	Hippocampus	Caudate-putamen
Acetylcholine	0.72 - 0.74	0.57 - 0.60	0.48 - 0.53	0.49 - 0.49	0.58 - 0.
Carbamylcholine	0.65 - 0.58	0.59 - 0.61	0.23 - 0.23	0.30 - 0.42	0.46 - 0.
Oxotremorine	0.64 - 0.66	0.65 - 0.66	0.19 - 0.18	∿ 0.1	∿ 0.1

The proportion of high affinity binding sites was evaluated from inhibition curves of binding of 2 nM (^{3}H)-4NMPB by agonists using nonlinear least squares regression procedure (11). Values given are those obtained from two separate experiments. In the hippocanpus and caudate-putamen, estimated values are given for oxotremorine.

According to these observations we therefore conclude that in the cortex, hippocampus and caudate-putamen agonist binding cannot be described solely in term of the binding of agonist to fixed receptor sites of high and low affinities. On the other hand, in the cerebellum and medulla-pons this explanation seems to fit well. We therefore suggest that agonist binding may be explained by at least two mechanisms:1) induced interconversion of the muscarinic receptors by agonists, reflected in differences in the ratio of high to low affinity binding sites for different agonists (e.g. in the cortex). In this respect it is important to note that interconversion between agonist sites has been inferred from agonist binding studies in mammalian brain (22)(23) and in *Torpedo* presynaptic membranes (11). 2) Different pre-existing states of muscarinic receptors result in marked regional differences in agonist binding (e.g. oxotremorine and carbamylcholine transferase (4) are cholinergic markers for presynaptic membranes, then their high levels in the medulla-pons (4)(26) would support this suggestion. Szerb _et al._ (27)(28) have presented evidence suggesting that hippocampal presynaptic muscarinic receptors differ from postsynaptic receptors. In _Torpedo_, muscarinic ligands affect presynaptic protein phosphorylation (10). In mammalian preparations receptor activation has been reported to affect phosphatidyl inositol breakdown (29), cGMP levels (30) and Ca^{2+} transport (31). Thus it is possible that the differences in affinity of the pre- and postsynaptic receptors are a manifestation of different physiological functions. It should be noted that a high ratio of high to low affinity binding sites would indicate the presence of presynaptic receptors, while a low ratio would indicate postsynaptic receptors. However, recent experiments in our laboratory indicate that interconversion of these sites, in addition to being mediated by guanine nucleotides, may also be dependent on other factors, such as pH, ionic strength and temperature. Further characterization of binding and the physiological responses of muscarinic ligands are required in order to determine the synaptic localization of muscarinic receptors in different brain regions and possible differences in function between pre- and postsynaptic muscarinic receptors.

Acknowledgements

Mrs. Ronit Galron provided excellent technical assistance.

REFERENCES

1. Kloog, Y. and Sokolovsky, M. Brain Res. (1977) 134, 167-172.
2. Kloog, Y. and Sokolovsky, M. Brain Res. (1978) 144, 31-48.
3. Kloog, Y. and Sokolovsky, M. Biochem. Biophys. Res. Commun. (1978) 81, 710-717.
4. Kloog, Y., Egozi, Y. and Sokolovsky, M. FEBS Lett. (1978) 95, 265-268.
5. Kloog, Y., Egozi, Y. and Sokolovsky, M. Mol. Pharmacol. (1979) 15, 545-558.
6. Birdsall, N.J.M. and Hulme, E.C. J. Neurochem. (1976) 27, 7-16.
7. Birdsall, N.J.M., Burgen, A.S.V. and Hulme, E.C. Mol. Pharmacol. (1978) 14, 723-736.

8. Birdsall, N.J.M., Burgen, A.S.V. and Hulme, E.C. In: Recent Advances in Receptor Chemistry. Gualtieri, Giannella, Melchiorre Eds. (Elsevier/North Holland Biomedical Press) (1979) pp. 71-95.

9. Kloog, Y., Michaelson, D.M. and Sokolovsky, M. FEBS Lett. (1978) 95, 331-334.

10. Michaelson, D.M., Avissar, S., Kloog, Y. and Sokolovsky, M. Proc. Natl.Acad. Sci. USA (1979) 76, 6336-6340.

11. Kloog, Y., Michaelson, D.M. and Sokolovsky, M. Brain Res. (1980) In press

12. Sokolovsky, M., Egozi, Y. and Kloog,Y. In Progress in Neural Sci. Vol. 7 (1980) In press.

13. Michaelson, D.M. and Sokolovsky, M. Biochem. Biophys. Res. Commun. (1976) 73, 25-31.

14. Michaelson, D.M. and Sokolovsky, M. J. Neurochem. (1978) 30, 217-230.

15. White, T.D. J. Neurochem. (1977) 29, 193-198.

16. Sachs, C. and Jonsson, G. Biochem. Pharmacol. (1975) 24, 1-8.

17. Kato, G., Carson, M.L., Kemel, J. Glowinski, J. and Giorguieff, M.F. Life Sci. (1978) 22, 1607-1614.

18. Descarries, L., and Saucier, G. Brain Res. (1972) 37, 310-316.

19. Galper, J.B., Klein, W. and Catterall, W.A. J. Biol. Chem. (1977) 252, 8692-8699.

20. Kloog, Y., Heron, D.S., Korczyn, A.D., Sachs, D.I. and Sokolovsky, M. Mol. Pharmacol. (1979) 15, 581-587.

21. Kloog, Y., Sach, D.I., Korczyn, A.D., Heron, D.S. and Sokolovsky, M. Biochem. Pharmacol. (1979) 28, 1505-1511.

22. Aronstram, R.S. and Eldefrawi, M.E. Biochem. Pharmacol. (1979) 28, 701-70

23. Hedlund, B. and Bartfai, T. Mol. Pharmacol. (1979) 15, 538-544.

24. Tsai, B.S. and Lefkowitz, R.J. Mol. Pharmacol. 16, 61-68.

25. Berrie, C.P., Birdsall, N.J.M., Burgen, A.S.V. and Hulme, E.C. Biochem. Biophys. Res.Commun.(1979) 87, 1000-1005.

26. Coyle, J.T. and Yamamura, H.I. Brain Res. (1976) 118, 429-440.

27. Szerb, J.C. and Somogyi, G.T. Nature (1973) 241, 121-122.

28. Szerb, J.C., Hadhazy, P. and Dudarm, J.D. Brain Res. (1977) 128, 285-291.

29. Michell, R.H.M., Jafferji, S.S. and Jones, L.M. FEBS Lett. (1976) 69, 1-5.

30. Matsuzawa, H. and Nirenberg, M. Proc. Natl. Acad. Sci. USA (1975) 72, 3472-3476.

31. Burgermeister, W., Klein, W.L., Nirenberg, M. and Witkop, B. Mol. Pharmacol. (1978) 14, 751-767.

Neurotransmitters and their Receptors
Edited by U.Z. Littauer, Y. Dudai, I. Silman,
V.I. Teichberg and Z. Vogel

Nicotinic Acetylcholine Receptors of the CNS, In Comparison to Peripheral Receptors

E.A. Barnard, R.I. Norman, B. Lang, K. Sumikawa and J.O. Dolly
Department of Biochemistry, Imperial College, London SW7, UK

Abstract

Post-synaptic α-toxins have been used as probes to compare nicotinic acetylcholine receptors from (a) brain (optic tectum), (b) various muscles, and (c) Torpedo electric organ. The toxin-binding receptors isolated from (b) and (c) by affinity chromatographic methods differ in the number and sizes of their subunits. The latter always have in common, however, a subunit of ~42,000 MW which carries the acetylcholine-binding site and the α-bungarotoxin binding site (in equal numbers, each at two sites per oligomeric molecule). In the case of (a), the optic tectum of lower vertebrates, where a functional synaptic nicotinic acetylcholine receptor blocked by this toxin again occurs, a number of important differences from (b) and (c) are found.

The nicotinic acetylcholine-binding receptor protein has been isolated from the optic tectum of the chick. Ultra-structural evidence shows a synaptic location of this receptor. Comparisons are made here between these central and peripheral acetylcholine receptors. Such comparisons can lead to the recognition of essential elements of nicotinic cholinergic transmission.

Receptors from Peripheral Sites: Principal Features

The nicotinic acetylcholine (ACh) receptor from peripheral sites in vertebrates is now a well-characterized molecular entity. It has been studied extensively in the membrane-bound state and in purified form, from fish electric organs (for reviews see (1) and the articles from many of the laboratories active in this field in (2)) and likewise from skeletal muscles (3-5). From both sources, the receptor can be extracted into non-ionic detergent media with full retention of its specific binding properties, and can be purified to homogeneity as a protein. For comparison with the CNS nicotinic ACh receptors, some of the salient features of the ACh receptors from mammalian skeletal muscles, as determined in our laboratory or that of Z. W. Hall (3-14), are summarized in (i) to (vi) below. In general, these apply also to the ACh receptors from fish electric organ as studied extensively elsewhere (1, 2).

(i) They can be isolated in detergent media, as a pure glycoprotein in each case, with isoelectric point near pH 5. They are devoid of possible contaminants such as acetylcholinesterase or actin.

(ii) They react specifically with elapid venom post-synaptic neurotoxins; with the 'long' (71- to 74- residue) post-synaptic toxins such as α-bungarotoxin (α-BuTX) the dissociation rate from the complex is so slow that the binding is pseudo-irreversible.

(iii) The specific binding of such a toxin occurs at saturation to the extent of about 1 molecule per 125,000 MW of the protein.

(iv) The receptor, both in the membranes and when isolated, binds nicotinic agonists or antagonists, with relative affinities parallel to those observed pharmacologically with the muscles in question. Each of these bindings and the toxin binding are mutually fully exclusive. This binding can be converted to a specific irreversible reaction (after -SS- reduction) using a maleimide affinity reagent (14) or using bromoacetylcholine (Fig.1) as the ligand (8,9).

(v) In the case of the bromoacetylcholine affinity reaction, there is (9) one such site for every toxin binding site, both in the membrane-bound and the purified muscle receptor. This holds true as well (Fig. 1) in the <u>Torpedo</u> receptor (despite earlier evidence (15,16) showing apparently only half that stoichiometric ratio there). The same has been shown to be true for the sites binding reversible ligands, which are equal in number to the toxin-binding sites (17).

(vi) The receptor exists in detergent media, when freshly extracted or when purified, as one hydrodynamic species, with sedimentation coefficient 9S. This is the form extracted from both innervated and denervated muscle.

The last point does not apply to the receptor from *Torpedo* electroplax membranes, which is, in contrast, obtained in the extracts as a mixture of 9S and 13S active species. The proportions of these are affected by the addition of thiols or by a pre-blocking of -SH groups in the membranes, suggesting that the 13S form is a native, disulphide-bridged dimer of the 9S form (18,19). It has not been proven that this dimer is the form of the receptor actually in the membrane, and this dimerization is not evident from negative-stained electron micrographs of these membranes (20,21) nor in freeze-etched views of the synaptic membranes in ultra-rapidly-frozen electric organ (22). The disulphide-binding dimerization of the receptor in solution cannot be induced in the muscle receptor by the treatment (18) with N-ethylmaleimide (blocking other thiols) which encourages it in the *Torpedo* receptor (11).

The 9S sedimentation coefficient of the isolated receptor, characteristic of all species so far investigated, corresponds to a molecular weight of about 260,000 daltons, as measured by several physical techniques (independent of bound detergent) with the electric organ purified ACh receptor (23, and refs. cited therein). The same size is shown by gel analysis after chemical cross-linking of it (24). Since the mammalian muscle receptor migrates with the *Torpedo* receptor in a sucrose density gradient and in agarose gel columns, we take it to be close to the same molecular weight.

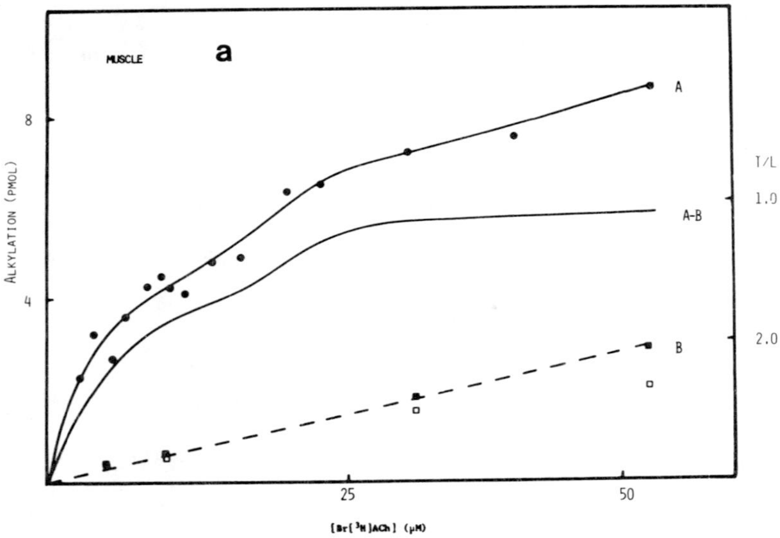

Fig. 1:

(a) Affinity alkylation of muscle receptor by bromoacetylcholine. The receptor purified from cat denervated leg muscles was reduced by dithiothreitol and alkylated by various concentrations of bromo[^{3}H]-acetylcholine as shown. Curve A (●), total bound reagent. Curve B, bound reagent, in equivalent control samples treated with (■) 5 μM α-BuTX or (□) 100 μM tubocurarine before and during the alkylation. The difference curve, A-B, represents the specific alkylation. All values are for a fixed concentration of receptor. T/L (right hand axis) is the ratio of the toxin-binding sites in the sample to the sites alkylated. Note that at the maximum of specific alkylation this ratio is 1:1, and that the two reactive sites per molecule react with different affinities in the alkylation. From Wolosin *et al*. (9).

(b) SDS gel electrophoresis of the cat muscle receptor after reduction and labelling with bromo[^{3}H]acetylcholine. (■) Calibration of molecular weight by standard proteins: The peak corresponds to an apparent molecular weight of 43,000. (o) A parallel control sample pretreated with 5 μM α-BuTX and then labelled as before. From Lyddiat et al. (8). The same peak was obtained after alkylation at low or at high bromo[^{3}H]acetylcholine concentrations (see a), and for the muscle ACh receptor in the membrane and in the purified state; the same concentration dependence curve, final ratio, and single α-subunit labelling were obtained with the *Torpedo* ACh receptor, in either state (9).

Subunit Structure of Peripheral ACh Receptors

When analysed by sodium dodecyl sulphate (SDS) gel electrophoresis, the purified ACh receptor from Torpedo has widely been reported to contain 4 subunit types, with the composition $\alpha_2\beta\gamma\delta$, with apparent molecular weights about 40,000 (α), 50,000 (β), 60,000 (γ) and 68,000 (δ) daltons, varying somewhat with the species of electric ray (and eel 25)) and the precise conditions of analysis (see reviews in (1 , 24). and an example in Fig. 2 (right)). Even the relative values of the subunit molecular weights determined in SDS gel electrophoresis are apparent only, since they vary with the degree of the gel cross-linking (5,8).

On the other hand, J.-P. Changeux and co-workers have reported a method of receptor isolation from highly purified Torpedo membranes, which avoids the usual affinity chromatography on immobilised toxin and yields a preparation of highly active ACh receptor comprising primarily the α-chain, with very much smaller proportions of the β and δ chains (only) which may not be intrinsic to the native ligand-binding unit (1,26,27). The significance of these differences from the other type of receptor preparation is at present an unresolved question (1,2,26,27). The δ chains can mutually cross-link by a disulphide bridge (19,24); this may explain the formation of the 13S dimer in the Torpedo receptor.

The ACh receptor purified from cat denervated muscle has subunits apparently of only one size in SDS gel analysis, 43,000MW (7,8) (Fig.2). However, two-dimensional subunit mapping (28) of muscle receptor proteins indicates that there are two types of these subunits, α and $\acute{\alpha}$ differing in charge but not resolvable by size alone in the usual polyacrylamide SDS gel system (29,30). In another gel system the cat muscle receptor migrates as a 46,000 MW subunit (Fig.2).

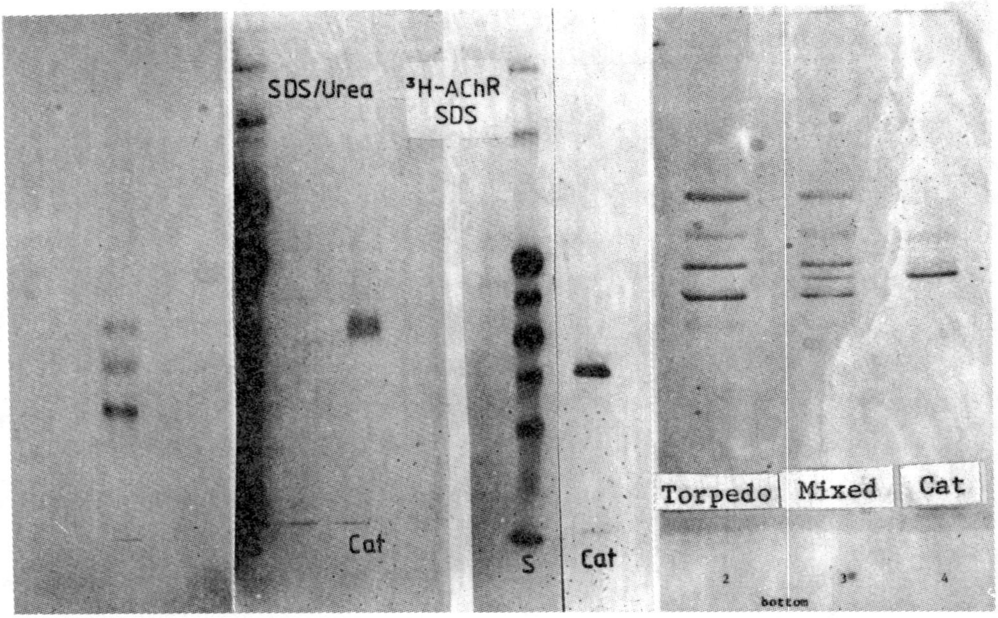

Fig. 2.

Right: SDS gel electrophoresis (with protein staining) of purified ACh receptor from Torpedo (track 2) cat muscle (track 4) and an equal mixture of the two (track 3). In the polyacrylamide system used here with only 0.08% bisacrylamide, the subunit of the cat receptor has an apparent molecular weight of 46,000 and is well resolved from the α-subunit of Torpedo receptor. Centre: Fluorograms after SDS gel electrophoresis of pure ACh receptor from cat denervated muscle (labelled by [^{3}H]propionylation after purification) in right-hand track, with 9 standard labelled proteins run in parallel (5). In left-hand tracks, the same standards and also the labelled, pure cat receptor, run in 0.1% SDS/9 M urea. Note that the positions of the standard has apparent molecular weight of 46,000 in the urea and 43,000 in its absence. It remains a single band in each, although broadened in the urea. Left: Fluorogram after gel electrophoresis in 0.1% SDS/9 M urea of similarly-[^{3}H]labelled pure ACh receptor from denervated chicken muscle. The migration time and gel length are less than in the gel for the cat receptor, and the lowest subunit seen is the α-subunit (which also labels specifically by bromo[^{3}H]acetylcholine after reduction), of 42,000 apparent molecular weight, the other subunits being at about 52,000 and 62,000.

The α-subunit is the site of bromoacetylcholine affinity labelling, and is the only species specifically labelled when the reaction is applied to the muscle itself (Fig. 1b). Hence it is a native, ligand-binding subunit.

Muscle ACh receptors purified from some other species studied, e.g. the chick (Fig. 2 , _left_), are found to contain two subunits in addition to the α-subunit, so the composition of the molecule apparently varies between different sources. The α-subunit is always the major one, its exact MW varying between species, from 40,000-46,000. When the _Torpedo marmorata_ ACh receptor is purified by the method which we use for the cat muscle preparation showing only the α-size subunit, then the same multiple subunit pattern is found (Fig. 2, _right_) as reported by others, namely $\alpha_2\beta\gamma\delta$ (by size).

The α-subunit from _Torpedo_ can be resolved in certain conditions of gel electrophoresis (8) from the α-subunits from muscle receptors (Fig. 2, _right_). Gel electrophoresis in the presence of SDS and 9M urea gives a clearer demonstration of the bands due to the subunits of muscle receptors (although the urea gives some broadening of these bands, and the molecular weight calibration by standard globular proteins becomes skewed). The difference between the α-subunits of the cat muscle receptor and the 3 subunits - α, β and a heavier (between γ and δ size) one - of the denervated chicken muscle receptor is clearly seen (Fig. 2). The receptors purified similarly from innervated or embryonic chicken muscles show the same triple subunit pattern (30). Again, the α-subunit in these chicken muscle receptors can be labelled, alone, by reduction and $\{^3H\}$ bromacetylcholine reaction, indicating that the α-subunits from the cat, chicken and _Torpedo_ receptors are equivalent structures despite the varying numbers of heavier subunits found with them.

Hall and co-workers (5,14,31) have purified the ACh receptor from rat muscles and found in SDS gels two major subunits, with apparent molecular weights 45,000 and 51,000, and several minor components. The 45,000 MW subunit (α_1) labels with the maleimide affinity reagent after reduction, but there is also a strong labelling in a minor subunit of 49,000 MW, but not the others seen (5,14). The significance of the apparent subunit structure differences between receptors of muscles from different species, prepared in different laboratories, is not yet clarified.

Since the molecular weight of the intact molecule is about 260,000, this agrees in the case of Torpedo receptors with the structure $\alpha_2\beta\gamma\delta$ based on the sizes of the subunits observed (Fig. 2) in the usual SDS gel analysis (23,32). Hence the molecule could be a pentameric structure, with two subunits (α) each carrying one ACh binding site. This assembly is presumed to contain the ion channel, opened by an allosteric change induced by the binding of 2 ACh per molecule.

For the receptor from cat denervated muscle, the molecular weight is about the same, and again there are two α subunits per molecule, which bind the ACh. However, the other (α') subunits, chemically different from α, are in this species the same apparent size in the usual SDS gel analysis. This would fit a hexameric structure, $\alpha_2\alpha'_4$, although we do not know whether the non-binding α' subunits are themselves all of one structure, and their exact number, 3 or 4, is as yet uncertain, since they are larger than α in some species; the anomalous behaviour in SDS gel electrophoresis may differ between these subunit types. Nevertheless, a general pattern of subunit structure similarity and difference between electric organ and muscle ACh receptors is apparent from the summary of information on them given here.

Binding sites in the vertebrate brain for post-synaptic neurotoxins.

The binding of toxins such as α-BuTX, in radioactive form, has been described by various authors at sites in vertebrate brains, spinal cord and autonomic ganglia (see reviews in 3, 33, 34). In general, however, no physiological blockade of synaptic transmission or associated receptor function has as yet been shown to be associated with this binding of the toxin, and, in fact, in a number of cases where tested by intracellular recording α-BuTX has been shown to cause no blockade of response in the conditions where the binding is observed (34). Likewise, Hunt and Schmidt (35) found that the development in the rat hippocampus of the α-BuTX binding sites is independent of cholinergic input, and that they are unaffected when cholinergic termination and acetylcholinesterase are absent due to lesion. Another differentiation between toxin binding and receptor activity was shown by Patrick and Stallcup (36), in cultured neurones previously shown to bind ^{125}I-α-BuTX in a saturable, cholinergic ligand-sensitive manner, and to respond to ACh by Na^+ permeability increase: α-BuTX did not block the response to an agonist, and those two phenomena were shown, by immunological methods, to be independent and to occur at different components on those cells. Pharmacological dissociation of the binding of α-BuTX from ACh excitation in neurones in culture has been made, also, by Carbonetto et al. (37).

When the post-synaptic toxin probe is used, it seems desirable to accept as a nicotinic ACh receptor only sites where the α-toxin binding is (a) saturable, at a high enough affinity to distinguish it clearly from non-specific binding; (b) sensitive to nicotinic cholinergic ligands at physiological concentrations; (c) exerted at sites where blockade of the physiological response can be demonstrated under the conditions of binding of the toxin; and (d) present to an extent, and with a regional distribution in the nervous system,which are not inconsistent with physiological evidence on the occurence of nicotinic types of synapse. While these are necessary criteria for the use of this probe, and (a) and (b) alone are inadequate, they will not identify all nicotinic ACh receptors, since at some locations synapses are known which are of the nicotinic type by pharmacological criteria but which are completely insensitive to α-BuTX (34,38).

There is evidence, however, at two types of central site, so far, for blockade by a post-synaptic toxin of a functional ACh nicotinic receptor. Firstly, at certain sites in the spinal cord, Miledi and colleagues have shown that two post-synaptic toxins from the venom of Dendroaspis viridis (D.v., a green mamba) can block the neurally-evoked response at synapses of nicotinic cholinergic character in the frog (39, 40). Other post-synaptic toxins, including α-BuTX, were ineffective there (38, 40). The most potent in this effect was the pure toxin D.v. 4.9.3 of Shipolini et al. (41), a long neurotoxin of 72 amino acid residues and with a high degree of sequence homology with α-BuTX, but differing at the usually invariant positions lysine-29 and glutamic acid-43 (39). The second toxin from the same venom active at this spinal cord synapse was D.v. 4.11.3, a 'short' neurotoxin (60 residues) which had much poorer blocking ability. The second type of toxin-sensitive site involves synapes in the optic tectum of lower vertebrates. There, Freeman and co-workers (42,43) have shown that application of α-BuTx to toad or goldfish optic tectum abolishes the activation of certain neurones by optic nerve stimulation. The synapses in question depend upon nicotinic ACh receptors, by pharmacological analysis (42,44, 45).

The latter results are particularly interesting, since the use of α-BuTX or cobratoxins as probes for the central nicotinic ACh receptor is arbitrary, depending upon their originally observed blocking potency on muscle, and distinct variations in the activities of snake venom post-synaptic toxins between different muscle types are known (46,47). It is to be expected, therefore, that such variation would be more pronounced when any sensitive central receptor is brought into comparision;

the latter receptor type may well have diverged from the structure to which α-BuTX is particularly adapted, whereas other such toxins may happen to fit it better. We have, therefore, examined the optic tectum binding of both α-BuTX and the D.v. toxins.

Properties of nicotinic ACh receptors in optic tectum membranes

The chick optic lobe contains a distinct set of specific α-BuTX binding sites, as measured by the binding of [^{3}H]monopropionyl-α-BuTX (3) or ^{125}I-α-BuTX (Table I). When the tectum layer is separated, the binding is found to be concentrated therein, and when fractionated the great majority of it is in the synaptosomal-mitochondrial fraction. The binding is saturable, showing a single class of sites in a Scatchard plot (3). The dissociation constant, K_D, obtained thus for the receptor-α-BuTX complex is 1 nM at 22°C, the binding being reversible (half-time for dissociation, 5¾ hr). A low proportion of lower affinity binding sites is not excluded by the data obtained. The binding is blocked by unlabelled α-BuTX competitively, and also by nicotinic ligands at low concentrations (Table II), but not by atropine, adrenaline or dopamine. Wang et al. (48) have deduced from ligand competition studies with optic lobe extracts that there is one specific ligand binding site per toxin site (as in the peripheral receptors: see above).

The concentrations of these sites in the tissue are shown in Table I). They decline notably with development of the animal, as has been reported in more detail previously (48,49) for the toxin binding of whole optic lobe Triton extracts. The mature frog (Rana pipiens) optic lobe contains about the same level of these sites as in the 2-day chick. The concentrations in the mammalian cortex or the rest of the brain, tissues which have been used in a number of toxin-binding studies (Table I), are much lower, even in the chick, and show much less decrease with age (49).

Table I

Concentrations of Binding Sites for α-BuTX in Brain Membranes

Source	pmoles/g wet weight[a]	Reference
Optic Lobe		
Chicks, 1 day	27.7 $\pm$ 2.7 (S.D.)	This work
3-4 weeks	4.8	
>3 months	3.7	
Cortex		
Chicks, 1 day	6	
> 3 months	4	
Rat	2 - 5	51, 55
Guinea pig	2.1	56
Whole Brain		
Chick, 1 day	7.5	57
Rat	2.3	52, 53
Mouse	1.7	58
Goldfish	1.1	54

[a]The binding of radioactive α-BuTX at saturation was measured either in the particulate fraction from a homogenate, or after extracting it in Triton X-10 medium, and was related to the wet weight of the original tissue.

The mamba toxin D.v.4.9.3 showed strong binding to these chick optic tectum sites (Table II), whereas D.v. 4.11.3 showed binding 100- to 1000- fold weaker than this (Fig.3). Both toxins were equally strong in binding to skeletal muscle receptor (Table II).

When reduced with dithiothreitol as in the case of muscle (8), there is no loss of the toxin binding activity, and reaction with bromoacetylcholine (as described above; cf. Fig.1) then blocks all of that binding, this reaction being as sensitive to cholinergic ligands as is the α-BuTX reaction. A specific affinity labelling is thus obtained as with the muscle and electroplax receptors (Fig.1), indicating a similarity in the binding site.

An active conjugate of α-BuTX with peroxidase (1:1) has been used to localise this binding in the whole optic tectum. Electron microscopy of the conjugate-stained chick tectum showed labelling at certain synapses, which is abolished by pre-treatment with α-BuTX (3).

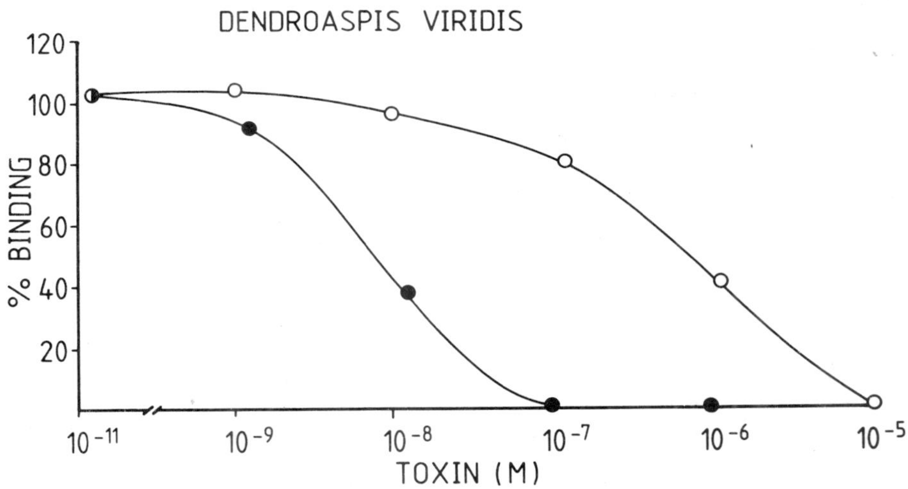

Fig.3

Binding isotherms at 22°C for 2 mamba toxins at chick optic tectum membranes. The displacement of [^{3}H]-α-BuTX at equilibrium by increasing amounts of the competing toxin was measured. The percentage change produced in the uptake by a fixed number of binding sites is plotted against the logarithm of the concentration of the competing toxin (o), D.v. toxin 4-9-3 (mean for 6 experiments); (o), D.v. toxin 4-11-3.

TABLE II Dissociation constants of ligands at α-BuTX binding sites in membranes

	Optic tectum (22°)[a]	Muscle (25°)	
	Chick	Cat[b]	Chick[c] embryo
	M	M	M
[^{3}H]α-BuTX	0.7×10^{-9}	$\sim 10^{-12}$	$\sim 10^{-12}$
D.v. toxin 4-9-3	4.5×10^{-9}	$<10^{-11}$	
toxin 4-11-3	6×10^{-7}	$<10^{-11}$	
Nicotine	2.5×10^{-7}		1.4×10^{-6}
d-Tubocurarine	2.9×10^{-6}	4×10^{-8}	2.1×10^{-7}
Decamethonium	7.1×10^{-6}	3×10^{-7}	2.3×10^{-8}
Atropine	$>10^{-3}$	$>10^{-3}$	
Adrenaline	$>10^{-3}$		
Hexamethonium	$>10^{-5}$	4×10^{-5}	4.7×10^{-5}

[a]Experiments of the type shown in Fig.3 were performed with each ligand, using the membrane fraction, and the data were treated to derive K_D. The medium was 50 mM Na phosphate, pH 7.6. For other data on ligand affinities (at 37°C) in extracts of o[illegible] lobe, see ref. 48.

[b]A receptor-rich membrane fraction from denervated cat leg muscle was used. From Barnard et al. (4), except for the toxin bindings.

[c]Data of Wang et al.(48), for solubilised chick embryo (13-day) leg muscles, crude extract in 0.1% Triton X-100: the protection constant at 37°C was measured.

These are in the layers corresponding to the physiologically-recorded nicotinic sites, but account for only a small fraction of the total synapses. The staining was conducted in the absence of metals which would stain post-synaptic densities, and control sections were devoid of the latter. Nevertheless, the specific staining seen was post-synaptic (3); only such a synaptic localisation of this binding component has been detected thus.

Properties of the isolated ACh receptor from optic cectum

The α-BuTX binding activity can be extracted in high yield (>80%) in each of several non-ionic detergents, in the conditions used (6) for muscle ACh receptor. The solubilised receptor shows a specific, reversible binding, with K_D 1.8 nM at 22°C, this being sensitive as before to nicotinic ligands. This receptor is a glycoprotein, binding well to both concanavalin A and *Lens culinaris* lectin, as for the muscle ACh receptor (7,12) and for the α-BuTX binding activity from rat brain cortex (50).

Purification of the optic tectum receptor has been achieved using the procedures summarised in Table III. Actin is removed by the DNase I affinity gel, and some other contaminating proteins by the GTP-Sepharose. α-BuTX is used as the immobilised ligand in the first affinity chromatography, due to the reversibility of the complex with this toxin (in contrast to the case of the electric organ or muscle receptor, where α-BuTX cannot be employed thus). The affinity chromatography on the lentil (*Lens culinaris*)lectin column can be used as for the muscle receptor (7).

The purified receptor is labelled with ^{125}I when finally concentrated in the sugar elution from the lectin colum. When examined thus, or as the native receptor complexed with [^{125}I]α-BuTX, it is seen to behave as essentially one species (Fig.4). The binding activity is totally destroyed by mild protease treatments. The purified receptor migrates as a single peak in sucrose density gradients, with sedimentation coefficient 8.6 S. This value is obtained (with 0.2% Lubrol PX present in the sucrose grdient, using either pure [^{125}I]receptor or assaying native receptor) when the initial extraction is performed in 5% Lubrol PX and the full pro-

TABLE III Purification procedure for optic tectum ACh receptor

Chick Optic Lobe[a]
↓
5% Lubrol PX + protease inhibitors[b] (1hr, 4°C)
↓
α-BuTX-gel (minimum 7 hr; 4°C; 74% bound)[c]
↓
1 M NaCl + buffer washes
↓
1 M carbamylcholine (25-30% eluted)
↓
G-25 gel filtration (removal of all carbamylcholine)
↓
GTP-Sepharose[d]
↓
DNase-Sepharose[d]
↓
lentil lectin gel[b] (100% bound)
↓
0.4 M glycosides[b] + EDTA (84% eluted)
↓
gel filtration or dialysis

---

[a] Homogenised and particulate fraction extracted.

[b] Details as in (7).

[c] All procedures from here onwards are in 0.2% Lubrol PX, buffered at pH 7.4.

[d] The solution is extracted with these gels and the soluble fraction processed further.

cedure of Table III is employed. When the initial extraction is in 2% Triton X-100 and the extractions with GTP-Sepharose and DNase-Sepharose are omitted, the density gradient (in 0.2% Triton X-100) gives, instead, a value of about 12 S (3). Values in the range 11.4 S - 12.9 S have been found by others for the α-BuTX-binding activity in whole brain crude extracts from rat (51-53) or goldfish (54). The higher value in the case of the chick optic tectum receptor is associated with the presence of additional subunits which are removable without activity loss to give the 8.6 S species and are therefore regarded as not integral to the receptor. Subunit analysis, as above, of the purified (8.6 S) tectum [^{125}I]receptor shows subunits of 53,000 and 58,000 daltons as present, while a subunit in the range 40-46,000 as found in muscle is definitely absent; however, further analysis is required to determine the stoichiometric subunit composition of this protein.

Most of the properties determined for the chick optic tectum receptor in crude extracts have been found, also, to be shown in extracts of the frog optic tectum, for which direct physiological evidence on toxin blockade exists.

Antibody raised to the pure receptor from cat denervated muscle shows a low but definite cross-reactivity with the chick optic tectum

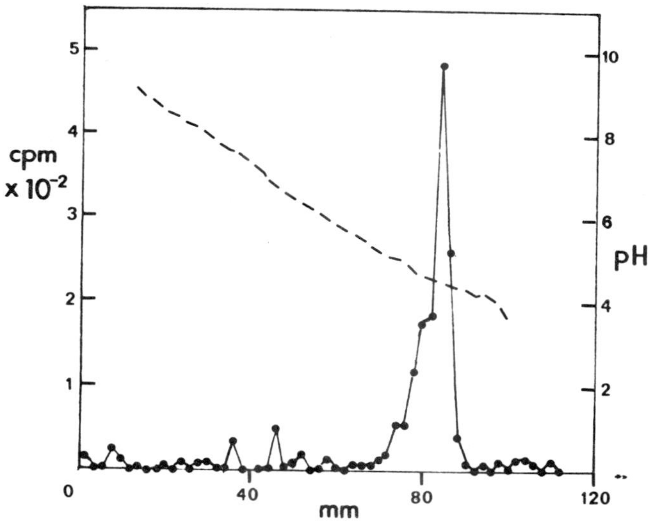

Fig.4 Purity of the isolated receptor from chick optic tectum. The receptor from 2-day chicks was purified as in Table II, radio-iodinated and analysed by isoelectric focussing (pH gradient, shown by broken line). The main component has an isoelectric point of 4.6 (cf. 4.9-5.0 for non-iodinated pure muscle and Torpedo receptors). The additional, more acidic species, not resolved, may be due to higher degrees of iodination.

receptor (E.Nockles and J.O.Dolly, unpublished data), as shown by immunoprecipitation assay. This cross-reactivity is about one-third that of innervated chick muscle receptor as antigen towards this antibody, and is of the same order as that for Torpedo receptor as the antigen, so this constitutes evidence for some degree of homology of the tectum and muscle receptors.

Similarities and differences

In summary, the ACh receptor from the optic tectum has clear similariti to the peripheral ACh receptor (Table IV). Its ligand affinities resemble those expected from the pharmacology of the neuromuscular junction, and not those (34) of the toxin-insensitive nicotinic cholinergic synapses at autonomic ganglia or the Renshaw cell. Thus, decamethonium and d-tubocurarine are strong ligands (though definitely weaker than in muscle) and hexamethonium is weak, in the case of the tectum receptors, whereas the opposite is true for the latter two types of synapse (34). Significant differences, however, have already emerged, as in the reversibility of the tectum toxin-receptor complex and the differential effects of the D.v. toxins. The stronger tectal interaction of nicotine is a difference generally found with central α-BuTX sites (48, 52, 55). The toxin sensitivity, bromoacetylcholine reactivity and the antibody cross-reactivity all suggest that basic molecular homologies do exist between the two classes of receptor compared here. It should be of value to pursue those similarities, in defining the essential molecular elements of the nicotinic receptor/ion channel assembly.

Acknowledgement The work of the authors was supported by a Programme Grant of the Medical Research Council.

TABLE IV Similarities in muscle and optic tectum ACh receptors

Property	Optic tectum	Muscle
1. Binding of α-BuTX (at 25°C) [a]	1 class of binding sites $k_{on} \sim 10^5$	1st class $\sim 10^5\ M^{-1}s^{-1}$
But	K_D=1	$\sim$ 0.001 nM
2. A protein, extracted in non-ionic detergent in active form	Yes	Yes
3. Binding to concanavalin A and lentil lectins	Strong	Strong
4. Sedimentation coefficient	8.6 S	9.0 S
5. Specific reaction with BrACh, after reduction	Yes	Yes
6. Cross-reactivity to antibody to cat muscle extra-synaptic ACh receptor (ratio, relative to chick innervated muscle receptor as antigen)	0.3	1 (chick)
7. Cholinergic ligand binding	Specific, and generally similar (see Table II)	

[a] The tectum binding sites are homogeneous in reaction in the membranes (3) and in extracts (48), as is the muscle 9 S receptor (10). k_{on} is the rate constant for the forward reaction with α-BuTX, and is 7 x $10^5\ M^{-1}\ s^{-1}$ for embryonic chick tectum extracts (48) and 2 x $10^5\ M^{-1}\ s^{-1}$ for cat denervated muscle 9 S receptor (10).

REFERENCES

. Heidmann, T. and Changeux, J.-P. (1978) Ann. Rev. Biochem. 43, 317-357.

. Ceccarelli, B. and Clementi, F. (editors) (1979). Advances in Cytopharmacology, Vol. 3 (Raven Press, New York).

. Barnard, E.A., Dolly, J.O., Lang, B., Lo, M. and Shorr, R.G. (1979). In ref. (1), pp.409-435.

. Barnard, E.A., Coates, V., Dolly, J.O. and Mallick, B. (1977). Cell Biol. Int. Rep. 1, 99-106.

. Nathanson, N.M. and Hall, Z.W. (1979). Biochemistry 15, 3392-3401.

6. Dolly, J.O. and Barnard, E.A. (1977). Biochemistry 16, 5053-5060.

7. Shorr, R.G., Dolly, J.O. and Barnard, E.A. (1978). Nature 274, 283-284.

8. Lyddiatt, A., Sumikawa, K., Wolosin, J.M., Dolly, J.O. and Barnard, E.A. (1979). FEBS Letts. 108, 20-24.

9. Wolosin, J.M., Lyddiatt, A., Dolly, J.O. and Barnard, E.A. (1980). Eur. J. Biochem. (in press).

10. Lo, M., Dolly, J.O. and Barnard, E.A. (1980). Eur. J. Biochem. (in press).

11. Barnard, E.A., Dolly, J.O., Lo, M. and Mantle, T. (1978). Biochem. Soc. Trans. 7, 649-651.

12. Brockes, J.P. and Hall, Z.W. (1975). Biochemistry 14, 2092-2099.

13. Brockes, J.P. and Hall, Z.W. (1975). Biochemistry 14, 2100-2106.

14. Froehner, S.O., Karlin, A. and Hall, Z.W. (1977). Proc. Natl. Acad. Sci. USA 74, 4685-4688.

15. Damle, V.N., McLaughlin, M. and Karlin, A. (1978). Biochem. Biophys. Res. Commun. 84, 845-851.

16. Moore, H.-P.H. and Raftery, M.A. (1979). Biochemistry 18, 1862-1867.

17. Neubig, R.R. and Cohen, J.B. (1979). Biochemistry 18, 5464-5475.

18. Chang, H.W. and Bock, E. (1977). Biochemistry 16, 4513-4519.

19. Hamilton, S.L., McLaughlin, M. and Karlin, A. (1977). Biochem. Biophys. Res. Commun. 79, 692-699.

20. Lo, M., Garland, P.B., Lamprecht, J. and Barnard, E.A. (1980). FEBS Letts. 111, 407-412.

21. Zingsheim, H.P., Neugebauer, D.-C., Barrantes, F.J. and Frank, J. (1980) Proc. Natl. Acad. Sci. USA 77, 952-956.

22. Heuser, J.E. and Salpeter, S.R. (1979) J. Cell Biol. 82, 150-173.

23. Reynolds, J. and Karlin, A. (1978). Biochemistry 17, 2035-2038.

24. Hucho, F., Bandini, G. and Suarez-Isla, B.A. (1978). Eur.J.Biochem. 83, 335-340.

25. Lindstrom, J., Cooper, J. and Tzartos, S. (1980) Biochemistry 19, 1454-1458.

26. Sobel, A., Weber, M. and Changeux, J.-P. (1977). Eur. J. Biochem. 80, 215-224.

27. Wennogle, L.P. and Changeux, J.-P. (1980). Eur.J.Biochem. 106, 381-393.

28. O'Farrell, P.H. (1975). J. Biol. Chem. 250, 4007-4021.

29. Merlie, J.P., Changeux, J.-P. and Gros, F. (1978). J.Biol. Chem. 253, 2882-2

30. Sumikawa, K., Dolly, J.O. and Barnard, E.A. (1980). In preparation.

31. Froehner, S.C., Reiness, S.G. and Hall, Z.W. (1977). J.Biol. Chem. 252, 8589-8596.

32. Vandlen, R.L., Wu, W.C.-S., Eisenach, J.C. and Raftery, M.A. (1979). Biochemistry 18, 1845-1854.

33. Lukas, R.S., Morimoto, H. and Bennett, E.L. (1979). Biochemistry 18, 2384-2394.

34. Brown, D.A. (1979). In ref (1), pp.225-230.

35. Hunt, S. and Schmidt, J. (1979). Neuroscience 4, 585-592.

36. Patrick, J. and Stallcup, B. (1977). Proc. Natl. Acad. Sci. USA 74, 4689-4692.

37. Carbonetto, S.T., Fambrough, D.M. and Muller, K.J. (1978). Proc. Natl. Acad. Sci. USA 75, 1016-1020.

38. Duggan, A.W., Hall, J.G.. Headley, P.M., Hendry, I.A. and Minchim, M.C.W. (1976). Neurosci. Lett. 3, 123-127.

39. Banks, B.E.C., Miledi, R. and Shipolini, R.A. (1974). Eur.J. Biochem. 45, 457-468.

40. Miledi, R. and Szczepaniak, A.C. (1975). Proc. R. Soc. Lond.(Biol.) 190, 267-274.

41. Shipolini, R.A., Bailey, G.S. and Banks, B.E.C. (1974). Eur. J. Biochem. 42, 203-211.

42. Freeman, J.A. (1977). Nature 269, 218-222.

43. Freeman, J.A., Schmidt, J.T. and Oswald, R.E. (1980). Neuroscience (in press).

44. Freeman, J.A. and Schmidt, J.T. (1980). Brain Res. (in press).

45. Chung, S.-H., personal communication.

46. Lee, C.Y. (1979). In ref. (2), pp.1-16.

47. Burden, S.J., Hartzell, H.C. and Yoshikami, D. (1975). Proc. Natl. Acad. Sci. USA 72, 3245-3249.

48. Wang, G.-K., Molinaro, S. and Schmidt, J. (1978). J. Biol. Chem. 253, 8507-8512.

49. Kouvelas, E.D. and Greene,L.A. (1976). Brain Res. 113, 111-126.

50. Salvaterra, P.M., Gurd, J.M. and Mahler, H.R. (1977). J.Neurochem. 29, 345-348.

51. Salvaterra, P.M. and Mahler, H.R. (1976). J.Biol. Chem. 251, 6327-6334.

52. Lowy, J., McGregor, J., Rosenstone, J. and Schmidt, J. (1976). Biochemistry 15, 1522-1527.

53. Moore, W.M. and Brady, R.N. (1977). Biochim. Biophys. Acta 498: 331-340.

54. Oswald, R.E. and Freeman, J.A. (1979). J. Biol. Chem. 254, 3419-3426.

55. Eterovic, V.A. and Bennett, E.L. (1974). Biochim. Biophys. Acta 362, 346-355.

56. Salvaterra, P.M. and Moore, W.J. (1973). Biochem. Biophys. Res. Commun. 55, 1311-1318.

57. Polz-Tejera, G., Schmidt, J. and Karter, H.J. (1975). Nature 258, 349-341.

58. Seto, A., Arimatsu, Y. and Amano, T. (1977). Neurosci. Letts. 4, 115-119.

Neurotransmitters and their Receptors
Edited by U.Z. Littauer, Y. Dudai, I. Silman,
V.I. Teichberg and Z. Vogel

Immunological Studies on the Nicotinic Acetylcholine Receptor of Rat Brain

S. Wonnacott, R. Harrison and G.G. Lunt
Biochemistry Department, University of Bath, Bath BA2 7AY, England

The nicotinic acetylcholine receptor (nAChR) is the best characterised synaptic receptor. Its isolation from the electric organs of Torpedo and Electrophorus and from vertebrate muscle and the subsequent characterisation of the isolated protein have been facilitated by specific neurotoxins, particularly α-bungarotoxin (1). The occurrence of nAChR in the CNS also has been inferred from the specific binding of radiolabelled snake α-toxins to mammalian brain (see 2). Although nicotinic-like responses have been recorded from the CNS, the characteristics of these responses often differ from the classical example of the neuromuscular junction (3); in particular, certain responses are not blocked by α-bungarotoxin (4,5). To date it has not been demonstrated that the specific α-toxin binding molecules in the CNS are related to a functional nAChR, except in the case of the chick optic tectum (6). Moreover, it is not clear either that all α-bungarotoxin binding sites correspond to nAChR molecules or conversely that all nAChR molecules in the CNS bind α-bungarotoxin.

Study of the nAChR of skeletal muscle has been prompted by its involvement in the autoimmune disease Myasthenia gravis, in which the muscle nAChR is an autoantigen and anti-AChR antibodies are found in the circulation (7). The CSF of myasthenic patients also contains these antibodies (8) and central disturbances, for example, an increased incidence of epilepsy (9) may accompany Myasthenia gravis. We have attempted to compare the immunology of central and peripheral nicotinic receptors by investigating their cross-reactivity with a view to establishing the functional significance of α-toxin binding molecules in the brain.

Distribution of α-bungarotoxin binding sites in rat brain

Subcellular fractions were prepared from cerebral cortices of adult male rats according to the procedure of Rodriguez de Lores Arnaiz et al(10), except that 0.5mM-phenylmethyl sulphonylfluoride and 0.1mM-benzethonium chloride were present in the media. Fractions were assayed for α-toxin binding sites as follows: the resuspended fractions (50-200μl) were incubated with ^{125}I-α-bungarotoxin (0.2 pmol; 600 Ci/mmol) in a total volume of 250µl (containing 10mM-phosphate, pH 7.4, 1% Triton X100, 0.1% BSA) for 20h at $4^{o}C$. Incubations were performed in the presence and absence of 2mM-benzoquinonium chloride. The samples were filtered and washed on Whatman DE 81 filters. The amount of α-toxin bound was linearly related to tissue concentration over at least a ten-fold range and similar results were obtained by $(NH_4)_2SO_4$ precipitation and filtration, or by centrifugation methods.

The binding of ^{125}I-α-bungarotoxin to subcellular fractions of rat cerebral cortex is shown in Table 1. Specific binding was that protected by benzoquinonium chloride; 1mM-d-tubocurare resulted in similar protection.

Specific binding sites were concentrated in the P_2 fraction. When this fraction was osmotically shocked and subjected to sucrose density gradient centrifugation the binding activity peaked in fractions B and C corresponding to synaptic membranes.

Immunological Cross Reactivity

(a) Absorption of rabbit anti-(rat muscle nAChR) antibodies by brain fractions.

TABLE 1. Binding of ^{125}I-α-bungarotoxin to subcellular fractions of rat cerebral cortex

	^{125}I-α-bungarotoxin binding sites (fmol/mg protein) Total	Specific	*Relative Specific Activity
Homogenate	24.2	11.8	11
P_1 (nuclei)	13.3	5.1	-
P_2 (crude mitochondria)	23.3	13.2	-
A(myelin)	26.4	4.3	0.1
B } nerve	73.1	63.5	2.7
C } ending	127.3	68.6	1.7
D } membranes	40.7	31.3	0.9
E (mitochondria)	24.5	7.4	0.1

$$*\frac{\%\ \text{specific binding sites recovered in fraction}}{\%\ \text{total protein recovered in fraction}}$$

Subcellular fractions (2ml representing 4 to 7-fold excess of α-bungarotoxin-binding sites relative to the antiserum added) were incubated with rabbit anti-(rat muscle junctional nAChR) serum (40μl, diluted 1:10 with control rabbit serum) for 90min at 20°C. The samples were then cooled, centrifuged at 100,000*g* and the antibody titre of the supernatant was assayed by using ^{125}I-α-bungarotoxin-labelled rat muscle nAChR.

The results are shown in Table 2. Incubation with homogenate decreased the antibody titre of the serum by 50%. Of the subcellular fractions tested, B and C were the most competent at removing anti-(rat muscle nAChR) antibodies. Control experiments were performed by incubating fractions with anti-(human IgG) serum. No decrease in anti-(human IgG) titre was observed, indicating that the decrease in anti-(rat muscle nAChR) titre reflects a specific adsorption of antibodies.

(b) Assay of anti-(rat muscle nAChR) antiserum with solubilised α-bungarotoxin-labelled molecules from rat brain as antigen.

Subcellular fractions from rat cerebral cortex were solubilised in 1% Triton X100. Samples of the supernatant (equivalent to 50fmol of α-toxin binding sites in the original fraction) were labelled with ^{125}I-α-bungarotoxin (0.5 pmol) and incubated with anti-(rat muscle nAChR) antiserum for 16h at 4°C, followed by addition of sheep anti-(rabbit IgG) antiserum and incubation for a further 16h at 4°C to precipitate the immune complexes. Determinations were performed in the presence and absence of 2mM benzoquimonium chloride. The results are given in Table 3. Homogenate and fractions B and C gave the highest titres. However these titres are less than 20% of the titre with rat muscle nAChR as antigen, despite a presumed excess of brain α-toxin binding sites. This may reflect low cross-reactivity between brain and muscle α-bungarotoxin binding components but alternative explanations are possible. Poor solubilisation from brain or the dissociation or inactivation of labelled species during the prolonged assay period would give low values. Dissociation of ^{125}I-α-bungarotoxin from CNS nAChR in Triton solution has been reported (6).

TABLE 2 Absorption of rabbit anti-(rat muscle AChR) antisera by subcellular fractions of rat cerebral cortex

Fraction	Homogenate	A	B	C	D	E
% Decrease in antibody titre	52.5	12.3	62.1	43.7	23.7	13.3

Conclusions

Rat brain binds α-bungarotoxin in a specific manner, protectable by nicotinic antagonists. Following subcellular fractionation, synaptic membrane fractions show the highest specific activity of α-bungarotoxin binding. These fractions are the most efficient at absorbing antibodies generated against muscle nAChR from the same species, indicating that up to 60% of the antibodies can cross-react with brain species. Experiments are in progress to determine if this is the maximum cross-reactivity. Solubilised ^{125}I-α-bungarotoxin binding molecules from brain fractions give low titres for rabbit anti-(rat muscle nAChR) antiserum; this may reflect (i) low cross-reactivity between brain and muscle ^{125}I-α-bungarotoxin binding molecules, (ii) instability of solubilised nAChR from brain, or (iii) the presence of cross-reacting species from brain which do not bind α-bungarotoxin under the conditions employed.

Acknowledgements

We are grateful to Ms. G. Edwards and Ms. T. Marengo for their assistance in this work, which is supported by the Medical Research Council and the Muscular Dystrophy Group of Great Britain.

TABLE 3 Rabbit anti-(rat muscle nAChR) antiserum titres comparing rat cerebral cortex fractions and rat muscle nAChR as antigen

Fraction	Homogenate	A	B	C	D	E	Muscle nAChR
Titre (10^{-9}M)	18.3	0	9.9	7.7	2.2	1.8	97.2

References

1. Heidmann, T. and Changeux, J-P, (1978) Ann. Rev. Biochem. 47, 317-357.
2. Morley, B.J., Kemp, G.E. and Salvaterra, P. (1979) Life Sci. 24, 859-872.
3. Krnjevic, K. (1974) Physiol. Rev. 54, 418-540.
4. Miledi, R. and Szczepaniak, A.C. (1975) Proc. Roy. Soc. Lond. B. 190, 267-27
5. Duggan, A.W., Hall, J.G. and Lee, C.Y. (1976) Brain Res. 107, 166-170.
6. Barnard, E.A., Dolly, J.O., Lang, B., Lo, M. and Shorr, R.G. (1979) Adv. in cytopharmacol. 3, 409-435.
7. Simpson, J.A. (1978) Muscle and Nerve, 1, 151-156.
8. Lefvert, A.K. and Pirksanen, R. (1977) The Lancet ii, 351-352.
9. Hoefer, P.F.A., Aranow, H. and Rowland, O.P. (1958) Arch. Neurol. Psychiat. 80, 10-17.
10. Rodriguez de Lores Arnaiz, G., Alberici, M. and De Robertis, E. (1967) J. Neurochem. 14, 215-225.

Neurotransmitters and their Receptors
Edited by U.Z. Littauer, Y. Dudai, I. Silman,
V.I. Teichberg and Z. Vogel

Studies of Nicotine-Like Binding Sites in Brain

Christer Larsson and Agneta Nordberg,

Department of Pharmacology, Box 573, S-751 23 Uppsala, Sweden

Abstract

Binding properties for the nicotinic antagonists labelled tubocurarine (^{3}H-TC) and α-bungarotoxin (^{3}H-Btx) and labelled nicotine (^{3}H-Nic) to crude synaptosomal fractions (P2) from mouse brain (hippocampus) have been studied. Scatchard plots of the binding data indicate two binding sites for ^{3}H-TC and one for ^{3}H-Btx. Experiments also indicate that unlabelled Nic and TC displace ^{3}H-Nic and ^{3}H-TC from their binding sites with a greater efficiency than ^{3}H-Btx indicating a greater preference for the ^{3}H-Nic and ^{3}H-TC binding sites than ^{3}H-BTx binding sites.

Introduction

The introduction of high affinity ligands of high specific radioactivities has accelerated the receptor binding studies during recent years. For in vitro binding sites studies of the nicotinic acetylcholine receptor (NAChR) α-bungarotoxin (Btx) has been used as radioindicator. It is well established that α-Btx binds to the NAChR on electric organ of electric eel and ray and skeletal muscle and functionally acts as a irreversible antagonist (for review see 1). Binding of α-Btx to sympathetic ganglion cells and membrane fragments from the brain has also been reported but it has not been proved that this binding is to a functional active NAChR binding site (2, 3, 4). It must be considered important to find an adequate radioindicator for NAChR in brain and ganglia. In the present study the nicotinic antagonists labelled TC (^{3}H-TC) and α-Btx (^{3}H-Btx) and labelled Nic (^{3}H-Nic) were used as radioindicators for titration of NAChR in the hippocampus of the mouse.

Materials and Methods

A crude synaptosomal fraction (P2) was prepared from the hippocampus of the mouse brain. Aliquots (0.1 ml; protein conc. 1-3 mg/ml) were pipetted into plastic microcentrifuge tubes containing 50 mM $NaKPO_4$ buffer (pH 7.4) and radioligand

(($(13^1-{}^3H)$-Tubocurarine chloride, dextro (16.48 Ci/mmol); (G-^3H) Nicotine d-bitartrate (3 Ci/mmol); (N-propionyl-^3H) α-Bungarotoxin (48 Ci/mmol)) giving a final volume of 1.02 ml. In the displacement studies unlabelled Nic and TC in increasing concentrations were added. The samples were incubated for 15 min (^3H-TC) or 60 min (^3H-Btx and ^3H-Nic) at 25 ^oC according to the technique previously described (5). Specific binding of the labelled ligands were calculated by substracting the values for non specific binding in the presence of 10^{-4}M unlabelled TC.

Results and Discussion

Saturation studies with increasing concentrations of ^3H-TC (1-10 nM) and ^3H-Btx (0.7-11nM) were performed in the hippocampus. Scatchard plots of the binding data show as seen in table 1, two binding sites for ^3H-TC and one for ^3H-Btx.

Table 1.

	B_{max} (pmol/g protein)	K_d (nM)
^3H-Btx	50	4
^3H-TC	75	2
	275	14

Figure 1 shows the inhibition of ^3H-TC binding with increasing concentrations of unlabelled TC. As seen in the figure the inhibition curve is very flat and has a shape which might indicate more than one binding site for TC.

The binding of ^3H-Btx,^3H-Nic and ^3H-TC can be blocked by increasing concentrations of unlabelled ligands. Table 2 shows the IC_{50} values for unlabelled Nic and TC obtained after incubation with ^3H-Btx, ^3H-TC and ^3H-Nic. The IC_{50} values are higher when using ^3H-Btx than using ^3H-TC and ^3H-Nic.

Table 2. IC_{50} values for TC and Nic when incubated with different radioindicators.

	IC_{50} (10^{-8}M)		
	^3H-Btx	^3H-TC	^3H-Nic
TC	170	3	30
Nic	200	70	80

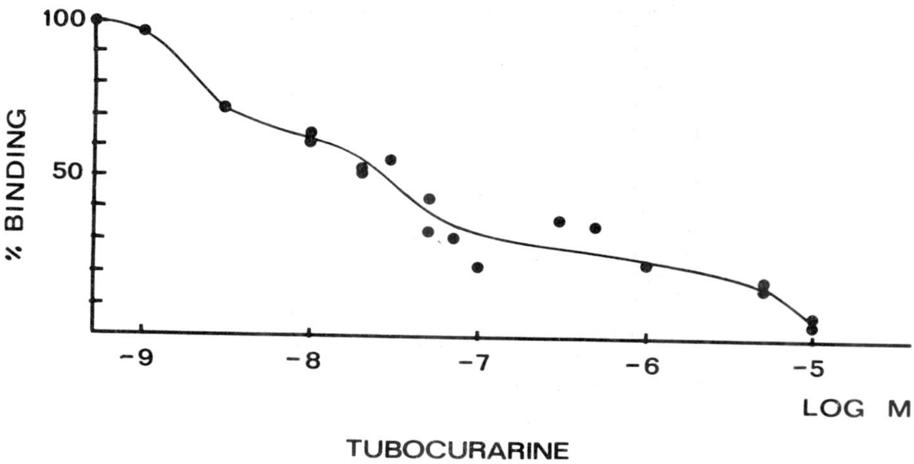

Fig. 1. Inhibition by TC of the specific binding of ^{3}H-TC (3 nM). Each point represents the mean value of 3 experiments. Data taken from Nordberg and Larsson (5).

To further analyse the displacement data, the inhibition of the radioindicators by the same serial dilution of the competitors is compared (fig. 2-4). Each point represents per cent inhibition of binding for two of the radioindicators by the same concentration of unlabelled TC and Nic. This is in accordance with the method described by Terenius and Wahlström for the opiate receptors (6). In the present study, chemical identical solutions were not prepared and the tests were not run simultaneously. Figure 2 shows the inhibition of ^{3}H-TC and ^{3}H-Nic by identical serial dilution of unlabelled Nic (10^{-8}-$0.5 \cdot 10^{-6}$M). At a certain concentration of unlabelled Nic the remaining binding of ^{3}H-TC and ^{3}H-Nic are the same. The points fall on a straight line indicating that Nic equally displace the radioindicators.

Figure 3 shows that both Nic and TC are less effective in displacing ^{3}H-Btx in comparison with ^{3}H-TC. A deviation from the straight line is obtained indicating a greater preference for the ^{3}H-TC binding sites than the ^{3}H-Btx binding sites. A similar curve is also obtained for unlabelled Nic when incubated with ^{3}H-Nic and ^{3}H-Btx.

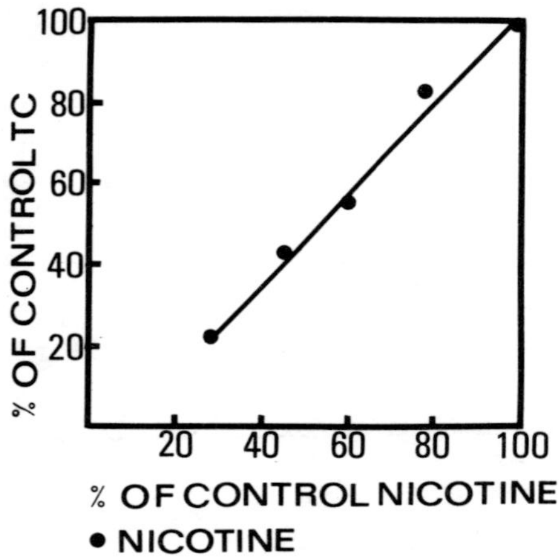

Fig. 2. Inhibition of ^{3}H-TC and ^{3}H-Nic binding to a P2 fraction by nicotine (10^{-6}-$0.5 \cdot 10^{-6}$M).

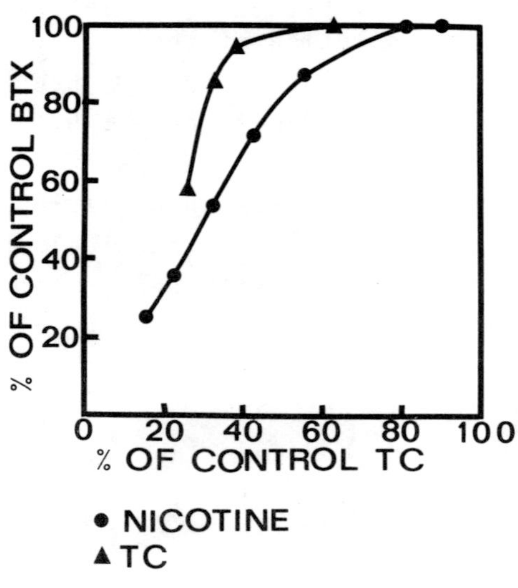

Fig. 3. Inhibition of ^{3}H-Btx and ^{3}H-TC binding to a P2 fraction by nicotine (10^{-8} -10^{-5}M) and TC (10^{-8} -10^{-6}M)

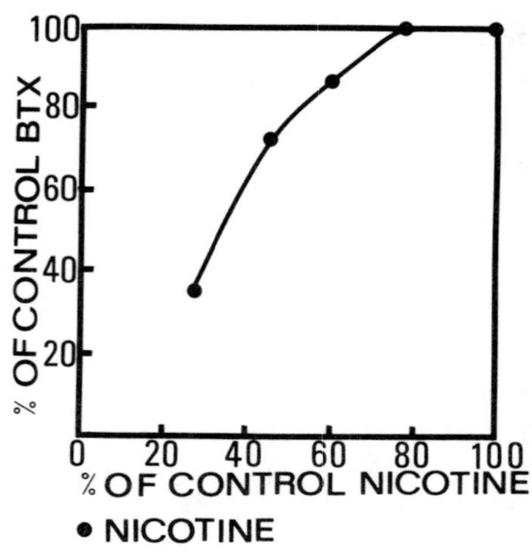

Fig. 4. Inhibition of ^{3}H-Btx and ^{3}H-Nic binding to a P2 fraction by nicotine (10^{-9}-$0.5 \cdot 10^{-6}$M).

To conclude: Displacement experiments with unlabelled Nic and TC indicate a greater preference for the ^{3}H-Nic and ^{3}H-TC binding sites than the ^{3}H-Btx binding sites. By saturation studies we have found two binding sites (a high and a low affinity site) for ^{3}H-TC and one binding site for ^{3}H-Btx. The binding constants (B_{max} and k_d) for the high affinity binding site of ^{3}H-TC are very similar with the values for the ^{3}H-Btx binding site which might indicate that the two radioindicators bind to an identical site. These findings are in agreement with the suggestion made by Carbonetto et al. (3) from their studies on chick sympathetic neurons.

References

1. Morley, B.J., Kemp, G.E. and Salvaterra,, P.: α-Bungarotoxin binding sites in the CNS. Life Sci., 24:859-872 (1979).

2. Patrick, J. and Stallcup, W.B.: Immunological distinction between acetylcholine receptor and the α-bungarotoxin-binding component on sympathetic neurons. Proc. Natl. Acad. Sci., 74: 4689-4692 (1977).

3. Carbonetto, S.T., Fambrough, D.M. and Muller, K.J.: Non-equivalence of α-bungarotoxin receptors and acetylcholine receptors in chick sympathetic neurons. Proc. Natl. Acad. Sci., 75: 1016-1020 (1978).

4. Ben-Barak, J. and Dudai, Y. : Cholinergic binding sites in rat hippocampal formation: properties and ontogenesis Brain res., 166: 245-257 (1979).

5. Nordberg, A. and Larsson, C.: Studies of muscarinic and nicotinic binding sites in brain. Acta Physiol. Scand. suppl. 479: 19-23 (1980).

6. Terenius, L. and Wahlström, A.: A method for selectivity analysis applied to opiate receptors. Eur. J. Pharmacol., 40: 241-248 (1976).

Neurotransmitters and their Receptors
Edited by U.Z. Littauer, Y. Dudai, I. Silman,
V.I. Teichberg and Z. Vogel

Drug Effects on Acetylcholine Receptor Function

M.A. Reis[1], A. Amir[2], A. Gamliel[1], S. Zangen[1], A. Shainberg[1], and P. Fuchs[2]

[1] *Department of Life Sciences, Bar-Ilan University, Ramat-Gan, Israel*

[2] *Israel Institute for Biological Research, Nes-Ziona, Israel*

Abstract

The effects of phencyclidine (PCP) type drugs on nicotinic acetylcholine receptor function were studied in skeletal muscle cells grown in culture. PCP and 4 PCP analogs were found to inhibit carbamylcholine induced ion fluxes with 50 percent inhibition at $2\text{-}6\times10^{-6}$M drug concentration. Ketamine was less effective with 50% inhibition at 10^{-4}M. ^{125}I-α-Bungarotoxin (α-BGT) binding was not affected by drug concentrations that cause 100% inhibition of ion fluxes. ^{3}H-PCP binding to intact cell monolayers was measured. 50 percent inhibition of ^{3}H-PCP binding by PCP was obtained at $6\text{-}8\times10^{-5}$M. The capacity of ^{3}H-PCP binding was 1000 fold higher than the number of α-BGT binding sites. It is concluded that PCP and analog drugs affect the acetylcholine receptor at a site other than the α-BGT binding site. At drug concentrations that cause 50% inhibition of agonist induced ion fluxes the amount of ^{3}H-PCP bound to the cells is ∿1000 fold larger than the amount of α-BGT binding sites.

Nicotinic acetylcholine receptor (AChR) levels are customarily measured by means of radiolabeled α-neurotoxins. This method, which is in fact a count of vacant antagonist binding sites, does not necessarily reflect the degree of receptor function. Post-synaptic nicotinic AChR function may be conveniently assayed in skeletal muscle cultures by agonist-induced cation fluxes as measured by ^{22}Na or ^{45}Ca uptake, or ^{42}K efflux following exposure to carbamylcholine. We examined the applicability of this system to the study of drugs suspected of interaction with AChR.PCP and similar compounds are potent psychotomimetics and are most popular drugs of abuse. Now a problem of major importance these drugs are under intensive study (Reviewed by Domino (1)). Several recent studies have suggested that PCP and related drugs interact with the ionic channel of the nicotinic receptors (2-6). PCP binds to the

---

This work was supported by grants from the Muscular Dystrophy Association of America and the U.S.-Israel Binational Science Foundation (BSF), Jerusalem.

nicotinic frog rectus abdominis AChR with a K_d of 2.4×10^{-7}M (7). However, whereas PCP antagonizes the contractile response of frog rectus abdominis to ACh with 50% inhibition (I_{50}) of 1.2×10^{-6}M, it does not affect ^{125}I-α-Bungarotoxin (α-BGT) binding to a Torpedo ocellata preparation at concentrations up to 10^{-3}M (2). This led to the suggestion that it interacts with the cholinergic ionophore. PCP inhibits the binding of ^{3}H-perhydrohistrionicotoxin to the ionic channel of the nicotinic receptor of frog sartorious muscle, but does not antagonize ^{3}H-ACh binding, which also led to the suggestion (3) that PCP blocks the ionic channel of nicotinic receptors. Binding of PCP to a membrane preparation from Torpedo electric organs showed a specific binding at the μMolar level, which was also interpreted as binding to the cholinergic ionophore (6).

The present study is an attempt to elucidate the effect of PCP and related drugs on the function of the nicotinic AChR of intact skeletal muscle cells grown in culture (8). This system allowed measurement of drug effects on agonist induced ion fluxes, direct drug binding and of drug effects on neurotoxin binding. All these tests were run on sister cultures of the same age.

The drugs tested were 1(1-phenylcyclohexyl) piperidine (PCP), 1-[1-(2-thremyl) cyclohexyl] piperidine (TCP), [1-(3-aminophenyl) cyclohexyl] piperidine (NH_2PCP), N-Ethyl 1 phenyl cyclohexylamine (PCE), the quaterinary PCP methiodide (PCPMeI) and Ketamine. TCP PCE and NH_2PCP are known to be more active than PCP in the mouse rotarod test (9,10) and in the rat discriminative stimulus test (10).Ketamine is a drug clinically related to PCP.

PCP, TCP, NH_2PCP, PCE and PCPMeI all inhibited the carbamylcholine (Carb) induced ^{45}Ca or ^{22}Na flux with I_{50} of $2\text{-}6 \times 10^{-6}$M. No significant differences were found between the inhibitory effects of the various PCP analogs. Ketamine was less efficient, with an I_{50} of 10^{-4}M. α-BGT inhibited these ion fluxes with an I_{50} of $\sim 5 \times 10^{-9}$M, indicating the nicotinic character of these ion fluxes. Preliminary tests of the inhibition by NH_2PCP of Carb induced ^{42}K efflux showed an I_{50} of about 7×10^{-6}, in agreement with the effects on ^{45}Ca and ^{22}Na influxes.

All the PCP analogs tested showed 100% inhibition (I_{100}) of ion fluxes at concentration of 10^{-4}M. Ketamine had an I_{100} of 10^{-3}M. However, ^{125}I α-BGT binding was not altered by any of these drugs even at concentrations corresponding to I_{100}, (Tab.1).

The binding of ^{3}H-PCP to muscle cells was performed on monolayer cell cultures in their dish. The total binding of ^{3}H-PCP to the muscle cells, measured at constant specific ac-

Table 1

Drug	Inhibition of AChR Function (a) I_{50}	I_{100}	%αBGT binding (d)
PCP	$2\text{-}5\times10^{-6}$ (a) 2.2×10^{-6} (b)	10^{-4} (a,b)	97
NH_2-PCP	$4\text{-}6\times10^{-6}$ (a) 3×10^{-6} (b) 7×10^{-6} (c)	10^{-4} (a,b,c)	98
TCP	$2\text{-}6\times10^{-6}$	10^{-4}	100
PCPMeI	$2\text{-}6\times10^{-6}$	10^{-4}	100
PCE	$2\text{-}5\times10^{-6}$	10^{-4}	94
Ketamine	10^{-4}	10^{-3}	100
α-BGT	4×10^{-9}	10^{-7}	-

a) ^{45}Ca influx induced by 10^{-3}M & 3×10^{-5}M carb
b) ^{22}Na influx " " " " "
c) ^{42}K efflux " " 3×10^{-5}M Carb
d) In presence of I_{100} concentration of the drug.

Tab.1. Experiments were carried out on rat myotubes differentiated in vitro 6-10 days after plating (8). Drug effects on influx of ^{45}Ca or ^{22}Na were measured as follows: Drugs were added to the growth medium and incubated at 37°C for 10 minutes. The medium was replaced by 0.5μCi radioisotope and the drug in 1ml buffer (pH7.4). Influx was induced by the addition of carbamylcholine (Carb) to a final concentration of 1mM. After swirling for 30 seconds at 22°C-25°C, the radioactive solution was removed by aspiration, cells were washed and collected for counting. ^{42}K efflux was measured after 3h of loading with ^{42}K in the growth medium. After 10' incubation with the drug, cultures were rinsed and exposed to buffer containing the drug and Carb. The buffer was then collected for counting. Controls underwent similar treatment without exposure to drugs. Any possible agonist effects of the drugs were tested by omitting addition of carb. ^{125}I-α-BGT binding was carried out in the presence of 10^{-4}M or 10^{-3}M of the drug under test following 10' preincubation in the growth medium. Unbound toxin was removed by rinsing the cultures x5 with 1ml of PBS. Bound activity was counted on a crystal γ counter.

tivity, was resolved into two binding components: A linear, non-saturable binding, determined in the presence of 10^{-3}M unlabeled PCP, and a saturable binding, calculated by subtracting the linear binding from total binding. The binding capacity of this saturable component was about 0.1 nMole per fMole α-BGT binding sites. Fig. 1 shows the inhibition of ^{3}H-PCP binding by PCP, TCP, NH_2PCP and by PCPMeI. TCP and NH_2PCP were as efficient as PCP in inhibiting the binding, with an I_{50} of $6\text{-}8 \times 10^{-5}$M, PCPMeI was much less efficient.

The total inhibition of agonist induced ion fluxes by drug concentrations that do not affect α-BGT binding, indicates that the PCP drugs affect the function of the AChR at a site different from the α-BGT binding site, possibly the cholinergic ionophore suggested previously (2), following experiments

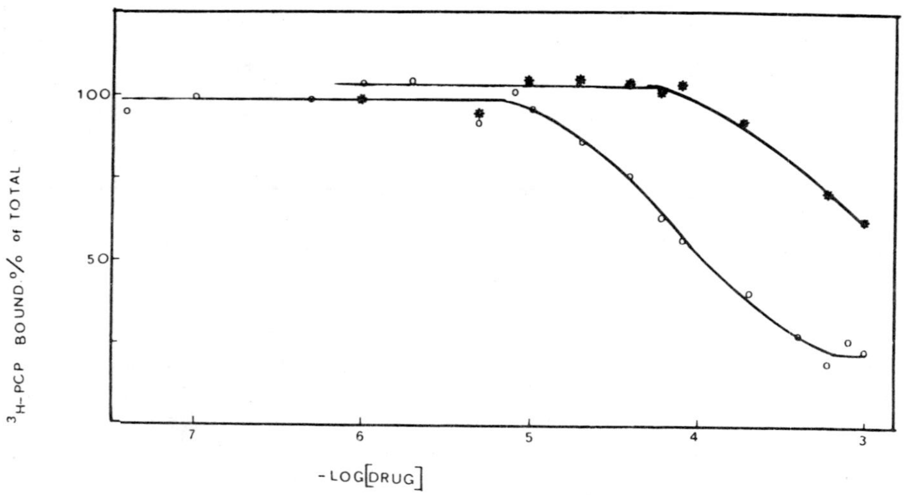

Fig. 1. Inhibition of ^{3}H-PCP binding. 40nM ^{3}H-PCP, containing 1.4×10^{16} CPM/Mole at our counting efficiency, were incubated with varying concentrations of PCP, TCP or NH_2PCP; **O**; or with PCPMeI:*; 100% binding was 40,000 CPM for plates containing cells with 50fMoles αBGT binding sites. Binding was assayed at 37°C by incubating cultures in 0.5ml buffer containing ^{3}H-PCP and the derived concentration of unlabeled liquid. After 5 minutes of incubation, the buffer was discarded and the plates were rinsed 3 times with 0.5 ml 0°C PBS. The washing procedure was completed within 10 seconds. The cells were then collected in 1% SDS for counting. The binding of ^{3}H-PCP to the collagen treated plates was less than 5% of the specific binding.

in which nicotinic receptor function, and effects on α-BGT binding were measured on two different preparations. Muscle cell cultures offer the advantage that the effects on AChR function and on α-BGT binding can be measured in the same system. ^{3}H-PCP binding studies on this preparation showed that the number of PCP molecules apparently bound to the cells greatly exceeds the number of α-BGT binding sites. At 4×10^{-6}M PCP, which is the I_{50} concentration for Carb induced ion fluxes, the concentration of apparently bound PCP is ~3 orders of magnitude greater than the number of α-BGT binding sites. The possibility of a nonsteric interaction with the AChR, occurring at a third hydrophobic site, should therefore be considered. Additional data is being gathered to test this possibility. The low affinity, and high capacity of PCP binding to whole cells, may indicate that these measurements reflect uptake and distribution of PCP into intracellular compartments in addition to specific receptor binding. Studies are in progress in an attempt to analyze the components of this binding.

This system of embryonic muscle cells, differentiated in vitro in the absence of nerve cells can serve as a good model for the study of direct effects of PCP drugs on muscle cells. Inhibition of nicotinic motor end plant receptors demonstrated in this study may be relevant to the understanding of motor effects as well as respiratory depression and arrest caused by PCP and similar drugs(1). The muscular component of the drug effect could also be important for the correct interpretation of behavioral experiments involving motor activity.

References

1. Domino, E.F. N.I.D.A. Research Monograph Series 21 18-43 (1973).
2. Kloog, Y., Gabrielevitz, A., Kalir, A., Balderman, D. Sokolovsky, M. Biochem. Pharmacol. 28:1447-50 (1979).
3. Tsai, M.-C, Aronstam, R.S., Eldefrawi, M.E.E., Eldefrawi, A.T. and Albuquerque, E.X. Fed. Proc. 38: 274 (1979).
4. Mittag, T.W., Cross, S.P., 7th Meeting Int. Soc. Neurochem. Jerusalem, Israel, Sept. 2-6 (1979) Abstract, p. 486.
5. Leprince, P., Hess, G.P., EMBO Meet. "Drug Receptors in the CNS", Feb. 10-14 (1980) Abstracts.
6. Kloog, Y., Kalir, A., Buchman, O., and Sokolovsky, M. FEBS Lett. 109: 125-128 (1980).

7. Kloog, Y., Rehavi, M., Maayani, S., Sokolovksy, M. Eur. J. Pharmacol. 45: 221-7 (1977).
8. Shainberg, A., Yagil, G., and Yaffe, D. Develop. Biol. 25: 1-29 (1971).
9. Kalir, A., Eur. J. Med. Chem. (1978) 13 17-24
10. Zukin, S.R., Zukin, R.S., P.N.A.S. 76 no. 10. p. 5372-5376 (1979).

Neurotransmitters and their Receptors
Edited by U.Z. Littauer, Y. Dudai, I. Silman,
V.I. Teichberg and Z. Vogel

Quaternary Structure of Elongated Forms of Electric Eel Acetylcholinesterase

L. Anglister[1], S.J. Leibovich[2], E. Roth[1], and I. Silman[1]

Departments of Neurobiology[1] and Membrane Research[2],

The Weizmann Institute of Science, Rehovot, Israel

ABSTRACT

Molecular forms of acetylcholinesterase (AChE) purified from fresh electric organ tissue of the electric eel are elongated structures in which a multisubunit head, containing the catalytic subunits, is connected to a collagenous tail. The principal form, 18S AChE, contains three subunit tetramers each, apparently, attached to one strand of a collagen triple-helix *ca.* 500 Å long. Within this structure half the catalytic subunits occur as disulfide-linked dimers, which are not covalently attached to the tail, while the remainder occur as pairs linked to the tail by disulfide bonds. Neither the subunit-subunit nor subunit-tail interchain disulfides are essential for maintaining the quaternary structure. Tryptic digestion degrades the tail, with concomitant release of discrete tetramers which contain a fragment of the tail. Pepsin digests the catalytic subunits, leaving intact the triple-helical section of the tail, while collagenase digests the distal part of the tail, leaving intact a residual section still capable of holding together the catalytic subunit tetramers.

INTRODUCTION

The main role of acetylcholinesterase (AChE) is believed to be the termination of impulse transmission by hydrolysis of the neurotransmitter acetylcholine. The highly specialized electrogenic tissue of electric fish is a particularly rich source from which AChE was first purified and characterized, thus permitting detailed studies on the molecular structure of this enzyme.

As originally purified from electric organ tissue of the electric eel, *Electrophorus electricus*, AChE was found to be a globular protein of sedimentation coefficient 11S (1). It was subsequently shown that 11S AChE is a tetramer of MW ∿330,000, containing four similar active-site-bearing subunits each of MW ∿80,000. These subunits are sometimes partially or completely degraded to species of 60,000 and 20,000 MW by prolonged autolysis or proteolysis, without any concomitant change in the overall molecular weight or activity of the AChE molecule. Moreover, in the intact molecule they are arranged as pairs of 160,000 dimers linked by disulfides (for reviews see refs. 2 and 3).

The 11S form of AChE is not, however, present in fresh electric organ tissue, from which three molecular forms can be extracted, with sedimentation coefficients of 18S, 14S and 9S (4). These forms, which aggregate reversibly at low ionic strength (4,5), are all converted by proteolysis or autolysis to the 11S form which does not aggregate at low ionic strength (5,6). Acrylamide gel electrophoresis reveals that these forms, like the 11S form, contain the 80,000 species as their principal component (7). Physicochemical and electron microscope studies on purified AChE preparations, however, revealed that all three forms obtained from fresh tissue are asymmetric structures containing a multisubunit head connected to an elongated tail (8-12), whereas the 11S tetramer is devoid of this tail. The physicochemical data are best rationalized by assuming that the 9S, 14S and 18S species contain respectively 1, 2 and 3 subunit tetramers attached to a tail of similar dimensions. Thus 18S AChE has a MW of 1.1×10^6, contains *ca.* 12 subunits in its head and has a tail about 500 Å long.

Various studies, both on electric organ tissue and skeletal muscle AChE, have indicated that a significant part of the enzyme is not tightly bound to the plasma membrane, and it was suggested that *in situ* AChE might be associated with the basal lamina (for literature, see ref. 3). McMahan *et al.* (13) have recently provided histochemical evidence for such association at the neuromuscular junction. The basal lamina contains collagen as one of its principal constituents (14). It was therefore proposed that the tail of the elongated forms of AChE is collagen-like, and serves to anchor the enzyme to the basal lamina of the synaptic cleft where it performs its biological function (3).

Three experimental approaches now provide strong evidence that the fibrous tail of the elongated forms of AChE is indeed collagen-like:

1) Amino acid analysis of the tailed forms of the enzyme reveals the presence of hydroxyproline and hydroxylysine, both of which are characteristic components of collagen (15-18). The amounts of these two amino acids are of the order to be expected if the tail were a collagen triple-helix of the length seen in the electron microscope (15). Furthermore, both these amino acids are absent from the 11S tetramer which is devoid of the tail.

2) Immunological cross-reactivity of elongated forms of AChE, but not of the tetramer, can be demonstrated with rat tail tendon collagen (19).

3) Collagenase releases AChE from electric organ tissue, and also specifically modifies the elongated forms of electric eel AChE (18,20-24). Thus 18S AChE is converted to a form of *ca.* 20S, and 14S AChE to a form of *ca.* 16S, and both the physicochemical data and amino acid analysis suggest that collagenase acts by digesting the distal half of the tail of the enzyme (18). Furthermore, SDS-polyacrylamide gel electrophoresis (SDS-PAGE) reveals that putative tail polypeptides of MW *ca.* 45K (17,18,24; see below) are converted to a new 30K species by the collagenase treatment (18).

The above evidence suggests that the tail observed in the electron microscope is indeed a collagen triple helix to which the catalytic sub-unit tetramers are attached, as shown schematically for 18S AChE in Fig.1. In the following, we will present experiments in which SDS-PAGE together with controlled modifications of the intact molecules, are used to elucidate the detailed molecular structure of the elongated forms of AChE.

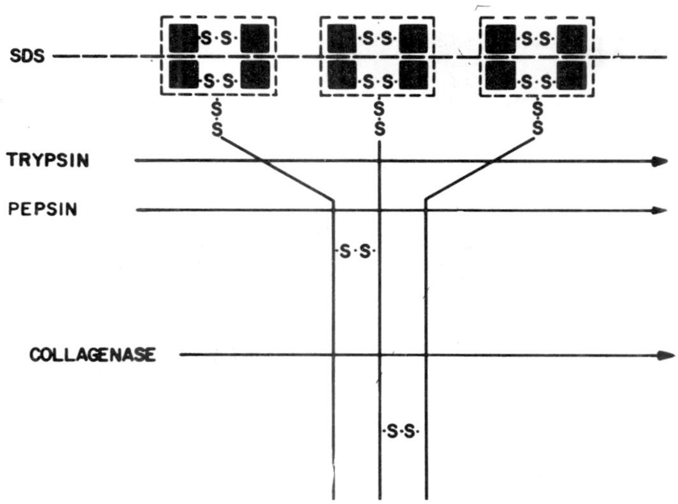

Fig. 1. Model of the 18S AChE molecule, showing points of cleavage by SDS, trypsin, collagenase and pepsin.

Polypeptide Composition and Quaternary Structure

As already mentioned, the principal polypeptide observed on SDS-acrylamide gel electrophoresis of 14S+18S AChE in the presence of reducing agent is the same 80,000 species, corresponding to the catalytic subunits, which is seen in the 11S tetramer. However, on electrophoresis in the absence of reducing agent a very different pattern is obtained. Whereas 11S AChE under such conditions contains the 160,000 dimer, with varying amounts of monomer also present (Fig. 2C), 14S+18S AChE contains two heavier components. As can be seen in Figure 2A, these additional species have apparent molecular weights of ∿360,000 and ∿460,000. Electrophoresis of separated samples of 14S and 18S AChE showed that the ∿360,000 component is derived exclusively from 14S AChE and the ∿460,000 component from 18S AChE (18,25). These two components are clearly visualized and resolved when SDS-PAGE is performed on 3.1% acrylamide gels as shown in Fig. 2. On

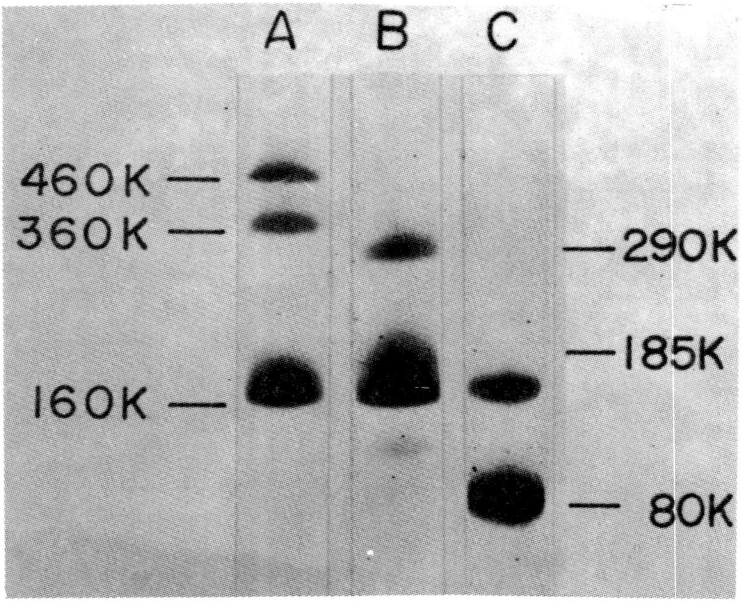

Fig. 2. SDS-PAGE of 14S+18S AChE, in the absence of reducing agent, before and after collagenase digestion. Electrophoresis was performed on 3.1% cylindrical gels and staining was with Coomassie Brilliant Blue R. A) 14S+18S AChE, control. B) 14S+18S AChE after digestion with collagenase. The enzyme (400 μg/ml) was digested with purified collagenase (20 μg/ml) for 1 hr at room temperature (18). C) 11S AChE.

5-20% acrylamide gradient slab gels (Figs. 3,4) they remain at the origin. These heavy components comprise close to half the protein applied to the gel (18), in agreement with earlier experiments using AChE labelled in its active sites with ^{3}H-diisopropylfluorophosphate (^{3}H-DFP), which showed that they accounted for *ca.* 40% of the catalytic subunits (11).

It seemed likely from these results that in the elongated AChE molecules half the subunits are in the form of disulfide-linked dimers, while the remainder occur in head-tail complexes in which they are linked by disulfide bonds to the putative tail polypeptides (see Fig. 1). In fact, qualitative experiments revealed that the 360,000 and 460,000 components both contained significant amounts of hydroxylysine, while this component was not detected in the 160,000 dimer.

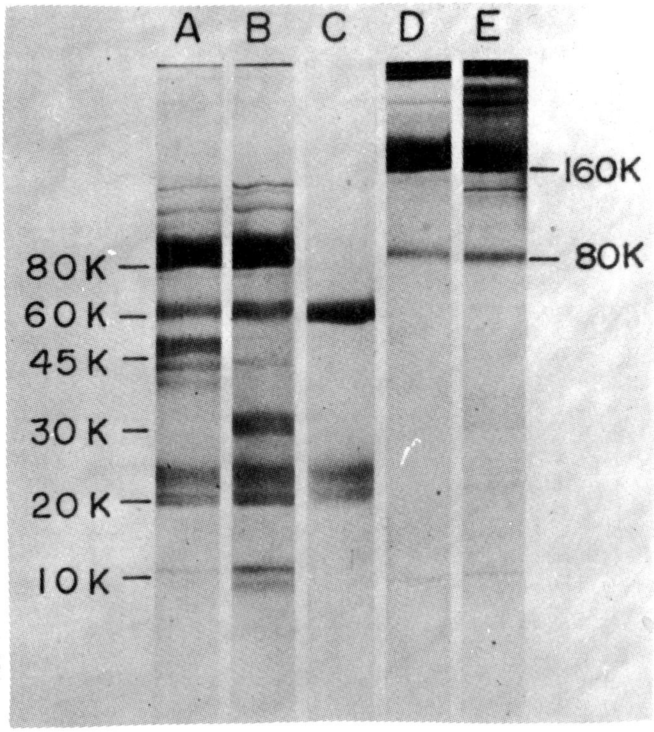

Fig. 3. SDS-PAGE of 14S+18S AChE, before and after collagenase digestion. Electrophoresis was performed on 5-20% acrylamide gradient slab gels in the presence (A-C) and absence (D-E) of β-mercaptoethanol. A,D) 14S+18S AChE. B,E) 14S+18S AChE incubated with collagenase as in Fig. 2B but for 30 min. C) 11S AChE.

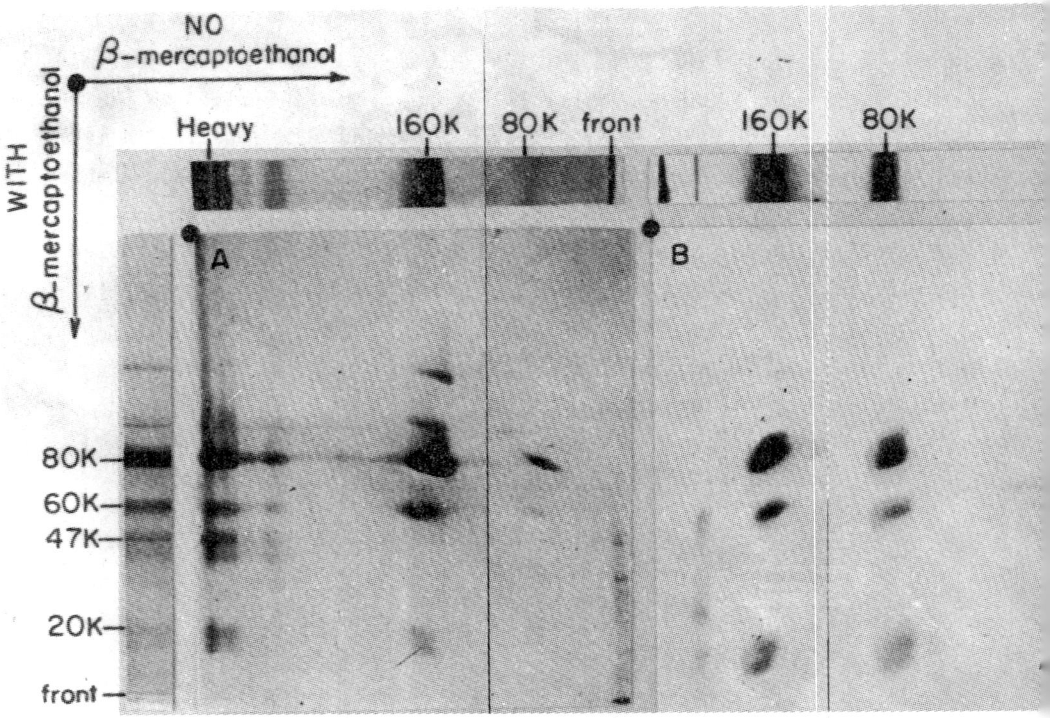

Fig. 4. Two-dimensional SDS-PAGE of A) 14S+18S AChE and B) 11S AChE. The first dimension was run on a 5-15% acrylamide gradient slab gel in the absence of reducing agent. One strip was stained for protein with Coomassie Brilliant Blue R; an adjacent strip was incubated for 15 min at 25°C in 0.05% β-mercaptoethanol- 1% SDS-10% glycerol 0.02M Tris, pH 6.8. The reduced strip was then implanted along the origin of a second 5-15% acrylamide gradient slab gel and set in place with 3% agarose. Electrophoresis in the second dimension was carried out in the presence of β-mercaptoethanol.

Collagenase Digestion Studies

The postulate that collagenase modifies the elongated forms of AChE by removing a portion of the fibrous tail is born out by examination of the products using SDS-PAGE. Controlled collagenase digestion was carried out under conditions which converted 14S+18S AChE to 16S+20S AChE (18). SDS-PAGE in the absence of reducing agent (Fig. 2B) reveals that it converts both the 360,000 and 460,000 species to two new species of MW ∿290,000 and 185,000 without attacking the 160,000 dimer. This again supports the view that these heavy components represent 'head-tail' complexes linked by disulfide bonds, and that collagenase partially digests the tail under the conditions employed.

As first reported by Rosenberry and Richardson (17) one or more polypeptides of apparent MW *ca.* 40-45,000 are present in 14S+18S AChE and absent in the 11S enzyme, and they suggested that these might be the putative collagen polypeptides of the tail. In agreement with these authors, we observe similar components (the principal one of apparent MW *ca.*45,000) in 14S+18S AChE on electrophoresis in the presence of β-mercaptoethanol (Fig. 3A), but not in its absence (Fig. 3D), and do not detect them in 11S AChE (Fig. 3C). These bands are specifically digested by collagenase under the conditions used for conversion of 14S+18S AChE to 16S+20S AChE (Fig.3B). Their disappearance is accompanied by the appearance of a new band of apparent MW *ca.* 30,000 and also of smaller polypeptides of apparent MW 10-13,000. This digestion experiment thus provides the first direct evidence that the putative tail polypeptides indeed contain collagen-like sequences.

Two-dimensional SDS-PAGE clearly demonstrates that the 45K polypeptides are associated with the heavy (360,000 and 460,000) species in the intact AChE molecule (Fig. 4A). They are not observed at all in the first dimension, run in the absence of reducing agent, and are clearly seen to be derived from the heavy components, and not from the 160,000 dimer, on development of the second dimension after reduction; nor are they seen in either dimension in 11S AChE (Fig. 4B). The 30,000 polypeptide which appears after collagenase digestion is presumably derived from the residual tail holding together the subunit tetramers of the head, since it is only seen on electrophoresis in the presence of β-mercaptoethanol (compare Fig. 3E with Fig. 3B).

As mentioned above, the tail of the elongated forms of AChE as visualized in the electron microscope, *ca.* 500Å long ; it can be calculated that if it had a triple-helical character it would contain about 500 amino acid residues (15), e.g. about 165 residues per polypeptide chain. Such a collagenous polypeptide should display on SDS-PAGE a mobility corresponding to that of a 'globular' polypeptide of MW *ca.* 19,000 (26). By the same criteria, it can be calculated that if the 45,000 component were a single strand it would contain *ca.* 390 residues. It is thus possible that this species, as well as the 30,000 fragment derived from it by collagenase digestion, contain two or more strands linked by non-reducible covalent linkages. Such covalent linkages, or interchain disulfides (27), might also provide a site at which collagenase digestion of the elongated forms is terminated under our digestion conditions, rather than proceeding to completion.

Pepsin Digestion Studies

While collagenase is believed to be able to attack collagen-like sequences in folded and unfolded regions of collagen fibrils, pepsin has been employed to digest non-collagenous telopeptide sequences and unfolded regions of collagen molecules, leaving intact the triple-helical regions (see, for example, refs. 28 and 29). It was, therefore, of interest to study its effect on the elongated AChE molecules. Both 14S+18S AChE and 11S AChE were digested with porcine pepsin at pH 4.4. SDS-acrylamide gel electrophoresis revealed that under the conditions employed all polypeptides appearing in the original electrophoresis pattern for 11S AChE were completely digested to yield products of MW below 12,000 (Fig. 5D). However, under the same conditions a 14S+18S AChE preparation (Fig. 5A) yielded,

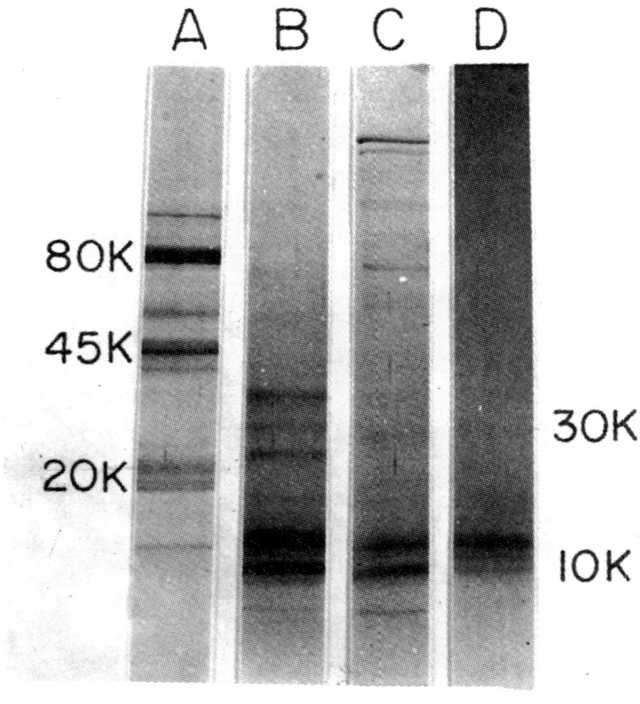

Fig. 5. Action of pepsin on AChE is observed by electrophoresis on 5-20% acrylamide gradient slab gels, in the presence of β-mercapto-ethanol, staining with Coomassie Brilliant Blue R. A) 14S+18S AChE. B) 14S+18S AChE (1 mg/ml) digested with porcine pepsin (7 μg/ml) for 16 hr at pH 4.5 and 25°C. C) 14S+18S AChE digested first with pepsin as in (B) and subsequently with collagenase as in Fig. 2B. D) 11S AChE digested with pepsin, conditions as in (B).

in addition, three new polypeptides of MW 25-30,000 (Fig. 5B). The fact that the new polypeptides are obtained from 14S+18S AChE, but not from 11S AChE, and their resistance to prolonged peptic digestion, both suggest that they represent triple-helical regions of the tail. This assignment is strongly supported by the observation that subsequent collagenase treatment of the peptic digest causes complete degradation of the 25,000-30,000 polypeptides (Fig. 5C). Thus, apparently pepsin digests the catalytic subunits and a non-ordered region of the tail, leaving intact a triple-helical region corresponding to rather more than half the tail. Electron microscope studies utilizing negative-staining, show that the peptic digest indeed contains rod-like structures, all of about the same length (∿300 Å) and thickness (10-20 Å), in agreement with this suggestion (Fig. 6). It is worth noting that from considerations similar to those given above for the intact tail, it is possible that the *ca.* 25-30,000 fragments seen on SDS-PAGE after pepsin digestion contain more than one polypeptide strand.

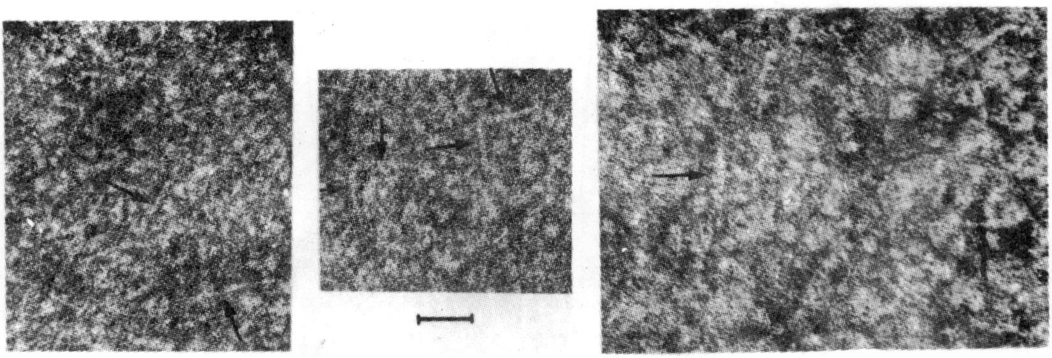

Fig. 6. Electron micrographs of preparations of 14S+18S AChE after peptic digestion as in Fig. 5B. Samples (50-100 μg/ml) in 1M NaCl-0.05M Tris, pH 7.5, were stained with 1% uranyl acetate. Finally magnification x 350,000. The bar represents 200 Å. The arrows point to rod-like structures.

Tryptic Digestion Studies

As mentioned above, both autolysis and tryptic digestion convert the elongated forms of AChE to the 11S species which appear to be globular tetramers devoid of the tail. On SDS-acrylamide gel electrophoresis in the absence of reducing agent this conversion could be followed by the disappearance of the heavy (*ca.* 360,000 and 460,000) components which are believed to represent disulfide-linked complexes of catalytic subunits and the tail (Fig. 7A). Initially, this leads to an 11S AChE preparation in which the principal components are 160,000 dimers (Fig. 7B). On continued tryptic digestion, gradual conversion of dimer to monomer is observed, even in the absence of reducing agent (Fig. 7C,D). This process proceeds rapidly until about 50% conversion has occurred, and much more slowly thereafter,

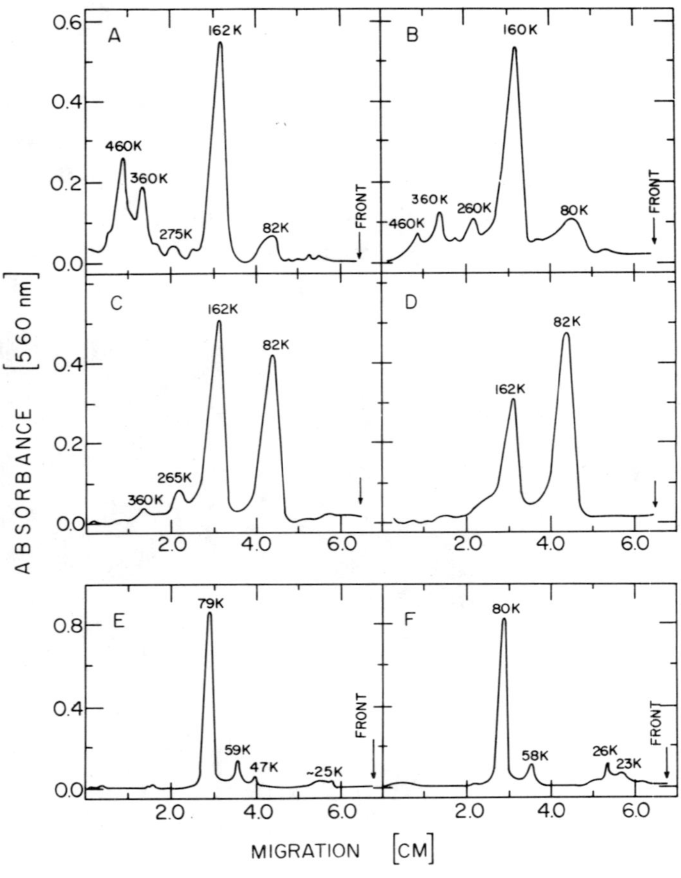

Fig. 7. Effect of trypsin on the polypeptide pattern of purified 14S+18S AChE. SDS-PAGE was performed on 3.1% cylindrical gels, in the absence of reducing agent (A-D) as in Fig. 2, and on 5-15% gradient slab gels, in the presence of β-mercaptoethanol (E,F) as in Fig. 3. The figures show densitometer tracings obtained after staining with Coomassie Brilliant Blue R. 14S+18S AChE (1 mg/ml) was incubated for 1 hr at 25°C with various trypsin concentrations. A,E) 14S+18S AChE control, without trypsin. B) with trypsin, 1 μg/ml. C) with trypsin, 6 μg/ml. D,F) with trypsin, 32 μg/ml.

as was shown by varying either the amount of trypsin or the time of incubation (Figs. 7,8); it seems, therefore, to involve preferential tryptic cleavage of one half of the 11S dimers. This does not involve proteolytic cleavage of the 80,000 subunit to 60,000 and 20,000 framents (see above) since this process does not occur under the conditions employed (Fig. 7E,F). Comparison of the 11S tetramer with the elongated forms indeed suggests that it should contain equal amounts of two types of dimers, one type derived from the dimers not attached covalently to the tail in the intact elongated molecule, and one type from the subunits originally attached by disulfides to the tail. The latter might, therefore, retain a fragment of the tail covalently bound to it. To investigate this point, the following experiment was performed: an 11S preparation containing 50% monomer was labelled in its active sites with ^{3}H-DFP, and a 14S+18S AChE preparation was similarly labelled with ^{14}C-DFP. SDS-acrylamide gel electrophoresis, followed by subsequent differential counting of ^{3}H and ^{14}C in gel slices, showed that the ^{3}H-dimer was distinctly heavier than the ^{14}C-dimer (Fig.9A). Since the ^{14}C-dimer represents the dimer which is not attached to the tail,

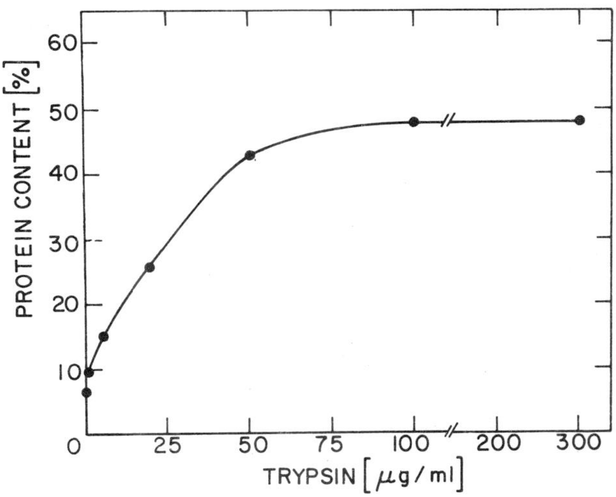

Fig. 8. Generation of catalytic subunit monomers by tryptic digestion of elongated forms of AChE. 14S+18S AChE samples were digested with trypsin for 1 hr at 25°C and electrophoresed on 5-15% gradient gels as in Fig. 3 in the absence of β-mercaptoethanol. The percentage of the monomer was determined by measuring its contribution to the total area under the densitometer tracing of gels stained as in Fig. 7, and is shown as a function of the trypsin concentration.

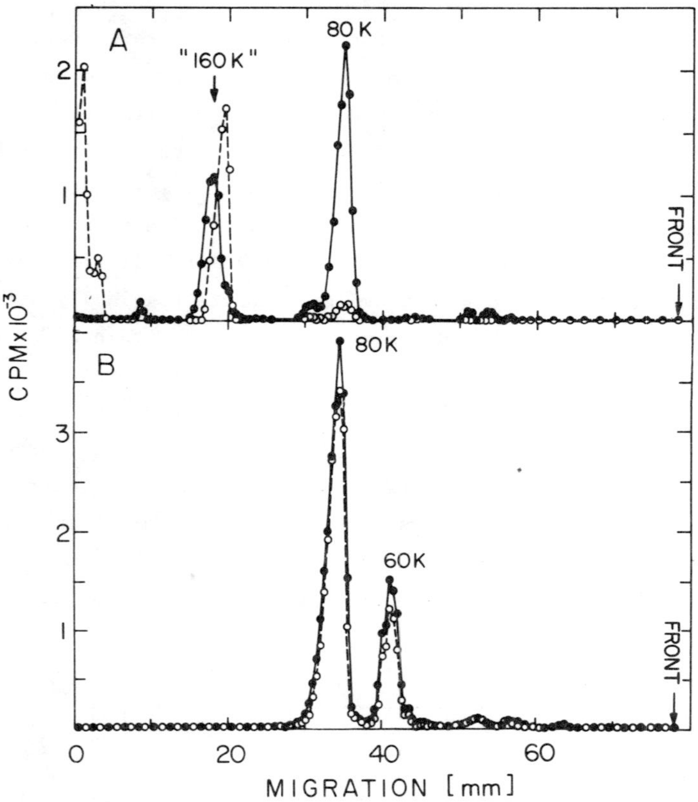

Fig. 9. Distribution of radioactivity upon coelectrophoresis of samples of 14S+18S AChE and 11S AChE labelled with radioactive diisopropylfluorophosphate. SDS-PAGE was performed on 5-15% gradient slab gels in the absence (A) and presence (B) of β-mercaptoethanol. 0.3 mm gel slices were cut in each lane and extracted with NCS (Amersham/Searle). ^{3}H and ^{14}C were counted simultaneously in a scintillation counter. A) Coelectrophoresis of ^{14}C-DFP-labelled 14S+18S AChE and of ^{3}H-DFP-labelled 11S AChE containing approximately 50% monomer. B) The ^{3}H-DFP-labelled 80,000 component derived from 11S AChE was extracted from a gel run as in (A), reduced with β-mercaptoethanol and mixed with a sample of ^{14}C-DFP-labelled 14S+18S AChE similarly reduced. The samples were electrophoresed as in (A) but in the absence of reducing agent.

this experiment indeed providesa strong indication that the 11S tetramer is an asymmetric structure in which one dimer contains a fragment of the tail. Since this is the species remaining after tryptic digestion, presumably the other dimer is preferentially converted to monomers by trypsin. It has been reported that there is only one intersubunit disulfide bond per catalytic subunit in AChE (2). If this is indeed the case, tryptic cleavage would be most easily explained by assuming that this disulfide bridge is at one end of the catalytic subunit polypeptide chain, and that tryptic cleavage occurs adjacent to it. This would mean that both the disulfide bridge and the cleavage point must be very close to the end of the chain, since no detectable difference in mobility is found when the ^{3}H-DFP-labelled 80,000 species is extracted from the gel in Fig. 9A, and run together with reduced ^{14}C-DFP-labelled 14S+18S AChE (Fig. 9B). Alternatively, the two subunits might be linked via a small peptide bridge in the same way as has been suggested for linkage of pairs of subunits to the tail (25) and experiments now underway are designed to clarify this point.

Selective Reduction of Interchain Disulfide Bonds

The data presented above demonstrate, in the intact elongated forms of AChE, the presence of both intersubunit disulfide bonds and subunit-tail disulfide bonds. Control experiments performed earlier excluded the possibility that these interchain disulfides are artefacts of solubilization and purification (18). Nevertheless, we were interested in knowing whether they are, in fact, necessary for maintaining the quaternary structure of the intact elongated molecules. It had earlier been shown that interchain disulfides could be selectively reduced by dithiothreitol in the absence of a denaturing agent (17). Fig. 10 shows that 10mM dithiothreitol, followed by excess N-ethylmaleimide in order to block the exposed sulfhydryls, completely eliminates both the 360,000 and 460,000 head-tail complexes and the 160,000 dimers, as visualized on SDS-PAGE without reducing agent (compare Fig. 10B,B' with Fig. 10C,C'); appearance of the 80,000 monomer and 45,000 'tail' polypeptides is observed concomitantly. It is of interest that this selective reduction does not even cleave an intrachain disulfide bond which bridges the 60,000 and 20,000 domains of the 80,000 subunit polypeptide, and holds them together even when the polypeptide itself has been cleaved (compare Figs. 10B' and A').

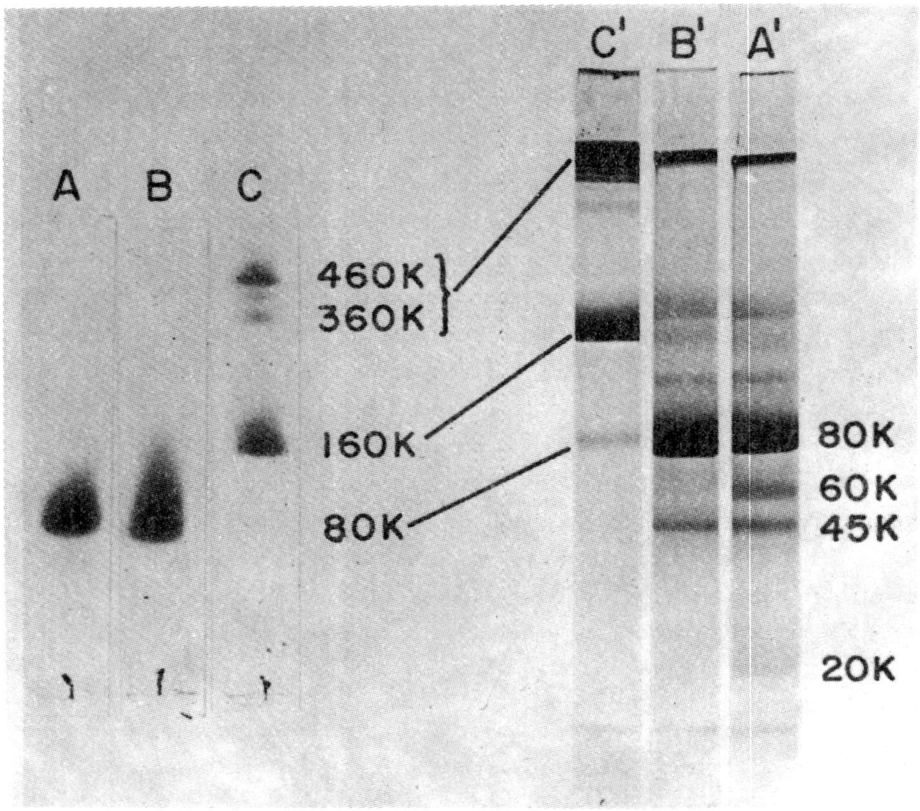

Fig. 10. SDS-PAGE of 14S+18S AChE before and after disulfide bond reduction Electrophoresis was performed in the absence of reducing agent on 3.1% acrylamide cylindrical gels (A,B,C) and on 5-15% acrylamide gradient slab gels (A',B',C'). A,A') Total reduction of disulfide bonds using 10 mM dithiothreitol in 1% SDS at 24°C for 40 min. B,B') Selective reduction of interchain disulfide bonds with 10mM dithiothreitol at 24°C for 40 min at pH 8.0. C,C') Control (no dithiothreitol). After reduction all samples were treated with a 4-fold excess of N-ethylmaleimide.

The mild reductive treatment has no significant immediate effect on catalytic activity, and sucrose gradient centrifugation reveals that cleavage of all interchain disulfides has little or no effect on the profiles obtained: the major 14S and 18S species are still present with essentially unaltered sedimentation coefficients (compare Figs. 11A and 11B). Furthermore, the capacity to aggregate reversibly at low ionic strength, characteristic of our purified preparations of elongated forms of AChE, is retained (Fig. 11C). Thus the quaternary structure of the elongated forms of AChE is maintained in the absence of covalent interchain linkages, suggesting a rather specific and intimate association of the fibrous tail with the cata-

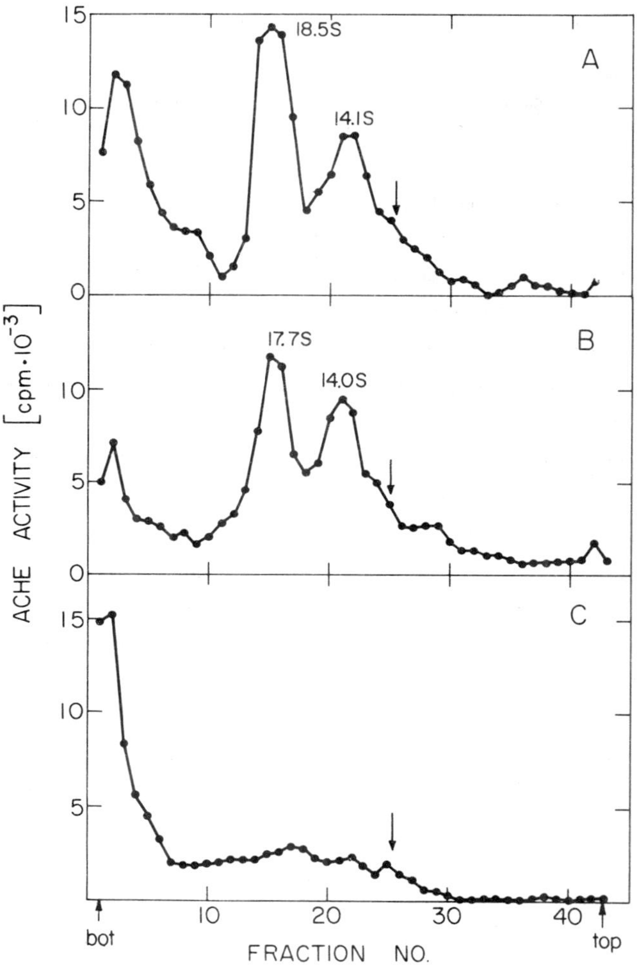

Fig. 11. Sucrose gradient centrifugation profiles of 14S+18S AChE before and after treatment with 10 mM DTT at pH 8.0. AChE activity was assayed radiometrically. A) Control. B,C) Selective disulfide bond reduction with 10 mM DTT as in Fig. 10B,B'. A,B) Centrifugation in 1M NaCl-0.01M phosphate, pH 7.0. C) Centrifugation in 0.1M NaCl-0.01M phosphate, 7.0. The arrow shows the catalase marker (11.4S).

Concluding Remarks

The experimental results discussed above can best be summarized and rationalized by reference to the scheme shown in Fig. 1, which displays the overall quaternary structure proposed for 18S AChE and the mode of attack by various agents. In this scheme three subunit tetramers are each attached to one strand of a collagen triple helix. However, half the 80,000 catalytic subunits, while linked to each other by disulfide bridges in the form of dimers, are not attached covalently to the tail and are detached from the intact structure by SDS. The remaining subunit pairs, in contrast, are linked to the tail by disulfide bridges. These disulfide bridges are not, however, essential for maintenance of the quaternary structure under non-denaturing conditions.

Trypsin cleaves the tail close to its point of attachment to the tetramers, releasing intact tetramers and, presumably, degrading the tail completely. Pepsin totally digests the catalytic subunits as well as part of the tail, leaving behind a rod-like fragment corresponding to the collagen triple helix. Collagenase digests the distal portion of the tail, removing about half the collagen sequence. As a result it produces a shortened structure in which the residual tail still holds the tetramers together.

Clarification of the chemical nature and origin of the tail, as well as elucidation of the type and arrangement of the various interchain linkages, whether tail-tail, tail-subunit or subunit-subunit, will be the object of future research: Obviously they are prerequisites for understanding the biosynthetic assembly of the intact elongated AChE molecules. This information in its turn, is essential for understanding the fashion in which the enzyme is anchored and localized in the mature synapse and the way in which its integration into the developing synapse is regulated.

ACKNOWLEDGEMENTS

The support of the Muscular Dystrophy Association of America is gratefully acknowledged.

REFERENCES

1. Kremzner, L.T. and Wilson, I.B. (1963). J.Biol.Chem. 235, 1714-1717.
2. Rosenberry, T.L. (1975). Adv.Enzymol. 43, 103-218.
3. Silman, I. (1976). Trends Biochem.Sci. 1, 225-227.
4. Massoulié, J. and Rieger, F. (1969). Eur.J.Biochem. 11, 441-455.
5. Dudai, Y., Silman, I., Kalderon, N. and Blumberg, S. (1972). Biochim. Biophys.Acta 268, 138-157.
6. Massoulié, J., Rieger, F. and Tsuji, S. (1970). Eur.J.Biochem. 14, 430-439.
7. Dudai, Y., Silman, I., Shinitzky, M. and Blumberg, S. (1972). Proc. Natl.Acad.Sci.USA 69, 2400-2403.
8. Dudai, Y., Herzberg, M. and Silman, I. (1973). Proc.Natl.Acad.Sci. USA 70, 2473-2476.
9. Bon, S., Rieger, F. and Massoulié, J. (1973). Eur.J.Biochem. 35, 372-379.
10. Rieger, F., Bon, S., Massoulié, J. and Cartaud, J. (1973). Eur.J. Biochem. 34, 539-547.
11. Silman, I. and Dudai, Y. (1975). Croatica Chim.Acta 47, 181-200.
12. Bon, S., Huet, M., Lemonnier, M., Rieger, F. and Massoulié, J. (1976). Eur.J.Biochem. 68, 523-530.
13. McMahan, U.J., Sanes, J.R. and Marshall, L.M. (1978). Nature, London, 271, 172-174.
14. Kefalides, N.A., Alper, R. and Clark, C.C. (1979). Internat.Rev.Cytol. 61, 167-228.
15. Anglister, L., Rogozinski, S. and Silman, I. (1976). FEBS Lett. 69, 129-132.
16. Lwebuge-Mukasa, J.S., Lappi, S. and Taylor, P. (1976). Biochemistry 15, 1425-1434.
17. Rosenberry, T.L. and Richardson, J.M. (1977). Biochemistry 16, 3550-3558.
18. Anglister, L. and Silman, I. (1978). J.Mol.Biol. 125, 293-311.
19. Anglister, L., Tarrab-Hazdai, R., Fuchs, S. and Silman, I. (1979). Eur.J.Biochem. 94, 25-29.
20. Dudai, Y. and Silman, I. (1974). J.Neurochem. 23, 1177-1187.
21. Johnson, C.D., Smith, S.P. and Russell, R.L. (1977). J.Neurochem. 28, 617-624.
22. Watkins, M.S., Hitt, A.S. and Bulger, J.E. (1977). Biochem.Biophys. Res.Commun. 79, 640-647.
23. Bon, S. and Massoulie, J. (1978). Eur.J.Biochem. 89, 89-94.
24. Webb, G. (1978). Can.J.Biochem. 56, 1124-1132.
25. McCann, W.F.X. and Rosenberry, T.L. (1977). Arch.Biochem.Biophys. 183, 347-352.

26. Freytag, W.J., Noelken, M.E. and Hudson, B.G. (1979). Biochemistry 18, 4761-4768.

27. Bruckner, P., Bächinger, H.P., Timpl, R. and Engel, J. (1978). Eur.J.Biochem. 90, 593-603.

28. Bellamy, G. and Bornstein, P. (1971). Proc.Natl.Acad.Sci.USA 68, 1138-1142.

29. Reid, K.B.M.(1976).Biochem.J. 155, 5-17.

Neurotransmitters and their Receptors
Edited by U.Z. Littauer, Y. Dudai, I. Silman,
V.I. Teichberg and Z. Vogel

Influence of the Ionic Strength upon Substrate Binding to Acetylcholinesterase

H.J. Nolte and E. Neumann

Max-Planck-Institut für Biochemie, D-8033 Martinsried, W. Germany

The binding equilibrium of the fluorescent dye N-methylacridinium, which is a competitive inhibitor of the natural substrate acetylcholine, with the neuroenzyme acetylcholinesterase has been studied by the relaxation kinetic technique. The observed high absolute value of the bimolecular association rate constant and its strong dependence on the ionic strength of the solution are discussed in terms of a diffusion controlled binding of the ligand that is caused by electrostatic interaction with a high effective charge on the enzyme active site.

Introduction

Acetylcholinesterase (AChE) catalyzes very efficiently the hydrolytic cleavage of the neurotransmitter acetylcholine at neuromuscular junctions and thus terminates the chemical signal flow across the synaptic cleft. Due to the fast subsequent hydrolysis the binding equilibrium with the natural substrate is not properly established and cannot be studied by relaxation kinetic methods. However, information about the electrostatic aspects of ligand association and about the ionic properties of the active site can be obtained with non-substrate ligands, if these are cations like acetylcholine, can be traced by optical methods and are not hydrolyzed in subsequent steps or can be maintained under steady state conditions. The N-methylacridinium (N-MAC) ion that competes with the natural substrate for the active site, meets these conditions; its fluorescence is completely quenched upon binding to the enzyme. Recent relaxation kinetic data have demonstrated the extremely rapid binding of cationic ligands to AChE (1); these studies are presently extended to the part of electrostatic effects that show up in ionic strength dependences (2).

Materials and Methods

Acetylcholinesterase (EC 3.1.1.7) was a 11S-preparation from the electric organ of the eel electrophorus electricus; the recrystallized perchlorate salt of N-methylacridinium was used as ligand.

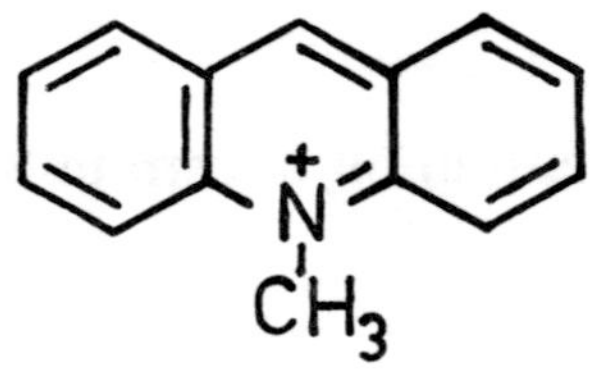

The reaction medium contained defined mixtures of Na^+- mono- and -dibasic phosphates in order to adjust the pH to 7.0. Solutions of different ionic strengths were prepared, varying between I_c= 1mM and I_c= 10mM.
In the T-jump experiments the temperature was raised by 3.3K to a final value of 298K. Whereas the enzyme concentration was adjusted to around 0.5μM, the concentration of the ligand varied in the fluorescence titrations from 0.1μM to about 10μM.

Results and Discussion

Since a single relaxation process was observed in the experimental range of ionic strengths, the interaction of AChE with N-MAC is discussed in terms of the simple reaction scheme

$$E + L \underset{k_{21}}{\overset{k_{12}}{\rightleftharpoons}} EL$$

The following observations have been made:

1. the relaxation is bimolecularly controlled under all experimental conditions;
2. the association rate constant assumes a very high value and strongly depends on the ionic strength of the solution;
3. the dissociation rate constant is not affected by a variation of the ionic strength ($k^o_{21} \approx 1.5 \cdot 10^2\ s^{-1}$).

The 11S-form of AChE isknown to carry four identical active sites; the Debye-Hückel-approximation was applied to the experimental data of figure 1 to evaluate the active site parameters and yields

k^o_{12}= $1.1 \cdot 10^{10} M^{-1} s^{-1}$; z_{AChE}=-6.3 (charge number on active site);
d = 0.91 nm (distance of least approach)

In a discussion of the reaction rate from diffusion considerations the simple reaction scheme has to be extended by introduction of an intermediate diffusional encounter complex E•L

$$E + L \underset{k_{-1}}{\overset{k_1}{\rightleftharpoons}} E \cdot L \underset{k_{-2}}{\overset{k_2}{\rightleftharpoons}} EL$$

Assuming steady state conditions for the intermediate, the

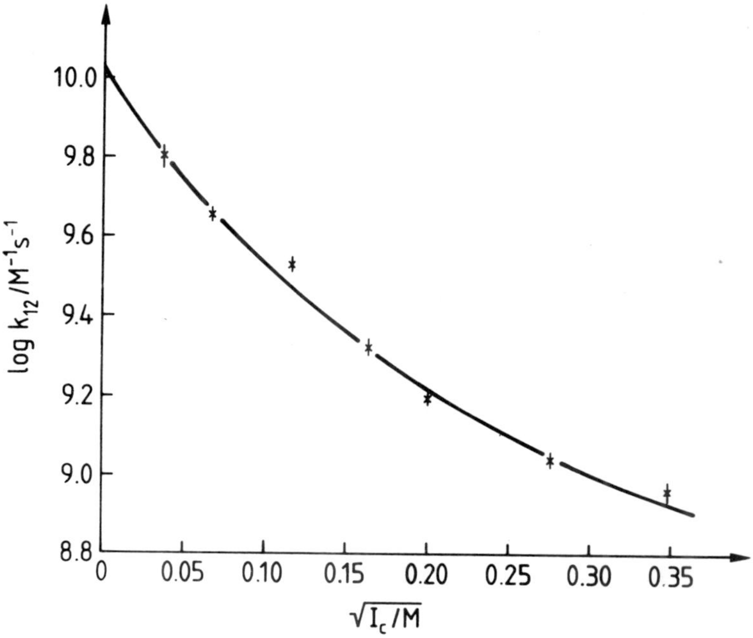

Figure 1: ionic strength dependence of the association rate constant between AChE and N-MAC

overall rate constants are given by $k_{12}=k_1k_2/(k_{-1}+k_2)$ and $k_{21}=k_{-1}k_{-2}/(k_{-1}+k_2)$, and the requirement for diffusion control can be expressed as $k_{-1} \ll k_2$. The diffusional rate constants in the presence of electrostatic interaction are calculated for the limit $I_c \to 0$

$$k_1^{\circ} = \frac{\Omega N_L}{10^3} \overline{D} \, d_{EL} \frac{\phi}{\exp(\phi)-1} = 1.7 \cdot 10^{10} M^{-1} s^{-1},$$

$$k_{-1}^{\circ} = \frac{1.5}{d_{EL}^2} \overline{D} \frac{\phi}{1-\exp(-\phi)} = 7 \cdot 10^7 s^{-1}, \quad \Omega = 2\pi;$$

N_L is Loschmidt's constant, $\overline{D}$ is the mean diffusion coefficient (= $10^{-5} cm^2 s^{-1}$) and ϕ is the ratio of electrostatic and thermal energy, here taken at distance d for bulk water and 298K. Comparison with the experimental values k_{12}° and k_{21}° (v.s.) yields $k_2^{\circ} \gg 10^8 s^{-1}$ and $k_{-2}^{\circ} \gg 4 \cdot 10^2 s^{-1}$; thus the requirement is fulfilled in the limit of vanishing ionic strength and the ligand association can be considered as diffusion controlled.

From the particular properties of AChE we can draw several conclusions:

1. AChE has evolved to a very efficient catalyst: notwithstanding the very high k_1°-value the enzymatic activity remains controlled by substrate diffusion in the range of physiological concentrations;

2. the high effective charge per active site accounts for the I_c-dependence of the association rate; a surface area larger than the active site itself should participate in trapping a cationic ligand;
3. in synapses AChE is unlikely to compete freely with the receptor-protein for the neurotransmitter; a sequential processing of ACh by the membrane proteins must be postulated.

References

(1) T.L.Rosenberry and E.Neumann Biochemistry 16,3870(1977)

(2) H.J.Nolte,T.L.Rosenberry and E.Neumann Biochemistry(1980) in press

EXCITATORY AMINO ACIDS

Neurotransmitters and their Receptors
Edited by U.Z. Littauer, Y. Dudai, I. Silman,
V.I. Teichberg and Z. Vogel

Excitatory Amino Acid Receptors in the Vertebrate Central Nervous System

J. Davies[1], R.H. Evans[2], A.A. Francis[2], A.W. Jones[2], and J.C. Watkins[3]

Department of Pharmacology, The School of Pharmacy, London WC1N 1AX[1], and Departments of Pharmacology[2] and Physiology[3], The Medical School, Bristol, BS8 1 TD, UK

ABSTRACT

On the basis of the effects of selective antagonists on responses to a range of excitatory amino acids, receptors for these excitants have been classified into three types. NMDA receptors in the amphibian and mammalian spinal cords are activated by the agonist N-methyl-D-aspartate (NMDA) and selectively blocked by a variety of antagonists, the most potent of which is 2-amino-5-phosphonovalerate (2APV). These receptors are also sensitive to low concentrations of Mg^{2+} and the transition metal ions, Co^{2+}, Ni^{2+} and Mn^{2+}. Quisqualate and kainate receptors are relatively insensitive to blockade by selective NMDA antagonists, both organic and inorganic. Quisqualate-induced responses in the cat spinal cord are selectively blocked by L-glutamic acid diethyl ester (GDEE) and can be distinguished from kainate-induced responses also by the antagonist γ-D-glutamylglycine (γDGG), which blocks the latter responses.

A strong correlation exists between the abilities of substances to block NMDA receptors and their abilities to block dorsal root-evoked synaptic excitation in the spinal cord. It is therefore likely that NMDA receptors are transmitter receptors activated physiologically by an excitatory amino acid transmitter. Quisqualate receptors may also be transmitter receptors, but more selective antagonists are required to further investigate this possibility. Although kainate receptors must also be considered as possible transmitter receptors, an extrasynaptic location of receptors for this amino acid has been demonstrated in some tissues.

The transmitter activating NMDA receptors is unknown, but studies with agonists of restricted conformational variability suggests a preference of these receptors for aspartate analogues or for glutamate analogues that possess or can adopt a conformation in which the carboxyl groups are less than maximally separated.

When one considers the relatively simple structures of the putative transmitters L-glutamate and L-aspartate, the acidic forms of which are shown in Fig. 1, it is perhaps a little surprising that nearly 100 compounds related to these amino acids are now known to possess qualitatively similar neuroexcitatory properties (1,2). For many years it was considered likely that all such excitatory amino acids acted on a single type of receptor. However, recent evidence strongly suggests the existence of a small number of different receptors each showing preferences for certain agonists over others, but accepting a certain range of structures, so that many agonists can be accommodated with varying efficacies by more than one receptor. The structures of three compounds, kainic acid, quisqualic acid and N-methyl-D-aspartic acid (NMDA), which have been particularly useful in the characterization of these different receptors are shown in Fig. 2.

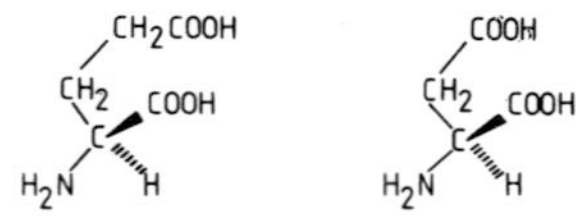

Fig. 1. Structures of L-glutamic and L-aspartic acids

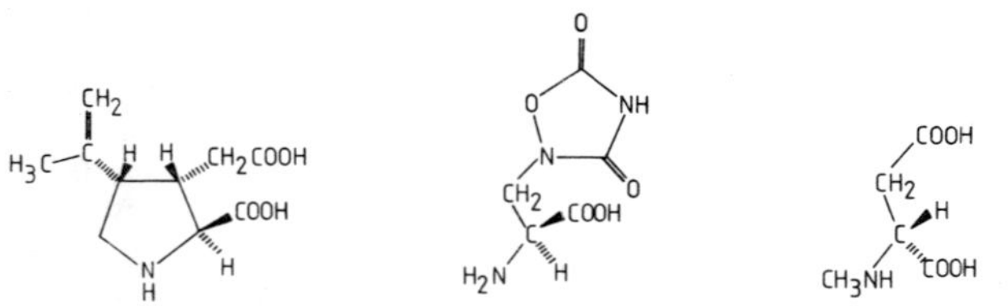

Fig. 2. Preferential agonists for different excitatory amino acid receptors

RECEPTOR DIFFERENTIATION

Using a range of techniques and tissues, including the isolated spinal cords of the frog and immature rat, and iontophoretic investigations *in vivo* in the cat and mouse spinal cords, we have identified a number of selective amino acid antagonists, the effects of which form the basis of the receptor classification to be described. The structures of some of these compounds are shown in Fig. 3, and their effects on responses evoked by a variety of excitants are summarized in Table 1. Thus, 2-amino-5-phosphonovalerate (2APV) is an extremely potent antagonist of NMDA-induced responses, but has little, if any, effect on responses induced in spinal neurones by quisqualate or kainate, either *in vitro* or *in vivo* (3). L-Glutamic acid diethyl ester (GDEE), when iontophoretically applied near cat spinal neurones, is a moderately effective antagonist of quisqualate-induced responses, but has no effect on kainate- or NMDA-induced responses (4,5). These two antagonists therefore suggest the existence of three different types of receptors, which for simplicity will henceforth be referred to as NMDA (or 2APV-sensitive) receptors, quisqualate (or GDEE-sensitive) receptors, and kainate (or 2APV- and GDEE-insensitive) receptors (2).

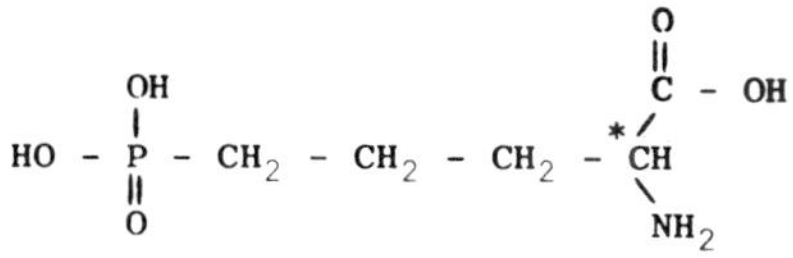

2 - AMINO - 5 -PHOSPHONOVALERIC ACID (2APV)

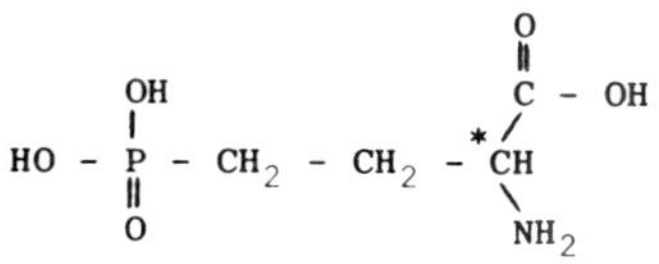

2 - AMINO - 4 - PHOSPHONOBUTYRIC ACID (2APB)

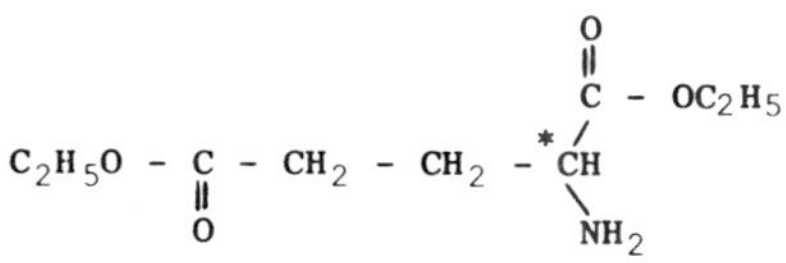

L - GLUTAMIC ACID DIETHYL ESTER (GDEE)

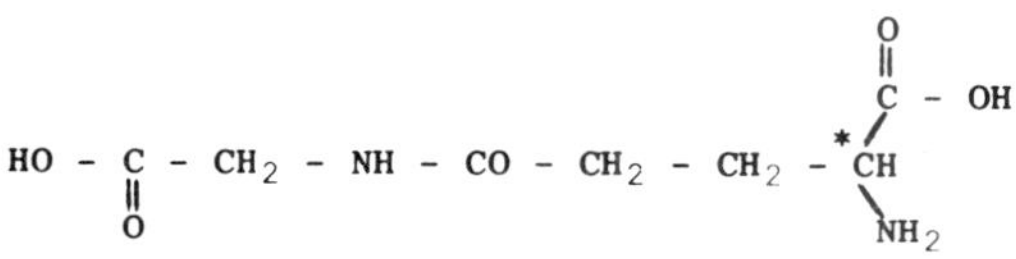

γ - D - GLUTAMYLGLYCINE (γDGG)

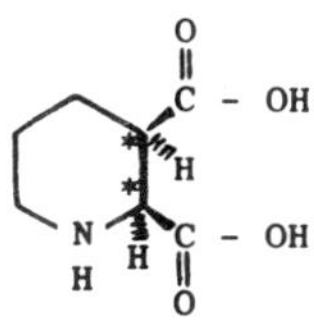

cis-2,3-PIPERIDINE DICARBOXYLIC ACID (cis-2,3-PDA)

Fig. 3. Structures of excitatory amino acid antagonists

Of the other antagonists whose effects are summarized in Table 1, γDGG is the next most selective (2,6). This substance distinguishes clearly between quisqualate- and kainate-induced responses, effectively antagonizing only the latter in the case of cat spinal neurones. However, this substance also blocks NMDA-induced responses. The other two antagonists are selective with respect to amino acid-induced vis à vis acetylcholine-induced responses, but show only limited selectivity with respect to different amino acid agonists. 2APB is relatively weak (100 times less effective as an NMDA-antagonist than the next higher homologue, 2APV), but nevertheless can be used effectively to block both NMDA- and kainate-induced responses, while quisqualate-induced responses are also relatively sensitive to this agent in the cat, but less so in the frog spinal cord (6). The cyclic aspartate analogue, cis-2,3-piperidine dicarboxylate (PDA), is also relatively non-selective with respect to the three 'specific' agonists, but is considerably more potent than 2APB as an amino acid antagonist (6). The main value of this compound (which also shows partial agonist activity) is that it is the most effective antagonist of quisqualate-induced responses that we have yet encountered.

Except for GDEE, none of these antagonists have significant depressant effect on acetylcholine-induced responses (3,4,5,6), although these responses are sometimes enhanced by cis-2,3-PDA, presumably because of its slight depolarizing action (6). In some regions of the CNS, GDEE also antagonizes amino acid-induced responses more than responses induced by acetylcholine, but this action is somewhat variable and in the case of Renshaw cells in the cat spinal cord GDEE does not differentiate effectively between these two types of excitation (4,5).

All of the substances block both L-aspartate- and L-glutamate-induced responses with varying degrees of discrimination, this partial selectivity usually being manifested better at lower doses of the antagonists. Several NMDA antagonists including 2APV, and the previously reported D-α-aminoadipate (DαAA) and D-α-aminosuberate (DαAS) (5,7), often discriminate effectively between L-aspartate- and L-glutamate-induced excitation of spinal neurones, responses to the former agonist being the more susceptible to blockade by these antagonists. GDEE discriminates in the reverse direction to a limited extent, usually depressing L-glutamate-induced responses more than those induced by L-aspartate (4,8). In general the pattern of effects of 2APV, GDEE and γDGG, coupled with those of other antagonists such as DαAA and DαAS, suggests that both L-aspartate and L-glutamate have mixed actions on different receptors, but that L-glutamate acts more effectively than L-aspartate on quisqualate receptors, while L-aspartate acts more effectively than L-glutamate on NMDA receptors.

The blockade of synaptic activity by these substances depends on the particular cells investigated and mode of testing employed. In the case of dorsal

SELECTIVE ANTAGONISM OF EXCITATORY AMINO ACID-INDUCED RESPONSES IN CAT SPINAL CORD

	ANTAGONIST				
AGONIST	2APV	GDEE	DγGG	2APB	PDA
NMDA	↓↓↓↓↓	o	↓↓↓	↓↓	↓↓↓
KAINATE	o	o	↓↓(↓)	↓↓	↓↓↓
QUISQUALATE	o	↓↓	(↓)	↓(↓)	↓↓↓
ACh	o	↓(↓)	o	o	o(↑)
L-ASP	↓↓↓	↓(↓)	↓↓	↓(↓)	↓↓↓
L-GLU	↓(↓)	↓↓	(↓)	↓(↓)	↓↓↓
DR-EVOKED (RENSHAW CELL SYN. EXCITATION)	↓↓↓	o	↓↓	↓	↓↓

Table 1. Effects of antagonists on chemical and synaptic excitation of spinal neurones

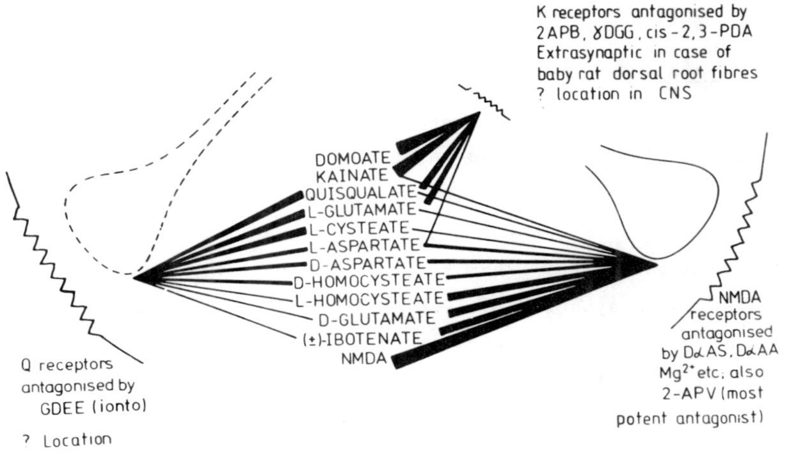

Fig. 4. Schematic representation of NMDA, kainate (K) and quisqualate (Q) receptors. The relative thicknesses of the lines directed from the agonists towards the receptors roughly indicates the relative extents of their actions at those receptors

root-evoked excitation of many spinal cells, including Renshaw cells, all NMDA antagonists effectively block synaptic activity, their relative potencies in producing this effect paralleling those for their NMDA antagonizing actions. This suggests that NMDA receptors are transmitter receptors on spinal neurones. In contrast, GDEE has little or no depressant action on synaptic activity of spinal neurones, suggesting that quisqualate receptors are not major transmitter receptors in the spinal cord, or that the synaptic drive at these sites is too intense to be antagonized by the relatively weak action of GDEE. The only compound of Table 1 that might provide a clue as to whether or not kainate receptors function as transmitter receptors is γDGG. Evidence relating to this possibility might be provided, for instance, by experiments in which the effect of γDGG on synaptic activity was tested after blocking NMDA receptors with 2APV. However, such studies have not yet been carried out.

Fig. 4 schematizes our present concepts regarding NMDA, quisqualate and kainate receptors. NMDA receptors are represented as transmitter receptors, in view of the striking correlation between NMDA antagonism and synaptic blocking activity of a large series of antagonists (1,2,5,7). Exogenous agonists preferentially acting on these receptors include ibotenate, D-glutamate and L-homocysteate, in addition to NMDA (4,5,7). An interesting feature of NMDA receptors is that their sensitivity is depressed by low concentrations of Mg^{2+} (threshold about 10 μM), this action not being reversible by raised $[Ca^{2+}]$ (9,10).

The location and function of GDEE-sensitive receptors is less clear. A feature of these receptors is that the agonists preferentially activating them (Fig. 4) all seem to be inactivated by rapid uptake into the tissue (7,11-14). Whether this underlies the apparent specificity of GDEE - only those agonists whose action is restricted by rapid uptake to the close proximity of the iontophoretic pipette being susceptible to the relatively weak action of GDEE, with other agonists that are not rapidly taken up activating receptors out of range of this antagonist (15) - has yet to be established. The role of GDEE-sensitive receptors in synaptic excitation is unknown, but the possibility that they are transmitter receptors which are different from NMDA receptors, but also activated physiologically by an excitatory amino transmitter, is gaining support. Thus, in certain higher regions of the CNS, GDEE has been shown to block synaptic excitation in addition to excitatory amino acid-induced responses (16-24) and such blockade of synaptic activity in the hippocampus appears to be selective (23,24) for those synapses at which an excitatory amino acid is favoured as the transmitter on neurochemical evidence (25,26). However, further elucidation of the specificity of GDEE with respect to both synaptic excitation and depolarizing responses induced by non-amino acid putative transmitters, such as amines and substance P, will be required before GDEE can be fully accepted as a pharmacological tool for identifying sites of amino acid-mediated synaptic excitation.

No information is yet available in relation to the role of kainate receptors in the CNS, but the possibility must be considered that their location is at least partly extrasynaptic. Thus, kainate and domoate (an analogue of kainate (27)) potently depolarize fibres in dorsal roots of immature rats (15). Quisqualate also depolarizes these fibres, but this action is weaker than on spinal neurones, whereas L-glutamate is considerably more potent on the fibre receptors than on neurones; however, L-aspartate is only weakly effective and NMDA inactive on these receptors at 1000 times the concentration necessary to depolarize motoneurones (15). Responses of dorsal root fibres to kainate and L-glutamate are antagonized by 2APB (15). Extrasynaptic kainate receptors have been identified in invertebrates (28), and have also been suggested as a possible explanation for the pattern of 'excitotoxic' lesions produced by kainate in the goldfish retina (29). Whether or not extrasynaptic kainate receptors do exist within the vertebrate central nervous system, the possibility cannot be excluded that other receptors for this amino acid are located sub-synaptically and, together with NMDA and quisqualate receptors, also play a role in synaptic excitation.

BINDING STUDIES

The results of binding studies with radioactive ligands provide support for the existence of different excitatory amino acid receptors in the mammalian CNS (30), although the correspondence between the conclusions drawn from these studies and those from electrophysiological investigations is far from complete. [^{3}H]Kainate binds with high affinity to rat brain membrane receptors that also have high and moderate affinity, respectively, for quisqualate and L-glutamate, but little or no affinity for ibotenate, DL-homocysteate, L-aspartate, D-aspartate and NMDA (31,32). Conversely, Snodgrass (33) has reported that [^{3}H]-NMDA binds with high affinity to cerebellar membranes of rat and mouse brain, the inhibition pattern of the binding of this amino acid being consistent with the results of electrophysiological studies. Thus, DL-homocysteate, D-glutamate and D-aspartate inhibit [^{3}H]NMDA binding more effectively than do L-glutamate and kainate, and the NMDA antagonist DL-α-aminoadipate is also an inhibitor of this binding. Similar effects have been observed with D-[^{3}H]aspartate (30). This ligand binds to receptors that also interact strongly with NMDA, to a lesser extent with L-glutamate and L-aspartate, and to a lower extent again with kainate. DL-α-Aminoadipate also inhibits D-[^{3}H]aspartate binding, suggesting that these sites may be the same as those binding [^{3}H]-NMDA.

The number of binding sites for L-[^{3}H]glutamate exceed those for kainate or NMDA ten fold or more (31-33) and in general these sites appear to resemble those classified on the basis of electrophysiological experiments as quisqualate (GDEE-sensitive) receptors rather than kainate or NMDA receptors. Thus, neither kainate nor NMDA were effective inhibitors of L-[^{3}H]glutamate binding to cerebellar membranes, whereas quisqualate was almost as effective as L-glutamate itself; however the preferential NMDA receptor agonists, ibotenate, *cis*-1-amino-1,3-dicarboxycyclopentane and D-glutamate (4,5,7,35) were also relatively effective inhibitors of this L-[^{3}H]glutamate binding, whereas GDEE inhibited only weakly (34). In a more limited study of the binding of L-[^{3}H]glutamate to hippocampal membranes (36), the main feature was again the lack of inhibitory effect of kainate and NMDA, indicating clearly that the main sites of L-glutamate binding differ from NMDA and kainate receptors. The binding of L-[^{3}H]glutamate to hippocampal membranes showed a cation dependency which may have functional significance (37), especially the enhancement by Ca^{2+} in the physiological range of concentrations. This supports previous suggestions that Ca^{2+} or other divalent metal ions may be an integral part of excitatory amino acid receptors (27,38-40). It may also be relevant in this respect that Michaelis has isolated a glycoprotein from synaptic membranes which binds

L-[^{3}H]glutamate in a very similar way to intact brain membranes, and which contains iron (41).

ELECTROPHYSIOLOGICAL CHARACTERIZATION AND LOCALIZATION OF NMDA RECEPTORS

The view that NMDA receptors are transmitter receptors activated physiologically by an excitatory amino acid transmitter is supported by a range of observations. In addition to the selective depression by NMDA antagonists of amino acid-induced responses, as already outlined, these substances show the following spectrum of activity.

1. Little or no action on depolarizing responses evoked by cholinomimetics (5,7, 42-46), amines (46) or substance P (46-48).
2. Antagonism of a) dorsal root evoked excitation of spinal neurones, including Renshaw cells (5,7,42-44,46,48,49); b) excitation of cortical neurones evoked by pyramidal tract stimulation (50); c) excitation of cochlear nucleus neurones evoked by auditory stimuli (51,52); d) excitation of neurones in the lateral geniculate nucleus evoked by visual stimuli (21); e) excitation of neurones in cuneate nucleus evoked by cortical stimulation (50); f) excitation of neurones in caudate nucleus evoked by cortical stimulation (50); g) excitation of granule cells in dentate gyrus of hippocampus evoked by stimulation of contralateral hippocampus (23); h) excitation of cerebellar Purkinje cells evoked by parallel fibre stimulation (but, with the relatively weak NMDA antagonist, DLαAA, used as the blocking agent, this depression of synaptic excitation is seen only if the firing of the cells is initially damped down by GABA) (53).
3. Parallel relative potencies of series of monoamino and diamino dicarboxylic acids when tested as NMDA-blockers and as antagonists of DR-evoked synaptic excitation in the frog spinal cord (7).
4. No action on the cholinergic synaptic excitation of Renshaw cells evoked by ventral root stimulation (5,42-44,49) or of rat superior cervical ganglion cells evoked by preganglionic stimulation (46).
5. No action on spinal dorsal horn neurones evoked by noxious stimuli (48), on neurones in the substantia nigra evoked by stimulation of the ipsilateral striatum (47), or on hippocampal granule cells evoked by perforant path stimulation (23). The former two pathways may use substance P as the transmitter and the latter pathway L-glutamate.

These observations indicate that the actions of NMDA antagonists are highly selective with respect to both synaptic and chemically-evoked excitation, and strongly suggest that these actions are mediated at specific transmitter receptors operated by an excitatory amino acid transmitter.

RELATIONSHIP BETWEEN THE EFFECTS OF ORGANIC AND INORGANIC NMDA ANTAGONISTS

The close similarity between the effects of low concentrations of Mg^{2+} and those of the organic NMDA antagonists raised the question of whether the actions of the organic and inorganic agents are mediated at the same sites. Comparison of dose-ratios for antagonism of NMDA-induced responses measured in the presence of separate and paired antagonists (54,55) indicated that whereas organic NMDA antagonists (DαAA and α,ε-diaminopimelate) acted at the same sites, Mg^{2+} acted at different sites. Other evidence suggests that the organic antagonists act competitively with NMDA at the receptors but that Mg^{2+} acts non-competitively (6). Co^{2+} and Ni^{2+} are even more potent than Mg^{2+} as NMDA antagonists but Mn^{2+}, which has more potent presynaptic actions than Mg^{2+} on transmitter release, is less potent than Mg^{2+} in blocking NMDA-induced responses (10). The specificity of the transition metal ions with respect to responses induced by non amino acid putative transmitters has not been investigated, but Mg^{2+} also has some effect (much less marked than on NMDA receptors) on cholinergic, adrenergic and substance P receptors in the spinal cord of the immature rat (10). It is possible that Mg^{2+} acts on the ionophore mediating the effects on membrane ionic permeability that result from the interaction of NMDA (especially) and some other putative transmitter agonists with their respective receptors (10,54-56). The marked effects on NMDA receptors of small changes in $[Mg^{2+}]$ has suggested the possibility that these ions function physiologically to regulate the sensitivity of NMDA receptors to the natural transmitter (46,55).

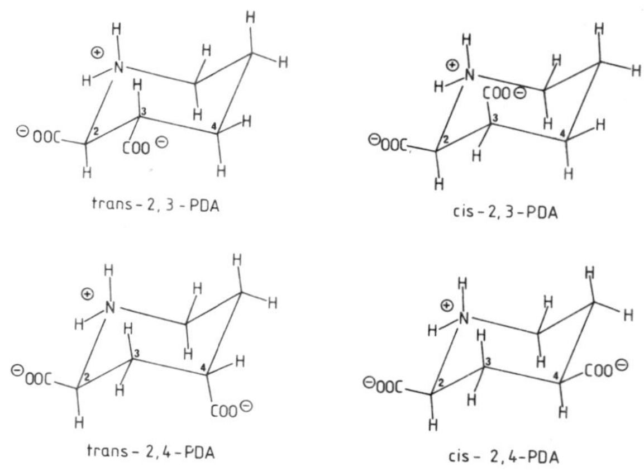

Fig. 5. Three dimensional structures of *cis*- and *trans*- isomers of 2,3- and 2,4-piperidine dicarboxylate (PDA)

CONFORMATIONAL STUDIES AT NMDA RECEPTORS

Compounds of restricted conformational variability and which superficially resemble either aspartate or glutamate with respect to the separation of charg groups have been used to assess the conformational requirements for NMDA agoni action. Progress in this sphere has been recently reviewed (2). The most important finding is that *trans*-2,3- and *trans*-2,4-piperidine dicarboxylates (Fig. 5) are both NMDA agonists of high potency, whereas the *cis*-2,3- isomer i an NMDA antagonist, with partial agonist activity, and the *cis*-2,4- isomer is relatively inactive. The 2,3- compounds are aspartate analogues, and the 2,4- compounds are glutamate analogues. However, with respect to the separation of the carboxylate groups, the inactive *cis*-2,4- isomer may be regarded as an 'extended' glutamate analogue and the *trans*-2,4- compound a 'partially folded glutamate analogue. Both the *trans*-2,3- and the *trans*-2,4- substances could provide an anionic oxygen atom from the C_3 and C_4 carboxyl groups, respectivel which could be almost isosteric, and thus able to interact effectively with t same active site in the receptor. It would therefore seem likely that in con- formity with theoretical arguments (57,58), the NMDA receptor is preferential activated by aspartate analogues or by glutamate analogues that possess, or a able to adopt, a conformation in which the two carboxyl groups are less than maximally separated.

THE TRANSMITTER AT NMDA RECEPTORS

The above considerations, coupled with the results of experiments with NMD antagonists, indicate that both L-aspartate and L-glutamate can interact with NMDA receptors. However, at least four antagonists often differentiate clear between L-aspartate- and L-glutamate-induced excitation in the mammalian spin cord, the former agonist being the more susceptible to blockade. These antag ists are 2APV, DαAA, DαAS, γDGG and α,ε-diaminopimelate (2,4-6, 42-44, 49). many instances these substances have failed to influence L-glutamate-induced excitation while almost abolishing excitation produced by L-aspartate. Hence L-aspartate must be considered the more likely transmitter at those synapses where such clear differentiation can be observed and where the synaptically-evoked excitation is also effectively blocked by the antagonist at the same as those that block L-aspartate-induced excitation. It is also relevant tha the basis of neurochemical evidence, L-aspartate has been favoured as the tr mitter in several regions where NMDA antagonists are effective as synaptic blockers. Thus, changes in aspartate levels correlate better than those of glutamate with regional neuronal loss in the spinal cord, following ischaemi

(59), in the dorsal column nuclei following dorsal column section (60), in the cochlear nucleus following auditory nerve section (61), and in the hippocampus following section of the commissural pathway (25,26). However, L-glutamate cannot be excluded as the transmitter acting at NMDA receptors, nor other possibilities such as a sulphur-containing amino acid or an as yet unidentified NMDA-like substance (1).

REFERENCES

1. Watkins, J.C. (1978). 'Excitatory amino acids', in Kainic Acid as a Tool in Neurobiology (Eds. E.G. McGeer, J.W. Olney & P.L. McGeer) pp.37-69, Raven Press, New York.

2. Watkins, J.C. (1980). 'Pharmacology of excitatory amino acid receptors' in Glutamate: Transmitter in the Central Nervous System (Eds. P.J. Roberts, J. Storm-Mathisen & G.A.R. Johnston) J. Wiley & Sons, London, in press.

3. Davies, J., Francis, A.A., Jones, A.W. & Watkins, J.C. (1980). '2-Amino-5-phosphonovalerate (2APV), a highly potent and specific antagonist at spinal NMDA receptors'. Br. J. Pharmacol. in press.

4. McLennan, H. & Lodge, D. (1979). 'The antagonism of amino acid-induced excitation of spinal neurones in the cat'. Brain Research., 169, 83-90.

5. Davies, J. & Watkins, J.C. (1979). 'Selective antagonism of amino acid-induced and synaptic excitation in the cat spinal cord'. J. Physiol. (Lond.), 297, 621-635.

6. Davies, J., Evans, R.H., Francis, A.A., Jones, A.W. & Watkins, J.C. unpublished observations.

7. Evans, R.H., Francis, A.A., Hunt, K., Oakes, D.J. & Watkins, J.C. (1979). 'Antagonism of excitatory amino acid-induced responses and of synaptic excitation in the isolated spinal cord of the frog'. Br. J. Pharmacol., 67, 591-603.

8. Hicks, T.P., Hall, J.G. & McLennan, H. (1978). 'Ranking of excitatory amino acids by the antagonists glutamic acid diethylester and D-α-aminoadipic acid'. Can. J. Physiol. Pharmacol., 56, 901-906.

9. Evans, R.H., Francis, A.A. & Watkins, J.C. (1977). 'Selective antagonism by Mg^{2+} of amino acid-induced depolarization of spinal neurones'. Experientia (Basel), 33, 489-491.

10. Ault, B., Evans, R.H., Francis, A.A., Oakes, D.J. & Watkins, J.C. (1980). 'Selective depression of excitatory amino acid-induced depolarizations by Mg^{2+} in isolated spinal cord preparations'. J. Physiol. (Lond.) in press.

11. Evans, R.H., Francis, A.A. & Watkins, J.C. (1978). 'Mg^{2+}-like selective antagonism of excitatory amino acid-induced responses by α,ε-diaminopimelic acid, D-α-aminoadipate and HA-966 in isolated spinal cord of frog and immature rat'. Brain Res., 148, 536-542.

12. Lodge, D., Curtis, D.R., Johnston, G.A.R. & Bernstein, J.C. (1980). '*In vivo* inactivation of quisqualate; studies in the cat spinal cord'. Brain Res., 182, 491-495.

13. Balcar, V.J. & Johnston, G.A.R. (1972). 'Glutamate uptake by brain slices and its relation to the depolarization of neurones by acidic amino acids'. J. Neurobiol., 3, 295-301.

14. Balcar, V.J. & Johnston, G.A.R. (1972). 'The structural specificity of the high affinity uptake of L-glutamate and L-aspartate by rat brain slices'. J. Neurochem., 19, 2657-2666.

15. Davies, J., Evans, R.H., Francis, A.A. & Watkins, J.C. (1979b). 'Excitatory amino acid receptors and synaptic excitation in the mammalian central nervous system'. J. Physiol. (Paris), 75, 641-645.

16. Haldeman, S., Huffman, R., Marshall, K.C. & McLennan,H. (1972). 'The antagonism of the glutamate-induced and synaptic excitation of thalamic neurones'. Brain Res., 39, 419-425.

17. Stone, T.W. (1973). 'Cortical pyramidal tract interneurones and their sensitivity to L-glutamic acid'. J. Physiol. (Lond.), 233, 211-225.

18. Stone, T.W. (1976). 'Blockade by amino acid antagonists of neuronal excitation mediated by the pyramidal tract'. J. Physiol. (Lond.), 257, 187-198.

19. Spencer, H.J. (1976). 'Antagonism of cortical excitation of striatal neurons by glutamic acid diethyl ester: evidence for glutamic acid as an excitatory transmitter in the rat striatum'. Brain Res., 102, 91-101.

20. Davies, J. & Watkins, J.C. unpublished observations.

21. Kemp, J.A. & Sillito, A.M. (1979). 'Action of excitatory amino acid antagonists on the retinal input to the cat lateral geniculate body'. J. Physiol. (Lond.), 292, 46P.

22. Segal, M. (1976). 'Glutamate antagonists in rat hippocampus'. Br. J. Pharmacol., 58, 341-345.

23. Hicks, T.P. & McLennan, H. (1979). 'Amino acids and the synaptic pharmacology of granule cells in the dentate gyrus of the rat'. Can. J. Physiol. Pharmacol., 57, 973-978.

24. Wheal, H.V. & Miller, J.J. (1980). 'Pharmacological identification of acetylcholine and glutamate excitatory systems in the dentate gyrus of the rat'. Brain Res., 182, 145-155.

25. White, W.F., Nadler, J.V., Hamberger, A., Cotman, C.W. & Cummins, J.T. (1977) 'Glutamate as a transmitter of hippocampal perforant path'. Nature (Lond.) 270, 356-357.

26. Nadler, J.V., White, W.F., Vaca, K.W., Perry, B.W. & Cotman, C.W. (1978). 'Biochemical correlates of transmission mediated by glutamate and aspartate' J. Neurochem., 31, 147-155.

27. Biscoe, T.J., Evans, R.H., Headley, P.M., Martin, M.R. & Watkins, J.C. (1976 'Structure-activity relations of excitatory amino acids on frog and rat spinal neurones'. Br. J. Pharmacol., 58, 373-382.

28. Takeuchi, A. & Onodera, K. (1975). 'Effects of kainic acid on the glutamate receptors of crayfish muscle'. Neuropharmacology 14, 619-625.

29. Yazulla, S. & Kleinschmidt, J. (1980). 'The effects of intraocular injection of kainic acid on the synaptic organization of the goldfish retina'. Brain Res., 182, 287-301.

30. Johnston, G.A.R. (1979). 'Central nervous system receptors for glutamic acid' in Glutamic Acid: Advances in Biochemistry and Physiology (Eds. L.J. Filer et al), pp.177-185, Raven Press, New York.

31. Simon, J.R., Contrera, J.F. & Kuhar, M.J. (1976). 'Binding of [^{3}H]kainic acid, an analogue of L-glutamate, to brain membranes'. J. Neurochem., 26, 141-147.

32. Johnston, G.A.R., Kennedy, S.M.E. & Twitchin, B. (1979). 'Action of the neurotoxin kainic acid on high affinity uptake of L-glutamic acid in rat brain slices'. J. Neurochem., 32, 121-127.

33. Snodgrass, S.R. (1979). 'In vitro binding studies with [^{3}H]-N-methyl-aspartate'. Soc. Neurosci. Abst., 5, 572.

34. Foster, A.C. & Roberts, P.J. (1978). 'High affinity L-[^{3}H]glutamate binding to postsynaptic receptor sites on rat cerebellar membranes. J. Neurochem., 31, 1467-1477.

35. Hall, J.G., Hicks, T.P., McLennan, H., Richardson, T.L. & Wheal, H.V. (1979). 'The excitation of mammalian central neurones by amino acids'. J. Physiol. (Lond.), 286, 29-39.

36. Baudry, M. & Lynch, G. (1979). 'Two glutamate binding sites in rat hippocampal membranes'. Eur. J. Pharmacol., 57, 283-285.

37. Baudry, M. & Lynch, G. (1979). 'Regulation of glutamate receptors by cations'. Nature (Lond.), 282, 748-750.

38. Curtis, D.R. & Watkins, J.C. (1960). 'The excitation and depression of spinal neurones by structurally related amino acids'. J. Neurochem., 6, 117-141.

39. Curtis, D.R., Phillis, J.W. & Watkins, J.C. (1961). 'Actions of amino acids on the isolated hemisected spinal cord of the toad'. Br. J. Pharmacol., 16, 262-283.

40. Watkins, J.C. (1965). 'Pharmacological receptors and general permeability phenomena of cell membranes'. J. Theoret. Biol., 9, 37-50.

41. Michaelis, E.K. (1979). 'The glutamate receptor-like protein of brain synaptic membranes is a metalloprotein'. Biochem. Biophys. Res. Comm., 87, 106-113.

42. Biscoe, T.J., Davies, J., Dray, A., Evans, R.H., Francis, A.A., Martin, M.R. & Watkins, J.C. (1977a). 'Depression of synaptic excitation and of amino acid-induced excitatory responses by D-α-aminoadipate, α,ε-diaminopimelic acid and HA-966'. Eur. J. Pharmacol., 45, 315-316.

43. Biscoe, T.J., Evans, R.H., Francis, A.A., Martin, M.R., Watkins, J.C., Davies, J. & Dray, A. (1977b). 'D-α-Aminoadipate as a selective antagonist of amino acid-induced and synaptic excitation of mammalian spinal neurones'. Nature (Lond.), 270, 743-745.

44. Biscoe, T.J., Davies, J., Dray, A., Evans, R.H., Martin, M.R. & Watkins, J.C. (1978). 'D-α-Aminoadipate, α,ε-diaminopimelic acid, and HA-966 as antagonists of amino acid-induced and synaptic excitation of mammalian spinal neurones *in vivo*'. Brain Res., 148, 543-548.

45. McLennan, H. & Hall, J.G. (1978). 'The action of D-α-aminoadipate on excitatory amino acid receptors of rat thalamic neurones'. Brain Res., 149, 541-545.

46. Evans, R.H. & Watkins, J.C. (1978b). 'Specific antagonism of excitant amino acids in the isolated spinal cord of the neonatal rat'. Eur. J. Pharmacol. 50, 123-129.

47. Collingridge, G. & Davies, J. (1978). 'An evaluation of D-α-aminoadipate and D- (and DL-)α-aminosuberate as selective antagonists of excitatory amino acids in the substantia nigra and mesencephalic reticular formation of the rat'. Neuropharmacology, 18, 193-199.

48. Davies, J. & Dray, A. (1979). 'Effects of D-α-aminoadipate on physiologically evoked responses of cat dorsal horn neurones'. Experientia, 35, 353-354.

49. Lodge, P., Headley, P.M. & Curtis, D.R. (1978). 'Selective antagonism by D-α-aminoadipate of amino acid and synaptic excitation of cat spinal neurones'. Brain Res., 149, 541-545.

50. Stone, T.W. (1979). 'Amino acids as neurotransmitters of corticofugal neurones in the rat: a comparison of glutamate and aspartate'. Br. J. Pharmacol., 67, 545-551.

51. Martin, M.R. & Adams, J.C. (1980). 'Effects of DL-α-aminoadipate on synaptically and chemically evoked excitation of anteroventral cochlear nucleus neurons of the cat'. Neuroscience, 4, 1097-1105.

52. Martin, M.R. (1980). 'The effects of iontophoretically applied antagonists on auditory nerve and amino acid evoked excitation of anteroventral cochlear nucleus neurons'. Neuropharmacology, in press.

53. Stone, T.W. (1979). 'Glutamate as the neurotransmitter of cerebellar cells in the rat: electrophysiological evidence'. Br. J. Pharmacol., 66, 291-296.

54. Evans, R.H. & Watkins, J.C. (1978a). 'Dual sites for antagonism of excitatory amino acid actions on central neurones'. J. Physiol. (Lond.), 277, 57P.

55. Davies, J., Evans, R.H., Francis, A.A. & Watkins, J.C. (1979a). 'Excitatory amino acid receptors and synaptic excitation in the mammalian central nervous system', in Advances in Pharmacology and Therapeutics, Vol. 2, Neurotransmitters (Ed. P. Simon) pp.161-170, Pergamon Press, Oxford.

56. Davies, J. & Watkins, J.C. (1977). 'Effects of magnesium ions on the responses of spinal neurones to excitatory amino acids and acetylcholine'. Brain Res., 130, 364-368.

7. Johnston, G.A.R., Curtis, D.R., Davies, J. & McCulloch, R.M. (1974). 'Spinal interneurone excitation by conformationally restricted analogues of L-glutamic acid'. Nature (Lond.), 248, 804-805.

8. McCulloch, R.M., Johnston, G.A.R., Game, C.J.A. & Curtis, D.R. (1974). 'The differential sensitivity of spinal interneurones and Renshaw cells to kainate and N-methyl-D-aspartate'. Exp. Brain Res., 21, 515-518.

9. Davidoff, R.A., Graham, L.T., Shank, R.P., Werman, R. & Aprison, M.H. (1967). 'Changes in amino acid concentrations associated with loss of spinal interneurones'. J. Neurochem., 14, 1025-1031.

0. Roberts, F. & Hill, R.G. (1978). 'The effect of dorsal column lesions on amino acid levels and glutamate uptake in rat, dorsal column nuclei'. J. Neurochem., 31, 1549-1551.

1. Wenthold, R.J. & Gully, R.L. (1977). 'Aspartic acid and glutamic acid levels in the cochlear nucleus after auditory nerve lesion'. Brain Res., 138, 111-123.

Neurotransmitters and their Receptors
Edited by U.Z. Littauer, Y. Dudai, I. Silman,
V.I. Teichberg and Z. Vogel

The Interactions of Excitatory Amino Acids with Brain Tissue: A Study of Amino Acid-Induced Ion Fluxes in Rat Striatal Slices

V.I. Teichberg, O. Goldberg*, N. Tal and A. Luini

Departments of Neurobiology and Organic Chemistry,*

The Weizmann Institute of Science, Rehovot, Israel

SUMMARY

We have studied the effects of glutamate and other neuroexcitatory amino acids on the efflux rate of $^{22}Na^+$, $^{36}Cl^-$ and $^{42}K^+$ from preloaded rat striatum slices. The desaturation curve of these ions does not follow a monoexponential kinetic behavior and after 15 min the efflux rates are stabilized with rate constants of 0.1 min^{-1} for $^{22}Na^+$, 0.065 min^{-1} for $^{42}K^+$. Glutamate causes a large increase in the $^{22}Na^+$ efflux rate while it increases only slightly the efflux rates of $^{42}K^+$ and $^{36}Cl^-$. These effects are dose-related. The increase of the $^{22}Na^+$ efflux rate is not produced by GABA and other non-excitatory agents and cannot be prevented by 10^{-7}M TTX, a high Mg^{++}/Ca^{++} ratio and low temperature. GABA however, increases the $^{36}Cl^-$ efflux rate in a process blocked by picrotoxinin. The changes in efflux rates of ions caused by glutamate are a reflection of its interactions with specific receptor-ionophore complexes that regulate the neuronal membrane permeability. An increase in $^{22}Na^+$ efflux rate can be elicited by a large number of excitatory amino acids and this effect is blocked by amino acid antagonists. These results are in excellent agreement with those obtained by electrophysiological techniques. They emphasize the validity of the tracer ion efflux assay for the study of excitatory amino acid receptors and demonstrate its usefulness in pharmacological investigations of brain areas that are not easily studied by conventional electrophysiological techniques.

INTRODUCTION

In recent years, an ever increasing attention has been devoted to the study of the excitatory actions of dicarboxylic amino acids in the nervous system and of their possible involvement in neurotransmission. Since the 1960s it has been known that L-glutamate and L-aspartate display an almost ubiquitous depolarizing (1) and neurotoxic action (2) in the mammalian central nervous system. However, the relevance of these effects to natural excitatory activity in brain is still a matter of contention. Recent pharmacological investigations involving the screening of a large number of acidic amino acids have led to the recognition of the existence of multiple excitatory amino acid receptor types (3,4). The function, the structure and cellular localization of these receptors as well as the identity of their natural ligands are now problems to be elucidated.

Most of the advances in the knowledge of amino acid receptors have been achieved through the use of electrophysiological methods. However, the qualitative nature of these methods presents an impediment to a more extensive analysis of the molecular interactions of excitatory amino acids with CNS tissue. Ligand binding studies with isolated membrane preparations can theoretically provide quantitative data concerning parameters of ligand-receptor interactions such as apparent affinity constants and Hill coefficients. However the assignment of the observed binding sites in brain to genuine receptors is often not convincingly established and remains dependent on the availability of probes of high specificity. The limitations of the electrophysiological and ligand binding methods create therefore the need for additional assay systems allowing quantitative studies of the functional interactions of excitatory amino acids with their neuronal receptors.

The above challenges led us to undertake a multidisciplinary research aiming at the development of new methods and of novel synthetic ligands for the investigation of the properties of functional receptors of amino acids in CNS neurons.

Assay of receptor-ionophore complexes of amino acids in brain slices

The method that we have developed is based on the measure of ion movements that result from the interaction of neurotransmitters with membraneous receptor-ionophore complexes. A method based on this principle has already been applied successfully to the study of acetylcholine receptors in microsacs from electric organ tissue (5) and muscle cultures (6) and of γ-aminobutyric acid (GABA) receptors in crayfish muscle (7).

In brain, the effects of glutamate and other excitatory amino acids on the influx of Na^+ ions have been studied by Mc Ilwain and his colleagues (8,9) who found that excitatory amino acid-receptor interactions are characterized by an increased membrane permeability to Na^+ ions. The measure of amino acid induced ion influxes presents however some technical problems. In particular the amplitude of the signal (amount of tracer ion taken up by brain tissue following the exposure to amino acids) depends on the amount of tissue used, and the signal/noise ratio is very small. Receptor assays based on such measurements cannot, therefore, be carried out in a routine way. We decided to study ion effluxes from preincubated brain slices. The following procedure was adopted: 300 μ thick slices from rat striatum are incubated at 37°C in an oxygenated Tris-buffered Krebs-Ringer solution containing traces of radioactive ions such $^{22}Na^+$, $^{86}Rb^+$, $^{42}K^+$, $^{36}Cl^-$ or $^{65}Cr^{+++}$. After a loading period of 30 minutes, the slices are transferred every minute, with the help of a basket shaped sieve, through a series of twenty tubes containing a non-radioactive Krebs-Ringer solution. They are then transferred every minute in successive wash-out tubes containing the excitatory ligand to be tested. The amount of radioactive tracer in the individual wash-out tubes is determined as well as that present in the slices at the end of the experiment. The tracer ion content of the tissue at any time t is calculated by adding the total radioactivity released after this time t to the radioactivity left in the tissue at the end of the experiment. The wash-out curve is expressed as the evolution of the specific efflux rate with time, where the specific efflux rate R is defined as $R = \frac{C_t - C(t + \Delta t)}{C_t \cdot \Delta t}$.

C_t is the tracer ion content of the tissue at time t and $C(t + \Delta t)$ is the content after Δt. This treatment of the data is very convenient since the specific efflux rate is independent of the amount of tissue used and of the actual number of radioactive counts released.

Figure 1 shows the evolution of the specific $^{22}Na^+$ efflux rate with time.

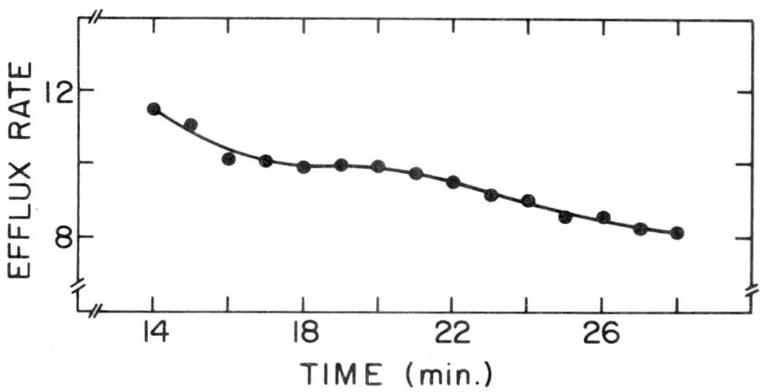

Figure 1: Evolution of the specific $^{22}Na^+$ efflux rate with time. 300 μ thick coronal sections from rat striata are placed within 4 minutes after sacrifice into basket shaped sieves (3 slices per sieve) kept in an oxygenated physiological medium (124 mM NaCl, 0.76 mM KCl, 1.24 mM KH_2PO_4, 1.3 mM $MgSO_4$, 2 mM $CaCl_2$, 10 mM glucose and 26 mM Tris HCl, pH 7.3) at 37°C. After being allowed to recover for 30-40 min, the slices are transferred and incubated for 20 min in a physiological medium containing 1-2 Ci/ml $^{22}Na^+$. The wash-out

of the radioactive tracer is then carried out by transferring the sieve every minute through a series of vessels containing a non-radioactive medium. The amount of radioactive tracer in each individual wash-out vessel is determined, as well as that present in the slices at the end of the transfers. The $^{22}Na^+$ content of the tissue at any time t is calculated by adding the total radioactivity released after this time t to the radioactivity left in the tissue at the end of the experiment. The wash-out curve is presented here as the evolution of the specific efflux rate, R with time

$$R = \frac{C_t - C_{(t+\Delta t)}}{C_t . \Delta t}$$

C_t is the $^{22}Na^+$ content of the tissue at time t and $C_{(t+\Delta t)}$ is the content after Δt.

The specific efflux rate (min^{-1}) has been multiplied by 100 fold.

It can be seen that efflux rate is stabilized around a value of 0.1 min^{-1} for the time period between 16 and 22 minutes. Figure 2 shows that if at t=20 min, the striatal slices are transferred into wash-out tubes containing L-glutamate, the efflux rate is rapidly increasing from a basal level of 0.1 min^{-1} to reach different maximal levels at t=22, depending on the concentration of L-glutamate (figure 2). Then, in spite of the continuous

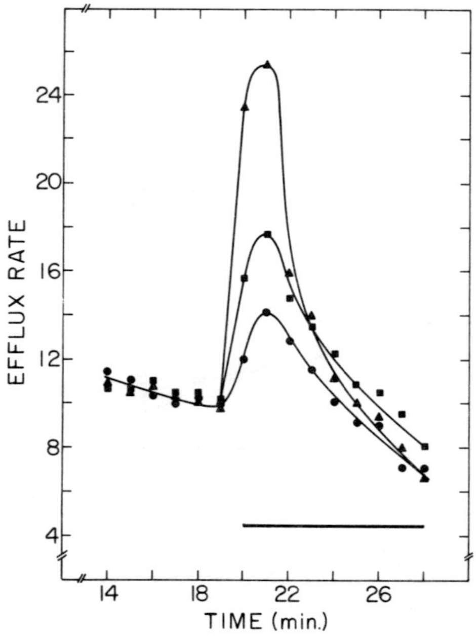

Figure 2:

Effect of increasing doses o L-glutamate on the specific $^{22}Na^+$ efflux rate from stria slices. The black horizonta bar indicates the time of exposure to L-glutamate at the following concentrations 0.3 mM (●), 1 mM (■), 3 mM (Δ). Specific efflux rate (min^{-1} x 100).

presence of L-glutamate, the efflux rate decreases to reach the basal level in 5-6 minutes. Qualitatively, similar results are obtained if the slices are exposed to L-glutamate at an earlier time than that needed for a stabilization of the basal $^{22}Na^{+}$ efflux rate. Experiments with inulin, a non permeating substance, indicate, that a complete wash-out of the extracellular space requires about 16 minutes. Accordingly, in order to optimize the signal/noise ratio the ligand-stimulated $^{22}Na^{+}$ efflux rates are best measured at times (> 16 min) when the $^{22}Na^{+}$ released from extracellular compartments does not mask anymore that released from intracellular pools.

<u>Glutamate increases $^{22}Na^{+}$ efflux rate by enhancing membrane permeability</u>

Theoretically, the glutamate induced increase in $^{22}Na^{+}$ efflux rate may involve a single, or a combination of the following processes.

a) activation of action potentials resulting in an increase of Na^{+} movements across the excitable membrane.

b) activation of Na^{+}/K^{+} activated ATPase following a glutamate-induced depolarization.

c) activation of polysynaptic pathways resulting in the release and subsequent interaction of various excitatory neurotransmitters with receptors triggering increases in membrane permeability to Na^{+} ions.

d) specific opening of Na^{+} channels (ionophores) linked to glutamate receptors.

The possible contribution of each of the above processes to glutamate-stimulated $^{22}Na^{+}$ effluxes was investigated. Table I summarizes the results. Three parameters are studied: the basal efflux rate which corresponds to the average specific rate measured during the two minutes preceding the glutamate stimulation, the stimulated efflux rate which represents the average value for the two first minutes of exposure of the slices to glutamate, and Δ which is a value representing the difference between these two averages. As seen in figure 2, Δ varies with glutamate concentration. However, inspection of the values of Δ in table I shows that this parameter does not vary under conditions preventing the activation of polysynaptic pathways (low $[Ca^{++}]/[Mg^{++}]$), of action potentials (tetrodotoxin (TTX)), and of Na^{+}/K^{+} activated ATPase (temperature).

The concentration of 10^{-7}M TTX was chosen as that needed to block the $^{22}Na^{+}$ efflux stimulated by veratridine, a neurotoxin known to maintain the Na^{+} action potential channel in an open state. Veratridine at 10^{-4}M increases at 37°C the basal efflux rate from 0.09 min^{-1} to 0.13 min^{-1}. TTX, a specific inhibitor of the action potential Na^{+} channel, abolished the veratridine effect at a concentration of 10^{-7}M.

			EFFLUX RATE (min^{-1} x 100)		
[Ca^{++}]/[Mg^{++}]	TTX(M)	T^{o}C	BASAL	STIMULATED	Δ
1.5	-	37	10.1±1.5	25.2±3.3	15.1
1.5	10^{-7}	37	9.3±1.1	23.7±2.1	14.4
0.05	-	37	10.3±2	26.3±1.6	16
0.05	10^{-7}	37	9.5±0.7	24.0±4.2	14.5
0.05	10^{-7}	15	6.7±0.5	22.1±3.2	15.4
0.05	10^{-7}	23	8.1±1.0	23.1±1.8	15.1
0.002	10^{-7}	23	8.3±0.9	23.8±1.2	15.5

TABLE I: Effects of temperature, [Ca^{++}]/[Mg^{++}] ratio and tetrodotoxin on the basal and glutamate-stimulated ^{22}Na^{+} efflux from rat striatal slices as well as on the difference (Δ) between their average values. L-glutamate concentration: 5 mM.

Inhibition of the Na^{+}/K^{+} activated ATPase was achieved by carrying out wash-out experiments at 15°C rather than at 37°C. The Na^{+}/K^{+} activated ATPa has a Q_{10}= 3 and therefore its activity at 15°C should be reduced to about 10% of that at 37°C (10). As seen in table I, temperature is the only parameter affecting the basal ^{22}Na^{+} efflux rate. This result is expected since the Na^{+}/K^{+} activated ATPase plays an important role in the turnover and removal of intracellular Na^{+} ions. The Δ values however are not temperature dependent.

On the basis of the results presented in table I, one can clearly disregard the contribution of three of the four processes mentioned above to the glutamate - stimulated increase in ^{22}Na^{+} efflux rate. It is accordingly proposed that the effects of glutamate on ^{22}Na^{+} efflux result from a increase in membrane permeability originating in the opening of Na^{+} channel associated with glutamate receptors. The following considerations strength this proposition. In the absence of any active process the unidirectional efflux of tracer ions measured in the above experiments is a function of th permeability of the membrane, the tracer ion intracellular concentration an the membrane potential (electric field factor) (see formula in Fig. 3). Mak the constant field assumption of Goldman (11) for the outward movement of Na^{+} ions, it is possible to calculate the theoretical contribution of the electric field factor for a depolarization by 30 mV [the maximal depolarization elicited by glutamate, (12)] of a membrane at a resting potential of

- 70 mV. One finds that the efflux of the tracer ions will be increased by two fold compared to that at the resting membrane potential. As seen in figure 2, glutamate stimulates the specific efflux of $^{22}Na^+$ from a basal level of 0.10 min^{-1} to a maximal level of 0.25 min^{-1}. Since the basal efflux of $^{22}Na^+$ originates in part from glia and glutamate-insensitive cells, the stimulation factor for glutamate-sensitive cells is probably larger than 2.5 and therefore, one may infer that glutamate increases $^{22}Na^+$ efflux via an increase in membrane permeability.. The contribution of the electric field factor to the undirectional efflux can be further demonstrated when the effects of glutamate are studied under conditions preventing depolarization. This is achieved by the removal of extracellular Na^+ ions [it is assumed that glutamate does not decrease K^+ permeability (see below)]. Experiments were carried out with striatal slices preincubated in $^{22}Na^+$ and subsequently transferred into a physiological solution in which Na^+ions were substituted with choline or Tris ions. We found that under such conditions, glutamate is capable of increasing by two fold the $^{22}Na^+$ efflux to a rate which is two thirds of that observed in the Na^+ containing medium (Figure 3).

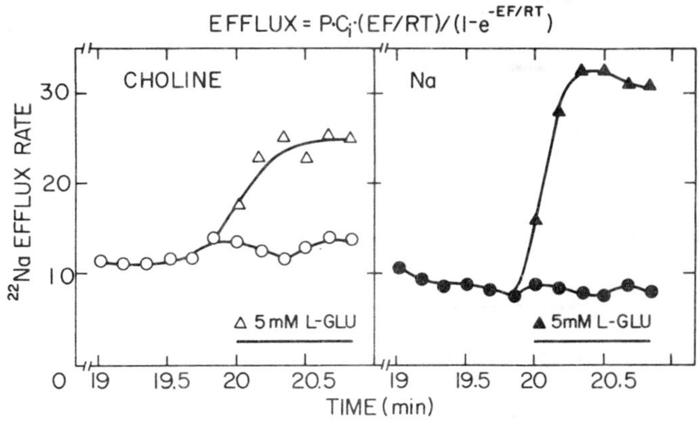

Figure 3: Glutamate-stimulated specific $^{22}Na^+$ efflux in a normal Krebs/Ringer medium (Na^+) and in a choline containing medium. Both solutions contain 10^{-7}M TTX, 0.2 mM Ca^{++}, 4 mM Mg^{++}. In the choline containing medium, no sodium was present, choline was used as a substitute of Na^+. Because of the deleterious long term effects of choline, the slices were incubated in this solution only for a short period before the transfers into glutamate containing solutions. The rate of transfer was 6/min. Specific efflux rate (min^{-1} x 100).

The existence of a glutamate enhanced $^{22}Na^+$ efflux in a Na^+ free medium is a clear proof that glutamate indeed increases membrane permeability. The objec tion can be made that Na^+ ions cannot be totally substituted with choline and therefore a small glutamate-induced depolarization can still take place. However, the theoretical considerations mentioned above indicate that the electric field factor will always be smaller than 2.0 if the amplitude of glutamate induced depolarizations is less than 30 mV. The observed differential action of glutamate in choline or Na^+ containing media is thus in agreement with theoretical considerations.

On the basis of these results and those mentioned in table I, we conclude that the increase in $^{22}Na^+$ efflux rate caused by glutamate originates mainly in its interaction with receptors which control the membrar ionic permeability.

To determine whether the glutamate-stimulated increase in membrane perme bility involves other ions besides Na^+ ions, we carried out experiments simil

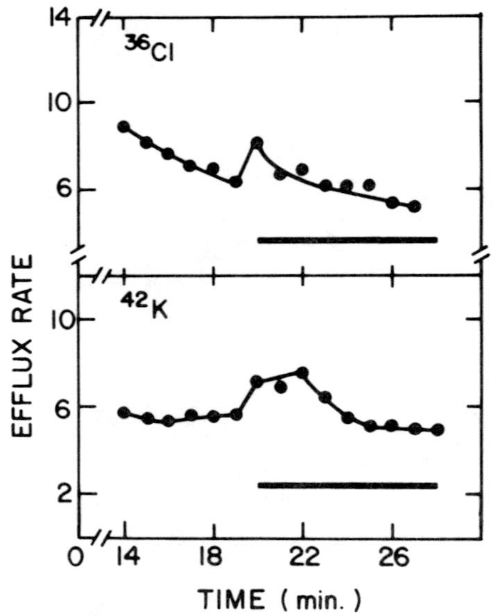

Figure 4:

Glutamate stimulated $^{42}K^+$ and $^{36}Cl^-$ efflux rate. The black horizontal bar indicates the time of exposure to 3 mM L-glutamate. Specific effluх rate (min^{-1} x 100).

to those described above, in which we substituted $^{22}Na^+$ with $^{42}K^+$, $^{36}Cl^-$ or $^{65}Cr^{+++}$. Figure 4 shows that glutamate has almost no effect on $^{36}Cl^-$ movements but can increase $^{42}K^+$ movements. The efflux of $^{65}Cr^{+++}$, however, is not at all affected by glutamate. The effect of glutamate on $^{42}K^+$ efflux rate i probably not due to a glutamate-induced depolarization since it remains almo unaffected in Na^+- free medium. This result and those described above suggest that glutamate increases the membrane permeability to both Na^+ and K^+ ions. However, it is not yet possible to determine whether these ions are translocated through common ionophores or whether receptors with different ionic specificities are involved.

Origins of the bell-shaped response to glutamate

As seen in figures 2 and 4, glutamate affects Na^+ and K^+ efflux rates in a bell-shaped fashion. In both cases the efflux rate is increasing for the first 2-3 minutes and then decreases. Several mechanisms can account for this phenomenon.

a) Desensitization of the glutamate receptors leading, after prolonged exposure to glutamate, to a closure of receptor-linked ionophores.

b) Depletion of radioactive tracer ions in glutamate sensitive cellular pools.

d) Diffusion-limited wash-out of tracer ions from the extracellular space.

We have examined the possibility of the existence of a desensitization of glutamate receptors by carrying out the experiments described in figure 5. Slices were preincubated with $^{22}Na^+$ and an experimental protocol in three steps was used.

1) Slices were exposed to a control dose of glutamate and the response observed was used as a reference. (panel A).

2) Slices were first exposed to a "desensitizing" dose of glutamate and subsequently transferred into wash-out tubes containing glutamate at a concentration higher than that used to "desensitize" (panel B).

3) Slices were first exposed to a "desensitizing" dose of glutamate, then washed into a glutamate free medium and finally transferred into wash-out tubes containing glutamate at a concentration higher than that used to "desensitize" (panel C). From figure 5, it can be seen that no recovery of the response was observed after "desensitization", either under conditions of panel B or C. Although these results can indeed be accounted for by the existence of a desensitization process, they can equally be interpreted on the basis of a selective depletion of tracer ions in glutamate-sensitive pools.

The possible contribution of a depletion process to the decrease in efflux rates can be examined using the model of Daniel (13) which assumes that the evolution of the tissue content of tracer ions with time, C_t, is the sum of exponentials $C_i e^{-k_i t}$ where k_i are rate constants with dimensions of time^{-1}, and C_i are coefficients representing compartment size ($C_{t=0}=1$). We have found that a simple two compartments model fully accounts for our results (figure 6).

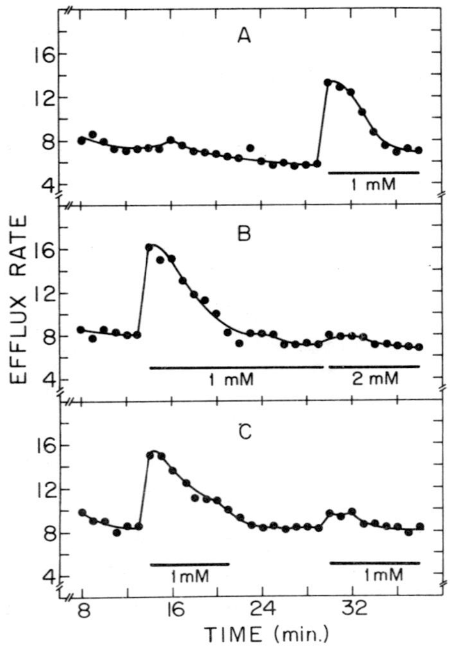

Figure 5: Effect of cumulative doses of L-glutamate on specific $^{22}Na^+$ efflux rate from rat striatum slices.
A. Control dose of 1 mM L-glutamate
B. Control dose of 1 mM L-glutamate followed by test dose of 2 mM L-glutamate
C. Control dose of 1 mM L-glutamate followed by 8 transfers into washing solution and exposure to test dose of 1 mM L-glutamate. Specific efflux rate (min^{-1} x 100).

The two compartments, C_1 which is sensitive to glutamate, and C_2 which is not, are preequilibrated with a radioactive tracer ion which subsequently comes out monoexponentially with respective rate constants k_1 and k_2. The total tracer content of the slices at any time t is $C_t = C_1\ e^{-k_1 t} + C_2\ e^{-k_2 t}$ and the specific efflux rate is $R = \frac{C_t - C_{(t + \Delta t)}}{C_t . \Delta t}$. If the rate constant k_1, is rapidly increased (as a result of the interaction of glutamate with C_1), while k_2 remains constant, the specific efflux rate will first increase as a result of an enhanced tracer release but will then decrease following the depletion of tracer ions from C_1. At the end of this process, R will be a reflection of the basal efflux rate from C_2 only. In figure 6, the evolution of specific $^{22}Na^+$ efflux rates R at two glutamate concentrations are compared with curves simulated according to the above mentioned model.
At high glutamate concentrations, the best fitted values of C_1 and C_2 at t= were 0.4 and 0.6 and those of k_1, k_2 were 0.7 min^{-1} and 0.06 min^{-1}

respectively. In the absence of glutamate and at 0.3 mM glutamate the values of k_1 were 0.12 min^{-1} and 0.33 min^{-1} respectively.

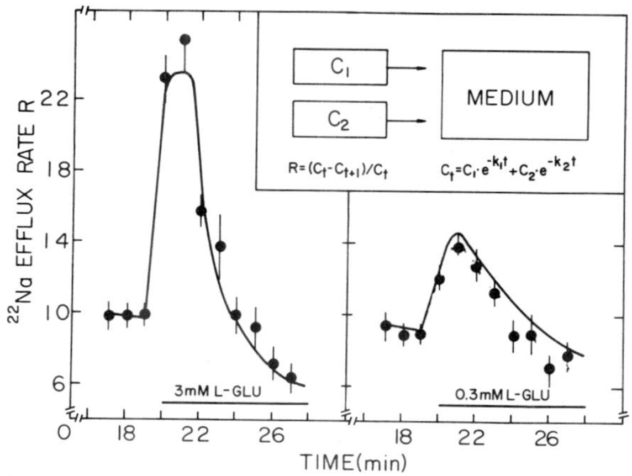

Figure 6: Simulation of glutamate dependent specific Na^+ efflux rates. The dots represent experimental points. The line represents the best fit of the experimental curve. At t=0, $C_{t=0}=1$ and $C_1=0.4$, $C_2=0.6$. The simulation was carried out for two values of the stimulated rate constant k_1. To simulate a high glutamate concentration (3 mM), k_1 was increased from a value of 0.12 min^{-1} to 0.7 min^{-1}. It was increased to 0.33 min^{-1} to simulate 0.3 mM glutamate. To account for the diffusion of glutamate into the slices, we assume that during the first minute of exposure to glutamate, half of C_1 is depleted at a rate of 0.12 min^{-1} whereas the other half is depleted either at a rate of 0.7 min^{-1} or at 0.33 min^{-1}. This correction for the diffusion rate of glutamate is used only for the first minute of exposure to glutamate.

The close correlation between the model and the experiment, particularly at high glutamate concentrations, indicates that the glutamate-induced decrease in specific efflux rates can probably be attributed to a depletion of tracer ions in glutamate sensitive compartments. At low glutamate concentrations, this correlation is not as good, (figure 6) and it is an appealing possibility that a desensitization of the glutamate receptor does indeed take place concomitantly with the depletion process. Such a desensitization could not be observed at high glutamate concentrations since a massive depletion of tracer ions from the glutamate sensitive compartments could mask the effect. Conflicting reports have appeared in the literature concerning the existence of a desensitization of the glutamate response (14,15) and our results, unfortunately do not contribute to the elucidation of this problem.

In any event, it is clear that one of the factors contributing to the glutamate-induced decrease in efflux rates is the depletion of tracer ions in glutamate sensitive compartments.

The existence of diffusional delays is another factor that can operate concurrently with the process of depletion to decrease stimulated efflux rates. The rate at which $^{22}Na^+$ ions are washed out from their cellular pools into the bathing medium depends not only on the intrinsic permeability of the membrane but also on the rate of diffusion of the released ions through the extracellular space. In a brain slice, the diffusion is affected by the tortuosity and the volume fraction (16). Furthermore, the average transit time needed for an ion to diffuse to a distance d, increases with d^2. On that basis, one can calculate that the efflux of Na^+ from the superficial layers of a slice ($d < 50\ \mu$) will not be limited by diffusion whereas the efflux from inner layers ($d < 150\ \mu$) will be affected by diffusional delays.

At this stage, the bell-shaped evolution of efflux rates in the presence of glutamate can be explained by the involvement of the following processes: a) increased permeability of the membrane leading to an enhanced release of tracer ions into the extracellular space, and b) depletion of ion pools and diffusion-limited wash-out of released ions from the extracellular space into the bathing medium. The first process is clearly the expression of a glutamate-specific response and represents the only relevant "signal" in a pharmacological assay. Since the increase in efflux rate is due to glutamate-induced changes in membrane permeability which are presumably mediated by glutamate receptors, one expects this process to be saturable.

Figure 7 shows the dose-response curve of L-glutamate obtained by measuring Δ as a function of concentration. A hyperbolic curve is observed and saturation is reached at 5 mM glutamate and $\Delta_{max} = 18$.

The question arises, however, whether this saturation reflects a full receptor occupancy or whether it indicates that the $^{22}Na^+$ wash-out rate has become limited by diffusion. A partial answer to this problem is obtained from the dose-response curve (figure 8) of another glutamatergic ligand, kainic acid, whose receptor is considered to be distinct from that of glutamate (4). Also in this case saturation is reached at a $\Delta_{max} = 18$. Since the density of kainic acid receptors is most probably different from that of glutamate receptors, one would expect the respective saturation of these receptors to be reached at different Δ_{max} values. Since identical Δ_{max} values are observed, it is plausible that this value does not reflect full receptor occupancy but is diffusion-limited. The relevant region in dose-response curves is therefore that of Δ values smaller than 10. From figure 7,

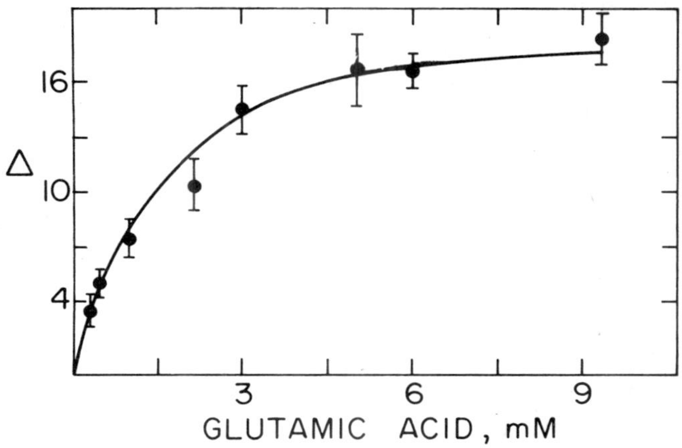

Figure 7: Dose-response curve of L-glutamate. The effect of L-glutamate is expressed here as the difference Δ between the averages of the specific efflux rates, measured and calculated as described in the legend to figure 1, for the two minutes preceding and those following the transfers into solutions of the ligand.

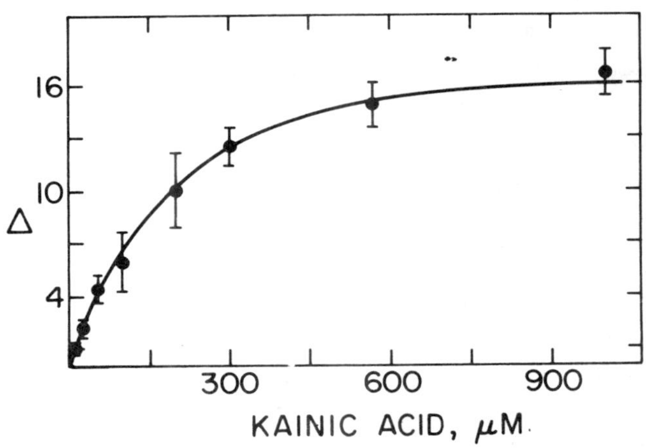

Figure 8: Dose-response curve of kainic acid.

it can be seen that glutamate elicits a response already at 0.3 mM. This concentration is similar to the minimal glutamate concentration (0.1 mM) needed to evoke excitation, found by electrophysiological techniques (17). Although this might appear to be a rather high concentration, one should keep in mind that glutamate is present in brain at a concentration of 10 mM and in the cerebrospinal fluid at 30 μM (18). Therefore, a relatively high threshold of activation might afford a margin of safety preventing fluctuations of the CSF concentrations of glutamate from giving rise to neuronal excitation. It may also be pointed out that the only dose-response curves of L-glutamate reported in the electrophysiological literature show apparent affinity constants in the mM range (19,20,21).

Figure 8 shows that kainic acid stimulates $^{22}Na^{+}$ efflux rate at concentrations lower than those of glutamate. This finding is also in line with electrophysiological data (3).

Pharmacological properties of excitatory amino acid receptors

We have studied a number of structural analogues and derivatives of glutamate in order to clarify the pharmacological properties of striatal excitatory amino acid receptors. All the compounds were tested at 0.1 mM and 1 mM for their ability to increase Na^{+} efflux rates from preloaded striatal slices. The results of this study are summarized in Table II. The most potent agonists were found to be N-methyl-D-aspartate >>DL-homocysteate> quisqualate>kainate>D-glutamate>L-glutamate>L-aspartate. The threshold concentration for stimulation by N-methyl-D-aspartate is around 5 μM. No reports have appeared yet on the relative potency of glutamate analogues in the depolarization of rat striatal neurons and therefore no direct comparison can be made. However the above sequence is quite similar to that found with frog spinal motoneurons or rat spinal interneurons (22,23).

In agreement with the literature (22) several compounds were found to be devoid of agonist properties. These include some antagonists of excitatory amino acids such as L-α-aminosuberate, diethyl glutamate, γ-D-glutamylglycine and 2-amino-5-phosphonovalerate (22). γ-Aminobutyric acid (GABA), used at 3 mM, was found to be unable to stimulate $^{22}Na^{+}$ efflux rate, but increased significantly $^{36}Cl^{-}$ specific efflux rate in a process blocked by 50 μM picrotoxinin. This result indicates that studies of GABA receptor-ionphore complexes are feasible by flux methods in brain slices. Table II lists also a series of kainate analogues that were synthesized in our laboratory. Their structures are shown in table III where their

N-Methyl-D-aspartate	80.0	D-Glutamate	1.2
DL-Homocysteate	11.6	N-Methyl-DL-aspartate	1.0
Kainate (1)	6.6	L-Glutamate	1.0
Quisqualate	6.4	L-Aspartate	0.6
Kainate-methyl ketone (3)	5.2	Dihydrokainate (2)	0.6
Allokainate-methyl ketone (4)	4.6	DL-α-Aminoadipate	0.2
Carboxy-kainate (5)	2.5	L-Proline	0.1
Carboxy-allokainate (6	2.3	L-Glutamate-γ-hydroxamate	0.1

TABLE II: Relative potency of structural analogues of glutamate on the specific $^{22}Na^+$ efflux rate from preloaded rat striatum slices. The order of potency was established by calculating, for each ligand, the inverse ratio between a concentration eliciting a response in the range between 20 and 70% of the maximal response and the concentration of L-glutamate eliciting the same response. All the compounds were tested at 2 concentrations, 0.1 mM and 1 mM. Values are means of triplicate determinations.

The following compounds were found to be devoid of agonist properties: DL-α-aminopimelate, LL-α,ε -diaminopimelic acid, L-α-aminosuberate, diethyl glutamate, DL-α-methylglutamate, glutarate, N-acetylkainate, GABA, γ-D-glutamylglycine and 2-amino-5-phosphonovalerate. The structures of compounds (1-6) are shown in table III.

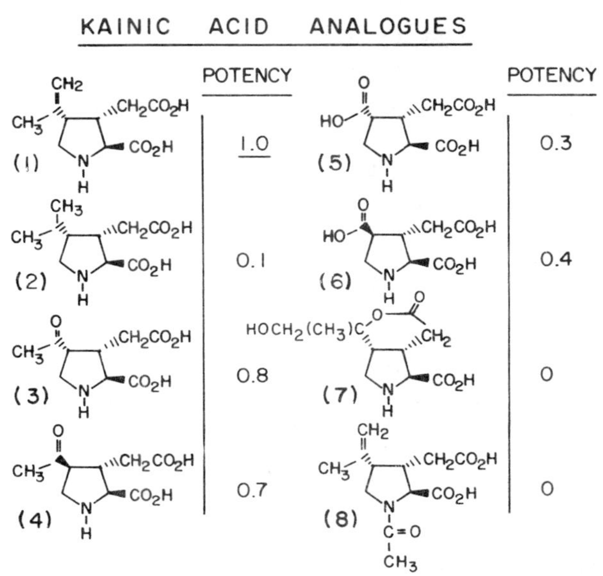

TABLE III: Structure of kainic acid analogues: their potency was tested as described in table II taking kainic acid as a reference.

agonist potency is compared to that of kainate. In agreement with the results of Johnston et al. (24), we find that dihydrokainate is much less potent than kainate. However, the potencies of the 3,4-cis-isomers of the methyl ketone-[(3)-table III] and carboxy-[(5)-table III] derivatives, are very similar to those of their respective 3,4-trans-isomers [(4) and (6)-table III]. This indicates, in distinction to an ealier suggestion (25), that the 3,4-cis-stereochemistry is not always essential for activity. Kainic acid-hydroxylactone [(7) in table III] and N-acetylkainic acid are devoid of agonist activity but the hydroxylactone derivative displays antagonist properties.

To further investigate the pharmacological properties of the excitatory amino acid receptors in the striatum, we have tested several compounds reported in the literature for their antagonism of amino acid-induced excitation in the frog or rat spinal cord. The structures of the antagonists used are presented in the paper of Davies et al. (22). Table IV summarizes the results. All agonists were tested at concentrations in the range between 20 and 70% of the maximal response. Clearly the most potent antagonist is 2-amino-5-phosphonovaleric acid (2APV) which at 50 μM, blocks significantly the response to 30 μM N-methyl-D-aspartic acid NMDA.

	Antagonist effect (% inhibition of agonist response)				
Agonist	DL-AA(3mM)	DL-AS(1mM)	γDGG(1mM)	2APV(1mM)	DEG(10mM)
NMDA(30μM)	93 ± 5 (76 ± 5)[a]	74 ± 7	95 ± 2 (72 ± 9)[b]	100 ± 1 (66 ± 11)[c]	9 ± 4
KA (100μM)	35 ± 4	7 ± 17	53 ± 14	0 ± 7	0 ± 5
QA (100μM)	30 ± 12	0 ± 15	0 ± 4	6 ± 3	0 ± 3
L-Glu(0.5mM)	22 ± 4	10 ± 18	29 ± 11	36 ± 3	33 ± 16
L-Asp(1mM)	17 ± 10	8 ± 10	40 ± 6	46 ± 7	23 ± 5

[a]1mM; [b]0.2 mM; [c]0.05 mM

TABLE IV: Antagonism of amino acid-stimulated $^{22}Na^{+}$ efflux rate from preloaded rat striatal slices. NMDA: N-methyl-D-aspartate, KA: kainate, QA: quisqualate, L-Glu: L-glutamate, L-Asp: L-aspartate, DL-AA: DL-aminoadipate, DL-AS: DL-aminosuberate, γDGG: γ-D-glutamylglycine, 2APV: 2-amino-5-phosphonovalerate, DEG: diethyl glutamate.

However a much higher concentration of this compound, (1 mM) is needed to partially block the response to L-glutamate (L-Glu) and L-aspartate (L-Asp). The responses to kainate (KA) and quisqualate (QA) remain unaffected at this 2APV concentration. These results as well as those obtained with γ-D-glutamylglycine are in complete agreement with the data presented by Davies et al. (22) which were obtained on a preparation of cat spinal cord. However, in contrast with these data, we find that diethyl glutamate, while affecting the response to L-Glu and L-Asp, does not inhibit the response to QA. The pattern of antagonism displayed by DL-aminosuberate (DL-AS) shows that this antagonist has a much higher affinity to the "NMDA-receptor" than to the other excitatory amino acid receptors. In contrast to DL-AS, DL-amino adipate (DL-AA), its shorter chain analogue, seems to display an equal affinity to all the receptors. We have also tested the properties of cis-2,3-piperidinedicarboxylic acid (PDA), a compound considered to display a non selective antagonism of amino acid-induced excitation (22). In the $^{22}Na^{+}$ efflux assay system, PDA was found to act as an agonist with a potency 20 fold lower than that of KA.

Based on the effects of selective antagonists on amino acid-induced excitation of cat spinal neurons the existence of three types of receptors has been inferred (22). These are classified as the NMDA, KA and QA receptors at which L-Glu, L-Asp and other agonists act to varying extents. Our results, however, cannot be accounted for by the sole involvement of these three receptors. The antagonist activity patterns displayed by 2APV and γDGG on the responses to L-Glu and QA cannot be rationalized without assuming the existence of distinct QA and L-Glu receptors. Also, the differences in the antagonism of the responses to NMDA and L-Asp suggest that these two agonists interact with distinct populations of receptors. Another indication of a heterogeneity of receptors is our finding that L-Glu increases the efflux rates of both $^{22}Na^{+}$ and $^{42}K^{+}$ whereas KA effects only the movements of Na^{+} ions. This leads to the conclusion that L-Glu and KA interact with differing receptor-ionophores complexes as already suggested by Hall et al.(26). Although our results indicate the existence of multiple receptors for excitatory amino acids, it is not yet clear whether these receptors indeed possess genuine functional or structural differences. The availability of a larger number of specific antagonists may be, at this stage, of great assistance. A further challenge is now to establish the identity of the natural excitatory ligands that interact with each class of amino acid receptors.

Acknowledgments: The authors thank Profs. I. Steinberg, R. Werman and S. Karlish for useful discussions. We are indebted to Prof. J.C. Watkins for sending us his manuscript before publication and for very generous gifts of glutamatergic anatagonists. A. Luini is on leave from the Istituto Mario Negri, Milan and is a recipient of an EMBO long-term postdoctoral fellowship. This research was supported by grants from the Délégation Générale à la Recherche Scientifique et Technique, the Israel Commission for Basic Research and the US.-Israel Binational Science Foundation.

REFERENCES

1. Curtis, D.R., Phillis, J.W. and Watkins, J.C. (1960). J. Physiol. 150, 656-682. The chemical excitation of spinal neurones by certain acidic amino acids.

2. Olney, J.W. (1969). J. Neuropath. Expl. Neurol. 28, 455-474. Glutamate-induced retinal degeneration in neonatal mice. Electron microscopy of the evolving lesion.

3. Watkins, J.C. (1978). in "Kainic Acid as a Tool in Neurobiology" (eds. McGeer, E.G., Olney, J.W. & Mc Geer, P.L.) 37-69 (Raven, New York).

4. Johnston, G.A.R. (1979). in "Glutamic acid: Advances in Biochemistry and Physiology" (eds. Filer, L.J. Jr., Garattini, G., Kare, M.R., Reynolds, W.A. & Wurtman, R.J.) 177-185 (Raven, New York).

5. Kasai, M. and Changeux, J.P. (1971). J. Memb. Biol. 6, 1-80. In vitro excitation of purified membrane fragments by cholinergic agonists. I. Pharmacological properties of the excitable membrane fragments II. The permeability change caused by cholinergic agonists III. Comparison of the dose response curves to decamethonium with the corresponding binding curves of decamethonium to the cholinergic receptor.

6. Catterall, W.A. (1975). J. Biol. Chem. 250, 1776-1781. Sodium Transport by the acetylcholine receptor of cultured muscle cells.

7. Ticku, M.K. and Olsen, R.W. (1977). Biochim. Biophys. Acta. 464, 519-529. γ-Aminobutyric acid-stimulated chloride permeability in crayfish muscle.

8. Bradford, H.F. and Mc Ilwain, H. (1966). J. Neurochem. 13, 1163-1177. Ionic basis for the depolarization of cerebral tissues by excitatory acidic amino acids.

9. Harvey, J.A. and Mc Ilwain, H. (1968). Biochem. J. 108, 269-274. Excitatory acidic amino acids and the cation content and sodium ion flux of isolated tissues from the brain.

10. Charnock, J.S., Cook, D.A. and Casey, R. (1971). Arch. Biochem. Biophys. 147, 323-329. The role of cations and other factors on the apparent energy of activation of (Na^+ + K^+) ATPase.

11. Goldman, D.E. (1943). J. Gen. Physiol. 27, 37-60. Potential, impedance and rectification in membranes.

12. Zieglgängsberger, W. and Puil, E.A. (1973). Expl. Brain Res. 17, 35-49. Actions of glutamic acid on spinal neurones.

13. Daniel, E.E. (1975). Methods in Pharmacology. 3, 699-721. Influx and efflux measurements.

14. Dostrovsky, J.O. and Pomeranz, B. (1977). Neurosciences Lett. 4, 315-319. Desensitization of glutamate responses; evidence for glutamate receptors in cat spinal cord.

15. Ransom, B.R., Bullock, P.N. and Nelson, P.G. (1977). J. Neurophysiol. 40, 1163-1177. Mouse spinal cord in cell culture III. Neuronal chemosensitivity and its relationship to synaptic activity.

16. Nicholson, C., Phillips, J.M. and Gardner-Medwin, A.R. (1979). Brain Res. 169, 580-584. Diffusion from an iontophoretic point source in the brain: role of tortuosity and volume fraction.

17. Curtis, D.R. and Watkins, J.C. (1965). Pharmacol. Rev. 17, 347-391. Pharmacology of amino acids related to aminobutyric acid (GABA).

18. Curtis, D.R. and Johnston, G.A.R. (1974). Ergebn Physiol (1974) 69, 97-188. Amino Acid transmitters in the Mannalian Central Nervous System.

19. Otsuka, M. and Konishi, S. (1977). in Substance P. (Euler, U.S. von and Pernow, B. editors) 207-214 (Raven

20. Konishi, S. and Otsuka, M. (1974). Brain Res. 65, 397-410. The effects of Substance P and other peptides on spinal neurons of the frog.

21. Otsuka, M., Konishi, S. and Takahashi, T. (1975). Fed. Proc. 34, 1922-1928. Hypothalamic Substance P as a candidate for transmitter of primary afferent neurons.

22. Davies, J. Evans, R.H., Francis, A.A., Jones, A.W. and Watkins, J.C. Excitatory amino acid receptors in the vertebrate central nervous system. (This book).

23. Davies, J. and Watkins, J.C. (1979). J. Physiol. 297, 621-635. Selective antagonism of amino acid induced and synaptic excitation in the cat spinal cord.

24. Johnston, G.A.R., Curtis, D.R., Davies, J. and Mc Cullock, R.M. (1974). Nature, 248, 804-805. Spinal interneurone excitation by conformationally restricted analogues of L-glutamic acid.

25. Biscoe, T.J., Davies, J., Dray, A., Evans, R.H., Francis, A.A., Martin, M.R. and Watkins, J.C. (1977). Europ. J. Pharmacol. 45, 315-316. Depression of synaptic excitation and of amino acid induced excitatory responses of spinal neurones by D- α-aminoadipate, α, ε-diaminopimelic acid and HA-966.

26. Hall, J.G., Hicks, T.P. and Mc Lennan, H. (1978). Neuroscience Lett. 8, 171-175. Kainic acid and the glutamate receptor.

Neurotransmitters and their Receptors
Edited by U.Z. Littauer, Y. Dudai, I. Silman,
V.I. Teichberg and Z. Vogel

Cerebellar Glutamate Receptors: Studies on their Stability, Susceptibility to Protein and Membrane-Modifying Agents, and Effects of Guanine Nucleotides

Najam A. Sharif and Peter J. Roberts

Department of Physiology and Pharmacology,
School of Biochemical and Physiological Sciences,
University of Southhampton, Southhampton, SO9 3TU, England

Abstract

Specific binding of L-^{3}H-glutamate to receptors on purified cerebellar membranes was substantially enhanced by sonication and pre-incubation of the membranes at 37°C, accompanied by extensive washings - the existence of an endogenous inhibitor or inhibitors is postulated. While binding was not maintained in frozen membranes, even in the presence of cryoprotectants, lyophilisation both preserved and enhanced binding properties. Protein modifying agents and lipid perturbants influenced specific binding. In contrast to adenine-based nucleotides, the guanine derivatives markedly reduced ^{3}H-glutamate binding - the possible modulatory role of these agents is discussed.

The specific binding of L-^{3}H-glutamate to a single population of high affinity sites on sonicated, highly-washed cerebellar synaptic membranes (K_d = 449 nM, B_{max} = 50.2 pmol/mg protein) has recently been reported (1). One of the major problems encountered in this study was the finding that approximately 80 per cent of the binding was lost following freezing of the synaptic membranes. Our primary objective in this study was to optimize conditions for the preservation of binding activity, and then to investigate the influence of a number of membrane-modifying agents on ^{3}H-glutamate binding.

Purified cerebellar synaptic membranes were prepared as described by Sharif and Roberts (2), after which they were either frozen (-30°C or -170°C), lyophilised, or used freshly-prepared, for the binding assay. Briefly, 0.5 ml membrane suspension (0.1 - 0.5 mg protein) were incubated for 10 min at 37°C with L-^{3}H-glutamate (25 nM), in the absence or presence of 1 mM unlabelled glutamate. The assay was terminated by rapid centrifugation, and the bound radioactivity determined by liquid scintillation counting. Calculation of specific binding was by subtraction from the total binding of that component which persisted in the presence of 1 mM glutamate.

Membranes were usually subjected to mild sonication during preparation, with a Kerry bath sonicator. Specific binding was increased with the duration of this process, and was enhanced approx. 30-fold after 180s. Pre-incubation at 37°C for 30 min, followed by extensive washings, always enhanced specific binding by over 50 per cent. Re-addition of post-incubation supernatant to control membranes resulted in a 70 per cent decrease in binding, implicating the presence of endogenous inhibitor(s). The striatum and cerebral cortex appear to have the highest concentrations of these endogenous substances.

Storage of membranes as suspensions or pellets, failed to maintain glutamate binding sites, and even addition of cryoprotectants did not confer stability. Lyophilisation of freshly prepared, osmotically-lysed membranes, not only preserved binding characteristics, but effected a pronounced enhancement. These membranes exhibited an approx. 300 per cent greater binding activity which was stable for up to six weeks. Kinetic analysis revealed that the enhancement following lyophilisation was almost entirely attributable to an increased number of binding sites (B_{max} increased from 117 $\pm$ 17 to 277 $\pm$ 48 pmol/mg protein), since the K_d was unchanged at approx. 300 nM. Pharmacological studies have shown that the specificity of the binding site in lyophilised membranes correlates well with that seen in the freshly prepared tissue. However, the majority of the glutamate receptor ligands exhibited an increased potency following membrane lyophilisation. We therefore postulate that the lyophilisation process may: (a) unmask receptors, thus effecting the increase in B_{max}, (b) lock receptors into an active conformation, (c) remove endogenous inhibitory agents that may normally modulate the availability and affinity of the binding sites, such as has been demonstrated for the GABA receptor (3,4).

The effects of a number of likely receptor-modifying agents were investigated using freshly-prepared membranes. These were incubated for 30 min with the test reagent, after which time, membranes were extensively washed and the standard ^{3}H-glutamate binding assay carried out. Tryptic digestion (20 μg/ml) and phospholipase A (20 μg/ml), both produced a 25 per cent decrease in binding; phospholipases C and D were inactive. The polyene antibiotics, amphotericin B and nystatin (200 μg/ml), which act as lipid perturbants, and extraction with acetone/water (50%) or Triton X-100, similarly produced marked reductions in specific glutamate binding. Reduction of disulphide bonds by dithiothreitol (DTT) (3 mM) inhibited binding, while N-ethylmaleimide (N-EM) (3-9 mM) produced approx. 100-150 per cent increase. Pre-incubation of membranes with DTT followed immediately by N-EM resulted in reversal of the effects of DTT with no overall change in binding being observed, thus indicating a common locus of action. Oxidation by 5,5'-dithiobis (2-nitrobenzoic acid) (DTNB) (10-25 mM) caused 20-60 per cent inhibition of binding. Since combined DTT and DTNB treatment resulted in a net 30 per cent increase in binding, we deduce that these randomly regenerated disulphide bridges cannot be identical with the original ones present. Alkylation of thiol groups by iodoacetamide (10-25 mM) produced a 25-50 per cent decrease in binding. The water-soluble carbodiimide derivative, 1-ethyl-3 (3-dimethylaminopropyl) carbodiimide (20 mM) which selectively interferes with carboxyl groups, increased binding by about 200 per cent.

In view of the finding that guanine nucleotides may regulate the sensitivity of a number of receptor systems, we have investigated the ability of various nucleotides to influence specific ^{3}H-glutamate binding, by their inclusion in the incubation medium during the assay. At a final concentration of 1 mM, the adenine-based nucleotides exhibited a small inhibitory effect. In contrast, the guanine derivatives produced approximately 70 per cent inhibition (5). Although these results yield no information on the mechanism of action of the guanyl nucleotides, it is probable that they alter the affinity of the receptor directly or indirectly , for its ligand. Since sonication may be producing everted, cleaved synaptic vesicles, we can speculate that the nucleotides may be interacting with an intracellularly localized guanylate cyclase effecting an allosteric modulation of ^{3}H-glutamate binding by negative co-operativity, thus producing negative feedback on the system. Alternatively, the purine binding site may be closely associated with the glutamate receptor protein. Experiments to delineate these possible mechanisms are currently in progress. It is, however, of some interest that the activation of guanylate cyclase by glutamate (6,7) may be involved in the synaptic actions of glutamate.

References

1. Foster, A.C. & Roberts, P.J. (1978) J. Neurochem. 31, 1466-1477.

2. Sharif, N.A. & Roberts, P.J. (1980) J. Neurochem. (In press).

3. Toffano, G., Guidotti, A. & Costa, E. (1978) Proc. Natl. Acad. Sci. U.S.A. 75, 4024-4028.

4. Greenlee, D.V., Van Ness, P.C. & Olsen, R.W. (1978) Life Sci. 22, 1653-1672.

5. Sharif, N.A. & Roberts, P.J. (1980) Eur. J. Pharmacol. 61, 213-214.

6. Garthwaite, J. & Balázs, R. (1978) Nature, Lond. 275, 328-329.

7. Foster, G.A. & Roberts, P.J. (1980) Br. J. Pharmacol. (In press).

Neurotransmitters and their Receptors
Edited by U.Z. Littauer, Y. Dudai, I. Silman,
V.I. Teichberg and Z. Vogel

Specific [^{3}H] Kainic Acid Binding in the Vertebrate CNS

H. Henke and M. Cuénod

Zurich, Switzerland

Specific [^{3}H]kainic acid binding was determined in various CNS regions of representatives of the different vertebrate classes in order to see whether there are regions with a high number of binding sites of the same types as those found in the rat CNS which have been linked to the neurotoxic effects of kainic acid. High binding values were measured in certain nonmammalian brain regions, e.g. the pigeon and trout cerebellum but kinetic and pharmacological studies indicated that the binding in these area is of a different type than that in the mammalian CNS. In the mammalian species examined, the kainic acid binding was stereospecific and L-glutamate had a high affinity for the binding sites. Three types of binding sites could be distinguished according to their app. affinity (K_d). In the telencephalic regions, a 'high' and a 'low' affinity site with K_d values of 1-4 and >20 nM were determined. In the cerebellum the affinity was between 10 to 20 nM. The binding was highest in the cortex, neostriatum and cerebellum and low in the brain stem and spinal cord. In the n. caudatus obtained postmortem from Huntington's disease (HD) patients the number of binding sites was reduced to a similar extend as in the rat neostriatum after kainate injections which further supports the validity of this animal HD model. Specific binding was not reduced in the cerebellum of Purkinje cell deficient mice mutants (pcd) when compared to control littermates. This may indicate a difference in the mode of kainic acid action between telencephalic regions and the cerebellum.

Specific kainic acid binding has first been described in the rat CNS (44). The binding sites are likely to be involved in the neurophysiological and neurotoxic effects of kainic acid. The neurotoxicity of kainic acid has become a widely used tool in neurobiology for it appears that kainic acid injections into the CNS cause destruction of neurons with their cell bodies in the injected area while afferent nerve terminals and fibres of passage are spared (32). Moreover, kainate injections into specific brain loci can induce changes similar to those observed in certain neurodegenerative disorders.

Best documented are the effects of kainate injections into the rat neostriatum which resemble the chemopathological, histological and possibly behavioral changes found in pati-

ents afflicted with Huntington's disease (8,14,27).
The experimental findings which indicate that the kainate toxicity is mediated by the kainic acid binding sites are: (i) parallel development of kainic acid toxicity and specific binding in young rat (7), (ii) correlation of toxic potency and amount of binding sites in the rat CNS (40) and chick retina (5) and (iii) simultaneous loss of toxicity (39) and affinity for the binding sites (9) after chemical modifications of the kainic acid molecule.
The striking specificity of kainate toxicity and the existence of specific, high affinity binding sites, which mediate this toxicty, rise the question whether kainic acid makes use of a physiological receptor. It was originally proposed that kainic acid acts as glutamate agonist at the glutamate binding site of the iontophoretically defined glutamate receptor (35, 36). However, present data strongly suggest that the binding sites for kainic acid and glutamate are separate although there is a functional interaction between the two substances in some cases (4,15,19,31,43,47).
Knowledge of the detailed mechanism of kainic acid action seems necessary to study the possibility of a physiological mechanism underlying the effects of kainic acid. Little is known at present about the mode of kainate action. The toxicity is intimately linked to the neuroexcitatory potency since subtle structural modifications of the kainic acid molecule which result in a loss of the excitatory action also abolish the neurotoxicity (42,49) and the affinity to the binding sites (9,17). The ability of certain narcotics to diminish the toxicity of kainic acid may be related to this excitatory action (52). In some regions, the toxicity depends on an excitatory input (4,26,31,47); there is some evidence that glutamate plays a special role in these afferents (10,13,16,25,30,37,45,46). Models of the neurotoxic mechanism have been proposed assuming an interaction between glutamatergic neurons and kainic acid (9,19,33,41). The strong effects of kainic acid on the flux of ions and water

as well as on the cellular ATP levels has led to the suggestion that depletion of the cellular energy stores is a reason for the cell destruction (3).

Presumably, further studies on the mechanism of kainic acid action are best undertaken in a brain region with a high amount of specific kainic acid binding sites. Using a constant concentration of ligand, we found that the amount of specifically bound tritiated kainic acid varies markedly between various CNS regions of representatives of the different vertebrate classes (table 1).

While the binding values in the mammals examined ranged from 10 to 550 fmol/mg protein, they were in general much higher in the nonmammalian species studied. Especially high binding values were found in the bird and the trout cerebellum and in the frog telencephalon. Another difference between mammals and nonmammals was that in the first the highest amounts of binding were usually measured in the cortex, neostriatum and cerebellum while the nonmammals showed the maximal values in the cerebellum and spinal cord.

After having established the presence of regions with a high amount of binding, the kinetic and pharmacological properties of the binding were measured in two such area, the pigeon and the trout cerebellum. The determination of these parameters was necessary since they should be similar to those of the rat binding sites which have been linked to kainate toxicity. In addition, these characteristics were determined too in several regions of the mammalian CNS and in the pigeon optic lobe where kainic acid toxicity is comparable to that in the rat CNS (10,47).

In the mammalian CNS, three types of binding sites could be distinguished according to their apparent affinity constant (K_d). The results are summarized in table 2. In the telencephalic regions a 'high' and a 'low' affinity type of binding site were present with K_d values of 1 to 4 nM and >20 nM respectively. These affinities correspond closely to those reported in the rat forebrain (29) and chick retina (5). In other brain regions, various groups have described specific

TABLE 1 SPECIFIC [^{3}H]KAINIC ACID BINDING AT 50 nM CONCENTRATION TO WASHED CRUDE MEMBRANE PREPARATIONS FROM DIFFERENT CNS REGIONS OF VARIOUS VERTEBRATES

SPECIES	CORTEX or TELENCEPHALON	NEOSTRIATUM	SUP. COLLICULUS or OPTIC LOBE	PONS + MEDULLA OBLONGATA	CEREBELLUM	SPINAL CORD
MEN (3)	154±29 (16)	145±7 (8)	56±14 (4)	24±7 (4)	155±33 (10)	10±6 (4)
CAT (2)	187±39 (8)	180±31 (8)	94±33 (7)	27±14 (6)	295±22 (8)	105±14 (8)
CALF (1)	398±47 (8)	210±45 (8)	73±21 (8)	n.d.	192±11 (8)	8±6 (8)
PIG (1)	204±14 (8)	270±51 (8)	43±26 (10)	n.d.	274±19 (8)	13±7 (8)
RAT (12)	256±62 (10)	405±37 (18)	188±39 (33)	125±44 (9)	225±41 (8)	101±18 (8)
MOUSE (6)	336±71 (6)	368±48 (8)	140±44 (6)	43±21 (6)	259±35 (6)	33±17 (8)
GUINEA PIG (3)	295±47 (8)	215±23 (6)	n.d.	68±9 (8)	238±51 (8)	32±17 (8)
HAMSTER (4)	554±101 (8)	n.d.	n.d.	228±25 (8)	484±89 (8)	109±24 (8)
PIGEON (62)	237±41 (23)		153±29 (105)	152±36 (10)	13134±1347 (62)	42±57 (9)
HEN (3)	375±52 (12)		1568±436 (9)	1412±92 (9)	14946±1943 (12)	3118±928 (12)
TURTLE (6)	978±86 (8)		654±105 (8)	1009±125 (8)	1555±102 (8)	3728±180 (9)
FROG (6)	51013±1100 (8)		3104±1403 (8)	2680±472 (6)	10367±2040 (2)	6782±90 (12)
TROUT (8)	686±108 (8)		18849±1310 (12)	6787±987 (11)	41980±2014 (12)	10194±1103 (12)

Frozen tissue was used for all membrane preparations. The values are given in fmol/mg prot. The number in parenthesis after the species name indicates the number of individual samples used. Data are the mean ± S.D. of (n) determinations done in quadruplet. n.d. = not determined. Specific binding is defined as the difference of binding in the presence of tritiated kainic acid alone minus the binding in presence of 0.1 mM unlabelled kainic acid. The species used were: rat: SIVZ; mouse: ICRZ; guinea pig: MZZ; hamster: LAKZ; pigeon: Columba livia; turtle: Pseudemys scripta elegans; frog: Rana esculenta; trout: Salmo lacustris.

TABLE 2 KINETIC CONSTANTS OF SPECIFIC [^{3}H]KAINIC ACID BINDING IN DIFFERENT CNS REGIONS OF VARIOUS VERTEBRATES

SPECIES	n	REGION	K_d (nM)	B_{max} (fmol/mg protein)	HILL COEFFICIENT
MEN	3	CORTEX	1.5 ± 0.4 / 20.2 ± 4.1	66 ± 13 / 103 ± 11	1.0 / 1.2
	3	N. CAUDATUS	1.9 ± 0.4 / 23.1 ± 1.8	61 ± 7 / 118 ± 4	0.9 / 1.2
	3	CEREBELLUM	16.2 ± 3.5	91 ± 17	1.1
RAT	3	CORTEX	2.7 ± 1.3 / 28.6 ± 7.2	83 ± 14 / 250 ± 24	1.0 / 1.0
	3	NEOSTRIATUM	1.4 ± 0.8 / 25.1 ± 3.8	132 ± 21 / 405 ± 33	0.9 / 1.2
	3	CEREBELLUM	17.7 ± 4.0	296 ± 37	0.9
GUINEA PIG	3	CORTEX	3.3 ± 0.7 / 24.6 ± 4.0	143 ± 21 / 200 ± 16	1.0 / 0.9
	3	NEOSTRIATUM	1.9 ± 1.1 / 27.2 ± 3.3	95 ± 13 / 182 ± 17	1.0 / 1.1
	3	CEREBELLUM	13.8 ± 4.7	242 ± 46	0.9
PIGEON	4	TELENCEPHALON	28.3 ± 4.2	341 ± 18	1.1
	7	OPTIC LOBE	30.0 ± 18.0	230 ± 58	1.0
	12	CEREBELLUM	30.0[a] / 330 ± 29	2600 ± 655 / 106000 ± 17000	1.0[a] / 2.2
TROUT	2	CEREBELLUM	50.0 ± 7.6	112000 ± 26000	1.1

[a] This value was set identical to the value found in the pigeon optic lobe and used for calculation.

Frozen tissue was used for all membrane preparations. The values are the mean ± S.E.M. of (n) separate determinations. All points were determined in quadruplets, the [^{3}H]kainic acid concentration was varied between 1 to 100 nM, higher concentrations were obtained by appropriate dilutions with unlabelled kainic acid. Specific binding as defined in legend figure 1.

kainic acid binding showing only one type of binding site with varying affinity (2,9,40,44,50). This discrepancy may in part be due to methodological differences. We have previously reported a K_d value of approx. 6 nM in the human caudate nucleus (18). However, using an extended range of ligand concentration, it became evident that the experimental data are best approximated by assuming two binding sites with a K_d value of 2 nM and 23 nM respectively (see figure 2). In the cerebellum, intermediate K_d values were measured, they ranged between 10 and 20 nM. The ratio between the different types of binding sites was constant in a given region but depended on the region and the species examined. This suggests that the differences in the binding affinities are more likely due to separate binding sites than to a single binding site of varying affinity. Also, the displacement curves in mammals were never bell shaped as in the pigeon cerebellum (see below) as this would be expected in the case of cooperative binding sites (1). In all regions studied, the kainic acid was bound stereospecifically as indicated by the relatively low affinity of L-α-allokainic acid, a stereoisomer of kainic acid (table 3). L-glutamate but not D-glutamate had a high affinity for the binding sites; this has also been found in the rat CNS and has been interpreted as an indication that the kainic acid binding site is not identical with the iontophoretically defined receptor glutamate binding site (17, 29) since there, L- and D-glutamate are of comparable excitatory potency (6,11). Numerous other substances, including neurotransmitters, transmitter agonists and antagonist as well as glutamate derivatives, had only little affinity for the binding sites (table 3). The displacement data show a high degree of specificity of the binding sites. The relatively high affinity of L-glutamate, which is well within the physiological range, opens the possibility that glutamate is a natural ligand of the kainic acid binding sites. In this case, glutamate may modulate the excitability of neuronal membranes carrying kainic acid bind-

TABLE 3 DISPLACEMENT POTENCY (IC_{50}) OF VARIOUS SUBSTANCES IN SOME REGIONS OF DIFFERENT VERTEBRATES

SUBSTANCE	MEN[a]		RAT[a]		PIGEON[a]	TROUT[a]
	N. CAUDATUS	CEREBELLUM	STRIATUM	CEREBELLUM	O. LOBE	CEREBELLUM
L-α-KAINIC ACID	0.026	0.031	0.035	0.029	0.006	0.087
L-GLUTAMATE	0.360	0.560	0.500	0.445	0.210	95.
L-α-ALLOKAINIC ACID	0.560	0.810	0.475	0.740	0.600	0.650
IBOTENIC ACID	100.	n.d.	45.	n.d.	10.	n.d.
L-GLUTAMIC ACID γ-MONOETHYL ESTER	120.	n.d.	n.d.	n.d.	40.	n.d.
L-GLUTAMIC ACID γ-MONOMETHYL ESTER	65.	n.d.	110.	n.d.	45.	n.d.
L-GLUTAMIC ACID γ-BENZYL ESTER	130.	95.	160.	180.	52.	n.d.
DL-α-AMINOADIPATE	560.	720.	130.	455.	140.	n.d.
L-GLUTAMIC ACID-DI-T-BUTYL ESTER HCl	n.d.	n.d.	n.d.	n.d.	140.	n.d.
D-GLUTAMATE	180.	240.	90.	330.	150.	200.
D-GLUTAMATE DIMETHYL ESTER	135.	n.d.	n.d.	n.d.	760.	n.d.
D-GLUTAMATE DIETHYL ESTER	140.	235.	250.	290.	900.	10^3

[a] Less than 10% inhibition of the binding was found at 1 mM concentration for: D-aspartate, L-aspartate, bicuculline, GABA, glycine, L-nuciferine, L-proline, strychnine.

Crude membrane preparations obtained from frozen tissue were used for the assay. The values are given in μM and indicate the concentration of substance at which 50% of the binding was inhibited. The [^{3}H]kainic acid concentration was 50 nM. For each determination at least 4 concentrations of displacer in the range of its IC_{50} value were used. The IC_{50} values were calculated from log-probit plots (28). Specific binding as defined in legend table 1, n.d. = not determined.

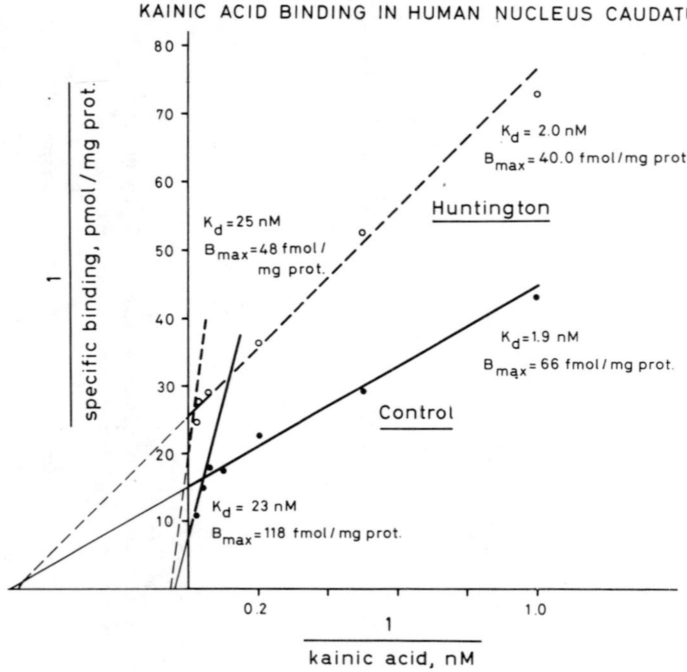

FIGURE 1 Displacement of bound [^{3}H]kainic acid (10 nM) by unlabelled kainic acid from pigeon cerebellar crude membrane preparations. Specific binding was determined as defined in legend table 1. The data were analysed using the formula:

$$y = B_1 \frac{(x+1)^{n_1-1}}{(K_1/d)^{n_1} + (x+1)^{n_1}} + B_2 \frac{(x+1)^{n_2-1}}{(K_2/d)^{n_2} + (x+1)^{n_2}}$$

x = unlabelled/labelled ligand concentration

y = specific binding

d = concentration of radioactive ligand

B_1, B_2 = maximal binding (B_{max}), system I,II

K_1, K_2 = apparent affinity constant (K_d), system I,II

n_1, n_2 = Hill coefficient, system I,II

r = standard error

Using only one type of cooperative binding site for approximation, the error was r = 4.7. Each point represents the mean of four determinations.

ing sites. Taken together, the similarity of kinetic and pharmacological properties between the binding sites found in the different mammalian species examined suggests that the same types of binding sites are present in all mammals. In the nonmammalian species at least the 'low' affinity type of binding site may be present too as the results in the pigeon optic lobe indicate. Here, the kinetic and pharmacological characteristics of the binding were very similar to those of the mammalian 'low' affinity system (see tables 2 and 3). Different types of binding sites seem to be present, however, in the trout and pigeon cerebellum. In the trout cerebellum, the K_d value was higher than in the mammalian cerebellum and in addition, both L- and D-glutamate exhibited only a low affinity for the binding site (tables 2 and 3). In the pigeon cerebellum, displacement curves were bell shaped, a sign for the presence of cooperative binding sites (1,12). A first evaluation of the data, assuming only one type of cooperative binding site, did not give a good correlation to the experimental data. Therefore, the results were reanalysed assuming two types of binding sites, a cooperative one and one with the same affinity as that found in the pigeon optic lobe. This approximation gave a good fit to the experimental data (figure 1). It is thus concluded that most of the kainic acid binding in the pigeon cerebellum is due to a cooperative binding site with a K_d value of approx. 330 nM. The pharmacological properties of this binding site were similar to those of the mammalian binding sites, except that the IC_{50} values were increased by a factor of 500 to 1000. Displacement curves with L-glutamate were comparable to those with kainic acid but the IC_{50} value was approx. 200 μM. Subcellular distribution studies showed that the binding is concentrated in the crude synaptosomal membrane fraction as it is in the rat CNS (44).

Thus, the pigeon cerebellum contains two types of binding sites for kainic acid. One is likely identical to that pre-

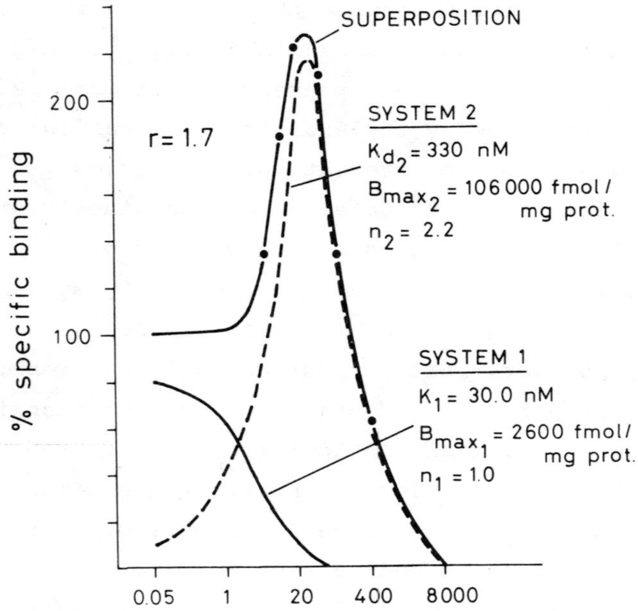

FIGURE 2 Double reciprocal plot of specific [^{3}H]kainic acid binding to crude membrane preparations obtained postmortem (8-14 h) from patients afflicted with Huntington's disease. Controls were from patients with no neurodegenerative disorder. The points are the mean of four experiments using samples from three (Huntington) or four (controls) individuals. Specific binding as defined in legend table 1.

sent in the pigeon optic lobe while the other type has not been observed in any other region examined. It shows, compared to the mammalian cerebellum, a low affinity constant and exhibits cooperative binding. In the rat CNS, there is a rough correlation between the number of binding sites and the toxic potency of kainic acid (7,40). If this correlation is also valid in the pigeon cerebellum, then a very high toxicity of kainic acid should be expected in the pigeon cerebellum. However, the toxic effect of kainate in the pigeon cerebellum is comparable to that in the rat cerebellum (48). This is consistent with the hypothesis that the toxicity in the pigeon cerebellum is mediated by the same type of binding site as found in the pigeon optic lobe and that the cooperative type of binding site is not involved in the toxicity. Nevertheless, it cannot be excluded that the two binding sites share common mechanistic properties and it is of interest to further study the cooperative type of binding site, especially since recent results have indicated that this binding site is exclusively localized in the molecular layer of the pigeon cerebellum (20).

It can thus be concluded that, although kainic acid binding is very high in the trout and the pigeon cerebellum, these regions cannot be used as model to study the toxic effects of kainic acid action because the high binding values are due to different types of binding sites.

In mammals, our data suggest, three different types of binding sites may be present. Their relative significance for the toxic effects of kainic acid remains to be established. The finding that only a 'low' affinity type of binding site is present in the pigeon optic lobe, where kainic acid toxicity is comparable to that in the rat telencephalon, may be taken as evidence that this type is more important for the toxicity than the 'high' affinity type. However, after kainic acid injections into the rat neostriatum, the number of both 'high' and 'low' affinity binding sites is reduced although the 'low' affinity type is slightly more affected (29). It is of interest that a comparable reduction in the number of the two binding sites could be demonstrated in the nucleus caudatus obtained postmortem from patients affected with Huntington's disease (figure 2). This further supports the hypothesis that kainate injections into the rat neostriatum provide a valuable animal model for Huntington's disease and indicates that the binding sites in the human telencephalic regions are of the same type as those observed in the other mammals.

Comparing the effects of kainic acid in the rat neostriatum and cerebellum certain peculiar similarities can be noted. In the neostriatum, the toxicity depends on the cortico-striatal input (14,31). There is evidence that glutamate may be used as neurotransmitter in this pathway (13,25,30,37,45). This agrees with the assumption that glutamate-receptive neurons are especially vulnerable to kainic acid. In the rat (23) and pigeon (48) cerebellum, the Purkinje cells are most sensitive to kainic acid. These cell receive an excitatory input from the parallel fibres for which there is also evidence that they use glutamate as transmitter (24,38,51). Although the K_d values in the neostriatum and the cerebellum of the rat are slightly different, it is tempting to assume that the mechanism of kainate toxicity is the same in both regions. As recent results from our laboratory indicate, this may however not be the case. In the rat neostriatum, the kainic acid binding sites are not affected by degeneration of the cortico-striatal pathway (17) but they are reduced after kainic acid lesion (29). The simplest explanation for these findings is that the binding sites are localized on those neurons which receive the excitatory cortical input (19). In analogy, it may be expected that the binding sites in the cerebellum are concentrated on the Purkinje cell membranes. In mice, there exists a cerebellar mutation (pcd) where the Purkinje cells are selectively missing at a certain stage of development (34). One may therefore expect a reduction in binding sites in the cerebellum of pcd mice mutants if the binding sites are localized on the Purkinje cell membrane. Yet, the binding in the cerebellum of pcd mutants was not different from that measured in control littermates (figure 3)(21).

Thus, in mammals, the mechanism of kainate toxicity in the telencephalic regions may be different from that in the cerebellum if not a species difference between the rodents rat and mice is assumed.

In summary, our studies on the kainic acid binding in the CNS of different vertebrates have shown that the binding varies markedly between the regions and species examined. Although very high binding values have been found in certain nonmammal brain area, the differences between the kinetic and pharmacological properties of the binding in these regions and the binding in the rat CNS indicate that these regions are not suitable for the study of the mechanism of kainic acid action. Within the mammals, the kinetic and pharmacological cha-

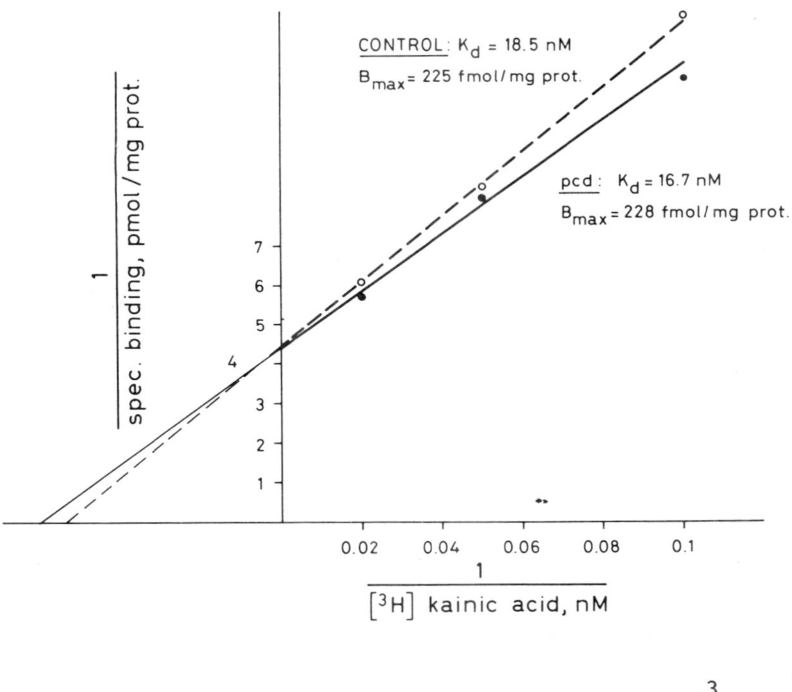

FIGURE 3 Double reciprocal plot of specific [^{3}H]kainic acid binding to cerebellar crude membrane preparations from pcd mice mutants (40-56 days old) and control littermates. Each point represents the mean of three separate experiments. Specific binding as defined in legend table 1.

racteristics are more uniform but there are differences between the brain regions too. Therefore, the mode of kainate action should best be studied in the telencephalic regions and the cerebellum separately, the mammalian species used for investigation, however, does not seem to be critical. An important finding is that the binding sites in the human CNS are likely identical to those in the other mammalian orders.

Acknowledgements: The authors thank R. Grieder, J. Gubler and M. Stella for excellent technical assistance.
This work was supported by Grants 3.506.79 and 3.505.79 from the Swiss National Science Foundation, the Dr. Eric Slack-Gyr-Foundation and the Emil Barell-Foundation.

LITERATURE

1 Akera, T. and Cheng, V.J.K., A simple method for the determination of affinity and binding site concentration in receptor binding studies, Biochem. Biophys. Acta, 470 (1977) 412-423.

2 Beaumont, K., Maurin, Y., Reisine, T.D., Fields, J.Z. Spokes, E., Bird, E.D. and Yamamura H.I., Huntington's disease and its animal model: Alterations in kainic acid binding, Life Sci., 24 (1979) 809-816.

3 Biziere, K. and Coyle, J.T., Effects of kainic acid on ion distribution and ATP levels of striatal slices incubated in vitro, J. Neurochem., 31 (1978) 513-520.

4 Biziere, K. and Coyle, J.T., Influence of corticostriatal afferents on striatal kainic acid neurotoxicity, Neurosci. Lett., 8 (1978) 303-310.

5 Biziere, K. and Coyle, J.T., Localization of receptors for kainic acid on neurons in the innernuclear layer of retina, Neuropharmacol., 18 (1979) 409-413.

6 Buu, N.T., Puil, E. and Van Gelder, N.M., Receptors for amino acids in excitable tissues, Gen. Pharmacol., 7 (1976) 5-14.

7 Campochiaro, P. and Coyle, J.T., Ontogenetic development of kainate neurotoxicity: Correlates with glutamatergic innervation, Proc. Nat. Acad. Sci. USA, 75 (1978) 2025-2029.

8 Coyle, J.T., McGeer, E.G., McGeer, P.L. and Schwarcz, R., Neostriatal injections: A Model for Huntington's Chorea. In E.G. McGeer, J.W. Olney and P.L. McGeer, (Eds.), Kainic Acid as a Tool in Neurobiology, Raven Press, N.Y., 1978, pp. 139-159.

9 Coyle, J.T., London, E.D., Biziere, K. and Zaczek, R., Kainic Acid Neurotoxicity: Insights into the Pathophysiology of Huntington's disease. In T.N. Chase, N.S. Wexler and A. Barbeau, (Eds.), Huntington's disease, Adv. in Neurology, 23, Raven Press, N.Y., 1979, pp. 593-608.

10 Cuénod, M. and Henke, H., Neurotransmitters in the avian visual system. In F. Fonnum, (Ed.), Amino Acids as Chemical Transmitters, Plenum Press, N.Y., 1978, pp. 221-239.

11 Curtis, D.R. and Watkins, J.C., The excitation and depression of spinal neurones by structurally related amino acids, J. Neurochem., 6 (1960) 117-141.

12 Davis, M.E., Akera, T., Brody, T.M. and Watson, L., Opiate receptor: Cooperativity of binding observed in brain slices, Proc. nat. Acad. Sci. USA, 74 (1977) 5764-5766.

13 Divac, I., Fonnum, F. and Storm-Mathisen, J. High affinity uptake of glutamate in terminals of corticostriatal axons, Nature (Lond.), 266 (1977) 377-378.

14 Fibiger, H.C., Kainic Acid Lesions of the Striatum: A Pharmcological and Behavioral Model of Huntington's Disease. In E.G. McGeer, J.W. Olney and P.L. McGeer, (Eds.), Kainic Acid as a Tool in Neurobiology, Raven Press, N.Y., 1978, pp. 161-176.

15 Hall, J.G., Hicks, T.P. and McLennan, H., Kainic acid and the glutamate receptor, Neurosci. Lett, 8 (1978) 171-175.

16 Henke, H., Schenker, T.M. and Cuénod, M., Effects of retinal ablation on uptake of glutamate, glycine, GABA, proline and choline in pigeon tectum, J. Neurochem., 26 (1976) 131-134.

17 Henke, H. and Cuénod, M., L-glutamate specific [^{3}H] kainic acid binding in the rat neostriatum after degeneration of the corticostriatal pathway, Neurosci. Lett., 11 (1979) 341-345.

18 Henke, H., Kainic acid binding in the human caudate nucleus: Effect of Huntington's disease, Neurosci. Lett., 14 (1979) 247-251.

19 Henke, H., Streit, P., Reubi, J.C. and Cuénod, M., Kainic acid toxicity and binding in the optic tectum. In M. Cuénod, G. Kreutzberg and F. Bloom, (Eds.), Development and Chemical Specificity of Neurons, Prog. in Brain Res., 51, Elsevier/North-Holland, Amsterdam, 1979, pp.497-503.

20 Henke, H. and Beaudet, A., in preparation.

21 Henke, H. and Changeux, J.P., in preparation.

22 Henke, H., unpublished results.

23 Herndon, R.M. and Coyle, J.T., Glutamatergic Innervation, Kainic Acid, and Selective Vulnerability in the Cerebellum. In E.G. McGeer, J.W. Olney and P.L. McGeer, (Eds.), Kainic Acid as a Tool in Neurobiology, Raven Press, N.Y., 1978, pp. 189-199.

24 Hudson, D.B., Valcana, T., Bean, G. and Timiras, P.S., Glutamic acid: A strong candidate as the neurotransmitter of the cerebellar granule cell, Neurochem. Res., 1 (1976) 73-81.

25 Kim, J.-S., Hassler, R., Haug, P. and Paik, K.-S., Effect of frontal cortex ablation on striatal glutamic acid level in rat, Brain Res., 132 (1977) 370-374.

26 Köhler, Ch., Schwarcz, R. and Fuxe, K., Perforant pathway transections protect hippocampal granule cells from kainate lesion, Neurosci. Lett., 10 (1978) 241-246.

27 Krammer, E.B., Lischka, M.F., Karobath, M. and Schönbeck, G., Is there a selectivity of neuronal degeneration induced by intrastriatal injection of kainic acid? Brain Res., 177 (1979) 577-582.

28 Litchfield, J.T. and Wilcoxon, F., A simplified method of evaluating dose-effec experiments, J. Pharmacol. exp. Ther., 96 (1949) 99-113.

29 London, E.D. and Coyle, J.T., Specific binding of [^{3}H]kainic acid to receptor sites in rat brain, Molec. Pharmacol., 15 (1979) 492-505.

30 McGeer, P.L., McGeer, E.G., Scherer, U. and Singh, K., A glutamatergic corticostriatal pathway? Brain Res., 128 (1977) 369-373.

31 McGeer, E.G., McGeer, P.L. and Singh, K., Kainate-induced degeneration of neostriatal neurons: dependency upon cortico-striatal tract, <u>Brain Res.</u>, 139 (1978) 381-383.

32 McGeer, P.L., McGeer, E.G. and Hattori, T., Kainic Acid as a Tool in Neurobiology. In E.G. McGeer, J.W. Olney and P.L. McGeer, (Eds.), <u>Kainic Acid as a Tool in Neurobiology</u>, Raven Press, N.Y., 1978, pp. 123-138.

33 McGeer, E.G., McGeer, P.L., Hattori, T. and Vincent, S.R., Kainic acid Neurotoxicity and Huntington's disease. In T.N. Chase, N.S. Wexler and A. Barbeau, (Eds.), <u>Huntington's disease</u>, <u>Adv. in Neurology</u>, 23, Raven Press, N.Y., 1979 pp. 577-591.

34 Mullen, R.J., Eicher, E.M. and Sidman, R.L., Purkinje cell degeneration, a new neurological mutation in the mouse, <u>Proc. Nat. Acad. Sci. USA</u>, 73 (1976) 208-212.

35 Olney, J.W., Ho., O.L. and Rhee, V., Cytotoxic effects of acidic and sulphur-containing amino acids on infant mouse central nervous system, <u>Exp. Brain Res.</u>, 14 (1972) 61-76.

36 Olney, J.W., Neurotoxicity of Excitatory Amino Acids. In E.G. McGeer, J.W. Olney and P.L. McGeer, (Eds.), <u>Kainic Acid as a Tool in Neurobiology</u>, Raven Press, N.Y., 1978, pp. 95-121.

37 Reubi, J.C. and Cuénod, M., Glutamate release in vitro from corticostriatal terminals, <u>Brain Res.</u>, 176 (1979) 185-188.

38 Sandoval, M.E. and Cotman, C.W., Evaluation of glutamate as a neurotransmitter of cerebellar parallel fibers, <u>Neurosci.</u>, 3 (1978) 199-206.

39 Schwarcz, R., Scholz, D. and Coyle, J.T., Structure-activity relations for the neurotoxicity of kainic acid, <u>Neuropharmacol.</u>, 17 (1978) 145-151.

40 Schwarcz, R. and Fuxe, K., ^{3}H-Kainic acid binding: Relevance for evaluating the neurotoxicity of kainic acid, <u>Life Sci.</u>, 24 (1979) 1471-1480.

41 Schwarcz, R., Köhler, Ch., Fuxe, K., Hökfelt, T. and Goldstein, M., On the Mechanism of Selective Neuronal Degeneration in the Rat Brain: Studies with Ibotenic Acid. In T.N. Chase, N.S. Wexler and A. Barbeau, (Eds.), <u>Huntington's disease</u>, <u>Adv. in Neurology</u>, Raven Press, N.Y., 1979, pp. 655-668.

42 Shinozaki, H., and Shibuya, I., Effects of kainic acid analogues on crayfish opener muscle, Neuropharmacol., 15 (1976) 145-147.

43 Shinozaki, H., Discovery of Novel Actions of Kainic Acid and Related Compunds. In E.G. McGeer, J.W. Olney and P.L. McGeer, (Eds.), Kainic Acid as a Tool in Neurobiology, Raven Press, N.Y., 1978, pp. 17-35.

44 Simon, J.R., Contrera, J.F. and Kuhar, M.J., Binding of [^{3}H]kainic acid, an analogue of L-glutamate, to brain membranes, J. Neurochem., 26 (1976) 141-148.

45 Spencer, H.J., Antagonism of cortical excitation of striatal neurones by glutamic acid diethyl ester: Evidence for glutamic acid as an excitatory transmitter in the rat striatum, Brain Res., 102 (1976) 91-101.

46 Storm-Mathisen, J., Glutamic acid and excitatory nerve endings: reduction of glutamic acid uptake after axotomy, Brain Res., 120 (1977) 379-386.

47 Streit, P., Stella, M. and Cuénod, M., Kainate induced lesion in the optic tectum: Dependency upon optic nerve afferents or glutamate, Brain Res., 187 (1980) 47-57.

48 Streit, P., unpublished results.

49 Ueno, Y., Nawa, H., Ueyanagi, J., Morimoto, R., Nakamori, R. and Matsuoka, T., Studies on the active compounds of Digenea Simplex Ag and related compounds: I. Studies on the structure of kainic acid, J. Pharmacol. Soc. Japan, 75 (1955) 807-811.

50 Vincent, S.R. and McGeer, E.G., Kainic acid binding to membranes of striatal neurons, Life Sci., 24 (1979) 265-270.

51 Young, A.B., Oster-Granite, M.L., Herndon, R.M. and Snyder, S.H., Glutamic acid: Selective depletion by viral induced granule cell loss in hamster cerebellum, Brain Res., 73 (1974) 1-13.

52 Zaczek, R., Nelson, M.F. and Coyle, J.T., Effects of anaestetics and anticonvulsants on the action of kainic acid in the rat hippocampus, Europ. J. Pharmacol., 52 (1978) 323-327.

GABA AND BENZODIAZEPINES

Neurotransmitters and their Receptors
Edited by U.Z. Littauer, Y. Dudai, I. Silman,
V.I. Teichberg and Z. Vogel

Gaba Modulates the Glycine-Receptor Interaction in Mauthner Cells Allosterically

Robert Werman

Neurobiology Unit, The Hebrew University of Jerusalem

Abstract: Membrane conductance measurements provide a delicate tool for determination of the stoichiometry of transmitter-receptor interactions. Using this approach quantitative measurements on acetylcholine and various amino acid receptors have been made in various isolated invertebrate and vertebrate preparations.

In the central nervous system such measurements are more difficult although some attempts have been made to assay both GABA and glycine induced conductance changes in cat motoneurons. The present study took advantage of the remarkable nature of the lateral dendrite of goldfish Mauthner cells. This structure is electrically inexcitable and antidromic action potentials passively conducted from the axon hillock can be used as a constant current source. Both GABA and glycine produced increases in chloride conductance (g_{Cl}). The maximal chloride conductance produced by glycine was four times as great as that produced by GABA while the half-maximal dose of glycine was only 60% of that of GABA. Both reactions were well described by an interaction of four molecules of amino acid with its receptor, involving infinite positive cooperativity:

$$Ng_a/g_{max} = 1/\{1 + (A_{0.5}/A)^4\}.$$

When steady-state responses to glycine were observed in the presence of a constant dose of GABA, the sigmoidal dose-response curve was shifted markedly to the left without any apparent change in the maximal response, nor in the limiting log-log slope. It thus appears that GABA can allosterically modify the glycine receptor so as to increase the affinity of glycine to its binding site without altering the cooperativity of the interaction. A similar but less well studied interaction of glycine with GABA sites was seen.

INTRODUCTION

For chemical synaptic actions of short (milliseconds to tens of milliseconds) and intermediate duration (tens to hundreds of milliseconds), the immediate electrical consequence of activation of a synaptic receptor by a neurotransmitter is a change - usually an increase - in conductance of one or more ion species across the membrane of the postsynaptic cell. Amino acids appear to generally act as synaptic transmitters through such conductance mechanisms, as demonstrated first in the CNS for glycine (1). Both GABA and glycine appear to increase postsynaptic Cl^- conductance.

If one assumes (2) that activation of single receptors results in a mean conductance increase that is normally distributed and that there is negligible interaction between neighboring receptors (3) - certainly true with low concentrations of transmitter - then the rule of parallel conductances tells us that activation of N receptors should produce N times the unitary conductance change. When the conductance change produced by a transmitter is related to transmitter concentration, the formulations of enzyme-substrate reactions, where conductance change is treated as if it were reaction product, the receptor as enzyme (more properly, as membrane bound enzyme) and the transmitter as substrate, appear to be valid (2, 4, 5,). Thus:

$$\Delta g = Ng_a = f(A), \qquad \ldots(1)$$

where Δg is the measured change in conductance; N, the number of receptors activated; g_a, the unitary conductance change produced by activation of a single receptor; and A, the concentration of transmitter. It is important to distinguish between synaptic conductance changes and others produced, for example, secondary to voltage changes (6). For this reason, voltage clamp techniques are frequently necessary (6). It is indisputable that measurement of conductance changes is preferable to all other measures, since these changes are the primary event in a complex chain involving non-linear operators which express themselves as voltage changes, firing rates and strength of contraction, etc. (2).

A reasonable steady-state description (2) of a multiple step interaction between transmitter molecules (A) and receptor subunits

(R) is given by:

$$A + R \rightleftharpoons AR, \qquad K_1 \qquad ...(2.1)$$
$$A + AR \rightleftharpoons A_2R, \qquad K_2 \qquad ...(2.2)$$
$$............ \qquad .. \qquad ....$$
$$A + A_{n-1}R \rightleftharpoons A_nR^* \qquad K_n \qquad ...(2.n),$$

where A_nR^* is the smallest complex that produces the conductance change and K_n, the dissociation constant of the nth step. (It is possible to add a separate final step representing the conformational change, $A_nR \rightleftharpoons A_nR^*$. Since the ratio A_nR^*/A_nR will be constant at steady-state, this additional step does not qualitatively alter the formulation.) If y is the fraction of receptors activated it will be related to the maximal conductance change, g_{max}, by the relationship:

$$y = Ng_a/g_{max} \qquad ...(3)$$

Furthermore it is also given by:

$$y = A^n/(A^n + K_nA^{n-1} + K_nK_{n-1}A^{n-2}...+ K_nK_{n-1}..K_nA + K_nK_{n-1}..K_2K_1 \qquad ...(4)$$

It can be shown (2) that the log-log slope of this relationship grows with decreasing transmitter concentration from zero to n (2), or

$$\lim A \rightarrow 0 \quad d(\log y)/d(\log A) = n \qquad ...(5)$$

and similarly,

$$\lim A \rightarrow 0 \quad d(\log Ng_a)/d(\log A) = n \qquad ...(5a)$$

Thus, a log-log plot of steady-state conductance change as the concentration of transmitter is lowered will give n as a limiting slope. It should be noted that equation (4) is a function of state (7) which gives information about the fraction of receptors in active form, and is not identical with the binding function used in biochemical studies. In general, n represents the minimal number of molecules of transmitter which will successfully activate the receptor (8).

ISOLATED PREPARATIONS

These formulations were first applied by Brookes and myself (7) to the inhibitory GABA-receptor interaction in leg muscles of the locust. This preparation was ideal for such measurements, showing no apparent desensitization and monotonically increasing conductance changes which grew to steady-state values with time. Voltage changes were minimal, ruling out membrane potential induced conductance changes.

Initial studies (7) showed that three molecules of GABA were necessary to activate the receptor. Moreover evidence was obtained against the <u>necessity</u> for a two state model to explain the results. The reaction was of high positive cooperativity and was described by:

$$Ng_a/g_{max} = A^3/(A^3 + K_3A^2 + K_3K_2A + K_3K_2K_1) \quad \ldots(6)$$

where K_1= 7.0 x10^{-4} M, K_2= 1.4 x10^{-4} M and K_3= 2.8 x10^{-5} M. It can be seen that the affinity increased five-fold in each successive step (7).

The stoichiometric analysis can also indicate how many antagonistic molecules are necessary to inhibit the GABA-receptor interaction. The strategy is to measure the conductance <u>decrease</u> produced by different concentrations of picrotoxin in the presence of a steady-state conductance change produced by a constant dose of GABA. When the results were plotted on a log-log plot, the limiting slope was clearly one. Thus one molecule of picrotoxin is sufficient to block the interaction requiring three molecules of GABA, with a dissociation constant of about 5.0x10^{-5} M (13, 14). These data may be interpreted as indicating that under the conditions of the experiment there are three and not more than three GABA-reacting subunits in the receptor and that occupation of one of them is sufficient to block a reaction requiring activation of all three subunits (but see 14, 10).

Furthermore, thermodynamic and kinetic measurements were also derived from these studies (9). Cooling increased the affinity of GABA for its receptor without significantly changing the cooperativity of the interaction. A van't Hoff plot showed more or less linear temperature behavior. The derived thermodynamic parameters indicate a standard enthalpy change, ΔH^o, of -64.3 $\pm$ 7.1 kcal/mole (standard error of estimate) and entropy change, S^o= -164 e.u./mole (15-23°C) (10). These high values are compatible with conformational changes in a multisubunit protein (9). The kinetic changes were much too slow to reflect GABA binding and apparently are a measure of conformational changes associated with synaptic conductance channel opening and closing. These findings also indicate the possible presence of occult desensitization (3, 5). Model analysis (11, 12) stresses the theoretical possibility of such desensitization as well as the fact that this desensitization will not invalidate steady-state stoichiometric formulations (3, 5).

Recent work indicates the existence of multiple states of aggregation of the GABA receptor in this preparation (10). Under different environmental conditions, particularly changes in external Mg^{2+} concentration, activation may involve two or four molecules (10) as well as the three indicated in earlier studies (7). In addition, differences in kinetic properties were also found to be associated with the observed changes in apparent cooperativity of the receptor (10).

STOICHIOMETRY IN THE CNS

The difficulties in quantitative studies in the CNS involving environmental change have been outlined elsewhere (15) and include control of concentrations, the presence of an isotropic extracellular space and complicated geometries. None-the-less there is some qualitative evidence that glycine (1, 2, 16) and GABA (16) interactions with cat spinal motoneurons require more than one molecule of ligand to activate their receptors. Mazliah and I used the lateral dendrite of the goldfish Mauthner cell as a possible structure for a quantitative analysis of GABA and glycine actions.

The Mauthner cell is a large, easily identified, paired cell found in the medulla of fish which sends an axon to the opposite side of the spinal cord. The lateral dendrite in goldfish is electrically inexcitable and the height of the antidromically evoked action potential which is electrotonically transmitted from the axon is a convenient and reliable constant current source for the measurement of conductance change (17), thereby eliminating the need for bridge measurements or the use of multiple intracellular electrodes. At the site chosen for recording, the dendrite approximates to a cylinder, 10 to 15 μ in diameter and the extracellular potential is sufficiently small and shifted in time so that it contributes negligibly to the intracellular monopolar recording. A rigid electrode assembly (1) was used with the tip of an intracellular recording electrode protruding 20-30 μ from the tip a parallel triple barrelled electrode containing concentrated solutions of GABA, glycine and NaCl. Iontophoretic currents through the amino acid barrels were controlled by constant current sources and were always delivered push-pull with respect to the NaCl barrel (18, 19, 20).

In order to obtain steady-state values for stoichiometric analysis, drug pulses of one minute were given throughout while stimulating antidromically at 1 Hz. Even from extracellular recordings it was clear that glycine was much more effective than GABA in shunting the antidromic response. These results were confirmed by intracellular recording (Table I): the maximum conductance change produced by glycine was 4.10 times that produced by GABA and the iontophoretic current producing a half-maximal glycine response was only 59.2% of that needed for GABA. Thus, on a current basis, glycine was 7.3 times more potent than GABA.

TABLE I

Glycine and GABA interactions with goldfish Mauthner cell lateral dendrite (20)

	Maximum Conductance Increase	Current Producing Half-Maximal Response ($A_{0.5}$)	
	Glycine/GABA	Glycine	GABA
Observed (n = 10)	$4.10 \pm 0.72^{*}$	$60.0 \pm 4.7^{**}$	101.3 ± 11.1
Calculated (n = 4)	$3.86 \pm 2.03^{+}$	$57.8 \pm 11.5^{++}$	117.6 ± 44.8

$^{*}p<0.0005$ $^{+}p<0.01$ $^{**}p<0.005$ $^{++}p<0.05$

Both mean ratio (±SEM) of maximal conductance changes (glycine/GABA) and mean currents (±SEM) necessary to produce half-maximal response in the same cell for each drug are shown. Calculated responses are based on a reaction of 4 amino acid molecules with their receptor showing infinite positive cooperativity.

Log-log plots of the increase in conductance produced by the amino acid dose showed slopes greater than three for both glycine and GABA. These consistent findings indicate that at least four molecules of each amino acid are needed to activate their respective receptors.

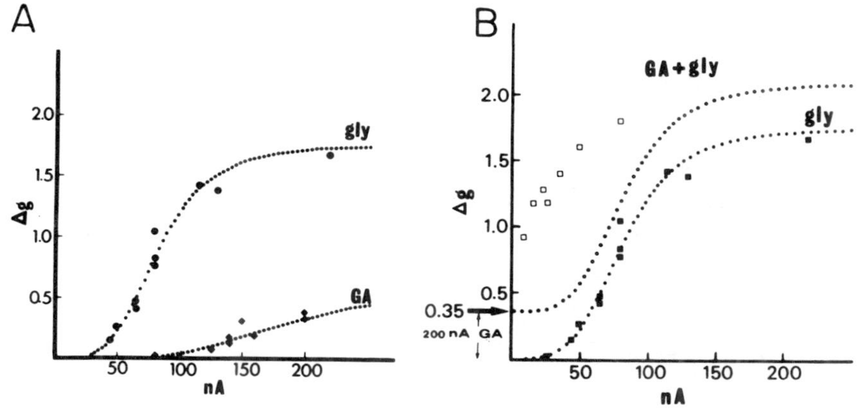

Figure 1. Four molecules of GABA (GA) and glycine (gly) are needed to activate their receptors in the goldfish Mauthner cell lateral dendrite; GABA modulates the glycine-receptor interaction allosterically. A. Dose-response curves for each amino acid in same cell. Calculated curves given by dotted lines assume interactions of infinite positive cooperativity of four molecules of amino acid with its receptor (14, 19). B. Dose-response curves for glycine in presence and absence of GABA in same cell. The lower curve and black squares are calculated and experimental responses to glycine alone. In presence of constant dose of GABA (arrow), algebraic sum of the responses is given by the intermediate curve, while the actual experimental values are shown by white squares (14, 19, 20).

Plotting the reciprocal of the conductance increase as a function of the reciprocal of the fourth power of the amino acid concentration showed straight lines which provided theoretical maximum responses as well as the dose ($A_{0.5}$) producing half-maximal response (Table I). Despite the simplifying assumption of infinite positive cooperativity given by the equation:

$$Ng_a/g_{max} = 1/\{1 + (A_{0.5}/A)^4\} \qquad \text{...(7)}$$

The fit of the theoretical curves to the data was remarkably good. Both the experimental data and the theoretical curves obtained were clearly sigmoidal, with the GABA curve shifted to the right and depressed with respect to the glycine curve (Fig. 1A). The value for the glycine/GABA maximum conductance increase ratio obtained from analysis was 3.86, while the half-maximal dose calculated for glycine was 49.2% of that for GABA. Thus, in terms of current, glycine was 7.9 times more potent than GABA (Table I). It can be seen that the results of analysis were in very good agreement with the experimental data in all respects.

For the activation of their receptors in the Mauthner cell, both GABA and glycine appear to utilize four binding sites to produce a unitary conductance change. Moreover, the strong positive cooperativity indicates that the energy barrier for binding the first amino acid molecule is appreciably higher than that of subsequent reactions for both amino acids. The action of glycine is appreciably greater than that of GABA, showing a higher affinity and a much greater maximal conductance change. Both amino acids produce conductance increases for Cl^- ions and the difference in maximal conductances might be the result of different open times for the Cl^- channels after receptor activation by the two amino acids. Kinetic studies, however, show that the rate of onset of the GABA reaction was consistently and significantly faster than that for glycine while the rate of offset was significantly slower. It thus appears likely that the density of glycine receptors is greater than that of GABA receptors in the Mauthner cell lateral dendrite.

GABA INTERACTS ALLOSTERICALLY WITH THE GLYCINE RECEPTOR IN THE MAUTHNER CELL

In order to measure possible amino acid interactions in the lateral dendrite of the Mauthner cell, dose-response curves for each amino acid were carried out in the presence of a constant dose of the second amino acid (3, 14, 20). When glycine was examined in the presence of a constant dose of GABA, the algebraic sum of the conductance changes produced by each amino acid was not obtained. Instead, the dose-response curve was markedly shifted to the left, the postsynaptic receptors becoming exquisitely sensitive to glycine (Fig. 1B). The shape of the glycine dose-response was not changed and the maximum response appeared to be that predicted by the algebraic addition of the maximal response produced by glycine alone and the constant conductance increase produced by GABA.

These results indicate that GABA acts directly on glycine receptors. Since the cooperativity of the glycine-receptor interaction was not affected, the action of GABA appears to be solely a lowering of the energy barrier for the binding of the first molecule of glycine to its receptor, thereby greatly increasing the affinity of glycine for its receptor. This conclusion was reinforced by double-reciprocal plotting of the conductance change against the fourth power of glycine concentration: the maximal response was not changed but the slope of the straight line relationship was markedly reduced.

From this finding it is clear that the GABA action is dual, both on its own set of receptors as well as an independent action on the glycine receptor. It is possible that the actions are identical in origin and that the GABA activation of its own receptor produces a change in nearby glycine receptors. This might be checked by examining the GABA effect after blockade of GABA receptors, but there is no guarantee that GABA binding to a non-synaptic receptor site near the glycine receptor would not be blocked by the same agent. Furthermore, we have already presented evidence for an appreciably greater density of glycine receptors than GABA receptors. The GABA action is not expressed as a conductance change; nor does it lower the cooperativity of the glycine receptor interaction which requires four glycine molecules for activation both in the presence and absence of GABA. The occult increase of glycine affinity produced by GABA appears to be a reaction on sites close to - but not identical with - the glycine recognition sites. This reaction reduces the energy barriers for the glycine-receptor interaction, probably for binding of the first glycine molecule which appears to be rate limiting. Such an interaction of GABA with the glycine receptor would therefore be allosteric in nature. The molecularity, n, of this GABA action has not been determined.

Since the GABA induced conductance change was so much smaller than the corresponding glycine response, it was difficult to determine the effect of glycine on the interaction of GABA with its Cl^- conductance activating receptor. In one cell, however, where GABA in large doses failed to produce a measurable conductance increase, the presence of a small background conductance evoked by a small constant dose of glycine, 32 nA, was sufficient to reveal a GABA response, even to relatively small doses. Glycine may have acted antagonistically with

GABA on the GABA receptor to reduce the cooperativity of the GABA receptor interaction or to increase the affinity of GABA to its receptor. It is also possible that the submaximal glycine response itself was increased by the allosteric action of GABA. It should be noted that the amount of glycine used was enough to activate less than 10% of the glycine receptors in the absence of glycine but more than 97% in the presence of a maximal GABA allosteric effect, in strong support of the last possibility.

These studies of glycine and GABA receptor interactions on an identified cell in the medulla of the goldfish are of great interest and provide a useful starting point for the quantitative evaluation of vertebrate CNS transmitter-receptor actions _in vitro_. In addition to the various direct implications of these results they must serve as a reference for the evaluation of binding studies in systems isolated from the CNS.

ACKNOWLEDGEMENTS

This work was partly supported by Grant NS-13935-03 from the U.S. Public Health Service.

REFERENCES

(1) Werman, R., Davidoff, R.A. and Aprison, M.H. The inhibitory action of glycine on spinal neurons in the cat. J. Neurophysiol. _31_: 81-95, 1968.

(2) Werman, R. An electrophysiological approach to drug-receptor mechanisms. Comp. Biochem. Physiol. _30_: 997-1017, 1969.

(3) Werman, R. Stoichiometry of transmitter-receptor interactions - the problem of desensitization. Adv. Pharmacol. Therapeut. _8_: 333-340, 1978.

(4) Werman, R. The transduction of chemical signals into electrical information at synapses. In: _Stability and Origin of Biological Information. Proceedings of the First Aharon Katzir-Katchalski Conference_, ed. I.R. Miller. John Wiley & Sons, New York, pp. 226-244, 1975.

(5) Werman, R. Desensitization and stoichiometry of transmitter receptor interactions. In: _Electrobiology of Nerve, Synapse and Muscle_, ed. J.P. Reuben, D.P. Purpura, M.V.L. Bennett & E.R. Kandel. Raven Press, New York, pp. 45-60, 1976.

(6) Werman, R. The reversal potential as a diagnostic tool in transmitter identification. In: Receptors for Neurotransmitters and Peptide Hormones, ed. G. Pepeu, M.J. Kuhar & S.J. Enna. Raven Press, New York, pp. 21-31, 1980.

(7) Brookes, N. and Werman, R. The cooperativity of γ-aminobutyric acid action on the membrane of locust muscle fibers. Mol. Pharmacol. 9: 571-579, 1973.

(8) Werman, R. The number of receptors for calcium ions at the nerve terminals of one endplate. Comp. gen. Pharmacol. 2: 129-137, 1971.

(9) Brookes, N., Blank, M. and Werman, R. The kinetics of the conductance increase produced by γ-aminobutyric acid at the membrane of locust muscle fibers. Mol. Pharmacol. 9: 580-589, 1973.

(10) Brookes,N. and Werman, R. Discrete states of responsiveness of a locust muscle GABA receptor: The influence of extracellular ion concentrations. Neuroscience, 1980 (in press).

(11) Spira, M.E., Armon, E. and Werman, R. A model for synaptic desensitization: steady-state. Israel J. Med. Sci. 11: 855-856, 1975.

(12) Armon, E., Spira, M.E. and Werman, R. A model for synaptic desensitization: kinetics. Israel J. Med. Sci. 11: 856, 1975.

(13) Brookes, N. and Werman, R. Use of conductance measurements in the study of drug-receptor interactions. Israel J. Med. Sci. 6: 322, 1970.

(14) Werman, R. Stoichiometry of GABA and glycine-receptor interactions: GABA modulates the glycine-receptor interaction allosterically in a vertebrate neuron. In: GABA---Biochemistry and CNS Functions, ed. P. Mandel & F.V. DeFeudis. Plenum Press, New York, Adv. Exper. Med. Biol. 123: 287-301, 1979.

(15) Werman, R. Criteria for identification of a central nervous system transmitter. Comp. Biochem. Physiol. 18: 745-766, 1966.

(16) Krnjević, K., Puil, E. and Werman, R. GABA and glycine actions on spinal motoneurons. Can. J. Physiol. Pharmacol. 55: 658-669, 1977.

(17) Diamond, J. The activation and distribution of GABA and l-glutamate receptors on goldfish Mauthner neurones: an analysis of dendrite remote inhibition. J. Physiol. (Lond.) 194:669-723, 1968.

(18) Mazliah, J. and Werman, R. The action of glycine and GABA compared in the same cell in vertebrates. Israel J. Med. Sci. 10: 556, 1974.

(19) Werman, R. and Mazliah, J. The actions of glycine and GABA compared on the Mauthner cell. Proc. Int. Union Physiol. Soc. 11: 149, 1974.

(20) Werman, R. and Mazliah, Y. The stoichiometry of glycine and GABA. Interactions with their receptors in a central neuron. In: _Iontophoresis and Transmitter Mechanisms in the Mammalian Central Nervous System_, ed. R.W. Ryall & J.S. Kelly, Elsevier/North Holland Biomedical Press, Amsterdam, pp. 400-402, 1978.

Neurotransmitters and their Receptors
Edited by U.Z. Littauer, Y. Dudai, I. Silman,
V.I. Teichberg and Z. Vogel

The Role of Gaba Receptors in the Genesis of Seizures

K. Krnjević

Anaesthesia Research & Physiology Departments,

McGill University, Montreal, P.Q. Canada. H3G 1Y6

ABSTRACT

A remarkable feature of the hippocampus is that it can be easily made to generate "seizure"-like discharges, either by the application of various drugs, or by repetitive stimulation of neural inputs at frequencies as low as 5-10/s. Perhaps the most important reason for this is the marked lability of the very powerful recurrent and other inhibitory mechanisms which normally suppress the effects of excitatory inputs. During such repetitive activation, a sharp reduction in this inhibitory action releases excitation. The consequent depolarization triggers a large Ca inward current that reinforces paroxysmal depolarization of the pyramidal cell bodies. Evidence will be presented that the initial loss of inhibitory efficiency may be triggered by reduced effectiveness of the probable inhibitory transmitter, GABA, owing to some form of desensitization.

INTRODUCTION

In a singularly perceptive paper, Hunt (10) in 1931 pointed out that epileptic seizures could result from an increase of an excitatory mechanism or the decrease of an inhibitory mechanism. He proposed specifically that Golgi Type I cells are excitatory ("erithic") and Golgi Type II cells inhibitory ("kolytic"). A loss of "kolytic" cells could therefore lead to convulsive manifestations. The idea that a weakening of inhibitory influences - arising in one way or another - is an essential, perhaps the essential cause of seizure phenomena is thus far from new and it has often been discussed (15,19,23). However, in the absence of any direct demonstration that inhibition is less effective in epileptic foci, other authors have placed greater emphasis on a possible abnormal enhancement of excitatory processes (4,17).

The experiments which are summarized here provide some new evidence that in the hippocampus - a structure that is notoriously susceptible to seizures (8) - the development of seizure activity coincides with a breakdown of the normally very powerful intrinsic inhibitory mechanisms. One aspect of this phenomenon is a reduction in the neurons' sensitivity to γ-aminobutyric acid (GABA), the probable physiological transmitter of inhibition (22).

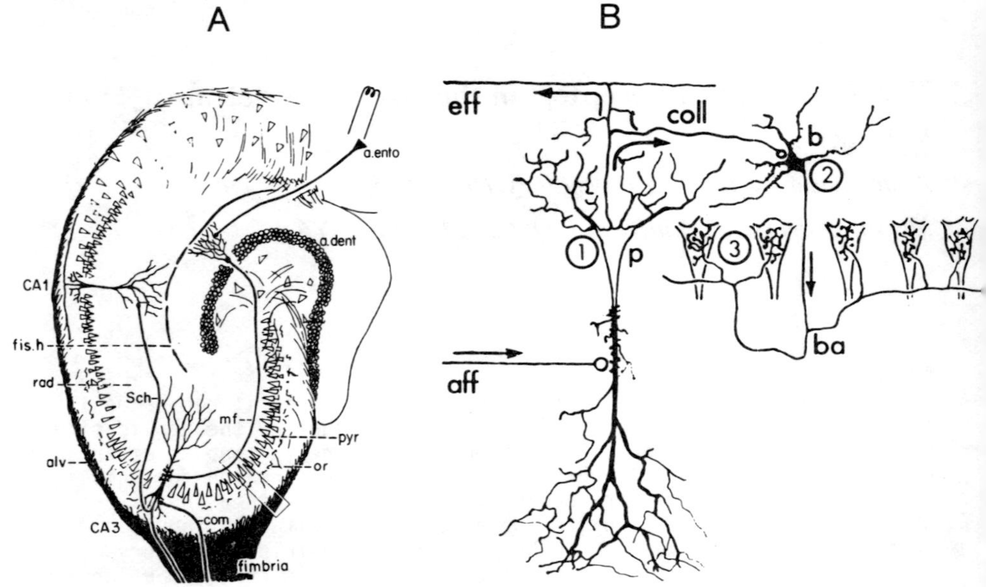

Fig. 1 A: diagram of hippocampal region based on horizontal section of rat brain. Abbreviations: a.dent, the dentate area; a.entor, entorhinal area; alv, alveus; com, commissural afferents; fis.h, hippocampal fissure; mf, mossy fibres; or, stratum oriens; pyr, stratum pyramidale; rad, stratum radiale; Sch, Schaffer collateral from CA3 pyramidal cell. (Part of Fig. 1 from Andersen et al., 1966.) B: diagram illustrating postulated pathway of inhibition in the hippocampus. An afferent volley (aff) excites a small number of pyramidal cells (p) and brings them to discharge along their axons (eff) (1). Via their axon collaterals (coll), they activate basket cells (2) which respond along with a short repetitive discharge. Terminals of the basket cell axons produce the IPSPs in the somata of a large number of pyramidal cells.

The hippocampus and some of its characteristics

Developmentally, the hippocampus has the same origin as the cortex. Originally the most medial portion of the pallium, it has been pushed inward and down into the lateral ventrical by the huge growth of the neocortex. Like the latter, it has a laminar organization, but in a simpler form: there is essentially only a single pyramidal layer, with the cell bodies well-aligned in a narrow band. The structural complexity of the hippocampus arises from a double folding, which has led to the superimposition of layers of pyramidal and granule cells (Fig. 1A).

From many parts of the forebrain pathways afferent to the hippocampus converge on the entorhinal cortex, where the cells of origin of the temporo-ammonic (or "perforant") tract are situated. The "perforant" fibres directly excite the granule cells in the most medial region, the dentate gyrus, as well as pyramidal cells of the other areas. Another important input is from the opposite hippocampus, via the hippocampal commissure (hence "commissural" pathway); this provides point-to-point connections between symmetrical areas of the two hippocampi. Other inputs come from the raphe nucleus, the locus coeruleus and the medial septum. The latter is probably cholinergic and probably plays an important role in the generation of the theta-rhythm, the characteristic 4-7/s electrical oscillations recorded from the hippocampus when an animal is alert and involved in motor activity.

Spencer and Kandel (21) were the first to demonstrate convincingly the existence of strong inhibitory mechanisms in the hippocampus. By removing all afferent inputs from the fornix, they were able to show that the large, and prolonged inhibitory synaptic potentials (IPSPs) evoked in the pyramidal cells of areas CA3 and CA1 by fornix stimulation must be produced by recurrent collateral branches of the pyramidal axons (Fig. 1B). Subsequent investigations have provided very strong evidence that this inhibition is mediated by the intrinsic "basket" cells (14), releasing GABA as their inhibitory agent (2,3,18,22).

A characteristic feature of the electrical responses of the hippocampus is their striking dependence on the frequency of stimulation. It has long been known (8) that repetitive stimulation at rates above 3-5/s is associated with a progressive change in the character of the evoked field, leading to a highly characteristic discharge in bursts in response to each stimulus (Fig. 2). If such stimulation is maintained or repeated several times (or if one stimulates at frequencies $\geq$ 10/s), desynchronized activity appears, signalling the onset of a "seizure", which persists for some seconds after the end of stimulation as an "after-discharge", or may develop into a massive shift in potential and total disappearance of on-going unit activity (a full seizure) that lasts several minutes.

The hippocampus' exceptional sensitivity to the rate of stimulation is of great interest for at least two reasons: on the one hand, it provides an outstanding example of a most reactive neural structure, showing a high degree of the "plasticity" expected of an organ involved in learning, laying down of memory traces, etc.; on the other hand, it is a most useful model for the study of seizures, especially since paroxysmal discharges are so readily elicited, without the need to apply special drugs.

Do we have any clues as to the mechanism of the characteristic progressive increase in excitation observed during repetitive stimulation? Clearly, this could be caused by a progressive facilitation of excitatory mechanisms; but in a tissue where inhibitory mechanisms are so preponderant, a reduction in the potency of inhibition could be just as effective.

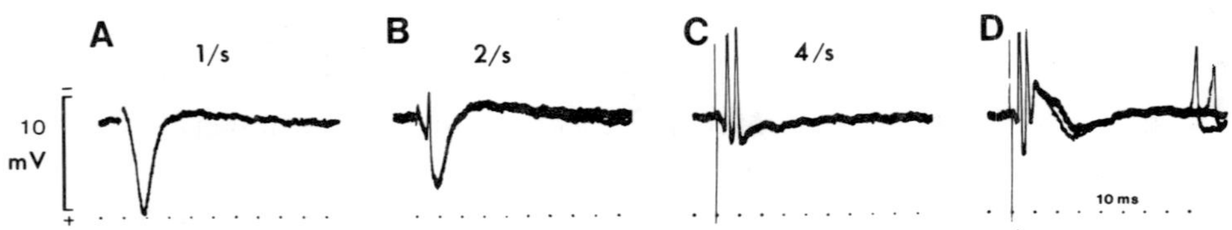

Fig. 2 Effect of increased frequency of fimbrial stimulation on the evoked field recorded in CA3 area at depth where maximal positive response was evoked by 1/s fimbrial stimulation (this corresponds to superficial pyramidal stratum). Repetitive fimbrial stimulation was at 1/s in A, 2/s in B and 4/s in C and D. B: note smaller positive field and appearance of early spike. C: within 5 s of onset of stimulation at 4/s; positive wave is largely replaced by a burst of two spikes; and D: 15 s later, spikes are now followed by prominent negative after-potential. (Part of Fig. 2 from Krnjević et al., 1980.)

Hippocampal inhibition during repetitive stimulation

Most of the observations (which are described in more detail elsewhere, Ben-Ari et al., 1979) were made from the CA3 and CA1 region of the hippocampus *in situ*, in rats under urethane anaesthesia. At very low rates of stimulation (< 3/s), extracellular recording shows in response to fimbrial stimulation (which activates the main afferent path antidromically and the commissural pathway orthodromically) a very predictable sequence of waves. In particular, there is a sharp positive wave strictly localized to the layer of pyramidal cell bodies, which is fully consistent with the preponderant IPSP observed intracellularly in response to this stimulation and the high density of inhibitory nerve terminals on the pyramidal cell bodies (2,18).

When the rate of stimulation is raised to 3-5/s, this positive wave diminishes and sharp population spikes appear. A spike is seen first near the start of the evoked response (Fig. 2B); as it grows larger, a second spike appears some 2 msec later (Fig. 2C,D) which may be followed by a third or even fourth spike when the burst is fully developed.

If intracellular recording is combined with regular tests of cell input resistance (by the application of series of known current pulses) the large IPSP evoked by fimbrial stimulation can be seen to be associated with large rise in membrane conductance (Figs. 3 and 4). Since this IPSP is essentially generated by a marked increase in permeability to Cl^- (as elsewhere in the CNS), it is highly sensitive to changes in internal Cl^- concentration: though normally a hyperpolarizing response, it soon becomes a depolarizing one if one records with Cl^--containing microelectrodes (as in the experiments illustrated in Figs. 3-5), but the change in polarity is <u>not</u> accompanied by any marked change in IPSP conductance.

With repetitive stimulation at higher frequency - which may or may not lead to overt seizure activity - the IPSPs diminish, and, most importantly, the associated conductance increase is sharply reduced. This is illustrated in Fig. 3: here one can see in A the large positive IPSP, accompanied by a major increase in conductance (indicated by the smaller responses to identical applications of 10 ms current pulses); after a very brief period of tetanic stimulation at 20/s, there is some depolarization, and the IPSP is greatly reduced, the conductance increment in particular being practically abolished (B); after progressive recovery over one minute, the IPSP shows quite substantial return of its initial properties (C). The graph below (D) illustrates the time course of these changes in more detail.

Many tests of this kind have consistently yielded comparable results. Repetitive stimulation at frequencies that lead to the generation first of activity in bursts and then seizures is regularly associated with a diminished potency of inhibition, most directly indicated by the reduction in IPSP conductance increment.

What would be the consequence of diminished inhibition? There is good reason to believe that under normal conditions, the inhibitory interneurones are continually active - presumably because of on-going afferent activity - and so they maintain the pyramidal cells in a relatively strongly inhibited state (this is indicated by the paucity of spontaneous and evoked firing, even in response to antidromic volleys, as well as by

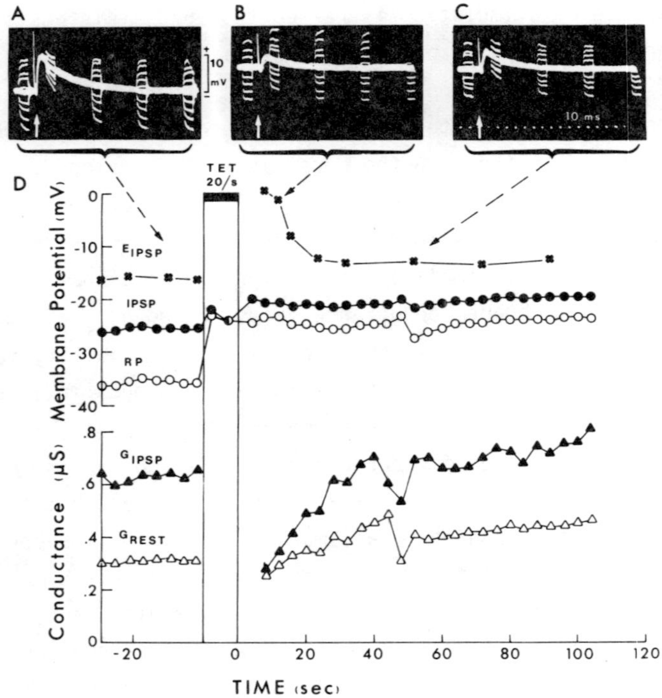

Fig. 3 Post-tetanic depression of IPSPs evoked in CA3 pyramidal neuron by stimulation of entorhinal cortex. Microelectrode contained 3 M KCl and therefore IPSP became positive. As illustrated in traces above (A-C), input conductance was measured with 10 msec pulses of both outward and inward current (-3 to +2 nA). Eight sets of pulses were applied: the first at the start of the trace, before the entorhinal stimulus (marked by arrow), one shortly after the peak of the IPSP and six more at subsequent intervals of 50 ms (only first 5 sets of pulses are shown in the figure). For each trace, ten IPSPs were superimposed during stimulation at 2/s. Initially, there was a marked increase in conductance near the peak of the IPSP, shown by the much smaller recorded voltage pulses, as well as their sharper time course indicating a shortening of membrane time constant. The corresponding values of input conductance are given in the graph below for the resting condition (open triangles) and near the peak of the IPSP only (closed triangles) (each being calculated from 10 voltage-current points and the corresponding lines-of-best-fit). The resting potential (open circles) and potential at the peak of the IPSP (closed circle) are also shown, as well as the reversal potential for the peak of the IPSP (crosses). Shortly after a 10 sec tetanus at 20/s, which caused some depolarization and conductance increase, there was a large reduction in resting conductance and especially in IPSP conductance (cf. also trace B, recorded about 15 sec after the end of the tetanus). Unlike the resting potential the IPSP conductance increase showed almost full recovery (cf. also trace C, recorded 1 min after tetanus). (Fig. 1 from Ben-Ari et al., 1979.)

a substantial rise in "background" cell resistance during stimulation at 2 or more per second). One can therefore postulate that as inhibition becomes weaker, the pyramidal cells become progressively more responsive to both antidromic and orthodromic stimulation, even repetitive firing becoming possible as recurrent inhibition diminishes. Moreover, with sufficient depolarization, a Ca^{2+} influx is triggered (20,25) which could greatly reinforce depolarization in two ways: by enhancing inward current and perhaps also by sharply lowering extracellular Ca^{2+} around the pyramidal cell bodies (where the Ca^{2+} influx appears to be limited)(12), and thus further diminishing the efficacy of inhibitory synapses.

Mechanism of Loss of Inhibitory Potency

Inhibition could become less effective in many quite different ways. The various possibilities can be grouped in two main categories: pre-synaptic and post-synaptic.

Presynaptic Changes

These include fatigue or inhibition of inhibitory interneurones, or a depression (presynaptic inhibition) of inhibitory transmitter release (not necessarily reflected in a change in interneuronal discharge). We have some evidence (11) that interneuronal firing can follow quite well rates of stimulation in the critical range (3-10/s), as long as major seizure activity does not develop: this leads to the disappearance of all unit activity, which is hardly surprising since at such time the extracellular K^+ activity rises to over 30 mM (12). Hence the limited evidence that is presently available does not indicate an early inactivation of inhibitory interneurones, so this is not very likely to be the initial cause of the reduction in inhibitory potency.

With regard to lowered efficacy of inhibitory synapses by depression of transmitter release, there is at present no relevant evidence. As already pointed out, the marked drop in extracellular Ca^{2+} (as well as increase in extracellular K^+) that follows the large Ca^{2+} influx triggered by bursting can be expected to depress inhibitory transmitter release; but this is a relatively late phenomenon, and there is initially only a minimal fall in extracellular Ca^{2+} level.

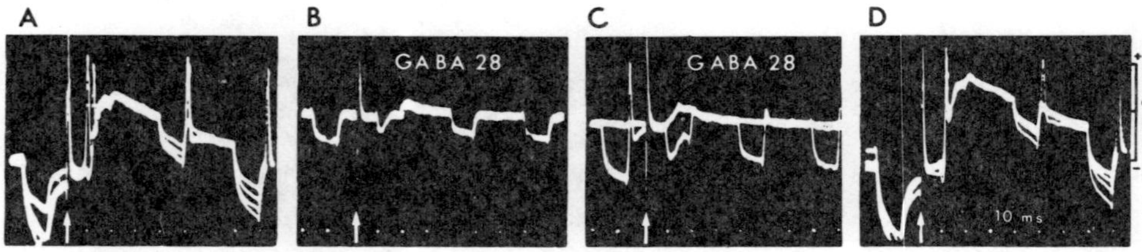

Fig. 4 GABA causes a large increase in conductance as well as marked depression of IPSPs. Oscilloscope traces (A-D) show several superimposed IPSPs evoked by entorhinal stimulation in a CA3 pyramidal neuron (at 2/s), while conductance was measured with 4 sets of hyperpolarizing pulses, regularly incremented in 10 equal steps within range -3 to 0 nA. In A (initial control, resting potential -77.9 mV) a large conductance increase is evident, especially at peak of the IPSP, subsequent pulses showing gradual recovery of resistance. In B, 10 s after starting release of GABA (28 nA), there is a marked depolarization (upward shift of trace, resting potential is now -52.4 mV) and large increase in resting conductance, indicated by the greatly reduced voltage deflections evoked by same current pulses. Ten seconds later (C), while maintaining GABA release at same intensity, there is partial repolarization and a clear fall in input conductance, especially at the peak of the IPSP. In trace D, 30 sec after end of GABA release, there is a nearly full recovery of resting potential (-72.0 mV), as well as of IPSP amplitude and conductance increase. (Part of Fig. 2 from Ben-Ari et al., 1979.)

Post-synaptic Changes

The inhibitory transmitter responsible for the large IPSPs generated by Cl^- increase is almost certainly GABA (22). In our own experiments, applications of GABA from a second, extracellular micropipette, produced very large increases in cell conductance (and corresponding potential changes) that were essentially indistinguishable from the changes observed during IPSPs (Fig. 4A and B). Since glycine was practically ineffective - glycine is the only other probable inhibitory transmitter that operates by increasing Cl^- permeability (24) - GABA is indeed very likely to be the physiological mediator of inhibition. An interesting feature of the action of GABA is that, as in the neocortex (7) and the spinal cord (13), it tends to "fade" markedly during a maintained application (note recovery of membrane potential and especially resistance in Fig. 4, cf. traces C and B). It is not known whether this "fading" is caused by a "true" receptor desensitization, an inactivation of Cl^- channels, or perhaps even acceleration of GABA removal (13). In the hippocampus, GABA not infrequently also caused a marked "fading" of the IPSP (and its conductance increment).

In view of this evidence that the action of GABA tends to wane it was necessary to investigate the possibility that repetitive activation might also in some way be associated with a comparable fading of transmitter action, which could explain the loss of inhibitory potency. By repeating identical applications of GABA at regular intervals, while stimulating the fimbria or the entorhinal cortex at various frequencies, we have been able to show that stimulation at rates of 3 or more per second leads to a diminished responsiveness to GABA, shown particularly clearly by a reduction or even practical disappearance of the normal conductance increase.

One experiment of this kind is illustrated in Fig. 5. When the stimulation rate was raised from 2 to 5/s, there was some diminution in IPSP conductance increase, and the effect of GABA was substantially reduced. The duration of such changes was rather variable: in Fig. 5, there was no obvious recovery of action of GABA one or two minutes after the return to a lower rate of stimulation; but in other cases practically full recovery was observed within 2-5 minutes. In general, there seemed to be a reasonable general correlation between the effectiveness of GABA and the "potency" of IPSPs; but because of the technical difficulties of these experiments, we do not yet have enough information to justify more than the tentative conclusion that repetitive stimulation at frequencies in the critical range <u>can</u> lead to a diminished responsiveness to GABA. Therefore a post-synaptic change causing fading of inhibitory synaptic action <u>could</u> explain the loss of inhibitory potency.

One can only speculate about the mechanism of such fading. It would be very remarkable if such low frequency activity caused a desensitization of inhibitory receptors: at the neuromuscular junction, desensitization cannot be produced by even high frequency junctional transmission (16). On the other hand, there is now much evidence for the presence in the synaptic membrane of an intrinsic modulator of GABA receptors, capable of greatly reducing their affinity for GABA (6). Although the precise nature of this modulator is still controversial, it may be "released" by the interaction of GABA and the post-synaptic membrane, thus providing a form of negative feedback. Alternatively, it may be released by some other agency, such as changes in ionic concentrations, or perhaps in a more selective manner by some other transmitter or "modulator" liberated by pathways that are activated particularly effectively by repetitive stimulation. Of course these agents could act directly on the GABA recep-

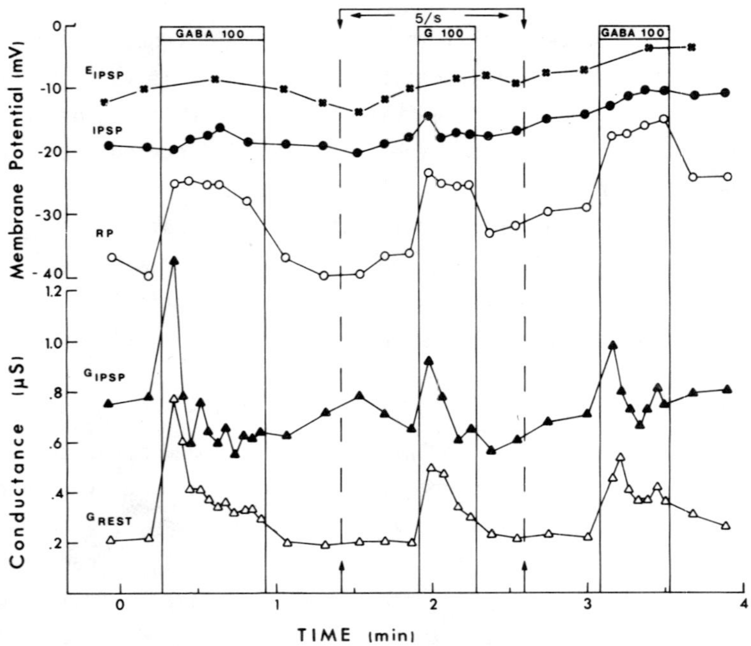

Fig. 5 Data recorded from another CA3 pyramidal neuron: membrane resting potential and IPSPs (respectively open and closed circles) as well as corresponding conductances (open and closed triangles). During initial and final portions of graph, fimbrial stimulation was at 2.5/s. Application of GABA caused a sharp depolarization and increase in conductance; latter decayed very rapidly, and at same time, peak level of IPSP conductance became clearly depessed. When frequency of stimulation was raised to 5 Hz, there was some minor depolarization, diminution in IPSP peak conductance and sharp reduction in conductance increase evoked by GABA. The IPSP conductance largely recovered after returning to stimulation at lower frequency, but the effectiveness of GABA remained diminished, possibly owing to the fall in resting potential. (Part of Fig. 2 from Ben-Ari et al., 1979).

tors and diminish their affinity without bringing into play an intermediary intrinsic modulator. Similarly, we cannot exclude a less specific inactivation of Cl^- channels, comparable to the blockage of Na^+ and K^+ channels produced by a variety of naturally occurring agents (9).

GENERAL CONCLUSIONS

These observations on hippocampal pyramidal cells have shown a surprising lability of the powerful inhibitory control, which is so evident at low rates of stimulation and appears to maintain much of the hippocampus in a shut-down state. A rapidly progressive diminution of inhibitory potency during stimulation at 3-5/s "releases" neuronal firing, typically in short, high frequency bursts. These are associated with large Ca^{2+} inward currents that may be important for "plastic" aspects of hippocampal function, and if excessive, may lead to full-blown seizures. The loss of inhibitory potency is probably due at least partly to a diminished responsiveness to GABA, whose mechanism, albeit obscure, indicates the possibility of a novel type of modulation of inhibitory control.

References

1. Andersen, P., Blackstad, T.W. and Lömo, T. 1966. Location and identification of excitatory synapses on hippocampal pyramidal cells. Exp. Brain Res. 1, 236-248.

2. Andersen, P., Eccles, J.C. and Løyning, Y. 1964. Location of postsynaptic inhibitory synapses on hippocampal pyramids. J. Neurophysiol. 27, 592-607.

3. Andersen, P., Eccles, J.C. and Løyning, Y. 1964. Pathway of postsynaptic inhibition in the hippocampus. J. Neurophysiol. 27, 608-619.

4. Ayala, G.F., Dichter, M., Gumnit, R.J., Matsumoto, H. and Spencer, W.A. 1973. Genesis of epileptic interictal spikes. New knowledge of cortical feedback systems suggests a neurophysiological explanation of brief paroxysms. Brain Res. 52, 1-17.

5. Ben-Ari, Y., Krnjević, K. and Reinhardt, W. 1979. Hippocampal seizures and failure of inhibition. Can. J. Physiol. Pharmacol. 57, 1462-1466.

6. Costa, E. and Guidotti, A. 1979. Molecular mechanisms in the receptor action of benzodiazepines. Ann. Rev. Pharmacol. Toxicol. 19, 531-545.

7. Dreifuss, J.J., Kelly, J.S. and Krnjević, K. 1969. Cortical inhibition and γ-aminobutyric acid. Exp. Brain Res. 9, 137-154.

8. Green, J.D. 1964. The hippocampus. Physiol. Rev. 44, 561-608.

9. Hille, B. 1976. Gating in sodium channels of nerve. Ann. Rev. Physiol. 38, 139-152.

10. Hunt, J.R. 1931. A theory of the mechanism underlying inhibition in the central nervous system and its relation to convulsive manifestations. Res. publ. Assoc. Res. Nerv. Ment. Dis. 7, 45-64.

11. Krnjević, K., Ben-Ari, Y. and Reinhardt, W. 1979. Hippocampal interneuronal activity during repetitive stimulation. Canada Physiol. 10, 174.

12. Krnjević, K., Morris, M.E. and Reiffenstein, R.J. 1980. Changes in extracellular Ca^{2+} and K^{+} activity accompanying hippocampal discharges. Can.J.Physiol.Pharmacol., in press.

13. Krnjević, K., Puil, E. and Werman, R. 1977. GABA and glycine actions on spinal motoneurons. Can. J. Physiol. Pharmacol. 55, 658-669.

14. Lorente de Nó, R. 1934. Studies on the structure of the cerebral cortex. II. J. Psychol. Neurol. (Leipzig), 46, 113-177.

15. Meldrum, B.S. 1975. Epilepsy and γ-aminobutyric acid-mediated inhibition. Int. Rev. Neurobiol. 17, 1-36.

16. Otsuka, M., Endo, M. and Nonomura, Y. 1962. Presynaptic nature of neuromuscular depression. Jap. J. Physiol. 12, 573-584.

17. Prince, D.A. 1978. Neurophysiology of epilepsy. Ann. Rev. Neurosci. 1, 395-415.

18. Ribak, C.E. Vaughn, J.E. and Saito, K. 1978. Immunocytochemical localization of glutamic acid decarboxylase in neuronal somata following colchicine inhibition of axonal transport. Brain Res. 140, 315-332.

19. Ribak, C.E., Harris, A.B., Vaughn, J.E. and Roberts, E. 1979. Inhibitory, GABAergic nerve terminals decrease at sites of focal epilepsy. Science, 205, 211-214.

20. Schwartzkroin, P.A. and Slawsky, M. 1977. Probable calcium spikes in hippocampal neurons. Brain Res. 135, 157-161.

21. Spencer, W.A. and Kandel, E.R. 1961. Hippocampal neuron responses to selective activation of recurrent collaterals of hippocampofugal axons. Exp. Neurol. 4, 149-161.

22. Storm-Mathisen, J. 1977. Localization of transmitter candidates in the brain: the hippocampal formation as a model. Progr. Neurobiol. 8, 119-181.

23. Ward, A.A., Jasper, H.H. and Pope, A. 1969. Clinical and experimental challenges of the epilepsies. In Basic Mechanisms of the Epilepsies, H.H. Jasper, A.A.Ward and A. Pope (Eds.). Boston, Little, Brown and Co., pp. 1-12.

24. Werman, R., Davidoff, R.A. and Aprison, M.H. 1968. Inhibitory action of glycine on spinal neurons in the cat. J. Neurophysiol. 31, 81-95.

25. Wong, R.K.S. and Prince, D.A. 1978. Participation of calcium spikes during intrinsic burst firing in hippocampal neurons. Brain Res. 159, 385-390.

Neurotransmitters and their Receptors
Edited by U.Z. Littauer, Y. Dudai, I. Silman,
V.I. Teichberg and Z. Vogel

The Regulation of Gaba Receptors as a Possible Mechanism for Gaba-1,4 Benzodiazepine Interactions

E. Costa, A. Guidotti, M. Massotti* and S. Mazzari

*Laboratory of Preclinical Pharmacology, National Institute of Mental Health, Saint Elizabeths Hospital, Washington, D.C. 20032 and *FDA Bureau of Drugs, Division of Drug Biology, 200 C Street, S.W,, Washington, D.C.*

Abstract: The view that the benzodiazepines act as anxiolytics by maximizing the function of GABAergic synapses is discussed. It appears that the site of action of benzodiazepine could be associated to the high affinity GABA receptors. The possibility that these high affinity GABA receptors are important in the regulation of the Cl^- fluxes in NB_{2a} cells is supported by the data presented. These data also show that the diazepam (10^{-6} - 10^{-8}M) facilitates the action of GABA receptor agonists to increase the Cl^- fluxes in NB_{2a} cells.

INTRODUCTION

The pharmacology of postsynaptic receptors includes two main categories of drugs: the agonists that mimic the transmitter and the antagonists that block the action of the transmitter on the receptors. Theoretically, both the antagonists and the agonists can act reversibly or irreversibly and directly or indirectly. When we transfer this paradigm to the clinical situation though in man reversibly acting drugs are preferred, because these drugs are given chronically, we are essentially confronted by a continuous and prolonged drug action which can directly or indirectly block or activate receptors. An antagonist acting indirectly is exemplified by reserpine which depletes the transmitter store, an agonist acting indirectly is exemplified by tyramine which continuously releases the transmitter. The salient feature shared by both agonists and antagonists given continuously for months or years is their ability to compete with nerve impulses for the control of the synapses. Under these drug regimens, the synapse can be either continuously activated or continuously inhibited, depending on the type of drug used. Since the brain functions as a network of feedback and feed forward neuronal circuits, during the persistent treatment with agonists and antagonists, the spontaneous rhythmicity of the synaptic activity is abolished, and a collateral neuronal loop will be activated in the attempt to compensate the damage induced by the drug. Important collateral loops may have taken over, and this results in a number of side effects.

If, as claimed, by the famous Dale's law, each neuron has one and only one transmitter, then there is no valid alternative to a direct attack of the neurotransmitter receptor in order to correct the defects in brain function due to a specific synaptic inadequancy. If synaptic blockade is the only alternative for a remedy then we must deal with a number of side effects deriving from the change in transmitter function that is imposed by the drug treatment. Recent data emerging from studies of neuropeptide location, using immunohistofluorescence, appear to indicate that in a neuron a primary transmitter may coexist with a neuropeptide (1) probably functioning as a cotransmitter (2). At the time of this writing we do not know whether every neuron contains a neuropeptide that functions as a cotransmitter and an amine or aminoacid that functions as a primary transmitter. Evidence obtained in the cholinergic synapses of adrenal medulla suggests that the neuropeptide that coexists in a neuron with the primary transmitter and functions as a cotransmitter acts after it is released extraneuronally and binds to specific receptors located in the membrane of the postsynaptic cells (2). Here the cotransmitter modulates the responsiveness of the primary transmitter receptor (3). The mechanisms participating in this modulation are not readily understood, some appear to involve enzymatic modifications of the lipids forming the phospholipid bilayers (4). Thus drugs that mimic or antagonize the action of a cotransmitter will act only when the primary transmitter is released and will never interfere with the transmission unless the primary transmitter has been released. They will just interfere with the fine tuning of the primary transmitter function. Since synaptic transmission will remain under the physiological control by the primary transmitter which is made, stored and released as if a drug were not present, it is possible that the extent and intensity of side effects which are triggered by the modification of the cotransmitter function will be less than those triggered when the primary transmitter function is reduced.

In neuroscience we tend to develop concepts from paradigms and this tendency has in several occasions delayed our progress because we instinctively become loathed to abandon schemes. To avoid repetition of past mistakes we should keep now an open mind about possible options available, and think that there are many ways to accomplish transfer of information through synpatic transmission and perhaps all the possible ways may be operative sometime and somewher in the several trillion synapses operative in the brain. Evidence that will be discussed in this report is consistent with the possibility that a number of GABAergic synapses in the brain possess a regulatory mechanism which in additio to GABA relies on another synaptic modulator (5). Whether this modulator is a polypeptide stored presynaptically it is difficult to assess at this time, however, we know that the activation of this physiological mechanism can be mimicked by the benzodiazepines (5).

Relationships between the benzodiazepines and brain neurotransmitters

A tenet of neuropharmacology indicates that drugs which modify behavior act on a synaptic function, selectively. When it became clear that benzodiazepines were effective in relieving anxiety it became important to know how these drugs act (6). The literature preceding 1974 contains indication that the benzodiazepines can affect cholinergic, dopaminergic, serotonergic and glycinergic synapses (7,8). However, these effects can be obtained for doses greater than those that modify the accepted behavioral models that predict an anxiolytic action in man (7). Hence we were forced to postulate that the benzodiazepines were acting on a mechanism which in turn could modify various neurotransmitter systems (6,7). In studying which neuronal mechanism was the primary target for the action of the benzodiazepines, our attention became polarized toward the GABAergic system (6). A previous report from Smith and colleagues (9) had already suggested that a facilitation of the GABAergic mechanism could explain the facilitation by benzodiazepines of the spinal cord depolarization elicited by the stimulation of the primary sensory afferent. We (6) and Haefely (7) studied the anticonvulsant action of benzodiazepines, their action on GABAergic transmission in several electrophysiological models, on the GABA mediated decrease of cerebellar cGMP and on behaviors that are facilitated by fear. These studies made it clear that a facilitation of the GABAergic transmission could be the unifying mechanism mediating the various actions of the benzodiazepines on behavior, neurochemistry and neurophysiology (6,7). When this concept was coming to fruition came the reports by two independent groups of investigators that the benzodiazepines selectively bind with high affinity to brain membranes (10,11). In a group of benzodiazepines the potency in displacing diazepam from specific binding sites relates to their muscle relaxant activity (10,11). Moreover the affinity of the binding sites for benzodiazepines is increased by the occupancy of GABA receptors (12,13). This finding indirectly suggests that a specific transmitter mechanism related to GABA transmission could be mimicked by the benzodiazepines. Hence GABAergic synapses could be considered as a possible site for the high affinity binding of benzodiazepines. At this point two questions become of importance: 1) are the benzodiazepines acting on presynaptic or on postsynaptic GABA mechanisms; and 2) are the benzodiazepines mimicking a neuromodulator (cotransmitter?) at the GABAergic synapses? Before answering these questions, it is in order a review of the current information on GABAergic mechanisms.

GABA as a neurotransmitter

Presynaptic regulation: Like any other synapse also the GABAergic synapse possesses a number of regulatory mechanisms (for review of GABA mechanisms see 14,15). Some are located presynaptically others are located postsynaptically. Presynaptically the uptake and synthesis of GABA maintain the steady state of the transmitter in the face of changing rates of utilization, during synaptic activity; this synthesis depends on glucose via glutamic acid decarboxylation. The quanta of GABA that are released by nerve impulses bind to receptors, the content of GABA at postsynaptic receptors and in the synaptic gaps is reduced by uptake mechanisms. There are two uptake mechanism which have different specificity: one is located on glial cells, the other in nerve terminals. The GABA taken up by glial cells, is degraded via transamination, probably insignificant amounts of transaminasis are present in the GABAergic terminals. There is still an insufficient degree of understanding of the operation and of the functional significance of some of these basic mechanisms. For instance, we do not understand whether the reuptake mechanism of GABA in glial cell functions continuously or is a sussidiary mechanism for the more important neuronal uptake of GABA. This might become functionally insufficient during high rates of GABA release, in fact, several authors maintain that there is no net uptake of GABA into the nerve terminals. That the two uptakes are different is supported by the selective blockade of neuronal uptake with nipecotic acid and the lack of activity of this drug on the GABA uptake by glia cells. That the neuronal uptake of GABA must be of a physiological importance is indirectly documented by reports showing that nipecotic acid can potentiate the effects that depend on GABAergic transmission. However, an additional cause of perplexity is the finding that inhibitors of GABA transaminase, which as mentioned above is preferentially located in glial cells, also potentiate GABAergic transmission. The reasons for such complexities and apparent discrepancies are not yet understood, they may well reside in the fact that GABA synapses are a less homogenous system that we would like to have. Maybe a uniform and well balanced scheme can not depict the function of an idealized GABAergic synapse, because there are several types of GABAergic synapses or because there are a number of subserving process that regulate GABAergic function. Because of these uncertainties, in our laboratory we evaluate the action of drugs on GABAergic transmission by measuring in vivo changes of the relative turnover rates of GABA in various brain nuclei (16).

There are a number of problems to be resolved before one can estimate the in vivo turnover rate of GABA. In addition to the usual problems encountered in the measurement of the in vivo turnover with other neurotransmitters, the estimation of GABA turnover involves specific problems: 1) glutamic acid, the immediate precursor of GABA, is an ubiquitous metabolite and a putative excitatory neurotransmitter, hence in certain tissue the dual function of glutamate may create problems; 2) the GABA metabolites can be recycled to form glutamic acid and GABA; 3) the decline in GABA content below certain levels causes convulsions, hence the use of perturbation of the steady state by injecting blockers of GABA synthesis is not a convenient tool to evaluate the turnover rate of GABA. The best available method to measure GABA turnover in vivo, is the constant rate of intravenous infusion with glucose labeled with the stable isotope ^{13}C and the change with time of the ^{13}C incorporated into glutamate and GABA (17). From the rate of change of the percent of incorporation of the label into the precursor and into the product, the GABA turnover can be estimated. Experience has shown that the areas which contain an abundant innervation with glutamatergic neurons represent a problem because after a few minutes of glucose infusion the percent of ^{13}C incorporation into GABA is greater than that in glutamate (17); thereby, invalidating a fundamental principle of precursor product relationship. It appears that the glutamate that functions as a neurotransmitter has a turnover rate slower than the glutamate that functions as a precursor, but the pool of the transmitter glutamate is larger than that of the glutamate that functions as a precursor of GABA. The pool size of glutamate functioning as the precursor of GABA in brain areas where numerous glutamatergic neurons are present, must represent only a small proportion of the total glutamate pool. The abnormal accumulation of the label in the GABA pool in tissues that have a large pool of glutamate functioning as a transmitter, can be minimized by increasing the rate of ^{13}C-glucose infusion and by killing the animals at short time intervals after the beginning of the infusion. Using this isotopic method, we have compared the turnover rate of GABA in various brain nuclei of rats given diazepam and muscimol. As shown in Fig. 1 muscimol and diazepam change the turnover of GABA only in some brain areas but the profile of the site of action is similar for the two drugs. This suggests that like muscimol also diazepam slows the turnover of GABA in those nuclei where the feedback regulation involves the presence of GABAergic synapses. This information can be interpreted to suggest that diazepam fails to act on presynaptic sites but can influence the turnover rate of GABA by an action on postsynaptic receptors (16).

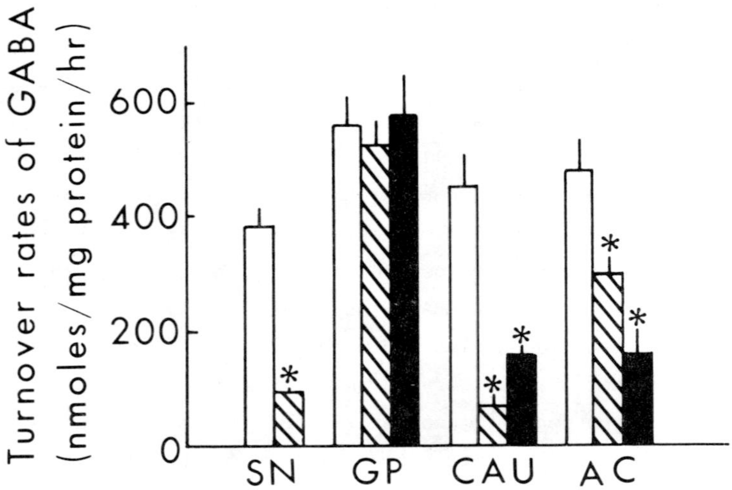

FIG. 1. Effects of muscimol and diazepam on GABA turnover rates in substantia nigra (SN), globus pallidus (GP), nucleus caudatus (CAU), and nucleus accumbens (AC). Muscimol (1.0 mg/kg, i.v.) was injected 40 min before beginning the infusion of ^{13}C-glucose. Diazepam (1.0 mg/kg, i.p.) injected 17 min before the killing. The ^{13}C-glucose infusion time and the killing times with respect to glucose infusion were the same (16). *$P<0.02$. ☐ Saline; ■ muscimol; ▨ diazepam (16).

GABA receptor regulation: Since the evidence discussed above excluded a presynaptic action of the benzodiazepines and indicated the possibility of an action of these drugs on GABA receptors, it became of interest to investigate whether benzodiazepines could mimic a specific neuromeodulator of GABA synapses. Enna and Snyder (18,19) have shown that fresh crude synaptic membranes prepared from mammalian brain, contained a significant number of binding sites for GABA, which had an affinity of about 200 to 300 nM for this ligand. They also reported that by freezing and thawing the crude synaptic membranes and by treating them with Triton X-100 (0.05%) at 25° to 30° for 15 minutes the number of binding sites increased by an extent greater than the change in protein specific activity due to a loss of membrane constituents as a result of the above mentioned manipulations. Moreover, also the quality of the binding was modified by the treatment. Two populations of binding sites could be distinguished, one with high affinity (20 to 30 nM) and one with low affinity (200 to 300 nM). Enna and Snyder (13) recommended that the preparation with two populations of binding sites was probably the one that was representative of the situation in vivo.

TABLE 1. Actions of Benzodiazepines on the Characteristics of GABA Binding Sites in Crude Synaptic Membrane (CSM) Preparations from Brain Cortex

	Specifically Bound (M) GABA							
	Fresh CSM				Frozen + Triton X-100 CSM			
Addition	Low Affinity		High Affinity		Low Affinity		High Affinity	
	Kd	Bmax	Kd	Bmax	Kd	Bmax	Kd	Bmax
Diazepam (10^{-8}M)	200	2.8	80	0.45	136	4.6	16	0.90
Diazepam (10^{-7}M)	180	3.2	70	0.55	140	5.1	18	0.85
None	220	2.5	ND	ND	130	4.9	15	0.75

ND = not detectable; Kd = nM; Bmax = pmole/mg protein. For details in membrane preparation see (20,21).

As shown in Table 1 when diazepam was added to fresh CSM it caused the appearance of high affinity binding sites that are normally absent in this preparation, in contrast, when diazepam was added to the frozen Triton X-100 membranes, it caused no change in the kinetic parameters of low affinity sites for GABA binding. Though the change caused by the benzodiazepines was marginal and smaller than that caused by repeated washings and freezing plus thawing, it was in the same direction.

TABLE 2. Inhibitors of High Affinity GABA Binding Present in Brain Homogenates

	Peak 1	Peak 2	GABA
Molecular Weight	15,000	400-1800	103
Thermostability	No	Yes	Yes
Tryptic Digestion	Yes	No	No
Pronase Digestion	Yes	No	No
Binds GABA	No	Yes	--
Binds BZD	No	Yes	--
Inhibits GABA Binding	Yes	Yes	Yes
Inhibits BZD Binding	Yes	Yes	Facilitates

The data were interpreted to indicate that the washing of the membranes was eliminating a modulator that inhibits the high affinity binding sites for GABA. After having attempted to evaluate the validity of this interpretation and having obtained a positive reinforcement from pilot experiments in this direction we proceeded in a thorough investigation of the various factors that can be solubilized from brain membranes which cause a change in the high affinity GABA binding to crude synaptic membrane preparations. The data reported in Table 2 summarize our present understanding of the phenomenon.

Some of the changes seen after washing the membranes are due to GABA. This contaminant can be eliminated from the supernatant of washed membranes by gel filtration in Biogel P-2 columns. Table 2 shows that inhibition of GABA binding due to GABA can be differentiated from the regulatory factor (Peak 1 of Table 2) that we have termed GABA-modulin (22) by 5 criteria: 1) molecular weight, 2) tryptic digestion, 3) pronase digestion, 4) thermostability and 5) effect on benzodiazepine binding. The latter is facilitated by GABA and inhibited by Peak 2. We are presently intrigued by another inhibitory factor (Peak 2 of Table 2) which we think is a peptide though it is not metabolized by trypsin and pronase. The factor is thermostable, is produced in large amounts during membrane manipulations (extraction with Triton X-100 0.05%) but binds GABA and benzodiazepines quite avidly. This factor appears to be produced during tryptic and pronase digestion of high molecular weight material extracted from brain membrane. This fact and the high binding capacity for GABA and benzodiazepines, makes this material of dubious physiological significance. We are presently attempting to complete the purification of peak 1 in order to prepare an antibody to proceed to a radioimmunoassay of the regulatory protein termed "GABA-modulin". While the total activity of the inhibitors of high affinity GABA binding is comspicuous, the amount of material responsible for peak 1 activity is small and therefore its purification is time consuming and difficult. The peak 1 inhibits GABA binding non competitively while it inhibits high affinity benzodiazepine binding competitively. Preliminary evidence appears to suggest that benzodiazepines displace the inhbitor from its binding site. Hence benzodiazepines could be mimicking the endogenous natural agonist that modulates the high affinity GABA receptors via an interaction with "GABA modulin" the latter appear to act on GABA binding allosterically. A working hypothesis which we are currently pursuing is that phosphorylation of certain sites increases the high affinity binding of GABA, in this scheme GABA-modulin would some how inhibit this phosphorylation.

Significance of high affinity GABA binding: The work discussed above emphasizes that the regulation of the high affinity site for GABA binding is a crucial point for the regulation of its physiological role in GABAergic synapses. But it is worth considering which is the evidence in support of this view. When a few years ago we first asked this question the evidence in support of the functional importance of high affinity GABA binding was inexistent. Now we can just mention two lines of independent evidence that support a role of high affinity GABA binding in GABAergic synaptic function. The first line comes from studies of substantia nigra denervation which were carried out in our (23) and in another laboratory (24). The terminals of the long axon GABAergic pathway that connects the nucleus caudatus to the pars reticulata of the substantia nigra presents a site for high density of GABAergic synapses. GABAergic synapses can be detected in the substantia nigra and GABA receptors of high and low affinity can be detected in frozen Triton X-100 treated membrane preparations prepared from this brain regions (23). The Bmax of GABA receptor has been reported to increase in the substantia nigra of patients with Huntington's chorea (25) or in rat substantia nigra after lesions of striatal nigral projections produced by intrastriatal injections of kainic acid (24). Having in mind to find a support for the view that the functional GABA receptors are those that are regulated by "GABA-modulin", it was studied whether following substantia nigra denervation there is a selective increase in the number of high or low affinity GABA receptors or whether both types of receptors change simultaneously (23). In rat brain the ratio of high and low affinity binding sites for GABA ranges from 0.14 in cerebellum to 1.3 in substantia nigra (23). Also the substantia nigra from human brain contains a high percentage of high affinity GABA receptor binding sites (26). Since the substantia nigra is one of the brain regions with the highest percentage of GABA synapses, we can observe that the density of low affinity GABA binding sites is small in substantia nigra suggesting that the high affinity receptor regulated by GABA-modulin are the ones that relate to GABAergic transmission. This is further substantiated by the finding that in substantia nigra after GABA receptor denervation, the density of low affinity binding sites fails to change whereas that of high affinity binding sites selectively increases by more than 2 fold (23).

The second line of evidence concerns the doses of GABA mimetics that are needed to regulate Cl^- ionophores located in cell membranes. A cloned neuroblastoma cells (NB_{2a}) possess Cl^- ionophores which can be opened by stimulation of GABA receptors. The doses of GABA and muscimol that increase Cl^- fluxes are of the order of magnitude of those required to saturate high affinity binding sites for GABA (this laboratory unpublished).

Function and supramolecular organization of GABA receptors and benzodiazepine action

We have discussed above the necessity of a specific molecular interaction to regulate the availability of high affinity GABA receptors and to mediate the action of benzodiazepines. However this inference were derived from studies on crude synaptic membrane preparations, where artefactual contamination are possible (27). We have investigated whether the NB_{2a} neuroblastoma line, which as mentioned above contains GABA receptors regulating Cl^- ion fluxes also contains "GABA modulin" or high and low affinity GABA receptors and high affinity benzodiazepine binding sites (22). These cells contain all the necessary features which we have attributed to the supramolecular organization of GABA receptors. We are presently identifying the molecular nature of the regulatory protein that is present in these membranes and assessing the functional role of benzodiazepine receptor in this molecular organization. Preliminary results indicate that benzo diazepines fail to facilitate Cl^- fluxes but in presence of inactive concentratio of GABA receptor agonists they can cause a facilitation of their action on Cl^- fluxes.

CONCLUSIONS

The experimental evidence available is consistent with the view that high affinity benzodiazepine receptors are an integral part of GABA receptor units. Their function is that of modulating availability of high affinity GABA binding sites via a competition with an endogenous inhibitory protein. In displacing this allosteric regulator of GABA binding benzodiazepines may be mimicking an endogenous "cotransmitter". However the molecular nature of this endogenous modulator is not known at this time.

REFERENCES

1. Hokfelt, T., Lundberg, J. M., Schultzberg, M., Johansson, O., Ljungdahl, A. and Rehfeld, J. (1980) Adv. in Biochem. Psychopharmacol. 22, in press.
2. Kumakura, K., Guidotti, A., Yang, H.-Y. T., Saiani, L. and Costa, E. (1980) Adv. in Biochem. Psychopharmacol. 22, in press.
3. Kumakura, K., Guidotti, A. and Costa, E. (1980) Nature 283, 489-492.
4. Dawson, D., McLawhon, R. and Miller, R. J. (1980) J. Biol. Chem. 255, 128-137.
5. Costa, E., Guidotti, A. and Toffano, G. (1978) Br. J. Pyschiatry 133, 239-248.
6. Costa, E., Guidotti, A., Mao, C. C. and Suria, A. (1975) Life Sci. 17, 167-186.

7. Haefely, W. E. (1978) In: Psychopharmacology: A Generation of Progress, edited by M. A. Lipton, A. Di Mascio and K. F. Killam, p. 1359, Raven Press, New York.

8. Guidotti, A. (1978) In: Psychopharmacology: A Generation of Progress, edited by M. A. Lipton, A. Di Mascio and K. F. Killam, p. 1349, Raven Press, New York.

9. Schmidt, R. F., Vogel, M. E. and Zimmerman, M. (1967) Naunyn Schmiedebergs Arch. Pharmacol. 258, 69.

10. Squires, R. F. and Braestrup, C. (1977) Nature 266, 732.

11. Mohler, H. and Okada, T. (1977) Science 198, 849.

12. Tallman, J. F., Thomas, J. W. and Gallger, D. (1978) Nature 274, 383.

13. Karobath, M., Placheta, P., Lippitsch, M. and Krogsgaard-Larsen, P. (1979) Nature 278, 749.

14. Roberts, E., Chase, T. N. and Tower, A. B., editors (1976): GABA in Nervous System Function. Raven Press, New York.

15. Krogsgaard-Larsen, P., Schael-Kruger, J. and Kopod, H., editors (1979) GABA-Neurotransmitters: Pharmacochemical, Biochemical and Pharamcological Aspects. Munksgaard, Copenhagen.

16. Mao, C. C. and Costa, E. (1978) In: Psychopharmacology: A Generation of Progress, edited by M. A. Lipton, A. Di Mascio and K. F. Killam, p. 307, Raven Press, New York.

17. Bertilsson, L., Mao, C. C. and Costa, E. (1977) J. Pharmacol. Exp. Ther. 200, 277.

18. Enna, S. J. and Snyder, S. H. (1975) Brain Res. 100, 81.

19. Enna, S. J. and Snyder, S. H. (1977) Mol. Pharmacol. 13, 442.

20. Toffano, G., Guidotti, A. and Costa, E. (1978) Proc. Natl. Acad. Sci. USA 75, 4024.

21. Costa, E., Guidotti, A. and Toffano, G. (1978) Br. J. Psych. 133, 239.

22. Baraldi, M., Guidotti, A., Schwartz, J. P. and Costa, E. (1979) Science 205, 821.

23. Guidotti, A., Gale, K., Suria, A. and Toffano, G. (1979) Brain Res. 172, 566.

24. Washington, J. L. and Cross, A. J. (1978) Nature 276, 618.

25. Enna, S. J., Bennett, J. P., Bylund, D. B., Snyder, S. H., Bird, E. D. and Iversen, L. L. (1976) Brain Res. 116, 531.

26. Olsen, R. W., Ness, P. C. and Tourtellotte, W. W. (1978) NINCDS Symposium on Huntington's Disease, San Diego, Calif., Nov. 16-18.

27. Guidotti, A., Toffano, G. and Costa, E. (1978) Nature 257, 553.

Neurotransmitters and their Receptors
Edited by U.Z. Littauer, Y. Dudai, I. Silman,
V.I. Teichberg and Z. Vogel

Modulation of Brain Gaba/Benzodiazepine Receptor Complex by the Pyrazolopyridines SQ 20009 and SQ 65396

Manfred Karobath, Porntip Supavilai, Peter Placheta* and Werner Sieghart,
Department of Biochemical Psychiatry and Institute of Pharmacology,*
University of Vienna, Vienna, Austria.

ABSTRACT

When brain membranes are incubated with ^{3}H-flunitrazepam and irradiated with UV-light, this radiolabeled benzodiazepine binds irreversibly to one major protein band with an apparent MW of 51,000 daltons (P_{51}) in cerebellum. In other brain regions P_{51} as well as additional protein bands are labeled by ^{3}H-flunitrazepam. Because of this apparent molecular heterogeneity of benzodiazepine receptors in other brain regions in this study cerebellar membranes were used for the investigation of benzodiazepine receptor binding. Binding of ^{3}H-flunitrazepam to cerebellar membranes can be modulated by GABA and other structural analogues including taurine. In addition, this binding is modulated by SQ 20009 and SQ 65396, two pyrazolopyridines with anxiolytic properties. Modulation of ^{3}H-flunitrazepam binding by these drugs is complex. Firstly, these drugs have a direct chloride ion-dependent stimulatory effect on ^{3}H-flunitrazepam binding which in turn appears to be modulated by the associated GABA receptor. Secondly, SQ 20009 has indirect effects on benzodiazepine receptor binding since it enhances the potency of GABA and taurine to stimulate ^{3}H-flunitrazepam binding. This second effect is caused mainly by an increase of the apparent affinity of GABA and taurine to stimulate ^{3}H-flunitrazepam binding.

In addition to the effects of SQ 20009 and SQ 65396 on benzodiazepine receptor binding, these drugs can also modulate GABA receptor binding. Both compounds increase ^{3}H-GABA or ^{3}H-muscimol binding more than 2-fold. This modulation is partially chloride ion-dependent, sensitive to Triton-X100 treatment and mediated through an increase of the apparent number of GABA binding sites. The results are compatible with a functional association between Na^{+}-independent GABA binding sites and the benzodiazepine receptor.

INTRODUCTION

Binding of benzodiazepines to membranes from mammalian brain can be enhanced by GABA or GABA-like drugs (1,2). Furthermore, there is some indication that SQ 20009 (1-ethyl-4-(isopropylidenehydrazino)-1H-pyrazolo-

[3,4-b] pyridine-5-carboxylic acid, ethyl ester, hydrochloride) and SQ 65396 (4-(butylamino)-1-ethyl-1H-pyrazolo[3,4-b]pyridine-5-carboxylic acid, ethyl ester), two new pyrazolopyridines with anxiolytic effects in animal test systems (3,4) can stimulate benzodiazepine receptor binding (4,5). This effect is chloride ion-dependent and inhibited by picrotoxin (6). To further characterize benzodiazepine receptor binding we investigated the effects of SQ 20009 and SQ 65396 and their interaction with GABA-like drugs as modulators of ^{3}H-flunitrazepam binding. In addition, the effects of SQ 20009 and SQ 65396 on Na^+-independent ^{3}H-GABA binding were investigated.

METHODS

Reversible ^{3}H-flunitrazepam binding and Na^+-independent ^{3}H-GABA or ^{3}H-muscimol binding was determined as described previously (7). Irreversible binding was performed by irradiation of membranes in the presence of ^{3}H-flunitrazepam with UV-light (8,9). Membrane proteins were solubilized and separated by electrophoresis on 10 % SDS-polyacrylamide slab gels (10). Proteins were stained, destained and fluorography was performed as described (11).

RESULTS

MOLECULAR HETEROGENEITY OF BENZODIAZEPINE RECEPTORS

Irreversible benzodiazepine binding was investigated in several regions of the rat brain. As can be seen in fig. 1, in cerebellum ^{3}H-flunitrazepam irreversibly binds to a single protein with an apparent molecular weight of 51,000 daltons (P_{51}). This P_{51} protein is found in the other examined brain regions too, and it seems to be identical to the labeled benzodiazepine receptor described previously (8). In other brain regions additional protein bands with apparent molecular weights of 55,000 (P_{55}), and 59,000 (P_{59}) are labeled with variable intensity (fig. 1). No labeling of protein bands was visible in incubations where 2 μM unlabeled diazepam was present during incubation and irradiation of membranes.

Control experiments suggest that these labeled proteins are not derived by differential degradation of a higher molecular weight

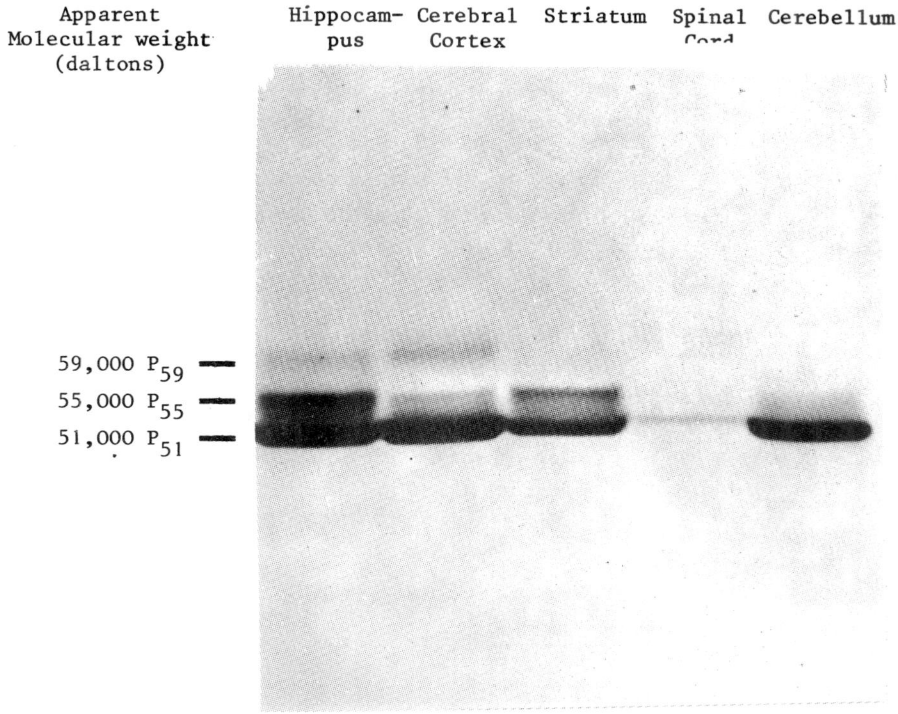

Figure 1: Fluorography, showing regional distribution of irreversible ^{3}H-flunitrazepam binding in rat brain.

Membranes from several rat brain regions derived from 6 mg tissue wet weight were incubated with 10 nM ^{3}H-flunitrazepam for 90 min at 0° C in 50 mM Tris-citrate buffer pH 7.1 and 150 mM NaCl. Samples were subsequently irradiated with UV-light (9) and subjected to electrophoresis on 10 % SDS-polyacrylamide slab gels and fluorography (11). All radioactive bands disappeared after treatment of the samples with pronase suggesting that the bands represent proteins. Apparent molecular weights were determined by calibrating the gel with standard proteins of known molecular weight (data not shown).

protein and that they are GABA receptor-associated benzodiazepine receptor sites or parts thereof which possess different pharmacological properties (Sieghart and Karobath, submitted for publication). In view of this regional molecular heterogeneity of benzodiazepine binding proteins subsequent pharmacological studies of benzodiazepine receptor binding were performed with cerebellar membranes which exhibit the least molecular heterogeneity and contain predominantly the P_{51} receptor protein.

MODULATION OF REVERSIBLE BENZODIAZEPINE RECEPTOR BINDING BY SQ 20009 AND SQ 65396

Specific reversible ^{3}H-flunitrazepam binding to cerebellar membranes was enhanced by SQ 20009 and by SQ 65396 in a concentration-dependent manner with half-maximal stimulation at 2 µM SQ 20009 and at 0.8 µM SQ 65396 (fig. 2). Maximal enhancement of ^{3}H-flunitrazepam binding was

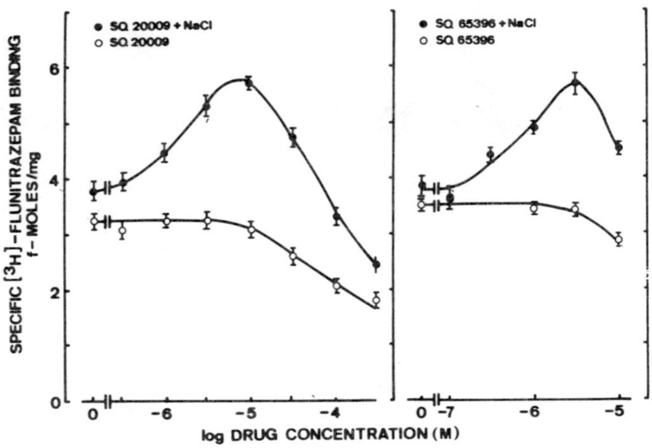

Figure 2: Concentration-effect curves of SQ 20009 and SQ 65396 on the binding of 0.25 nM ^{3}H-flunitrazepam to rat cerebellar membranes in the presence or absence of 150 mM NaCl.

observed at approximately 10 µM SQ 20009 and 3 µM SQ 65396 and in higher concentrations of both compounds stimulation was inhibited. In contrast, SQ 20006 (1-ethyl-4-hydrazino-1H-pyrazolo [3,4-b] pyridine-5-carboxylic acid, ethyl ester, hydrochloride), a structural analogue without CNS activity, did not stimulate but inhibited binding in higher concentrations (3 µM) (data not shown). SQ 20009 and SQ 65396 enhanced ^{3}H-flunitrazepam binding by increasing the affinity of the binding sites (data not shown). The effect of these drugs was completely dependent on the presence of chloride ions. Thus, in the absence of chloride, concentrations of SQ 20009 and SQ 65396 up to 1 µM had no effect, and in higher concentrations inhibition of ^{3}H-flunitrazepam binding was observed (fig. 2). Other anions such as bromide and iodide, but not fluoride, phosphate, acetate or sulfate could substitute for chloride (data not shown).

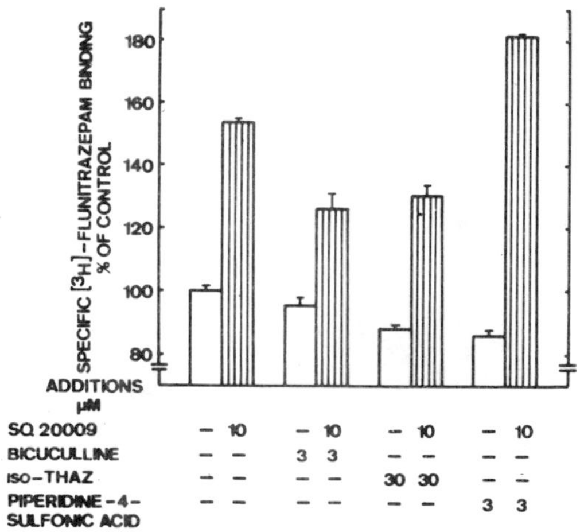

Figure 3: Stimulation of the specific binding of 0.25 nM ^{3}H-flunitrazepam to cerebellar membranes by SQ 20009 and its modulation by drugs which act on the GABA receptor.

Stimulation of specific ^{3}H-flunitrazepam binding by SQ 20009 was modulated by drugs which influence GABA receptor binding (fig. 3). Thus, the effect of SQ 20009 on ^{3}H-flunitrazepam binding was enhanced by the GABA-mimetic compound (12) piperidine-4-sulfonic acid (PSA), and was depressed by bicuculline. Iso-THAZ (5,6,7,8-tetrahydroisoxazolo[3,4-d] azepin-3-ol), a new structural analogue of GABA which *in vivo* exhibits weak GABA antagonist properties and which interferes with Na^+-independent ^{3}H-GABA binding with low potency (13), depressed SQ 20009-stimulated ^{3}H-flunitrazepam binding. All three drugs slightly depressed unstimulated ^{3}H-flunitrazepam binding.

In addition to this direct halide ion-sensitive stimulation of ^{3}H-flunitrazepam binding by SQ 20009 and SQ 65396, these drugs modulated GABA stimulation of benzodiazepine receptor binding. Thus, SQ 20009 enhanced the effect of GABA by decreasing GABA concentrations necessary for half-maximal stimulation of ^{3}H-flunitrazepam binding (fig. 4a). This effect was observed in chloride-free incubation media (fig. 4b) and was enhanced in the presence of chloride ions. Chloride alone had no significant effect on the EC_{50} value for stimulation of ^{3}H-flunitrazepam binding by GABA.

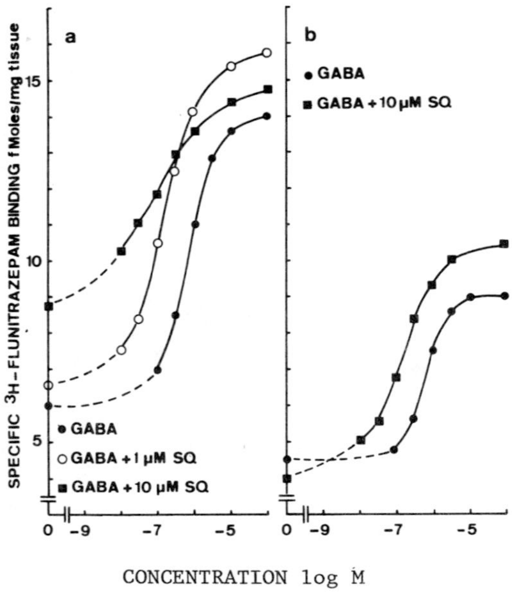

Figure 4: Effect of SQ 20009 and chloride ions on the stimulation of specific binding of 0.25 nM ^{3}H-flunitrazepam to rat cerebellar membranes by GABA. In "a" 150 mM NaCl was present, but not in "b".

Taurine, a structural analogue of GABA, seems to be a partial agonist at the GABA recognition site which mediates the stimulation of benzodiazepine receptor binding. Thus, taurine enhanced ^{3}H-flunitrazepam binding in high concentrations, but the maximal stimulation obtained was less than that observed with GABA (data not shown). This effect was blocked by bicuculline-methiodide. However, taurine in high concentrations inhibited GABA stimulation of ^{3}H-flunitrazepam binding (data not shown). 1 μM SQ 65396 potentiated the effect of taurine by decreasing taurine concentrations necessary for half-maximal stimulation of ^{3}H-flunitrazepam binding from 308 μM to 130 μM. In addition, in the presence of SQ 65396 the maximal stimulation of ^{3}H-flunitrazepam binding by taurine was enhanced and reached approximately those values which were observed with saturating concentrations of GABA alone (data not shown).

MODULATION OF GABA RECEPTOR BINDING BY SQ 20009 AND SQ 65396

For these experiments membranes from rat cerebral cortex were used since the modulation of GABA receptor binding was most pronounced in this brain region. Incubation of membranes with either SQ 20009 or SQ 65396 (30 min at 0° C) markedly increased GABA receptor binding. This effect was concentration-dependent (EC_{50} values: 3 μM and 5 uM for SQ 20009 and SQ 65396, respectively) and demonstrable with Na^+-independent ^3H-GABA binding (fig. 5a) as well as ^3H-muscimol binding (data not shown) assays. Maximal increase of ^3H-GABA or ^3H-muscimol binding was more than 2-fold with either drug used. Pretreatment of the membranes with the detergent Triton-X100, followed by washing, markedly attenuated the effect of SQ 20009 (and SQ 65396) on Na^+-independent ^3H-GABA binding. SQ 20006, the structural analogue which lacks CNS activity in animal models, did not affect ^3H-GABA binding in concentrations up to 1 mM.

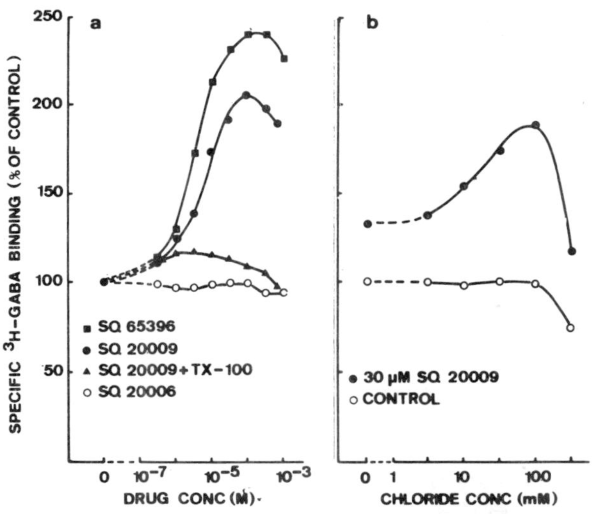

Figure 5: Effect of SQ 20009 and SQ 65396 on Na^+-independent ^3H-GABA binding.

Rat cerebral cortex membranes (2.5 mg tissue) were used at 5 nM ^3H-GABA. a. Concentration-effect curves of SQ-compounds in the presence of 100 mM chloride. "TX-100" indicates pretreatment with 0.05 % Triton-X100 (30 min at 37° C). b. Effect of chloride on stimulation of ^3H-GABA binding by 30 μM SQ 20009.

The enhancement of GABA receptor binding was partially chloride dependent, as shown in fig. 5b. SQ 20009 at 30 μM increased Na^+-independent ^{3}H-GABA binding in the absence of chloride ions. Addition of chloride up to 100 mM further increased GABA receptor binding with an EC_{50} of about 30 mM chloride. At higher concentrations chloride inhibited the effect of SQ 20009. In contrast, there was no stimulation of ^{3}H-GABA binding by chloride in the absence of SQ 20009. Similar results were obtained with SQ 65396 (data not shown).

The *in vitro* modulation of GABA receptor binding by SQ 20009 and SQ 65396 was reversible since incubation with either compound, subsequent washing and resuspension of the membranes in drug-free buffer abolished the increase of GABA receptor binding.

Kinetic analysis of ^{3}H-muscimol binding demonstrated that SQ 20009 as well as SQ 65396 increased the apparent number of GABA binding sites without significantly affecting the affinity for the ligand (table).

Effect of SQ 65396 and chloride on ^{3}H-muscimol binding

Addition	B_{max} (pmoles/g tissue weight)	K_d (nM)
none	2.7	8.4
30 μM SQ 65396	4.2	8.4
30 μM SQ 65396 + 100 mM Cl'	6.1	8.4

B_{max} and K_d were determined by Scatchard analysis of the binding of ^{3}H-muscimol (0.5 - 50 nM, 30 min at 0° C) to rat cortex membranes.

DISCUSSION

Several lines of evidence suggest the existence of more than one type of benzodiazepine receptor. Thus, thermal inactivation experiments and pharmacological studies with the novel triazolopyridazine CL 218 872 have led to the concept that in brain at least two distinct benzodiazepine receptors exist (14). We presently report evidence for a molecula heterogeneity of benzodiazepine receptors in rat brain. Since the differences in the molecular composition could possibly be related to functional and pharmacological differences of the benzodiazepine binding sites, it is reasonable to study benzodiazepine receptor binding under conditions where only one type of receptor protein is examined. Therefore in this study we used cerebellar membranes in which binding of ^{3}H-flunitrazepam occurs mainly to the P_{51} benzodiazepine binding protein.

An important dynamic property of benzodiazepine receptor binding is the modulation by GABA and GABA-like compounds which indicates a functional link between GABA receptors and benzodiazepine receptors (1,2). The present results suggest that this GABA/benzodiazepine receptor complex contains an additional modulatory site upon which SQ 20009 and SQ 65396 act and which differs pharmacologically from the GABA recognition site linked to the benzodiazepine receptor. The pharmacological differences include: (i) SQ 20009-induced stimulation of ^{3}H-flunitrazepam binding is absolutely dependent on chloride, bromide or iodide ions whereas GABA-induced stimulation is only partially dependent on the presence of these ions; (ii) SQ 20009-induced stimulation is potentiated by PSA, whereas GABA-induced stimulation of benzodiazepine receptor binding is inhibited by PSA (15).

In addition to these <u>direct</u> effects of SQ 20009 on benzodiazepine receptor binding which occur in the absence of GABA and GABA agonists, there are <u>indirect</u> effects which comprise a partially halide ion-dependent sensitization of the GABA/benzodiazepine receptor complex towards GABA and its analogues.

In order to better understand the mechanism by which SQ 20009 and SQ 65396 enhance GABA stimulation of benzodiazepine receptor binding, we investigated their actions on Na^+-independent GABA binding. It was interesting to note that GABA receptor binding to brain membranes was enhanced by these drugs via an increase of the apparent number of GABA binding sites. Of all brain regions studied this effect was most pronounced in cerebral cortex; therefore this tissue was thoroughly investigated. However, parallel experiments with cerebellar membranes showed qualitatively similar results. There were striking similarities between the effects of the SQ-compounds as modulators of GABA-stimulation of benzodiazepine receptor binding and of GABA receptor binding: (i) SQ 20009 and SQ 65396 which are CNS active compounds in animals, but not their centrally inactive congener SQ 20006, displayed modulatory effects on both benzodiazepine and GABA receptor bindings; (ii) these modulations were in part dependent on halide ions and sensitive to treatment with Triton-X100; (iii) the magnitude of the effect of SQ 20009 on Na^+-independent GABA binding appeared to parallel the regional distribution of benzodiazepine receptors more closely than that of GABA receptors (Placheta and Karobath, submitted for publication). Thus, the SQ-compounds may enhance the sensitivity of the GABA/ benzodiazepine receptor complex by reversibly unmasking Na^+-independent GABA binding sites. The present results are compatible with the hypothesis of a GABA receptor complex which consists of a recognition site for the neurotransmitter GABA, two drug receptors (for benzodiazepines and SQ-compounds) and the associated ion conductance mechanisms.

Acknowledgements: We thank Martina Scherer and Margit Lippitsch for excellent technical assistance, Eva Kotai for drawing the graphs and Jutta Reisenhofer for preparation of the manuscript. We thank S. J. Lucania for the donation of SQ 65396, SQ 20009 and SQ 20006 and P. Krogsgaard-Larsen for the gift of PSA and iso-THAZ. This work was supported by "Fonds zur Förderung der wissenschaftlichen Forschung in Österreich".

REFERENCES

1. Karobath, M., and Sperk, G., Proc. natn. Acad. Sci. USA, 76, 1004 (1979)
2. Tallman, J. F., Thomas, J. W., and Gallager, D. W., Nature 274, 383 (1978)
3. Beer, B., Chasin, M., Clody, D. E., Vogel, J. R., and Horovitz, Z. P Science 176, 428 (1972)
4. Beer, B., Klepner, C. A., Lippa, A. S., and Squires, R., Pharmacol. Biochem. Behav. 9, 849 (1978)
5. Williams, M., and Risley, E. A., Life Sci. 24, 833 (1979)
6. Supavilai, P., and Karobath, M., Europ. J. Pharmacol. 60, 111 (1979)
7. Placheta, P., and Karobath, M., Brain Res. 178, 580 (1979)
8. Möhler, H., Battersby, M. K., and Richards, J. G., Proc. natn. Acad. Sci. USA, in press (1980)
9. Battersby, M. K., Richards, J. G., and Möhler, H., Europ. J. Pharmac 57, 277 (1979)
10. Laskey, R. A., and Mills, A. D., Europ. J. Biochem. 56, 335 (1975)
11. Krueger, B. K., Forn, J., and Greengard, P., J. biol. Chem. 252, 2764 (1977)
12. Krogsgaard-Larsen, P., Falch, E., Schousboe, A., Curtis, D. R., and Lodge, D., J. Neurochem., in press (1980)
13. Arnt, J., and Krogsgaard-Larsen, P., Brain Res. 177, 395 (1979)
14. Klepner, C. A., Lippa, A. S., Benson, D. F., Sano, M. C., and Beer, B., Pharmacol. Biochem. Behav. 11, 457 (1979)
15. Braestrup, C., Nielsen, M., Krogsgaard-Larsen, P., and Falch, E., Nature, 280, 331 (1979)

Neurotransmitters and their Receptors
Edited by U.Z. Littauer, Y. Dudai, I. Silman,
V.I. Teichberg and Z. Vogel

Solubilization of a Benzodiazepine Receptor from Calf Cortex

Rivka Sherman-Gold and Yadin Dudai

Department of Neurobiology, The Weizmann Institute of Science, Rehovot, Israel.

ABSTRACT

A benzodiazepine-binding macromolecule has been solubilized from calf cortex by the use of a detergent, sodium deoxycholate (DOC). The solubilized receptor retained its high affinity for [^{3}H]flunitrazepam ([^{3}H]FNZ). The order of potency of various drugs, including benzodiazepines and xanthine derivatives, was also not altered. The ability of GABA to increase the affinity of the receptor for benzodiazepines was retained in the DOC-solubilized receptor although the magnitude of the effect was smaller than in the particulate state. The solubilized receptor displayed a sedimentation coefficient of about 11S. Photoaffinity labeling of a particulate preparation with [^{3}H]FNZ followed by SDS-polyacrylamide gel electrophoresis revealed a component with a molecular weight of about 50 K. Our data suggest that the benzodiazepine receptor is a multimer of about 200 K daltons, bearing distinct sites for benzodiazepines and GABA and composed of several subunits of which at least part are of about 50 K daltons.

INTRODUCTION

Mammalian brain contains specific receptors for benzodiazepines (1,2), which appear to be associated with GABAergic mechanisms (3,4). These receptors presumably mediate the potent pharmacological action of the benzodiazepines *in vivo* (5). Calf cortex is a rich source of benzodiazepine receptors and may therefore serve as a suitable tissue for studying their molecular properties (6,7,8). In the following, we report the solubilization of benzodiazepine receptors from calf cortex and describe some of their properties.

MATERIALS AND METHODS

Fresh calf brain was obtained from a local slaughterhouse. The entire cortex was removed, cut into cubes and homogenized (20% W/V) in ice-cold 0.32 M sucrose in a Sorvall Omni-Mix. The homogenate was centrifuged at

650Xg for 10 min. The pellet was discarded and the supernatant collected and frozen at -70°C. For preparation of a crude membrane fraction, the frozen homogenate was thawed, homogenized in 1:1 v/v of ice cold 0.32M sucrose in a glass-Teflon homogenizer and centrifuged at 30,000Xg for 30 min. The supernatant was discarded and the pellet was rehomogenized in double-distilled water, frozen for approximately 2 hr at -20°C, thawed and centrifuged again at 30,000Xg for 30 min. The resulting pellet was homogenized in a 0.06M NaCl, 0.025M Tris-Cl, pH 7.4 (=buffer 1) and centrifuged again as above. The latter procedure was repeated and the resulting pellet was homogenized in the original homogenate volume, to yield a crude membrane preparation (=M).

For preparation of the solubilized receptor, 2% of sodium deoxycholate (DOC) in buffer 1 was added to an aliquot of the M preparation to a final concentration of 0.5% DOC. The mixture was briefly homogenized and incubated with stirring at 4°C for 1 hr, followed by centrifugation at 100,000Xg for 1 hr. The resulting supernatant was referred to as the solubilized preparation.

Binding of [^{3}H]FNZ (84.3 Ci/mmol, New England Nuclear) to the solubilized preparation was determined as follows: Aliquots of receptor preparation were incubated at 0°C and the reaction was started by addition of [^{3}H]FNZ. The reaction was terminated after 60 min by addition of ice-cold 100% saturated, neutralized ammonium sulfate to a final concentration of 40% saturation, followed by rapid dilution with 2.5 ml ice-cold 40% saturated, neutralized ammonium sulfate and vacuum filtration on a glass fiber (GF/C) filter. The filter was than rapidly washed 3 times with 2.5 ml portions each of ice-cold 40% saturated neutralized ammonium sulfate, dried, and counted by liquid scintillation spectrophotometry. Specific binding was defined as total binding minus the binding observed in the presence of 10^{-5}M diazepam.

RESULTS AND DISCUSSION

In preliminary experiments we have determined the ability of various potential solubilizing agents to release [^{3}H]FNZ-binding sites from the particulate fraction (=M) into the high speed supernatant. The results are summarized in Table I. Several detergents were found effective. Nonionic detergents often yielded high blanks in the ammonium sulfate binding assay. DOC was reproducibly effective in solubilizing the

TABLE I: Effect of detergents and ions on the subcellular distribution of benzodiazepine receptors in calf cortex

Medium	M	$P_{100,000}$	$S_{100,000}$
Buffer	100	103	0
1% Triton X-100	70	76	13
1% NP40	103	64	22
1% Tween 80	74	103	0
1% Brij 35	114	124	0
1% Digitonin	92	66	3
0.5% DOC	118	37	35
1% DOC	76	44	32
1% Taurocholate	79	76	27
0.5% Tauro DOC	57	32	20
1% Cholate	62	55	3
0.1% SDS	102	85	2
1% NP40 + 0.5% DOC	99	43	40
2M NaCl	100	87	0
2M NaBr	21	29	0
2M $NaNO_3$	49	50	0
2M NaI	0	0	0
IM $NaClO_4$	0	0	0

Aliquots of a particulate preparation (=M) were incubated for 2 hr at 4°C with the appropriate detergent in Buffer 1 and then subjected to 100,000Xg centrifugation for 1 hr to yield a supernatant fraction (=$S_{100,000}$) and a pellet. The latter was resuspended in the original volume of the treated sample to yield $P_{100,000}$. The results are expressed as percent of total specific [^{3}H]FNZ bound in each fraction, where 100% is the binding level in M in the presence of Buffer 1 alone.

[^{3}H]FNZ-binding sites and did not markedly interfere with the assay under the conditions employed. This detergent was thus chosen for further work. Concentrations of 0.3% - 0.5% DOC were routinely used. Addition of 0.5M KCl was found to markedly stabilize the [^{3}H]FNZ-binding activity in the DOC-extracted preparation. Thus the number of [^{3}H]FNZ-binding sites in a DOC-solubilized preparation decreased when stored at 4°C with a half-life of about 30 hr in the absence of KCl and with a half-life of about 100 hr in the presence of KCl.

The solubilized preparation was found to contain a single-class of [^{3}H]FNZ-binding sites, with high affinity for [^{3}H]FNZ and other benzodiazepines (Table II). The order of potency of various benzodiazepines and other drugs in displacing [^{3}H]FNZ from the receptor was similar to that revealed in the particulate preparation (4,7). When assayed in parallel, the affinity of [^{3}H]FNZ-binding sites was consistently higher by about 30 - 40% in the presence than in the absence of 10^{-5}M GABA (Table II). This is a smaller effect than that induced by GABA in a particulate calf cortex preparation (4,7).

TABLE II: Affinity of various ligands for the DOC-solubilized benzodiazepine receptor.

Ligand	K, M
[^{3}H]FNZ	(1.5±0.2) x 10^{-9}
[^{3}H]FNZ+10^{-5}M GABA	(1.1±0.2) x 10^{-9*}
diazepam	(1.5±0.6) x 10^{-8}
chlorodiazepoxide	(6.8±0.8) x 10^{-7}
RO-5-4864	> 10^{-5}
IBMX	(1.6±0.2) x 10^{-4}
Theophylline	(5.9±0.7) x 10^{-4}
Inosine	(1.2±0.1) x 10^{-3}

The apparent K_d for [^{3}H]FNZ were calculated from Scatchard plots. Apparent K_i of other ligands were estimated from competition experiments as described in Ref. 7. Values are presented as mean ± SEM.

*Significantly different ($P < 0.05$) from the affinity of [^{3}H]FNZ in the absence of GABA, two-tailed t-test.

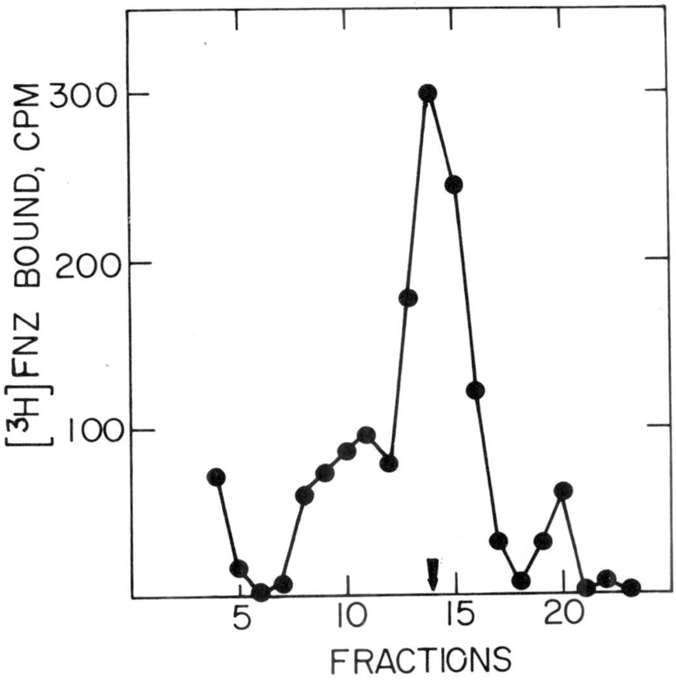

Fig. 1. Preparative sucrose gradient centrifugation of a DOC-solubilized calf cortex [^{3}H]FNZ receptor. A gradient of 5-20% sucrose in buffer 1 containing 0.2% DOC was layered on a 60% sucrose cushion. Centrifugation was carried out at 26,000 rpm for 17 hr in a SW27 rotor. Aliquots of each fraction were assayed for specific [^{3}H]FNZ-binding by the ammonium sulfate precipitation method. The bottom of the gradient is on the left hand side and the arrow indicates the position of catalase run as a marker.

The DOC-solubilized receptor displayed a major component of (10.9±0.4)S on sucrose gradient centrifugation (Fig. 1). Additional components with smaller size (e.g. 4S) or larger size (16-20S) were also often observed (Fig. 1). Aliquots isolated from the ∿ 11S peak again displayed a high-affinity for [^{3}H]FNZ and a GABA-induced increase in binding.

SDS-polyacrylamide gel electrophoresis of an aliquot of particulate calf-cortex preparation after photoaffinity labeling with [^{3}H]FNZ (9) revealed a major polypeptide of (52±2)K in the presence of β-mercaptoethanol and (58±2)K in the absence of β-mercaptoethanol.

Taken together, our data indicate that a putative [^{3}H]FNZ receptor can be solubilized from calf cortex as a multimer of about 200-250,000 K daltons which bears distinct recognition sites for benzodiazepines and GABA. It is possible that DOC specifically affects the GABA site or switches the receptor into a conformation that can be only slightly further affected by GABA, since the GABA-induced modulation seems to be smaller in the solubilized preparation when compared to the particulate preparation. The receptor appears to be composed of subunits of which at least part are of about 50K daltons and bind benzodiazepines. It is not yet clear whether the GABA recognition site(s) and the benzodiazepine binding site(s) reside on the same subunit; the existence of several types of subunits in the 11S component cannot yet be excluded.

The observation that receptors for benzodiazepines can be solubilized with no apparent change in affinity makes it possible to study in detail the molecular mechanisms that underlie the action of these potent tranquillizers in brain.

ACKNOWLEDGMENTS

This work was supported by a grant from the Israel Academy of Science, Jerusalem. Y.D. is incumbent of the Barecha Career Development Chair.

REFERENCES

1. Braestrup, C. and Squires, R.G., Specific benzodiazepine receptors in rat brain characterized by high-affinity [^{3}H]diazepam binding, Proc. Natl. Acad. Sci USA, 74 (1977) 3805-3809.
2. Möhler, H. and Okada, T., Benzodiazepine receptor: Demonstration in the central nervous system, Science, 198 (1977) 849-851.
3. Tallman, J.F., Thomas, J.W. and Gallager, D.W., GABAergic modulation of benzodiazepine binding site sensitivity, Nature, 274 (1978) 383-385.

4. Dudai, Y., Modulation of benzodiazepine binding sites in calf cortex by an endogenous factor and GABAergic ligands, Brain Res., 167 (1979) 422-425.

5. Randall, L.O., Schallek, W., Sternbach, L.H. and Ning, R.Y., Chemistry and pharmacology of 1.4-benzodiazepines, in Psychopharmacological agents, Vol. 3, pp. 175-281 Academic Press, New York, (1974).

6. Nielsen, M., Breaestrup, C. and Squires, R.F., Evidence for a late evolutionary appearance of brain specific benzodiazepine receptors: an investigation of 18 vertebrate and 5 invertebrate species, Brain Res., 141 (1978) 342-346.

7. Dudai, Y. and Sherman-Gold, R., Studies on the properties of benzodiazepine-binding sites from calf cortex, Progr. Biochem. Pharmacol. 16 (in press).

8. Sherman-Gold, R. and Dudai, Y., Solubilization and properties of a benzodiazepine receptor from calf cortex, submitted to Brain Res.

9. Battersby, M.K., Richards, J.G. and Möhler, H., Benzodiazepine receptor: Photoaffinity labeling and localization, Eur. J. Pharm. 57 (1979) 277-278.

N E U R O P E P T I D E S

Neurotransmitters and their Receptors
Edited by U.Z. Littauer, Y. Dudai, I. Silman,
V.I. Teichberg and Z. Vogel

Postsynaptic Excitatory Action of Fragments of Gastrin and Cholecystokinin in Mammalian Cerebral Cortex

J. S. Kelly and Jane Dodd

Department of Pharmacology, St. George's Hospital, Medical School, London SW17 ORE

ABSTRACT

The recent introduction of radioimmunoassay has led to the discovery, in many regions of the brain and peripheral nervous system, of peptides which were previously regarded as hormones of the gastrointestinal system. The presence of several of these peptides in the vicinity of the large pyramidal cells of the rat hippocampus has allowed the examination of their postsynaptic action on cortical neurones thought to be innervated by specific peptidergic pathways. Quantities (fmolar per sec) of each peptide applied by pressure ejection from a multibarrelled micropipette placed in the vicinity of an intracellular microelectrode showed somatostatin, vasoactive intestinal polypeptide, bombesin, enkephalin and fragments of gastrin cholecystokinin to be potent excitants of pyramidal cells. Brief applications of the biologically active, tetra- and octapeptide, C-terminal fragments of cholecystokinin evoked abrupt and rapidly reversible depolarizations which were accompanied by marked increases in excitability. Comparison of the actions of these peptides with those of glutamate and acetylcholine, released from the same multibarrelled micropipette, showed that the rate of onset of the cholecystokinin-evoked response was similar to that of the response evoked by glutamate and very much faster than that evoked by acetylcholine. The desulphated form of the cholecystokinin octapeptide was inactive, as was Substance P, a peptide not normally found in the hippocampus.

INTRODUCTION

In 1975, Vanderhaeghen, Signeau & Gepts[1] demonstrated the presence of a peptide in nervous tissue which was smaller than gastrin-17 but cross-reacted with an antibody raised against gastrin. On the basis of experiments with six different sequence-specific gastrin antisera, Dockray[2] suggested that the immunoreactivity present in the brain may represent the C-termina fragment of the gastrointestinal hormone cholecystokinin, whose C-terminal pentapeptide sequence is identical to that of gastrin. Later, Rehfeld[3] using a number of cholecystokinin sequence-specific antibodies was able to show the peptide present in the brain did indeed appear to be the C-terminal octapeptide fragment of cholecystokinin. Cholecystokinin immunoreactivity appeared to account for almost all that previously reported as being due to the presence of gastrin in the central nervous system[4]. High levels of cholecystokinin immunoreactivity have been found in the neocortex, hippocampus,amygdala, hypothalamus[5,6] and spinal cord. In the spinal cord the location of the immunoreactivity in the substantia gelatinosa is reminiscent of the distribution of Substance P in the fibres thought to be involved in nocioception. In the peripheral nervous system, cholecystokinin immunoreactivity is found in mesenteric ganglia, in both Meissner's and Auerbach's plexuses. in the walls of the colon and in the nerves to the pancreatic islet cells.

Gel chromatography of nervous tissue homogenates[5] confirmed the presence of the parent triacontatetrapeptide CCK-33 and at least 3 C-terminal fragments dodeca-(CCK-12), octa-(CCK-8) and tetra-(CCK-4) peptides. The two smallest peptide fragments, CCK-8 and CCK-4 account for 77% of the total immunoreactivity present in the nervous tissue.

Subcellular fractionation has shown CCK-8 and CCK-4 present in the rat cerebral cortex or hypothalamus to be concentrated in the vesicular fraction[7]. In slices of these tissues depolarizing stimulii evoke a calcium-dependent release of the fragments.

On the isolated perfused porcine pancreas, Rehfeld and colleagues[8] have shown the tetrapeptide to be highly potent and a specific releaser of insulin, glucagon, somatostatin and pancreatic polypeptide and suggest that the tetrapeptide may be the neurotransmitter of the nerves which innervate the pancreatic islet cells.

On the frog spinal cord, Phillis & Kirkpatrick[9] have shown the application of cholecystokinin to the isolated hemisceted toad spinal cord to cause a tetrodotoxin sensitive depolarization of both roots. On this preparation the effect of cholecystokinin on the primary afferent terminals and motoneurones resembles that of Substance P. In the gut[10] caerulein, a cholecystokinin analogue, causes a rapid depolarization of pancreatic acinar cells which in many ways resembles that evoked by ACh and bombesin. Although only the ACh mediated response is blocked by atropine, all 3 responses can be mimicked by the intracellular injection of calcium[11]. The responses to all 3 secretogogues have a similar reversal level and latency. Because of the structural similarity between their C-terminal peptide sequences of CCK, gastrin and caerulein[12,13] are believed to share a common receptor on the acinar cell membrane.

The aim of the present study was to determine the action of CCK-8, CCK-8 less the sulphated group on the second amino acid from the N-terminal end Tyr (CCK-NS), CCK-4, gastrin 13 and 14 and caerulein, on pyramidal cells of the CA1 region of the rat hippocampus, using intracellular electrodes. On the same cell the characteristics of these responses were compared with the response to glutamate and acetylcholine, released from adjacent barrels of the same multi-barrel micropipette[14]. In the rat hippocampus the cholecystokinin immunoreactivity appears to be concentrated in the nerve terminals which innervate the cell body layer and proximal dendrites of the pyramidal cells.

RESULTS

1. Actions of CCK-8 and CCK-4

Effects on excitability

CCK-8 and CCK-4 were found to be potent excitants of CA1 pyramidal cells when applied to 55 CA1 pyramidal neurones in 21 slices of the rat hippocampus, using on average a pressure of 647 KPa, resulting in the release of fmolar quantities of CCK-8 per second. In no case was inhibition observed. Although on 40 cells, CCK was excitatory on 97 occasions, on 7 cells, which had been shown to be excited by glutamate, applied iontophoretically from the same multibarrelled pipette, CCK-8 had no effect. Similarly, CCK-4 was excitatory on 7 cells on 26 occasions, yet had no effect on 1 cell, excited by glutamate.

On 12 cells which had already been shown to be excited by CCK-8 or CCK-4, a further 19 doses had no effect. On a number of these cells, the sensitivity to cholecystokinin returned when subsequent doses were tested less frequently, at intervals of about 5 minutes.

A more detailed examination of the excitation evoked by CCK-8 and CCK-4 was carried out on 9 cells with a mean resting potential of -71mV and 4 cells with a mean resting membrane potential of -61mV.

Effects on membrane potential

Both CCK-8 and CCK-4 evoked depolarizations of similar magnitude to those evoked by glutamate on the same cells. Both the onset and the rate at which the CCK-8 evoked depolarization developed were as fast as those evoked by glutamate. However, on average the actions of CCK-4 appeared to develop sooner and faster.

Effects on membrane resistance

On 9 occasions CCK casued a clear decrease in membrane resistance on 6 cells from a control level of 65 $\pm$ 6MΩ to 48 $\pm$ 6MΩ. On four occasions on 3 cells in which the mean resting membrane potential resistance was 41 $\pm$ 5MΩ, CCK-4 evoked a mean decrease of 9.5 $\pm$ 1MΩ. An increase in resistance was never observed. In contrast glutamate on the same cells evoked either no change or a small increase in membrane resistance[14].

Reversal potential of the cholecystokinin effects

Using the single pulse method of Ginsborg[15], the mean reversal potential of the action of CCK-8 on 8 cells determined on 9 occasions was 21 $\pm$ 1.0mV depolarizing with respect to the resting membrane potential, and was not significantly different from that of CCK-4 estimated on 3 cells to be 38 $\pm$ 13mV.

Apparent desensitization

As mentioned earlier, the termination of an application of either CCK-8, or CCK-4 caused the membrane potential and the excitability of the cell to rapidly return to the resting level. However, in a number of neurones the membrane potential and excitability of the cell and the membrane resistance returned to resting levels prematurely and the remainder of the dose was ineffective. In addition, on 9 occasions on 12 cells a subsequent application of CCK-4 or CCK-8 failed to evoke a response. Some times this apparent desensitization could be overcome by delaying the next application of the peptide to the cell for at least 5 minutes. During the apparent desensitization the membrane potential and resistance remained constant and the response evoked by glutamate appeared to be unaltered.

(ii) Effects of CCK-related peptides

(a) Non-sulphated CCK-8 (CCK-NS)

One interesting feature of naturally occurring cholecystokinin and caerulin is the presence of the HSO_3 group on tyrosine and the isolation of both sulphated and unsulphated forms of gastrin. For instance, CCK-8 is 5-8 times as active as the parent molecule as a stimulant of the guinea-pig gall bladder, and the non-sulphated forms of CCK-8 and caerulein appeared to be 300 times less active. (cf. review by Thomson[16]).

On 32 out of 35 occasions on 10 cells CCK-NS was totally inactive, even although on the same cell glutamate applied from the same multibarrelled micropipette was excitatory. Cn 3 occasions on 3 cells is was excitatory. One cell on which CCK-NS was inactive on 5 occasions was readily excited by CCK-8 applied from an adjacent barrel of the same multibarrelled micropipette.

b. Fragments of gastrin (G-13 and G-14)

Gastrin-13 and Gastrin-14, the C-terminal sequences of the larger gastrointestinal hormone, gastrin-34, were synthesized by Dr. Brian Williams at the Molecular Biology Laboratory, in Cambridge, as the lucine analogues.

Both contain the C-terminal pentapeptide sequence of CCK. However, the tyrosine residue was nonsulphated and lay one amino acid sequence nearer to the C-terminal end of the peptide. Although 9 cells were strongly excited by either G-13 or G-14, one cell was unaffected by 5 separate applications of

G13, even although it was readily excited by glutamate, applied by microiontophoresis from an adjacent barrel of the same multibarrelled micropipette. On 2 cells, 3 doses of G-13 and 14 were ineffective, although earlier and later doses from the same micropipette were excitatory. On 3 cells, the actions of G-13 and G-14 were indistinguishable when applied to the same cell from the same multibarrelled micropipette.

Effects on membrane potential

Both gastrins evoked a substantial depolarization with a mean value of 13 $\pm$ 6mV. On 9 occasions on 4 cells the mean latency of the depolarization evoked by either gastrin was not significantly different from that evoked by glutamate on the same cells. However, on 9 other occasions, on 5 different cells, the onset was very much slower.

Attenuation of the response to gastrin before the termination of the application was rarely observed and recovery was usually delayed when compared to that following glutamate on the same cell or CCK-8 and CCK-4 on other cells. On several occasions the cells appeared to recover quickly, but then went on to display intermittent bursts of depolarization and increased excitability for up to 5 min after initial recovery. This phenomena was never observed to follow excitations evoked by glutamate on the same cells, or CCK-4 or CCK-8 on other cells.

c. Caerulein

Caerulein is a decapeptide found in the skins of some South American and Australian amphibians and it was first isolated from the skin of Hyla caerula. Both natural and synthetic caerulein exhibit the entire range of CCK activity on vascular and extravascular smooth muscles, gastric secretion, amylase secretion from the pancreas and gall bladder contractility[17]. The structure of caerulein is very similar to that of CCK-8. It contains the pentapeptide sequence common to both gastrin and CCK and the HSO_3 grouping on the tyrosine which appears to be essential for CCK-like activity.

Caerulein applied by pressure ejection, on 4 out of 4 occasions was excitatory on 2 cells and the effects appeared to be

(iii) Controls

a. Omission of glutamate from pipettes

CCK-8 excited 6 cells when applied by pressure ejection from single and multibarrelled pipettes which did not contain glutamate or any other known excitatory substance. The excitation evoked by CCK-8 was indistinguishable from that evoked by CCK-8 released from pipettes with a glutamate-containing barrel.

b. Pressure ejection of peptide-free vehicle solutions

The effect of pressure application of peptide-free vehicle solution from an adjacent barrel of the peptide containing multibarrelled pipette was examined on 50 occasions, on 12 cells which were shown to be excited by one or other of the peptides or not affected by CCK-NS, or Substance P, applied with pressures of similar magnitude to those used to eject the peptide.

On no occasion did this procedure have any effect on the electrical characteristics of the cell under study.

DISCUSSION

In the gastrointestinal tract all the various actions of gastrin are possessed by the C-terminal peptide, TRP-MET-ASP-PHE-NH_2 and therefore shared with cholecystokinin and caerulein. Of the four amino acids present in the gastrin C-terminal peptide, only ASP is essential for activity, and even in this situation substitution is possible. In the same system optimal cholecystokinin-like activity requires a longer peptide and the TYR-0-SO_4 residue at position 8 ensures optimal activity. However, the 3 N-terminal amino acids of CCK-8 appear to be essential for contraction of the gall bladder[20] and the 5-8 tetrapeptide is inactive.

In the brain, therefore, the excitatory actions of the gastrin tetrapeptide, the cholecystokinin octapeptide, caerulein, and gastrin G-13 and G-14 on pyramidal cells could be due to the interaction of the peptide with a specific receptor. Since indistinguishable from those evoked by CCK-8.

d. Bombesin

Bombesin, a tetradecapeptide originally isolated from extracts of the skin of the frog, Bombina Bombina, has been shown to depolarize pancreatic acinar cells in a manner very similar to caerulein[10], the two yielding almost identical reversal potentials. However, bombesin does not bear any obvious structural similarity to caerulein and it has been postulated that, although they share a final common pathway in the acinar cells, the actions of bombesin and caerulein are mediated by different receptors[18,19]. Bombesin was applied to 2 neurones and on 4 out of 6 occasions it was escitatory. On one cell, an initial excitation evoked by the first application of bombesin was ineffective on 2 subsequent occasions, even although glutamate remained excitatory. Later, the response to bombesin recovered. Although the increase in excitability evoked by bombesin was accompanied by a clear depolarization, there was no detectable change in membrane resistance.

The time course of the response to bombesin differed from those of CCK-4 and CCK-8, described earlier on other cells and to the application of glutamate on the same cell.

e. Substance P

Substance P was applied by pressure ejection to a total of 16 neurones and on 49 separate occasions was without effect. When applied by iontophoresis Substance P was excitatory on 4 occasions on 2 cells, when the ejecting current exceeded 400nA. On 17 other occasions, on 7 cells, Substance P applied by iontophoresis was without effect. Pressure application of Substance P had no effect on 28 occasions on 6 cells on which glutamate was repeatedly shown to excite when ejected iontophoretically from an adjacent barrel of the same multibarrelled pipette.

The same cells are also excited by bombesin, the receptor can also be said to resemble that of the pancreatic acinar cells, which are activated by both caerulein and bombesin. Like the pancreatic acinar cells, the pyramidal cells of the hippocampus also respond to acetylcholine[14]. The failure of pyramidal cells to respond to Substance P is also interesting since this region of the brain appears to be devoid of Substance P. In other regions of the brain, such as the amygdala, a number of authors have correlated the high levels of Substance P with the ability of iontophoretically-applied Substance P to excite cells[21,22,23] Thus, despite a certain sequence nomology, the hippocampal receptor would appear to distinguish between Substance P and bombesin. In the salivary glands, for instance, Galagher & Petersen[24] were able to show Substance P, but not caerulein or bombesin to cause a marked increase in membrane conductance. Since hippocampal cells also appear to be excited by at least two more unrelated peptide sequences, vasoactive intestinal peptide (VIP)[25] and somatostatin[26], the failure of the cells to respond to Substance P is of added significance.

Since in a number of preliminary experiments we have been able to show the excitation evoked by CCK-4 to be unaffected by a medium containing sufficient atropine to block the excitation of the same cell by acetylcholine, we can exclude the possibility that the peptides act indirectly to cause the release of acetylcholine from adjacent nerve terminals.

ACKNOWLEDGEMENTS

We are grateful to George Marschall for technical support, Jens Rehfeld for immuno-assays, Drs. Morley and deCastiglione for supplies of peptides. Jane Dodd is indebted to the MRC for a scholarship. Jane Dodd's present address is: Department of Neurobiology, Harvard Medical School, Boston. The majority of the experimental work was carried out in the MRC Neurochemical Pharmacology Unit, Hills Road, Cambridge.

REFERENCES

1. Vanderhaeghen, J.J., Signeau, J.C., & Gepts, W., (1975). Nature 257, 604.

2. Dockray, G.J., (1976) Nature 264, 568.

3. Rehfeld, J.F., (1978a) J. Biol. Chem. 253, 4016.

4. Rehfeld, J.F., (1978b) J. Biol. Chem. 253, 4022.

5. Larsson, L-I., Rehfeld, J.F., (1979) Brain Res. 165, 201.

6. Innis, B.R., Correa, F.M.A., Uli, G.R., Schneider, B., & Snyder, S.H.,(1979) Proc. Natl. Acad. Sci., 76, 521.

7. Rehfeld, J.F., Coltermann, N., Larsson, L-I., Emson, P.M., & Lee, C.M., (1979) Federation Proc. 38, 2325.

8. Rehfeld, J.F., Larsson, L-I., Coltermann, N., Schwartz, T.W., Holst, J.J., Jensen, S.L., Morley, J.S., (1980). In preparation.

9. Phillis, J.W., & Kirkpatrick, J.R., (1969) Canadian J. of Physiol. & Pharmacol., 57, 887.

10. Petersen, O.H. & Philpott, H.G., (1979) J. Physiol. 290, 305.

11. Iwatsuki, N. & Petersen, O.H., (1979) Nature 268, 147.

12. Morley, J.S., Tracey, H.J., & Gregory, R.A., (1965) Nature 207, 1356.

13. Anastasi, A., Erspamer, V., & Endean, R., (1968) Archs. Biochem. Biophys. 125, 57-68,

14. Kelly, J.S., Dodd, J., & Dingledine, R., (1979). Prog. in Brain Res. 49, 251.

15. Ginsborg, B.L. (1967) Pharmacol. Rev. 19, 289.

16. Thomson, J.C., (1973) in "Pharmacology of Gastrointestinal Motility and Secretion", Ed. P. Holton, Internat. Encyclopedia Pharmacol. & Ther. Section 39A, 261.

17. Erspamer, V., Bertaccini, G., de Caro, G., Endean, R., & Impicciatore, M., (1967) Experimentia 23, 702.

18. Deschodt-Lanckman, M., Robberecht, P., de Nect, P., Lammens, M., & Christophe, J., (1976) J. Clin. Invest. 58, 891-898.

19. Petersen, O.H., & Iwatsuki, N., (1978) Ann. N.Y. Acad. Sci., 301, 599.

20. Rubin, B., (1973) In: Nobel Symposium XVI, Frontiers in Gastrointestinal Hormone Research. Almquist & Wiksell, Uppsala, Sweden.

21.Henry, J.L., (1976) Brain Res. 114, 439.

22.Le Gal La Salle, G., Ben-Ari, Y., (1977) Brain Res. 135, 174-179.

23.Guyenet, P.G., & Aghajanian, G.K., (1977) Brain Res.136, 178.

24.Gallagher, P.V., & Petersen, O.H., (1980) Nature 283, 393.

25.Dodd, J., Kelly, J.S., & Said, S.I., (1979) Br.J.Pharmacol. 60, 125P.

26.Dodd, J., & Kelly, J.S., (1978) Nature 273, 674.

Neurotransmitters and their Receptors
Edited by U.Z. Littauer, Y. Dudai, I. Silman,
V.I. Teichberg and Z. Vogel

The Contribution of the C-Terminal Heptapeptide and the N-Terminal Tetrapeptide of Substance P to its Biological Activities

Shmaryahu Blumberg and Vivian I. Teichberg

Departments of Biophysics and Neurobiology, the Weizmann Institute of Science, Rehovot, Israel

Summary

Synthesis of a series of C-terminal and N-terminal partial sequences of Substance P (SP) has yielded a class of compounds for evaluating the contribution of the different segments of the SP molecule to its biological activity. The C-terminal heptapeptide displays smooth muscle contracting activity much higher than the shorter C-terminal tri-, tetra- and pentapeptides but comparable to the longer C-terminal octapeptide. Its activity is as high or even higher than that of the native undecapeptide, depending on the smooth muscle examined. The differential response to SP and to its partial sequences is attributed to the existence of two types of SP receptors. The rate of inactivation of SP by rat brain homogenate or particulate fractions is significantly slower than that of the C-terminal heptapeptide suggesting that the N-terminal tetrapeptide sequence of SP is important for its stability. A post-proline cleaving peptidase present in bovine brain was found to cleave the SP molecule into an N-terminal tetrapeptide and a C-terminal heptapeptide raising the possibility that this enzyme may be involved in the turnover of SP and/or in its conversion into two active species. SP or its N-terminal tetrapeptide enhances the phagocytic activity of phagocyte cells. This property is consistent with the presumed role of SP in axon reflexes. The combination of the properties displayed by the N-terminal tetrapeptide and the C-terminal heptapeptide allows SP to play a role both in sensory neurotransmission and in inflammatory processes of neural origin.

Introduction

The undecapeptide Substance P (SP) was discovered in 1931 by von Euler and Gaddum in extracts of brain and intestine (1). For many years, the peptide was known primarily for its hypotensive, vasodilatory and smooth muscle contracting properties. In the 1950's,SP was found to be present in the dorsal roots of the spinal cord at concentrations much higher than that found in the ventral roots. This observation led Lembeck to propose, in 1953,that SP might be the natural neurotransmitter of primary sensory neurons (2). It was, however, only in 1971 that Chang, Leeman and Niall found the amino acid sequence of the peptide and opened the door to studies of SP on the molecular level (3).

The structure of SP is shown below:

Arg^{1}-Pro^{2}-Lys^{3}-Pro^{4}-Gln^{5}-Gln^{6}-Phe^{7}-Phe^{8}-Gly^{9}-Leu^{10}-Met^{11}-NH_2

Elucidation of the structure of the peptide and its first synthesis (4) led to the establishment of a radioimmunoassay (5,6) and the use of SP antisera in immunohistochemical mapping of SP(7-9).

The histochemical studies revealed that SP is present in the skin, around blood vessels and near smooth muscles (9). What is the physiological role of SP in these regions is not completely understood. Nevertheless,the main properties of SP in the peripheral nervous system, vasodilation and smooth muscle contraction,give probably relevant cues to its function. Recently, a release of SP in the eye could be demonstrated following the stimulation of the ophthalmic branch of the trigeminal nerve (10). This observation strongly support the view that SP might be the transmitter released during antidromic stimulations or in the related axon reflex phenomenon (9-11).

In the central nervous system,SP is unevenly distributed, being highly concentrated in the dorsal horn of the spinal cord, in the trigeminal nucleus and in the substantia nigra (12-14). It appears that 20%-25% of the cells in dorsal roots ganglia contain SP (8,9). The peptide is present in synaptic vesicles from where it can be released by a Ca^{2+}-dependent mechanism (15). In the last few years,it became possible to demonstrate a stimulus-evoked release of SP from slices of spinal cord (16) and of different brain areas (17-19). The peptide is a potent depolarizer of spinal cord motoneurons (20) and it also excites or facilitates the response of cells sensitive to noxious stimuli (21). The distribution of SP is remarkably similar to that of the enkephalins. This observation raises the possibility that the functions of these two types of peptides are interrelated (22). Recently, Jessell and Iversen found that the release of SP from the trigeminal nucleus is suppressed by opiates including enkephalin (18). They proposed that there exist presynaptic receptors for enkephalins on SP neurons. If indeed SP is a transmitter of pain,then,its suppressed release by enkephalins could be the basic mechanism for the analgesic action of opiates. This view has been supported by the work of Mudge, Leeman and Fischbach who found that the release of SP from dorsal root ganglion cells in culture is inhibited by enkephalins via a blockage of Ca^{2+} channels (23).

All the above properties of SP collectively suggest that the peptide plays a role in sensory neurotransmission. SP, however, does not meet yet all the criteria needed to identify it as a genuine neurotransmitter. A thorough understanding of its physiological role will await the solution of the following problems:

1) Characterization of SP receptors and their localization in the postsynaptic membrane.
2) Establishment of the ionic basis of SP depolarization.
3) Finding of specific antagonists.
4) Elucidation of the mechanism of SP inactivation.
5) Regulation of the synthesis and storage of SP.
6) Identification of the various molecular targets of SP outside the central nervous system.
7) Mechanism of dendritic release of SP.

We have addressed ourselves to the study of some of these problems and the purpose of this chapter is to summarize the results that we obtained so far.

The Size of the Peptide Combining Site of the Substance P Receptor on the Guinea Pig Ileum: The Substance P Receptor Interacts with the C-Terminal Heptapeptide

We have synthesized SP, its partial sequences as well as many analogs and blocked derivatives. The peptides were checked for purity by thin layer chromatography, high performance liquid chromatography or high voltage paper electrophoresis and characterized by their optical rotation, elemental analysis (C,H,N,S) or amino acid analysis. All compounds were routinely examined for their activity using the well known guinea pig ileum contraction bioassay. Each peptide was characterized by a dose-response curve and an ED_{50} value, corresponding to drug concentration which causes 50% of the maximal contracting response. Fig 1 summarizes the results of a study on the potencies of C-terminal

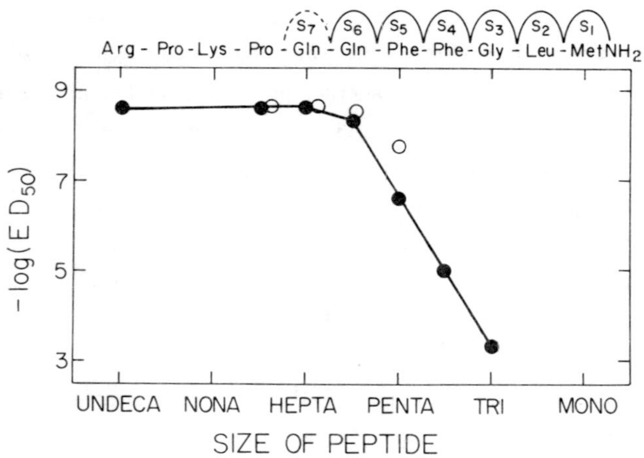

Fig. 1. Effect of the peptide chain length on the guinea pig ileum contracting potency of C-terminal partial sequences of Substance P. Experiments were carried out at 37°C in Tyrode solution (137 mM NaCl; 2.7 mM KCl; 1.8 mM $CaCl_2$; 1.1 mM $MgCl_2$; 0.4 mM NaH_2PO_4; 11.9 mM $NaHCO_3$; 5.5 mM glucose). Dose-response curves were constructed for each peptide and ED_{50} values were evaluated. The variation in the ED_{50} values with the elongation of the peptide chain of the free (●) and Boc (O) SP fragments implies that the Substance P receptor on the ileum can interact with 6-7 amino acid residues in sites designated S_1,S_2,S_3 etc.

partial sequences of SP, free at the amino terminus and blocked with the tert-butyloxycarbonyl blocking group, Boc (24,25). We found that even the small tripeptide Gly-Leu-Met-NH_2 can elicit a full contracting response although at very high peptide concentrations (ED_{50}= $5x10^{-4}$M). The potency of the peptides increases progressively on increasing the peptide chain length, until it reaches an optimum ED_{50} value of ∿ $2x10^{-9}$M at the hepta-peptide level. The octapeptide and SP have about the same potency as the heptapeptide. The observation that even the short tri-, tetra- and pentapeptides can display full contracting response, albeit at higher peptide concentration then SP, is rather unusual in view of the fact that larger segments of other biologically active peptides are often needed for the expression of the full biological response. This observation is also of importance for the design of SP antagonists since extensive substitutions of the fourth and fifth amino acids from the C-terminus (Phe^7, Phe^8) can be carried out and longer peptide chains may not be needed.

As seen in Fig. 1 the blocking of the N-terminal residue with Boc resulted, in a substantial increase in the potency of the pentapeptide and in a slight effect on the potency of the hexapeptide but had virtually no effect on the potencies of the hepta- and octapeptide. These results, taken together with those of other structure-function studies of SP using various bioassays (26-29), indicate that the SP receptor only interacts with the six or seven amino acid residues corresponding to the C-terminal part of the eleven amino acid SP molecule. They also suggest that the hexa-,hepta- and octapeptides or their N-blocked derivatives are the simplest probes of the receptor of SP.

The Activity of Substance P is Modulated by the N-Terminal Sequence

Measurements of SP activity were not only performed using the guinea pig ileum bioassay but were extended to other smooth muscles as well (30). This work was done in collaboration with Dr. S. Cohen. Fig 2A shows that the rat colon behaves similarly to the guinea pig ileum. There

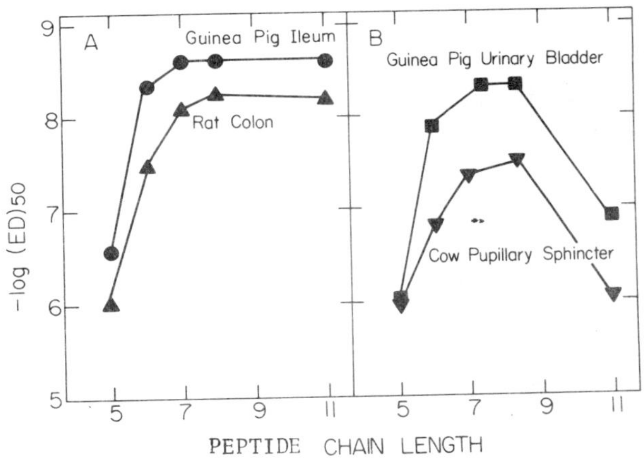

Fig. 2. Effect of the peptide chain length on the muscle contracting potency of C-terminal sequences of Substance P. Experiments with all four muscles were carried out in Tyrode solution at 37°C. In the case of the cow pupillary sphincter, the tyrode solution contained also 4.2 mM glutamate, 3.9 mM pyruvate and 4.4 mM fumarate.

is a great increase in the potency of the peptides on going from the C-terminal penta- to the C-terminal hepta- and octapeptides but there is no change on going further to SP. Fig. 2B shows the behavior of the guinea pig urinary bladder and the pupillary sphincter of the cow. Again, there is an increase in potency on going from the penta- to the hepta- and octapeptides but there is a substantial decrease in potency, by an order of magnitude in ED_{50} values, on going further to SP. The presence of 10^{-5}M of synthetic N-terminal tetrapeptide, Arg-Pro-Lys-Pro, in the assay mixture has no effect on the ED_{50} values of the peptides, indicating that the receptor does not possess an independent binding site for the N-terminal tetrapeptide.

On the basis of the above findings, we conclude that the SP receptors on the guinea pig ileum and the rat colon are of different nature than those present on the guinea pig urinary bladder and the cow pupillary sphincter. We have designated the first two receptors, type A receptors and the latter two receptors, type B receptors. In all four muscles, the highest contracting potency is displayed by the C-terminal hepta- or octapeptides. In this respect, the binding sites of all these receptors share the capacity to accommodate probably only seven amino acids (24). The additional N-terminal sequence does not affect the interaction with type A receptors but is responsible for the decreased activity of SP on the type B receptors. Thus, type B receptors are similar to type A receptors but contain an additional component that weakens the strength of interaction with SP.

This component may be fortuitously associated with the SP receptor but it may also play a role in a mechanism of regulation of SP activity. In this case, the additional component would be associated with type B receptors in order to render it responsive to only high concentrations of SP. While the necessity for such a regulation mechanism is so far unclear, in the case of the pupillary sphincter, it is conceivable that it could have a physiological role. Since SP has been shown to be released in the eye upon nerve stimulation (10) and to cause a contraction of the pupil and vasodilation of the capillaries of the iris (10,31) its involvement in the oculopupillary axon reflex has been suggested (10,31). Our results with the isolated pupillary sphincter showing that the miotic response to SP has a relatively high threshold (Fig. 2) suggest that this property might prevent weak stimulations of the trigeminal nerve from eliciting the axon reflex. An alternative possibility is that the peptide which actually interacts with the receptor is not SP but a shorter and more active fragment e.g. the C-terminal heptapeptide, which would be obtained by a specific enzymic cleavage of SP. In this regard, it is noteworthy that many tissues contain a post-proline cleaving enzyme (32-34) that can remove the N-terminal tetrapeptide from SP to yield the more active and more degradable C-terminal heptapeptide (vide infra).

Degradation of Substance P and its Partial Sequences by Rat Brain Enzymes: Effect of Blocking Groups on Peptide Stability

Since the C-terminal hexa- to- octapeptides or their N-blocked derivatives display optimal activity, we have compared their stability in order to find suitable ligands of the SP receptor that would display both high affinity and high resistance to degradation (24,25). Fig 3

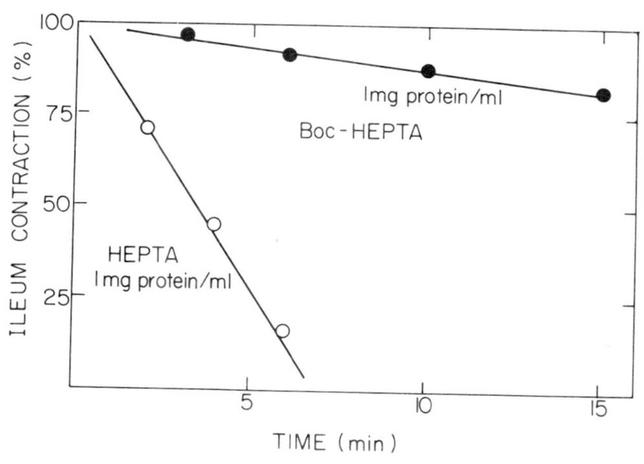

Fig. 3. Degradation of free and Boc C-terminal heptapepide sequence of Substance P by crude synaptosomal fraction of rat brain. The crude synaptosomal fraction was obtained from whole brain homogenized in 0.32 M sucrose, by collecting the 20000xg pellet (20 min) obtained after removal of the 1000xg pellet (10 min). Incubation of synaptosomal fraction with peptide, $2x10^{-7}$M, was carried out by suspending the pellet in 136 mM NaCl, 2.7 mM KCl, 1.47 mM KH_2PO_4, 1mM ethylene glycol-bis(β-aminoethyl ether)-N,N'-tetraacetic acid, 1mM dithioerythritol, pH 7.4 at 24°. Degradation of peptide was followed by the removal of samples at intervals and assay of the remaining activity using the guinea pig ileum. The sample size was chosen to be equivalent to a volume that yields 2-3 times the ED_{50} of the peptide in the assay mixture at the beginning of the experiment. Ileum contraction at time zero was normalized to 100%.

shows the degradation of the C-terminal free heptapeptide, Gln-Gln-Phe-Phe-Gly-Leu-Met-NH_2 and the corresponding Boc-heptapeptide by a crude synaptosomal fraction of rat brain. In these experiments, peptide concentration was $2x10^{-7}M$. This is the highest peptide concentration that one would employ in receptor binding experiments when the dissociation constant for the receptor-peptide complex is of the order of magnitude of $\sim 10^{-9}M$. Such a concentration of peptide would lead to full receptor occupancy and may be of the order of magnitude of the concentration of peptide released in the synaptic cleft. However, $2x10^{-7}M$ is expected to be well below the K_m for any proteolytic enzyme acting on the peptide. Hydrolysis of the peptide by a single specific enzyme would follow first order kinetics and the rate constant should reflect the k_{cat}/K_m value. As can be seen in Fig. 3, the rate of hydrolysis of the free peptide is $\sim$ 12-fold higher than that of the Boc peptide. The stabilizing effect of the blocking groups is due, in part, to the prevention of aminopeptidase(s) action. Such enzymes are metalloenzymes and their involvement in the degradation process is suggested by the fact that the addition of the ion chelator 1,10-phenanthroline at $10^{-3}M$, reduces the rate of hydrolysis of the free heptapeptide 3-fold while it does not affect the rate of hydrolysis of the Boc-heptapeptide. In addition, it is probable that the blocking group interferes with the recognition of the peptide by endopeptidase(s).

Table I summarizes the results of the hydrolysis of the various free

Table I. Half-life of Substance P in Crude Synaptosomal Fraction of Rat Brain

C-TERMINAL PEPTIDE	FREE PEPTIDE [a] t/2(min)	Boc-PEPTIDE STABILITY RATIO BLOCKED/FREE
(6-11) Hexapeptide	1.5± 0.5	8
(5-11) Heptapeptide	2 ± 0.5	12
(4-11) Octapeptide	5 ± 2	6
Substance P	5 ± 2	-
IPP-Heptapeptide [b]	-	15

[a] Peptide at a concentration of 2×10^{-7} M was incubated with 1 mg protein/ml.

[b] IPP-Heptapeptide is the heptapeptide blocked with Bolton-Hunter N-blocking group 3-(4-hydroxy-5-iodophenyl)propionyl.

and blocked peptides. The second column shows the half-life of the free peptides upon incubation with a synaptosomal fraction at 1 mg protein/ml. The stability of the Boc-peptides relative to the corresponding free peptides is indicated in the third column. The blocked hepta- and octa-peptides are significantly more stable than the corresponding free peptides and SP itself. The stabilizing effect of the blocking group is not limited to Boc but applies to other blocking groups examined such as Ac and Glp. The last compound presented in the table IPP-heptapeptide is the heptapeptide blocked with the Bolton-Hunter iodine-containing group (35) that can be made radioactive to a high specific activity. On the basis of these results one can suggest that blocked derivatives or their Nle^{11} analogs, which are more stable to oxidation, may be suitable compounds to use in binding studies of the SP receptor.

<u>Substitution of Gln^6 and Activity of Substance P Analogs</u>

SP belongs to the family of the tachykinins (36). These peptides have identical C-terminal residues, Gly-Leu-Met-NH_2 and share a Phe residue at the fifth amino acid from the C-terminus. In all tachykinins, the fourth amino acid from the C-terminus, Phe, Tyr, Ile or Val is hydrophobic. Thus, the five C-terminal amino acids have been well preserved through evolution. Since we found that the receptor of SP in the guinea pig ileum interacts with six to seven amino acids from the C-terminus, the question arised as what would be the effects of substituting the sixth amino acid. Table II shows that adding Gln to the C-terminal pentapeptide Phe-Phe-Gly-Leu-Met-NH_2 increases the activity

Table II. Substitution of Gln^6 and Activity of Substance P Analogs

PEPTIDE	$p(ED)_{50} \pm 0.2$
Substance P	8.6
| |-Phe-Phe-Gly-Leu-MetNH_2	6.6
|Gln|-Phe-Phe-Gly-Leu-MetNH_2	8.3
|Glp|-Phe-Phe-Gly-Leu-MetNH_2	8.6
| Ac|-Phe-Phe-Gly-Leu-MetNH_2	7.9
|Boc|-Phe-Phe-Gly-Leu-MetNH_2	7.7
|IPP|-Phe-Phe-Gly-Leu-MetNH_2	8.4

by almost two orders of magnitude whereas the addition of a pyroglutamyl residue,Glp,enhances it to the level of SP. Blocking groups which are not amino acids can also interact with the receptor. The ED_{50} value of the acetylpentapeptide is 7.9 while that of the Boc derivative is slightly lower probably because of steric hindrance. The pentapeptide blocked with the Bolton-Hunter group 3-(4-hydroxy-5-iodophenyl) propionyl (IPP) is almost as active as SP. These results show that the sixth amino acid from the C-terminus interacts with the receptor and suggests that affinity and photoaffinity labels of the receptor can be made by introducing suitable reactive moieties as blocking groups of the C-terminal pentapeptide or heptapeptide. In the first case,the reactive group may react with the receptor recognition site. In the other,the reactive group is likely to react outside the recognition site of the receptor.

Substitution of Gly^9 and Activity of Substance P analogs

In the structure of SP,the Gly^9 residue separates the molecule into two hydrophobic moieties Leu-Met-NH_2 and Phe-Phe. The question can be asked as whether peptide analogs with small structural changes in this Gly^9 residue can interact effectively with the SP receptor. Table III shows the activities of a series of Boc-hexapeptide analogs. It

Table III. Substitution of Gly^9 and Activity of Substance P Analogs

PEPTIDE	$-p(ED)_{50}\pm0.2$
Substance P	8.6
Boc-Gln-Phe-Phe-| Gly|-Leu-MetNH$_2$	8.5
Boc-Gln-Phe-Phe-| Ala|-Leu-MetNH$_2$	8.5
Boc-Gln-Phe-Phe-|DAla|-Leu-MetNH$_2$	7.0
Boc-Gln-Phe-Phe-|βAla|-Leu-MetNH$_2$	7.0
Boc-Gln-Phe-Phe-| Sar|-Leu-MetNH$_2$	8.4

can be seen that Ala can substitute for Gly whereas the D isomer, DAla, as well as βAla, which is longer than Gly by one methylene group, cannot.

The activities of these two derivatives are lower by almost two orders of magnitude than that displayed by native derivatives. Sar can also substitute for Gly. Such substitution could be the basis for the synthesis of highly active and more stable analogs than the native sequences.

The N-Terminal Segment of Substance P Stabilizes the Molecular Towards Enzymic Degradation

Many biologically active peptides contain proline residues in their N-terminal or C-terminal parts. These residues are not only important determinants of molecular structure but also may confer a resistance towards enzymic inactivation. The N-terminal sequence of SP, Arg^1-Pro^2-Lys^3-Pro^4,has two proline residues that can in principle provide such a protection, particularly against aminopeptidase(s) action. Table I shows the half-life of the C-terminal partial sequences of SP and of SP itself in crude synaptosomal fraction of rat brain. Although the hexa- and heptapeptides are about as active as SP,when tested in the guinea pig ileum contraction assay,they are significantly less stable than the native peptide. This indicates that the N-terminal part of the molecule is important for its stability (24).

Cleavage of Substance P to an N-terminal Tetrapeptide and C-Terminal Heptapeptide by Post-Proline Cleaving Enzyme from Bovine Brain:

The data of Table I also shows that the C-terminal octapeptide is virtually as stable as SP. However, SP is longer than the octapeptide by the sequence Arg^1-Pro^2-Lys^3. This sequence is expected to be quite resistant to the action of most aminopeptidases. One can therefore assume that the rate determining step in the inactivation of SP must be a cleavage by an endopeptidase of a peptide bound between the Pro^4 residue and the C-terminus of the peptide. Such cleavages by brain enzymes could occur near the Phe residues or near the Leu residue (37,38). Another appealing possibility involves a specific post-proline cleaving enzyme, a serine enzyme which cleaves peptide bonds on the carboxyl side of proline residues (32). This enzyme is distributed in many tissues (34) and was recently purified from bovine brain by our colleagues Drs. J.F. McKelvy and L.B. Hersh who showed that it can inactivate the neuropeptides Thyrotropin Releasing Hormone and Luteinizing Hormone Releasing Hormone (33). Together with them and Dr. J.L. Charli,we examined the effect of the enzyme on SP (39,40). Using high performance liquid chromatography, high voltage paper electrophoresis and various SP fragments obtained by synthesis as markers, we could identify the cleaved peptides and the site of cleavage of SP at the Pro^4-Gln^5 bond. Amino acid analysis of these peptides showed their unequivocal correspondance to the N-terminal tetrapeptide Arg-Pro-Lys-Pro and the C-terminal heptapeptide Gln-Gln-Phe-Phe-Gly-Leu-Met-NH_2 (40).

In order to further characterize the enzymic reaction, we examined the inhibition by SP of the hydrolysis of a synthetic substrate of the enzyme Z-Gly-Pro-para-nitroanilide (40). From these experiments, one could derive a dissociation constant for the enzyme-SP complex of 1.1 μM. This unusually low value might suggest a specific role of the enzyme in the degradation of the peptide. Since the C-terminal heptapeptide is easily degradable by brain fractions (Table I), the inactivation of the SP molecule could possibly proceed in two steps involving first the post-proline cleaving endopeptidase then aminopeptidases cleaving the resulting heptapeptide. It should be noted that with a K_m of 1.1 μM and an estimated k_{cat} value between 10 and 100 sec^{-1} found for the kidney post-proline cleaving enzyme acting on a variety of synthetic substrates (32), the enzyme would have a k_{cat}/K_m value of 10^7-$10^8 M^{-1} Sec^{-1}$. This value reflects a most efficient hydrolytic reaction. Detailed micro-regional distribution studies would now be required to better clarify the possible involvement of brain post-proline cleaving enzyme in the turnover of SP.

Substance P and its N-Terminal Tetrapeptide Enhance Phagocytosis

The cleavage of SP by the post-proline cleaving enzyme to yield a fully active C-terminal heptapeptide and an N-terminal tetrapeptide important for stability and for modulation of activity, raises the question whether the tetrapeptide may have other functions as well. Recently, it has been reported that SP, by virtue of its N-terminal tetrapeptide, increases cAMP levels and induces neurite extension in cultures of both neuroblastoma cells and embryonic chick dorsal root ganglia (41,42). These effects, however, were obtained only with high concentrations of SP (10^{-4}M-10^{-5}M) which, compared to the concentration of Nerve Growth Factor (10^{-10}M) needed to obtain similar neurite outgrowth, shed some doubts on the biological significance of these observations. They led us, however, to search for analogous functions of the N-terminal tetrapeptide.

Our colleagues Drs. Z. Bar-Shavit, R. Goldman, Y. Stabinsky, P. Gottlieb and M. Fridkin have been studying for some time another tetrapeptide, Tuftsin, Thr-Lys-Pro-Arg(43) which is present in blood and is known for its capacity to enhance the phagocytosis activity of phagocyte cells. The structures of the N-terminal tetrapeptide of SP and of Tuftsin are quite similar, both peptides having two basic amino acid residues separated by a proline residue. Together with them, we have examined the effect of SP and its N-terminal tetrapeptide on macrophages and polymorphonuclear leukocytes (44). We found that both SP and its N-terminal tetrapeptide enhance the phagocytosis activity of mouse macrophages in a dose-dependent manner with an half maximal effect at $\sim$ 20 nM peptide. The C-terminal hepta- and octapeptides as well as the dipeptides Arg-Pro and Lys-Pro were virtually without effect. Similar results were also obtained using human polymorphonuclear leukocytes. To further characterize this effect, we carried out competitive binding experiments using radioactive Tuftsin. SP and its N-terminal tetrapeptide were found to compete with labeled Tuftsin in binding to macrophages with the same efficiency as unlabeled Tuftsin, suggesting that these three peptides bind at identical sites with the same affinity. The question whether SP acts as an undecapeptide or has to be cleaved first to the N-terminal tetrapeptide has to await further investigation.

The newly found activity of SP and its N-terminal tetrapeptide is entirely consistent with other properties of SP in the peripheral nervous system and its possible involvement in axon reflexes (9-11). Fig. 4 shows the physiological basis of an axon reflex. An injury in the skin causes a sensory nerve stimulation which is propagated both orthodromically to the central nervous system and antidromically to blood vessels to cause vasodilation and inflammation. If indeed SP is the transmitter released in the axon reflex, then, it could cause vasodilation by virtue of its C-terminal heptapeptide and activate invading phagocyte cells by virtue of its N-terminal tetrapeptide. SP may also stimulate the release of histamine from mast cells (11,45) and thereby contribute to an amplification of the inflammatory response. This latter effect is probably also governed by the basic N-terminal sequence. In the eye, an axon reflex causes not only vasodilation but also a constriction of the iris sphincter. This is a reflection of another property of the C-terminal portion of SP-smooth muscle contraction.

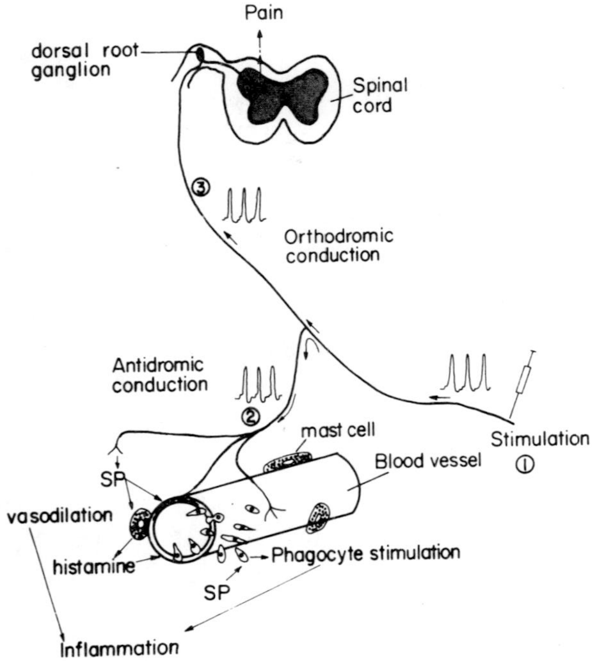

Fig. 4. Diagram of axon reflex and the presumed targets of the released transmitter (Substance P). The nerve stimulation (1) leads to the generation of action potentials travelling antidromically (2) and orthodromically (3). The antidromic conduction leads to the release of Substance P which causes vasodilation of blood vessels, degranulation of mast cells and activation of phagocyte cells, giving rise to an inflammatory response. The orthodromic conduction leads to the release of Substance P in the spinal cord and the stimulation of pain centers.

Conclusion

We have provided in this work evidence for the existence of individual properties of the N-terminal tetrapeptide and the C-terminal heptapeptide portions of the SP molecule. The fact that various activities of SP can be attributed to separate sequences of the molecule shows SP to be a versatile neurotransmitter particularly suitable for being released at the central and peripheral endings of sensory nerves.

Acknowledgements

We thank Mrs. Zofia Tauber and Mr. Israel Jacobson for their assistance in the preparation of the peptides. Support from the Israel Commission for Basic Research and from the Délégation Générale á la Recherche Scientifique et Technique is gratefully acknowledged. S.B. is the incumbent of the Mildred and William Levine Career Development Chair.

References

1. von Euler, U.S. and Gaddum, J.H.: An unidentified depressor substance in certain tissue extracts. J. Physiol (London) *72*, 74-87 (1931)

2. Lembeck, F.: Zur Frage der Zentralen Übertragung Afferenter Impulse. III Mitteilung. Das Vorkommen Und die Bedeutung der Substanz P in den Dorsalen Wurzeln des Rückenmarks. Naunyn-Schmiedeberg's Arch Pharmacol. *29*, 197-213 (1953).

3. Chang, M.M., Leeman, S.E. and Niall, H.D. Amino-acid sequence of Substance P. Nature, New Biol. *232*, 86-87 (1971).

4. Tregear, G.W., Niall, H.D., Potts Jr. J.T., Leeman, S.E. and Chang, M.M. Synthesis of Substance P. Nature New Biol. *232*,87-89 (1971).

5. Powell, D., Leeman, S., Tregear, G.W., Niall, H.D. and Potts, Jr.J.T. Radioimmunoassay for Substance P. Nature New Biol.*241*, 252-254 (1973).

6. Nilsson, G., Pernow, B., Fischer, G.H. and Folkers, K. Presence of Substance P - like immunoreactivity in plasma from man and dog. Acta Physiol. Scand. *94*, 542-544 (1975).

7. Nilsson, G., Hökfelt, T. and Pernow, B. Distribution of Substance P-like immunoreactivity in the rat central nervous system as revealed by immunohistochemistry. Med.Biol.*52*,424-427 (1974).

8. Hökfelt, T., Kellerth, J.-O., Nilsson, G. and Pernow, B. Experimental immunohistochemical studies on the localization and distribution of Substance P in cat primary sensory neurons. Brain Res. *100*, 235-252 (1975).

9. Hökfelt, T., Johansson, O., Kellerth, J.-O., Ljungdahl, A., Nilsson, G., Nygårds, A. and Pernow, B. Immunohistochemical distribution of Substance P. in Substance P (von Euler, U.S. and Pernow, B. eds) Raven Press, New York, pp 117-145 (1977).

10. Bill, A., Stjernschantz, J., Mandahl, A., Bradin, E. and Nilsson, G. Substance P:Release on trigeminal nerve stimulation, effects in the eye. Acta Physiol. Scand. *106*, 371-373 (1979).

11. Lembeck, F. and Holzer, P.: Substance P as neurogenic mediator of antidromic vasodilation and neurogenic plasma extravasation. Naunyn-Schmiedeberg's Arch.Pharmacol. *310*, 175-183 (1979).

12. Takahashi, T. and Otsuka, M.: Regional distribution of Substance P in the spinal cord and nerve roots of the cat and the effect of dorsal root section. Brain Res. *87*, 1-11 (1975).

13. Brownstein, M.J., Mroz, E.A., Kizer, I.S., Palkovits, M. and Leeman, S.E.: Regional distribution of Substance P in the brain of the rat. Brain Res. *116*, 299-305.

14. Kanazawa, I. and Jessell, T.: Post mortem changes and regional distribution of Substance P in the rat and mouse nervous system. Brain Res. *117*, 362-367 (1976).

15. Schenker, C., Mroz, E.A. and Leeman, S.E.: Release of Substance P from isolated nerve endings. Nature, *264*, 790-792 (1976).

16. Otsuka, M. and Konishi, S.: Release of Substance P-like immunoreactivity from isolated spinal cord of newborn rat. Nature, *264*, 83-84 (1976).

17. Iversen, L.L., Jessell, T. and Kanazawa, I.: Release and metabolism of Substance P in rat hypothalamus. Nature, *264*, 81-83 (1976).

18. Jessell, T. and Iversen, L.L.:Opiate analgesics inhibit Substance P release from rat trigeminal nucleus. Nature, *268*, 549-551 (1977).

19. Jessell, T.: Substance P release from the rat substantia nigra. Brain Res. *151*, 469-478 (1978).

20. Konishi, S. and Otsuka, M.: The effects of Substance P and other peptides on spinal neurons of the frog. Brain Res. *65*, 397-410 (1974).

21. Henry, J.H.: Effects of Substance P on functionally identified units in cat spinal cord. Brain Res. *114*, 439-451 (1976).

22. Hökfelt, T., Ljungdahl, A., Terenius, L., Elde, R. and Nilsson, G.: Immunohistochemical analysis of peptide pathways possibly related to pain and analgesia: Enkephalin and Substance P. Proc. Natl. Acad. Sci. USA *74*, 3081-3085 (1977).

23. Mudge, A.W., Leeman, S.E. and Fischbach, G.D.: Enkephalin inhibits release of Substance P from sensory neurons in cultures and decreases action potential duration. Proc. Natl. Acad. Sci. USA. *76* 526-536 (1979).

24. Blumberg, S. and Teichberg,V.I: Biological activity and enzymic degradation of substance P analogs: Implications for studies of the Substance P receptor. Biochem. Biophys. Res. Commun. *90*, 347-354 (1979).

25. Teichberg, V.I. and Blumberg, S.:Substance P and analogs:Biological activity and degradation. in "Endogenous Peptides and Centrally Acting Drugs" (Levi, R., Heldman, E., Vogel, Z. and Gutman, Y. eds.) Progr. Biochem. Pharm. Vol. *16*, Karger (1980) in press.

26. Bergmann, J., Bienert, M., Niedrich, H., Mehlis, B. and Oehme, P.: Über den Einfluss der Ketlenlange bei C-terminalen sequenzen der substanz P - in vergleich mit analogen physalaemin-und eledoisin-peptiden- auf die wirksamkeit am meerschweinchen-ileum. Experientia *30*,401-403 (1974).

27. Bury, R.W. and Mashford, M.L.:Biological activity of C-terminal partial sequences of Substance P. J. Med. Chem. *19*,854-856 (1976).

28. Yanaihara, N., Yanaihara, C., Hirohashi, M., Sato, H., Iizuka, Y., Hashimoto, T. and Sakagami, M.:Substance P. analogs:Synthesis, and biological and immunological properties.in Substance P (von Euler, U.S. and Pernow,B. eds.) Raven Press, New York, pp. 27-33 (1977).

29. Otsuka, M. and Konishi, S.:Electrophysiological and neurochemical evidence for Substance P as a transmitter of primary sensory neurons. in Substance P (von Euler, U.S. and Pernow,B. eds.) Raven Press, New York, pp. 207-214 (1977).

30. Teichberg, V.I., Cohen, S. and Blumberg, S.:The activity of Substance P is modulated by the N-terminal segment. (submitted).

31. Cohen, S., Duzman, E., Ben-Sira, I., Teichberg, V.I. and Blumberg, S.: Isolated preparation of bovine pupillary sphincter: Pharmacological characterization of the Substance P receptor. Proc. ARVO p. 220 (1980).

32.Walter, R. and Yoshimoto, T.:Postproline cleaving enzyme:Kinetic studies of size and stereospecificity of its active site. Biochemistry, *17*, 4139-4144 (1978).

33. Hersh, L.B. and McKelvy, J.F.:Enzymes involved in the degradation of thyrotropin releasing hormone (TRH) and luteinizing hormone releasing hormone (LH-RH) in bovine brain. Brain Res. *168*, 553-564 (1979).

34. Yoshimoto, T., Ogita, K., Walter, R., Koida, M. and Tsuru, D.:Post proline cleaving enzyme.Synthesis of a new fluorogenic substrate and distribution of the endopeptidase in rat tissues and body fluids of man . Biochim. Biophys. Acta. *569*, 184-192 (1979).

35. Bolton, A.E. and Hunter, W.M.:The labelling of proteins to high specific radioactivities by conjugation to a ^{125}I-containing acylating agent. Biochem. J. *133*, 529-539 (1973).

36. Erspamer,V., Erspamer, G.F. and Linari, G.:Occurrence of tachykinins (physalemin or Substance P-like peptides) in amphibian skin and their actions on smooth muscle preparations. in Substance P (von Euler,U.S. and Pernow,B.eds.) Raven Press,New York,pp.67-74 (1977).

37. Benuck, M. and Marks, N.: Enzymatic Inactivation of Substance P by a partially purified enzyme from rat brain. Biochem. Biophys. Res. Commun. *65*, 153-158 (1975).

38. Benuck, M., Grynbaum, A. and Marks, N.:Breakdown of somatostation and Substance P by cathepsin D purified from calf brain. Brain. Res. *143*, 181-185 (1977).

39. Blumberg, S., Teichberg, V.I., Charli, J.L., Hersh, L.B. and McKelvy, J.F.:Cleavage of Substance P to an N-terminal tetrapeptide and a C-terminal heptapeptide by a post-proline cleaving enzyme. Fed. Proc. *38*, 350 (1979).

40. Blumberg, S., Teichberg, V.I., Charli, J.L., Hersh L.B. and McKelvy, J.F.:Cleavage of Substance P to an N-terminal tetrapeptide and a C-terminal heptapeptide by a post-proline cleaving enzyme from bovine brain. Brain Res. (1980) in press.

41. Narumi, S. and Fujita, T.: Stimulatory effects of Substance P and nerve growth factor (NGF) on neurite outgrowth in embryonic chick dorsal root ganglia. Neuropharmacology *17*, 73-76 (1978).

42. Narumi, S. and Maki, Y.: Stimulatory effects of Substance P on neurite extension and cyclic AMP levels in cultured neuroblastoma cells. J. Neurochem. *30*, 1321-1326 (1978).

43. Nishioka, K., Constantopoulos, A., Satoh, P.S. and Najjar, V.A.: The characterization, isolation and synthesis of the phagocytosis stimulating peptide Tuftsin. Biochem. Biophys. Res. Commun. *47*, 172-179 (1972).

44. Bar-Shavit, Z., Goldman, R., Stabinsky, Y., Gottlieb, P., Fridkin, M., Teichberg, V.I. and Blumberg, S.:Enhancement of phagocytosis - A newly found activity of Substance P residing in its N-terminal tetrapeptide sequence. Biochem. Biophys. Res. Commun. (1980) in press.

45. Johnson, A.R. and Erdös, E.G.: Release of histamine from mast cells by vasoactive peptides. Proc. Soc. Exp. Biol. Med. *142*, 1252-1256 (1973).

Neurotransmitters and their Receptors
Edited by U.Z. Littauer, Y. Dudai, I. Silman,
V.I. Teichberg and Z. Vogel

Direct and Modulatory Actions of Thyrotropin-Releasing Hormone (TRH) in Sensorimotor Cortex

D.J. Braitman, C.R. Auker and D.O. Carpenter

Neurobiology Department, AF RRI, Bethesda, MD 20014 USA

Abstract

Ionophoretic application of TRH caused a direct inhibition or excitation of some neurons in sensorimotor cortex of cat. In addition, TRH specifically potentiated the excitatory action of acetylcholine and histamine in the absence of any direct action on spontaneous activity. Also, TRH down-modulated the excitatory action of glutamate on other neurons. These modulatory actions were distributed differentially among pyramidal tract and nonpyramidal tract neurons, suggesting that the receptors coupled to these different effects are located on different cell types.

Thyrotropin-releasing hormone (TRH), a three-amino acid peptide (pGlu-His-Pro-NH_2), is present throughout the mammalian CNS (1,2). Its predominant direct effect when applied to CNS neurons is inhibitory (3-8), although some excitatory actions have been demonstrated (5,8). Yarbrough (7) has reported that TRH modulates (potentiates) the excitatory action of acetylcholine on cerebral cortical neurons, but Winokur and Beckman (6) and Renaud et al. (9) have not been able to replicate his results. We have studied the variety of both direct and modulatory actions of TRH on pyramidal tract (PT) and nonpyramidal tract (NPT) neurons in sensorimotor cortex of the cat. We found that TRH may have either direct excitatory or inhibitory actions on different cortical neurons and may also modulate the response to other putative neurotransmitters. We have found the modulatory action of TRH different for different transmitters and the receptors mediating this modulation to be distributed differentially among PT and NPT neurons (10).

The center barrel of a 5- or 7-barrel micropipette (Glassblowing Unit, Division of Research Services, National Institutes of Health) was used to record extracellular action potentials from neurons in the sensorimotor cortex (area 4) of chloralose-anesthetized cats (70 mg/kg, i.v.). In each electode the center barrel was filled with 2 M NaCl, and each of the other barrels was filled with ACh (1 M), histamine (1 M), glutamate (1 M), or TRH (10 mM) for microionophoretic application. One other barrel was filled with NaCl (0.5 M) for current control. A constant voltage ionophoretic device was used to deliver the drugs (11). In most experiments PT neurons were identified by antidromically stimulating the medullary pyramids with a bipolar electrode.

Of 38 identified neurons examined, two PT and three NPT neurons were directly excited by ionophoretic application of TRH (Fig. 1A). Two other NPT neurons were inhibited by TRH (Fig. 1B). In four of the neurons that were directly affected by TRH and also excited by ACh, sequential application of TRH and ACh did not result in modulation of the ACh response but only summation of action of the two transmitters.

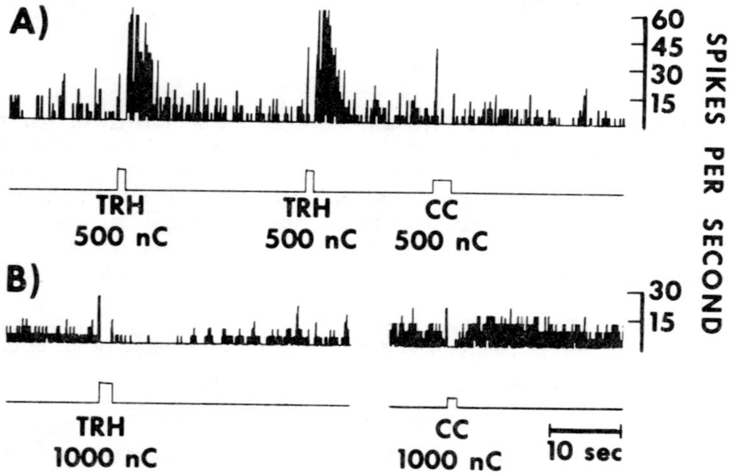

Fig. 1. Ratemeter records from two different cortical neurons showing direct effects of TRH. Each deflection represents frequency of firing of the cell calibrated in spikes per second on right. Labeled bars represent charge in nanocoulombs (nc) used to apply drugs. Width of bar indicates duration of drug delivery. (A) Fast excitation of pyramidal tract neuron (conduction velocity = 83 m/s). (B) Inhibitory action of TRH on nonpyramidal tract neuron. Depression of activity during current pulse is due to rapid passage of positive current. During current controls (CC) in both (A) and (B), it can be seen that this depression terminates immediately upon cessation of current.

We found that TRH did potentiate the excitatory action of ACh in 5 of 23 neurons in which the ionophoretic application of TRH and ACh were paired. Four (of 12) of these were PT neurons, and 1 (of 2) was a cell not tested by stimulation of the pyramids. Potentiation of the excitatory ACh response by TRH was not found in experiments on nine NPT neurons (Fig. 4B). The potentiation of the ACh response typically lasted for several minutes and was never accompanied by a direct effect of TRH alone. In 12 neurons tested, TRH did not similarly potentiate the excitatory action of glutamate even when the ACh response was potentiated (Fig. 2B). TRH potentiated the excitatory response to histamine in one of two NPT neurons (Fig. 3). The time course of this histamine response and its modulation was similiar to that of the ACh response on PT cells.

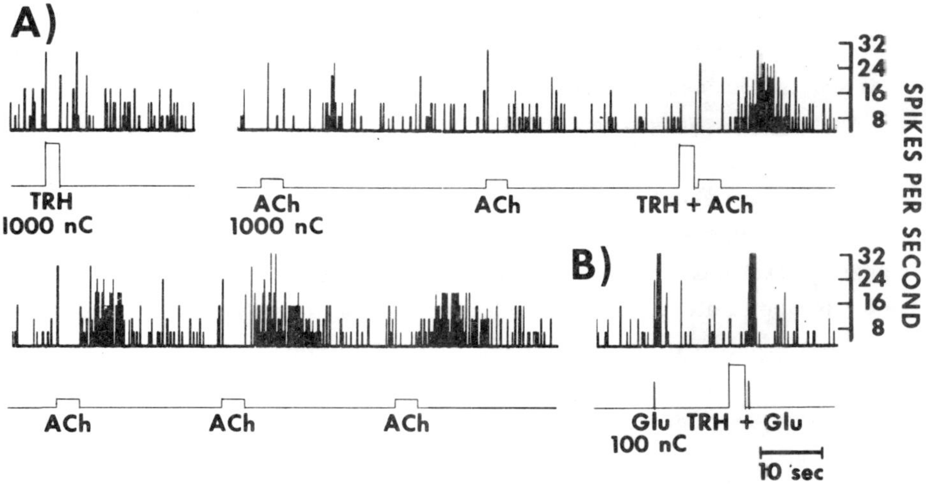

Fig. 2. Ratemeter records from pyramidal tract neuron (c.v. = 74 m/s) illustrating (A) Potentiation of a weak acetylcholine (ACh) response by pairing with TRH. TRH and ACh are shown applied alone and then paired with each other. Lower trace is continuous with upper trace. Other breaks in the records indicate noncontinuity. (B) The exitatory effect of glutamate (Glu) on this cell is not affected by pairing with TRH, demonstrating that TRH did not cause a subthreshold depolarization and that its effects are specific for ACh. (For detailed explanation, see Fig. 1.)

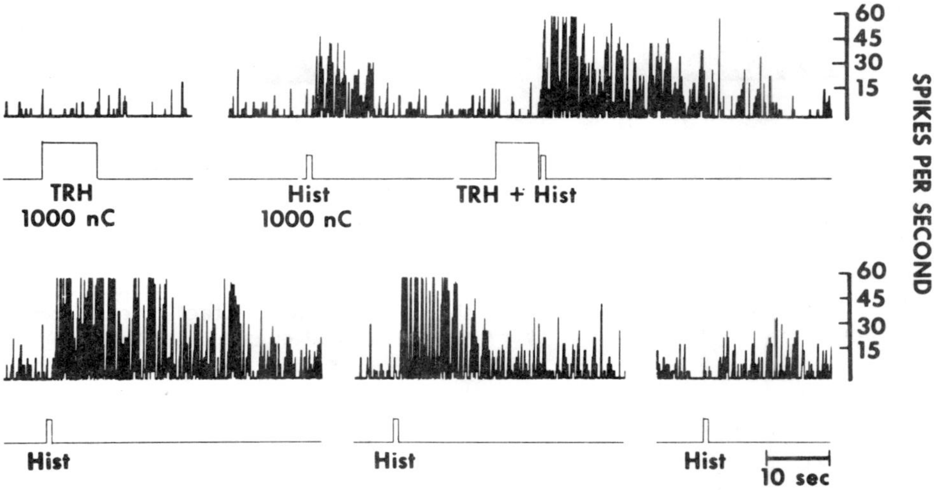

Fig. 3. Potentiation of an excitatory histamine (Hist) response by pairing with TRH (nonpyramidal tract neuron). Lower trace is continuous with end of upper trace. It should be noted that TRH had no effect on spontaneous activity as in Figs. 2 and 4. (For detailed explanation, see Figs. 1 and 2.)

We have also observed a depression of the excitatory glutamate response by TRH in four of eight NPT neurons and in one of four PT neurons. However, due to the low spontaneous neural activity one often encounters in anesthetized animals, it was usually not possible to determine if the depression of glutamate activity was a result of a direct inhibitory effect of TRH or a specific down-modulation. In the experiment illustrated in Figure 4, we found that TRH specifically down-modulated the excitatory glutamate response (Fig. 4A) on this NPT neuron while having no effect on the excitatory ACh response (Fig. 4B). These results are consistent with those of Renaud et al. (10), who recorded from somatosensory cortex of rat. Our results differ from theirs in that we did find potentiation of the ACh response, though only on PT cells. Since Renaud et al. (9) did not identify PT neurons, the apparent discrepancy between their results, those of Yarbrough (7), and the present studies may be due to sampling of different populations.

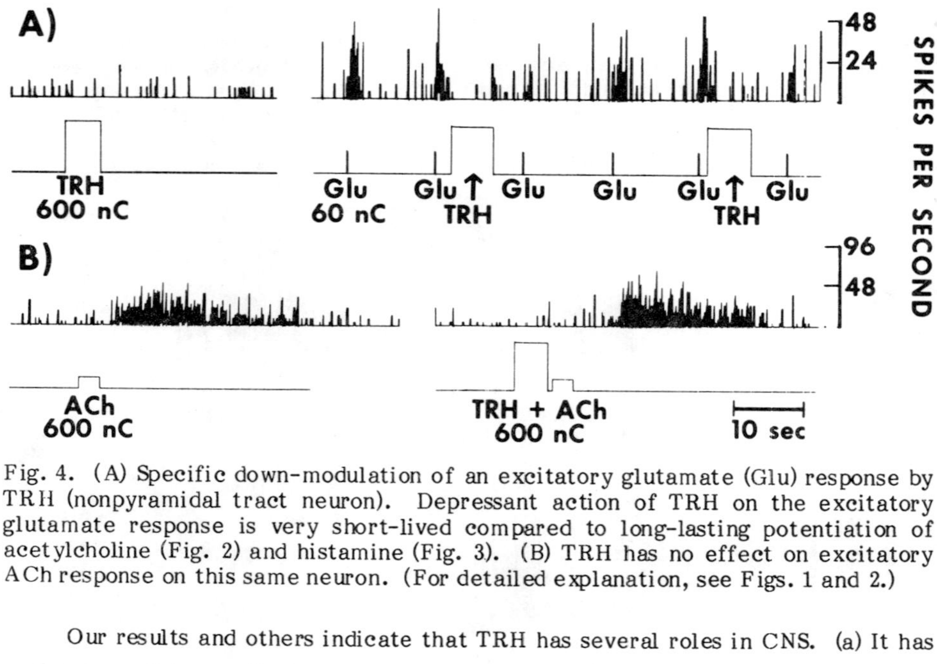

Fig. 4. (A) Specific down-modulation of an excitatory glutamate (Glu) response by TRH (nonpyramidal tract neuron). Depressant action of TRH on the excitatory glutamate response is very short-lived compared to long-lasting potentiation of acetylcholine (Fig. 2) and histamine (Fig. 3). (B) TRH has no effect on excitatory ACh response on this same neuron. (For detailed explanation, see Figs. 1 and 2.)

Our results and others indicate that TRH has several roles in CNS. (a) It has a direct excitatory effect on neurons in cat sensorimotor cortex as well as other neurons (5,8). (b) TRH inhibits some cortical as well as some subcortical neurons (3-8). (c) TRH can cause a specific long-lasting potentiation of the response to some neurotransmitters on neurons in which it has no effect on spontaneous activity (6). We have demonstrated potentiation of the excitatory response to ACh and histamine but not to glutamate. Of clearly identified cells, potentiation of ACh responses occurred only on PT neurons. The excitatory action of ACh was never found to be potentiated by TRH on NPT neurons. This may explain why Winokur and Beckman (6) were unable to find potentiation of ACh by TRH in their study since they were recording rostral to the site of PT neurons. (d) TRH can cause a specific down-modulation of the excitatory glutamate response on some cortical neurons (9). Our finding that TRH potentiated ACh only on PT neurons while TRH depressed glutamate responses primarily on NPT neurons suggests that the receptors coupled to different effects are probably located on different cell types. These results demonstrate that TRH has multiple functions in CNS and that these actions are not randomly distributed.

REFERENCES

1. Hokfelt, T., Fuxe, K., Johansson, O., Joffcoate, S. and White, N. (1975) European J. Pharmacol. 34: 389-392.

2. Winokur, A. and Uteger, R. D. (1974) Science 185: 265-267.

3. Dyer, R. G. and Dyball, R. E. J. (1974) Nature 252: 486-488.

4. Renaud, L. P. and Martin, J. B. (1975) Brain Res. 86: 150-154.

5. Moss, R. L. (1977) Fed. Proc. 36: 1978-1983.

6. Winokur, A. and Beckman, A. L. (1978) Brain Res. 150: 205-209.

7. Yarbrough, G. G. (1978) European J. Pharmacol. 48: 19-27.

8. Ishibashi, Y., Oomura, Y. and Okajima, T. (1979) Physiol. and Behav. 22: 785-787.

9. Renaud, L. P., Blume, H. W., Pittman, Q. J., Lamour, Y. and Tan, A. T. (1979) Science 205: 1275-1277.

10. Some of the research reported here has been accepted for publication in Brain Research.

11. Willis, J. A., Myers, P. R. and Carpenter, D. O. (1977) J. Electrophysiol. Tech. 6: 817-824.

Supported by Armed Forces Radiobiology Research Institute, Defense Nuclear Agency, under Research Work Unit MJ 60103. The views presented in this paper are those of the authors. No endorsement by the Defense Nuclear Agency has been given or should be inferred.

Neurotransmitters and their Receptors
Edited by U.Z. Littauer, Y. Dudai, I. Silman,
V.I. Teichberg and Z. Vogel

Pain Sensitivity and Endogenous Opiates in Hypertension

N. Zamir, M. Segal, D. Ben-Ishay* and R. Simantov**

*Departments of Isotope Research and Genetics**, The Weizmann Institute of Science, Rehovot, Israel.*

Department of Internal Medicine, Hadassah University Hospital, Mount Scopus, Jerusalem, Israel*

Abstract

Genetically and experimentally hypertensive rats as well as essential hypertensive humans were found to be less sensitive to noxious stimuli than normal controls. Hypertensive rats exhibit high levels of opioid peptides in the spinal cord. Decreased binding of ^{3}H Naloxone to opiate receptors was found in the dorsal horn and hippocampus of hypertensive rats. It is suggested that blood pressure and pain control systems are interrelated.

Central blood pressure and pain regulatory mechanisms are closely associated. Anatomically, the two control systems partially overlap; the nucleus locus coeruleus, the raphe nuclei, nucleus tractus solitarius and the nucleus of the vagus nerve have been implicated in regulation of both blood pressure and pain (1-4). Monoamines as well as opioid peptides and receptors have been found in relatively high concentrations in these structures (5,6). Furthermore, monoaminergic drugs that modulate blood pressure also affect pain sensitivity (7). We have measured pain sensitivity, opiate activity and opiate receptor binding in brain of renal hypertensive SABRA rats, in two strains of rats selected from the SABRA strain on the basis of their sensitivity (H) or resistance (N) to hypertension induced by DOCA-salt treatment.

The mean systolic pressure and the paw-lick latency were similar in all groups prior to the operation (Fig. 1). The renal hypertensive rats exhibited a gradual increase in both blood pressure and latency to paw-lick in the hot-plate test. Excision of the stenotic kidney of the renal hypertensive rats was done on day 20. Five days later there was a

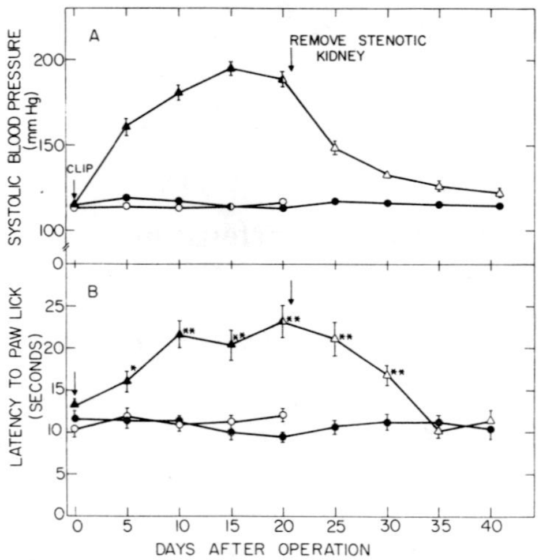

Fig. 1. The course of systolic blood pressure (A) and paw-lick latency (B) after unilateral constriction of a renal artery and following removal of the constricted kidney (day 20). Systolic blood pressure was monitored by means of a pulse transducer in the tail (6). Renal hypertension was induced by applying a solid silver clip on the left renal artery leaving the right kidney untouched. Two control groups were used; a sham operated control that underwent the same operative procedure without a clip on the artery, and a control group in which the renal artery was occluded following the application of the clip. Analgesia was measured by the hot-plate test (12). Stenotic kidney (- ▲ - ▲ -, n = 49); stenotic kidney removed (- Δ - Δ -, n = 17); sham operated control (- o - o -, n = 25); atrophic kidney control (- ● - ● -, n = 36). Values are mean ± S.E.M. Statistical significance * $p < 0.01$; ** $p < 0.001$ compared with atrophic kidney control (t - test).

substantial fall in blood pressure while the paw-lick latency remained high. Twenty days after the unilateral nephrectomy, both phenomena were completely reversed (Fig. 1). In the Randall-Selitto paw-pinch test we found that renal hypertensive rats were significantly less sensitive than controls to paw-pinch (158 ± 9 g, n = 12 and 103 ± 5 g, n = 19, respectively). Although naloxone had no effect on blood pressure it reversed the hypoalgesia found in renal hypertensive rats. Blood pressure and pain sensitivity were measured in H, N and the SABRA strain. The systolic and diastolic blood pressures of genetically hypertensive rats (H strain) were significantly higher than N and SABRA strains (systolic/diastolic 127 ± 3 mmHg/97 ± 5 mmHg, n = 10 vs. 108 ± 5 mmHg/74 ± 5 mmHg, n = 10, and 109 ± 2 mmHg/86 ± 4 mmHg, n = 11, respectively). Both H and N rats were significantly less responsive in the hot-plate test than rats of the SABRA strain. The mean paw-lick latencies of the SABRA rats were 11 ± 1.0 sec (n = 25) whereas that of the H and N rats were 24.9 ± 3.4 sec (n = 25) and 21.0 ± 3.1 sec (n = 25) respectively. This difference was also reflected in the paw-pinch test. The rats of the SABRA strain had a threshold of 101 ± 3.0 g (n = 25) and the H and N strains had a threshold of 198 ± 10 g, n = 25 and 219 ± 8 g, n = 25, respectively.

We have also measured blood pressure and responsiveness to tooth pulp stimulation in 55 unmedicated males (16 - 61 yrs old from Hadassah Hospital, Jerusalem).

Sensory and pain thresholds were significantly higher in the hypertensive subjects compared to normotensive controls (Table 1).

The human data corroborate the animal data and indicate that the relation between blood pressure and pain is likely to be a general phenomenon. Moreover, it indicates that the change in responsiveness to pain may take place already at the sensory end of the neuraxis and is not caused by a motor deficit.

The opioid activity in several brain areas and pituitary gland was measured in the renal hypertensive rats 20 days after the induction of hypertension and in H and N rats. There was a significant elevation (45%) in opioid content in the cervical spinal cord of the renal hypertensive rats compared to normotensive control rats (Table 2). The H and N rats had a significantly higher levels of endogenous opioids in the cervical spinal cord, hypothalamus and pituitary than the SABRA strain. There were no differences in the other brain areas tested (Table 2).

The higher opiate levels may underly the lower sensitivity to painful stimuli. There are only a few cases where such a correlation is established (8). The opiate activity is a presynaptic marker. For a postsynaptic marker we have selected to measure the density of ^{3}H-Naloxone binding sites in various brain areas. There was a significant decrease in ^{3}H-Naloxone binding in the dorsal horn, hippocampus and caudate nucleus of renal hypertensive rats compared to atrophic kidney controls (dorsal horn: 57.9 ± 4.7 pmole ^{3}H-Naloxone bound/mg protein (n = 12), for the hypertensive vs. 73.1 ± 5.3 pmole ^{3}H-Naloxone bound/mg protein (n = 10), for their controls; Hippocampus; 90.2 ± 5.3 ^{3}H-Naloxone bound/mg protein (n = 10), vs. 124.9 ± 5.4 pmole ^{3}H-Naloxone bound/mg protein (n = 8); and caudate nucleus; 111.7 ± 6.3 pmole ^{3}H-Naloxone bound/mg protein (n = 10) vs. 139.8 ± 11.8 pmole ^{3}H-Naloxone/mg protein (n = 8), respectively). Similar results were obtained in H strain when compared to the SABRA strain (unpublished observation). The present experiments

Table 1. Comparison of arterial pressure and pain perception of normotensive and hypertensive human subjects. Blood pressure was measured from the brachial artery with a sphygmomanometer. Sensory and pain thresholds were measured using pulp tester (Vita pulp, Pelton and Crane Company) which applied 600 Hz, 0.1 msec monophasic pulses to the tooth pulp.
*** $p < 0.001$ statistical significance compared with normotensive controls.

Group	Age	weight (kg)	systolic blood pressure (mmHg)	diastolic blood pressure (mmHg)	sensory threshold (volts)	pain threshold (volts)
Normotensive	32.3 ± 1.8 (34)	73.3 ± 1.9 (34)	118.7 ± 1.7 (34)	76.8 ± 1.0 (34)	33.0 ± 3.3 (34)	50.1 ± 4.0 (34)
Hypertensive	33.6 ± 2.8 (21)	76.7 ± 2.4 (21)	151.7 ± 2.2*** (21)	95.5 ± 1.6*** (21)	76.4 ± 5.9*** (21)	97.1 ± 6.4*** (21)

Table 2. Distribution of opioid activity in brain regions and pituitary gland in renal hypertensive and atrophic kidney control SABRA rats, 20 days after clipping (left), and in H, SABRA and N rats (right). Opioid activity was measured by the radioreceptor assay (6) and expressed as nmole met enkephalin equivalents per g tissue (mean ± S.E.M.).

* $p < 0.02$, ** $p < 0.01$, *** $p < 0.001$ compared with the SABRA rats.

Region	Atrophic Kidney control	Renal Hypertension	H	Sabra	N
cervical spinal cord	1.72 ± 0.18 (18)	2.50 ± 0.24* (19)	3.26 ± 0.20** (8)	1.89 ± 0.22 (13)	3.68 ± 0.32**
medulla oblongata	2.07 ± 0.27 (10)	2.35 ± 0.35 (12)	2.28 ± 0.29 (10)	1.94 ± 0.18 (16)	1.68 ± 0.15 (8)
Pons-midbrain	1.22 ± 0.10 (15)	1.34 ± 0.10 (12)	1.18 ± 0.13 (10)	1.14 ± 0.08 (21)	0.96 ± 0.06 (8)
hypothalamus	3.79 ± 0.28 (29)	3.49 ± 0.21 (32)	5.96 ± 0.43** (10)	4.29 ± 0.28 (28)	6.10 ± 0.66** (16)
hippocampus	1.12 ± 0.15 (12)	0.98 ± 0.06 (9)	-	1.05 ± 0.15 (13)	1.64 ± 0.29 (8)
Pituitary	357 ± 79 (9)	333 ± 63 (11)	604 ± 143* (10)	326 ± 46 (16)	583 ± 76** (16)

demonstrate an association between blood pressure and pain sensitivity in rats and humans. Hypertensive rats and humans were less sensitive to noxious stimuli.

There is ample evidence that correlates opioid peptides and pain processes (9,6). These peptides are abundant in the dorsal horn of the spinal cord where they were implicated in gating mechanisms of pain messages (5). It is therefore interesting to note that in renal hypertensive rats, the place where a profound rise (45%) in opioid activity was found is the spinal cord. This, of course, does not exclude possible changes that take place elsewhere in the brain upon hypertension, but does indicate that the spinal cord might participate in the observed changes in pain reactivity.

The role of opioids in blood pressure regulation is still controversial (6,10,11). Morphine caused hypotension and bradycardia, yet naloxone had no effect, in our hands and others, on blood pressure in normal rats (11) and in anesthetized hypertensive rats (6). This does not exclude possible roles of opioid peptides in regulation of blood pressure under stressful physiological conditions (11,12). Further experiments are needed to untangle the intricate interrelations among the blood pressure and pain regulatory systems.

References

1. Akil, M. and Liebeskind, J.C., Monoaminergic mechanisms of stimulation-produced analgesia, Brain Research 94 (1975) 279-296.

2. Chalmers, P.J., Brain amines and models of experimental hypertension, Circ. Res. 36 (1975) 469-480.

3. Mayer, D.J. and Price, D.D., Central nervous system mechanisms of analgesia, Pain 2 (1976) 379-404.

4. Scriabine, A., Clineschmidt, B.V. and Sweet, C.S., Central noradrenergic control of blood pressure, Ann. Rev. Pharmacol. Toxicol. 16 (1976) 113-122.

5. Fields, H.L. and Basbaum, A.I., Brain stem control of spinal pain transmission neurons, Ann. Rev. Physiol. 40 (1978) 217-248.

6. Zamir, N., Simantov, R. and Segal, M., Pain sensitivity and opioid activity in genetically and experimentally hypertensive rats, Brain Research 184 (1980) 299-310.

7. Paalzow, L., Analgesia produced by clonidine in mice and rats, J. Pharm. Pharmacol. 26 (1974) 361-363.

8. Madden, IV,J., Akil, H., Patrick, R.L. and Barchas, J.D., Stress induced parallel changes in central opioid levels and pain responsiveness in the rat, Nature (Lond.) 265 (1977) 358-360.

9. Belluzi, J.D., Grant, N., Garsky, V., Sarantkis, D., Wise, C.D. and Stein, L., Analgesia induced in vivo by central administration of enkephalin in the rat, Nature (London) 260 (1976) 625-626.

10. Laubie, M., Schmitt, M., Vincent, M. and Remond, G., Central cardiovascular effects of morphinomimetic peptides in dogs, Europ. J. Pharmacol. 46 (1977) 67-71.

11. Faden, A.I. and Holaday, J.W., Opiate antagonists: A role in the treatment of hypovolemic shock, Science 205 (1979) 317-318.

12. Zamir, N. and Segal, M., Hypertension-induced analgesia: changes in pain sensitivity in experimental hypertensive rats, Brain Research 160 (1979) 170-173.

Neurotransmitters and their Receptors
Edited by U.Z. Littauer, Y. Dudai, I. Silman,
V.I. Teichberg and Z. Vogel

Lesions of the Lateral Hypothalamus Potentiate Morphine- But Not Naloxone-Induced Anorexia

Micah Leshem and Hanan Frenk
Depts. Psychology, Haifa University and Tel Aviv University

Morphine, like fenfluramine but unlike amphetamine, caused a more potent anorexia in hypothalamically lesioned rats than in unlesioned controls. Tolerance to the anorexic effect developed more slowly in laterals than in controls. Naloxone was equipotent in causing anorexia in these groups. The possibility that serotonin plays a role in morphine anorexia is discussed.

The anorexic properties of morphine (1, 2, 3) and its antagonists (1, 2, 3, 4) are well established. The lateral hypothalamus contains relatively high concentrations of endogenous opioids (5) and opiate receptors and this structure is known as the site where a number of feeding-related neural systems converge. Lesions of the lateral hypothalamus attenuate amphetamine-induced anorexia in rats (6, 7) but appear to enhance fenfluramine anorexia (8, 9). These findings indicate that whereas the hypothalamus is implicated in amphetamine-induced anorexia, fenfluramine exerts its anorexic influence via extrahypothalamic systems, possibly serotonergic (10).

The present study attempted to determine whether the lateral hypothalamus is involved in anorexia induced by morphine and its antagonist naloxone, or maybe in only one of these drugs, using the same paradigm effective in answering this question for fenfluramine and amphetamine.

METHODS

Locally bred Charles Rivers city strain rats were maintained on a normal light/dark cycle (light on from 7 am to 19 pm). Half of the animals were prepared with small bilateral hypothalamic lesions ("laterals") under ether anaesthesia. Control animals ("controls") underwent the same surgical procedures as the laterals save penetration of brain tissue. Routine histological examination at the end of the experiment confirmed that the lesions in the laterals were typically centered in the far lateral hypothalamus at the level of the descending columns of the fornix, immediate below the zona incerta and encroaching upon the internal capsule. Drug tests were started when all surviving laterals were maintaining or increasing body weight on standard laboratory food.

Procedure: Subjects were maintained on a cyclical feeding regimen with food present *ad lib* from 9 am until 13 pm the following day. The animals were then deprived of all food until 9 am the next day, and the cycle was repeated. The feeding regimen was introduced 10 days before drug tests started and was maintained for the entire duration of the experiment. Drugs administered in these experiments were dissolved in water and injected intraperitoneally in a volume of 1 ml/kg. Drugs tested were dl-amphetamine sulphate (1.75 mg/rat), (+)fenfluramine hydrochloride (5 mg/kg), morphine hydrochloride (5, 10, or 15 mg/kg), and naloxone hydrochloride (2 or 5 mg/kg). Saline solution in matched volumes served as control injections. Drugs were administered 20 min before food was presented on test days. Food intake was measured 1, 4, and 24 h after the food was presented. Each drug trial was preceded by a saline test day to establish feeding baselines and was separated by at least seven days from other drug tests sessions.

RESULTS AND DISCUSSION

Both amphetamine and fenfluramine suppressed feeding in controls and laterals. However, amphetamine anorexia was significantly less severe in laterals 1-4 h after feeding started ($p < .01$), whereas fenfluramine anorexia was significantly more severe during the first hour of feeding in laterals ($p < .05$). These results replicated previous observations (6, 7, 8, 9) and provided a reference model in this experiment for the anorexic effects of morphine and naloxone.

The influence of morphine (15 mg/kg) on feeding over time was triphasic. Morphine reduced food intake during the first hour after injection both in controls and laterals ($p < .01$) as reported previously for drinking (3). A facilitation of feeding was observed in both groups at the 1-4 h interval (controls 291% of baseline, $p < .02$; laterals 322% of baseline, $p < .02$). During the subsequent 4-24 h interval severe anorexia was seen (controls 60% of baseline, $p < .01$; laterals 73% of baseline, $p < .01$). A significantly more severe anorexia was apparent in the laterals when compared to controls during the first hour of feeding after injection ($p < .02$). Morphine's facilitatory effect on ingestion has also been noted with fluid consumption, but as a function of dose rather than a function of time after injection (3). The facilitation in feeding observed in the present experiment is unlikely to be entirely attributable to "rebound eating", since it occurs at lower doses when there is no preceding anorexia during the first hour (Leshem and Frenk, in preparation). Repeated injection of the 15 mg/kg dose of morphine with several weeks separating the trials demonstrated that on a second and third test morphine failed to cause anorexia in controls during the first hour after injection, though in laterals on the second test severe anorexia occurred (24% of baseline, $p < .02$). Morphine failed to induce anorexia in laterals during the first hour following injection on the third test. These results indicate that morphine becomes less anorexogenic with repeated injection both in controls and laterals. However, the difference in degree of anorexia between laterals and controls during the first hour of feeding was fully replicable on the second test ($p < .02$), and a non-significant difference existed on the third test as well.

Naloxone reduced food intake at both doses tested (2 and 5 mg/kg). The 5 mg/kg dose reduced food intake significantly in controls and laterals ($p < .01$) and no difference between these groups in the degree of anorexia was observed. The 2 mg/kg dose attained significance only when the data from both experimental groups were pooled ($p < .01$). There were no differences from baseline tests after the first hour of feeding following the injection of naloxone.

It was attempted to reverse the anorexic effects of morphine (15 mg/kg) with naloxone (2 mg/kg). Naloxone reversed completely the anorexic effect of morphine during the first hour of feeding in the laterals but only partially in the controls and a slight anorexic effect remained in these animals (73% of baseline, $p < .01$). The facilitation of feeding observed 1-4 h after morphine injection was antagonized in both groups, but the reduction in feeding during the 4-24 h interval was maintained (87% of baseline in both groups, $p < .01$).

In the present experiment morphine, like fenfluramine but not like amphetamine, caused more severe anorexia in laterals than in controls. This effect was replicable and also appeared in the slower rate of tolerance with repeated injections in laterals. The enhanced morphine anorexia in laterals was reversible by naloxone. It may therefore be concluded that morphine anorexia is not mediated by the lateral hypothalamus or pathways passing through this structure. Naloxone was equipotent in causing anorexia in laterals and controls. This indicates that naloxone anorexia, like the anorexia caused by morphine, is not mediated by the lateral hypothalamus. However, the observation that morphine anorexia in laterals is enhanced when compared to controls whereas naloxone anorexia is not, argues that the mechanisms of producing anorexia are different for the two drugs.

The enhanced morphine anorexia ressembles fenfluramine anorexia.This may suggest that serotonergic mechanisms are not only implicated in the action of fenfluramine (10) but in morphine anorexia as well. Serotonin has been implicated in other morphine-induced behaviors such as analgesia (11), locomotion (12), tolerance (13), and tonic immobility (14). Morphine effects 5-HT levels in the brain (13). However, direct evidence for a role of 5-HT in the anorexic action of morphine remains to be acquired.

ACKNOWLEDGEMENTS

This study was supported by grants from the Israel Trustees of the Ford Foundation, the Israel Academy of Science and Yissum Applied Research Company. We thank Mssrs. D. Teucher, A. Weinstein, and T. Lahav for their help. We are indebted to Endo Laboratories, Garden City, NY. for naloxone, and to Abic Ltd., Israel, for fenfluramine.

REFERENCES

1. Frenk, H. and G.H. Rogers. Behav. Neur. Biol. 26:23-40, 1979.
2. Holtzman, S.G. Life Sci. 16:1465-1470, 1975.
3. Maickel, R.P., M.C. Braude, and J.E. Zabik. Neuropharmac. 16:863-866, 1977.
4. Frenk,H.and J.B. Rosen. Pharmac. Biochem. Behav. 11:387-390, 1979.
5. Yang, H-Y., J.S. Hong, and E. Costa. Neuropharmac. 16:303-307, 1977.
6. Ahlskog, J.E. Brain Res. 82:211-240, 1974.
7. Carlisle, H.F. J. Comp. Physiol. Psychol. 58:47-54, 1964.
8. Blundell, J.E. and M. Leshem. Postgrad. Med. J. 51 (Suppl. 1):45-54, 1974.
9. Carey, R.J. and E.B. Goodal. Neuropharmac. 14:827-834, 1975.
10. Garrattini, S., W. Puezko, A. Jori, and R. Samanin. Postgrad. Med. J. 51 (Suppl. 1):27-35, 1975.
11. Lee, R.C., R.D.E. Sewell, and P.S.J. Spencer. Eur. J. Pharmac. 47:251-253, 1978.
12. Oka, T. and E. Hosoya. Psychopharmac. 47:243-248, 1976.
13. Haubrich, D.R. and D.E. Blake. Biochem. Pharmac. 22:2753-2759, 1973.
14. Wallnau, L.B. Dissert. Abstr.Int. 38:2928B, 1977.

Neurotransmitters and their Receptors
Edited by U.Z. Littauer, Y. Dudai, I. Silman,
V.I. Teichberg and Z. Vogel

On the Inactivation of Enkephalin by Enkephalinase

Miriam Altstein and Zvi Vogel

Department of Neurobiology,

The Weizmann Institute of Science, Rehovot, Israel

ABSTRACT

Enkephalinase is an endopeptidase which cosediments with the synaptosomal membranes and cleaves Leu-enkephalin into Tyr-Gly-Gly and Phe-Leu. It also cleaves (D-Ala^2)Met-enkephalinamide, although at a lower rate. The enzyme is inhibited by thiol compounds and metal chelating reagents, as well as by several barbiturates. Secobarbital, pentobarbital, phenobarbital and barbital inhibit the hydrolysis of Leu-enkephalin with an IC_{50} of 8.0×10^{-6} M, 2.0×10^{-5} M, 7.0×10^{-5} M and 1.0×10^{-4} M, respectively. The N-1-methyl substituted barbiturates tested (methohexital and hexobarbital) as well as the non-sedative barbituric acid have little or no inhibitory activity. The inhibition by secobarbital is reversible and shows reaction kinetics of a mixed noncompetitive-competitive type with K_I^S of 2.0×10^{-5} M and K_I^I of 6.0×10^{-5} M. The enkephalin-degrading aminopeptidase and the endopeptidase enkephalinase B are not inhibited by barbiturates.

INTRODUCTION

Administration of the opioid peptides Leu- or Met-enkephalin into the brain produces only a transient and weak analgesia (1, 2) and is followed by the rapid degradation of the injected enkephalins (3, 4). Several laboratories have reported that the most rapid enzymatic attack on these enkephalins *in vitro* occurs at the Tyr-Gly peptide bond, releasing Tyr as the main hydrolysis product (3, 5). This result is in line with the increased stability and analgesic effect of enkephalin analogs having D-amino acids in position 2 (1, 6). On the other hand, the *in situ* data indicate that enzymatic attack occurs initially at the Gly-Gly and/or Gly-Phe peptide bond to yield Tyr-Gly-Gly and/or Tyr-Gly, while the cleavage of the N-terminal tyrosine occurs only later (4).

Enzymes having the appropriate cleavage specificity for yielding the above-mentioned degradation products have been identified in the brain.

They include: 1) Puromycin-sensitive aminopeptidase (3,7,8,9,10); 2) Enkephalinase, an endopeptidase which cleaves enkephalin at the Gly-Phe peptide bond into Tyr-Gly-Gly and Phe-Leu (11, 12); 3) Enkephalinase B, an endopeptidase recently discovered by Gorenstein and Snyder, which cleaves the enkephalin at the Gly-Phe peptide bond, releasing Tyr-Gly (13).

It is not clear which, if any, of these enzymes is involved in the physiological degradation of endogenous enkephalin at the synaptic cleft. The enzyme enkephalinase is a likely candidate since its regional distribution in the brain is in good correlation with that of the opiate receptors and its activity is regulated by morphine treatment (11, 14).

The activities of the other two enzymes, aminopeptidase and enkephalinase B, are not regulated by morphine treatment and their distribution does not correlate well with that of the opiate receptors (11,13,14).

In the following we describe some of the properties of the enzyme enkephalinase, with special emphasis on screening for specific inhibitors which might be used to distinguish between the activities of the various enzymes and serve eventually as a tool for studying enkephalin degradation *in vivo*.

MATERIALS AND METHODS

Enkephalin-degrading enzyme preparations

Striata (0.5 g) of adult male Sprague-Dawley rats or C57BL/6J male mice were homogenized in 15 ml of cold 0.3 M sucrose containing 10 mM Tris-HCl, pH 7.5 (Tris). The supernatant of a 10 min spin at 1000 x g was recentrifuged at 17,300 x g for 30 min. The resulting crude mitochondrial pellet was hypotonically lyzed by homogenization in 30 ml of 5 mM Tris, and the supernatant obtained following a 30 min spin at 48,000 x g was used as the soluble aminopeptidase preparation. The pellet of the last centrifugation step, containing the crude synaptosomal membrane, was dissolved and brought to a final volume of 60 ml of 36% sucrose (w/w) containing 5 mM Tris. The membranes were further purified by a modification of the flotation-sedimentation discontinuous sucrose gradient centrifugation of Jones and Matus (15), as follows: Each centrifuge tube contained 20 ml of the crude synaptosomal membrane preparation in 36% sucrose, overlayed respectively by 8 ml, 8 ml and 3 ml of 34%, 28.5% and 10% sucrose (w/w), all in 5 mM Tris. These discontinuous sucrose gradients were spun for 120 min at 56,000 x g in an SW27 rotor using a Beckman ultracentrifuge. The purified synaptosomal membranes were collected from the interphase between the 34% and 28.5% sucrose layers, diluted 10-fold with 5 mM Tris, and pelleted for 60 min at 56,000 x g. The pellet was dissolved in 5 mM Tris, frozen in aliquots, and used as the stock enkephalinase preparation.

Enzymatic hydrolysis of Leu-enkephalin by enkephalinase

Aliquots of rat striatal synaptic membranes (2-4 μg protein) were incubated for 40 min at 30°C with 50 nM [Tyr-^{3}H]Leu-enkephalin (Amersham Radiochemical Centre) in 100 μl of 10 mM Tris-HCl (pH 7.5), 0.1 mg bovine serum albumin/ml and 0.1 mM p-hydroxymercuribenzoate (PHMB) (to inhibit the residual aminopeptidase still present in the washed synaptic membrane preparation). PHMB and the other inhibitors used (see under Results) were added to the enzyme-containing mixture 15 min before adding Leu-enkephalin. Reactions were stopped by boiling and the hydrolysis products filtered through columns of Porapak Q (7, 8).

RESULTS AND DISCUSSION

Figure 1 presents the procedure used for the preparation of purified synaptosomal membranes from rat or mouse striatum. The specific activity of the enkephalin-degrading aminopeptidase and enkephalinase were tested during the various steps of the membrane purification. It was found (see ref. 12) that the aminopeptidase was present in the soluble fraction of the striatal homogenate. Some aminopeptidase cosedimented with the crude synaptosomal membranes, but its specific activity was drastically reduced by hypotonic lysis and upon washing the membranes through a sucrose gradient. The enkephalinase was associated with the particulate fraction and its specific activity was increased through the process of membrane purification.

Figure 2 presents thin-layer chromatography of the reaction products obtained by the incubation of [Tyr-^{3}H]Leu-enkephalin with rat striatal purified synaptosomal membranes. The results show the appearance of: 1) a tripeptide which comigrated with Tyr-Gly-Gly; 2) a material which comigrated with the aminoacid tyrosine and seemed to be a product of the residual aminopeptidase activity still present in these purified synaptosomal membranes. The formation of Tyr could be inhibited by the addition of 0.1 mM puromycin or 0.1 mM PHMB. This process is analogous

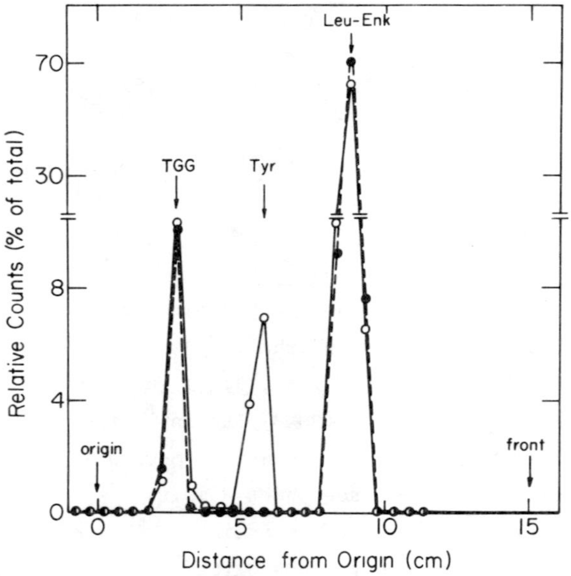

Fig. 1.
Preparation of purified synaptosomal membranes from rat or mouse striatum (for details see Methods).

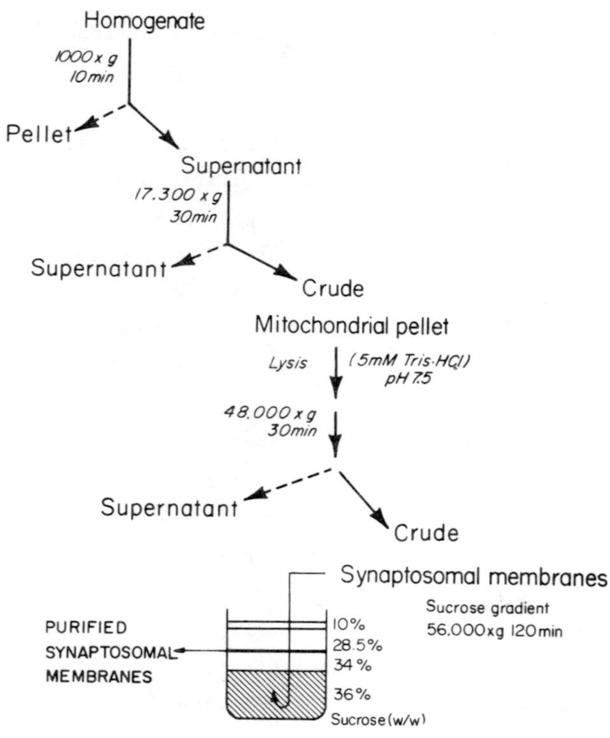

Fig. 2.
Thin-layer chromatography (silica plates in ethyl-acetate-isopropanol-acetic-acid-water, 40:40:1:19) of the reaction products obtained following a 20 min incubation of labeled Leu-enkephalin with 2.1 μg of rat striatal synaptic membranes in the absence (o——o) or presence (●---●) of 0.1 mM PHMB. Markers were visualized by fluorescamine spray as previously described (7).

to the inhibition of the soluble aminopeptidase activity by these materials (8, 11). The formation of Tyr-Gly-Gly was not affected by these drugs (Fig. 2 and refs. 11, 12). High-voltage paper electrophoresis of the reaction products of [Leu-^{3}H]Leu-enkephalin revealed the formation of the carboxy dipeptide moiety Phe-Leu (12, 16). The Tyr-Gly-Gly was therefore formed by an endopeptidase cleavage and did not result from the sequential action of carboxypeptidases.

Figure 3 shows the Lineweaver-Burk plot of the enkephalinase activity of rat striatal washed synaptic membranes. The K_m for the

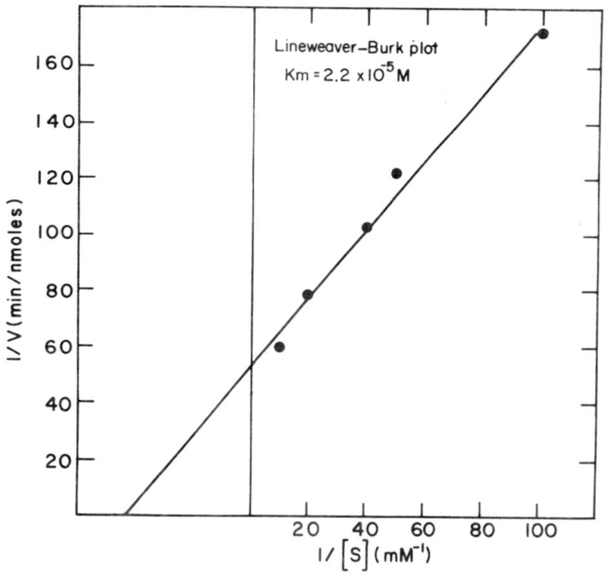

Fig. 3. Lineweaver-Burk plot of the hydrolysis of [Tyr-^{3}H]Leu-enkephalin by the enkephalinase present in washed synaptic membranes.

hydrolysis of Leu-enkephalin was 2.2 x 10^{-5} M and the V_{max} was 2 nmol x min^{-1} per mg protein (12). These values differ from those reported by Malfroy *et al*. (K_m = 9.0 x 10^{-8} M, V_{max} = 850 fmole x min^{-1} per mg protein) (11). However, the K_m value is in agreement with the value reported more recently by the same group (17).

Table 1 summarizes the effects of various compounds on the activity of enkephalinase in hydrolyzing Leu-enkephalin. The enzyme was sensitive to Thiol compounds: β-mercaptoethanol inhibited the enzyme by 50% at a concentration of 800 μM. Dithiols were much more effective: 2,3-dimercapto-1-propanol inhibited the enzyme by 50% at 2 μM, and dithio-

Table 1. Effects of various inhibitors on the activity of enkephalinase

Thiol compounds	IC_{50} (μM)
β-Mercaptoethanol	800
Dithiothreitol	8
2,3-Dimercapto-1-propanol	2
Chelating reagents	
EDTA	400
EGTA	200
o-Phenanthroline	100
Z-Aminoacid hydroxamates	0.04-1*

* Values depend on the specific aminoacid (see ref. 19).

The thiol compounds were incubated with mouse washed synaptic membranes (3.3 μg) for 60 min at 0°C in the absence of PHMB. Under these conditions the residual aminopeptidase showed negligible activity (see ref. 12). The effect of the other inhibitors was tested as described in Methods.

threitol at 8 μM. Neither the mercaptoethanol nor the dithiothreitol had any effect even at millimolar concentrations on the activity of the enkephalin-degrading aminopeptidase (18). Metal chelating agents also inhibited enkephalinase activity: EDTA, EGTA and o-phenanthroline inhibited activity by 50% at 400 μM, 200 μM, and 100 μM, respectively. We also found that the benzyloxycarbonyl aminoacid hydroxamates were very effective reversible inhibitors of enkephalinase, with an IC_{50} of 0.04 - 1.0 μM, depending on the aminoacid (19). This result is in line with the recent finding that peptide hydroxamic acids are strong reversible inhibitors of the metalloenzyme endopeptidase thermolysin (20), thus suggesting that enkephalinase contains a heavy metal ion in the active site.

The effect of unlabeled Tyr and Tyr-containing peptides from the N-terminal region of the enkephalin molecule on the rate of hydrolysis of Leu-enkephalin by enkephalinase is shown in Table 2. The affinity of the dipeptide Tyr-Gly to the enzyme was higher than that of tyrosine by almost two orders of magnitude, increasing the length of the peptide chain did not result in a further increase in affinity. The IC_{50} value of

Table 2. The effect of Tyr, enkephalins and peptides from N-terminus of enkephalin on the hydrolysis of Leu-enkephalin by the enkephalinase.

Compound tested	IC_{50} (μM)
Tyr	1000
Tyr-Gly	17
Tyr-Gly-Gly	17
Tyr-Gly-Gly-Phe	15
Leu-enkephalin	10
(D-Ala^2)Leu-enkephalin	7
Met-enkephalin	3
(D-Ala^2)Met-enkephalin	1

Tyr-Gly was similar to those obtained with Tyr-Gly-Gly, Tyr-Gly-Gly-Phe and Leu-enkephalin. On the other hand, the dipeptide Tyr-Arg (kyotorphin) had a much lower affinity to the enzyme (IC_{50} = 2.0 x 10^{-4} M, data not shown). Thus, the first two aminoacids of the enkephalin molecule, although not at the site of cleavage, were recognized by the enzyme.

In agreement with results reported by Fournie-Zaluski et al., we found that the affinity of Met-enkephalin to the enzyme was higher than that of Leu-enkephalin (17). Substituting D-Ala for Gly in position 2 increased the affinity. This result contradicts the findings of Malfroy et al. that the D-Ala^2 enkephalins are not recognized by the enzyme (11). Moreover, we have shown that the enkephalin analog D-Ala^2-Met-enkephalin-amide is hydrolyzed by the enkephalinase, but is completely resistant to hydrolysis by the soluble enkephalin-degrading aminopeptidase (12). The question of whether deamination precedes the hydrolysis at the Gly-Phe peptide bond or whether the enzyme is capable of removing the Phe-Met-NH_2 has not been resolved.

It has been reported that the administration of either D-Phe (21) or Tyr-Arg (22) induces analgesic effects in mice. Our results demonstrated that neither compound effectively inhibited enkephalinase activity (IC_{50} of 2.0 x 10^{-3} M and 2.0 x 10^{-4} M, respectively). Thus, the mechanism of action of these analgesic compounds does not seem to be related to the inhibition of enkephalin degradation by enkephalinase.

Vivante et al. reported that the narcotic antagonist nalorphine antagonized the respiratory effects of pentobarbital (23). Similarly, the administration of the opiate antagonist naloxone delayed the onset and decreased the duration of pentobarbital-induced loss of righting reflex (24). These experiments hint at the possibility that some of the effects of the barbiturates are accompanied by changes in the concentrations of endogenous opioid substances. We therefore investigated the effects of barbiturates on the enzymatic degradation of the enkephalins (25). Fig. 4 shows that both pentobarbital and phenobarbital inhibit the degradation of enkephalin by the enzyme enkephalinase. On the other hand, the activity of the rat-striatum aminopeptidase was not significantly affected by these drugs (5-10% reduction in activity in the presence of 1 mM pentobarbital or phenobarbital); nor was the activity

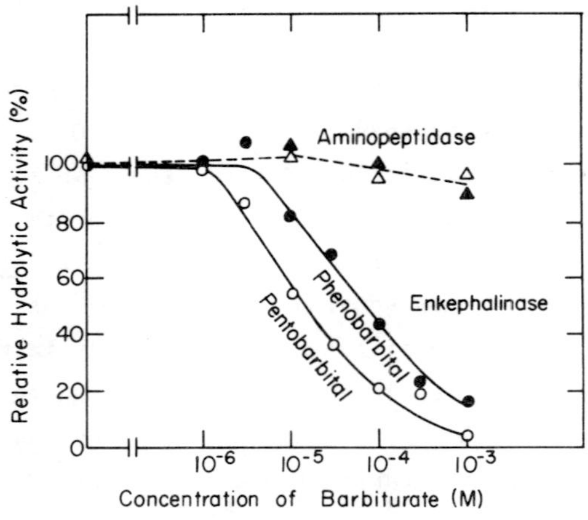

Fig. 4. The effects of pentobarbital and phenobarbital on the hydrolysis of Leu-enkephalin by rat striatal soluble aminopeptidase (1.3 μg, 10 min at 30°C, in the absence of PHMB) and rat striatal enkephalinase (as described in Methods). The extent of enkephalin hydrolyzed in the absence of barbiturates was equivalent to 0.61 and 1.82 pmoles respectively. Thin-layer chromatography revealed the formation of Tyr-Gly-Gly and Tyr as the major reaction products (> 95%) of the endopeptidase and aminopeptidase, respectively.

of the brain enzyme, enkephalinase B, affected by 0.1 mM of either pheno- or pentobarbital (25).

The barbiturates differ in their inhibitory potency toward the enzyme enkephalinase. Table 3 presents the IC_{50} values of various barbiturates towards this enzyme. The inhibitory activity was increased when the side chains on position 5 of the barbiturate ring were elongated. This order of activity correlated well with the central depressant potency of these drugs (26). The N-1-methyl substituted barbiturates (i.e., methohexital

Table 3. Effects of various barbiturates on the hydrolysis of Leu-enkephalin by enkephalinase

Compound	IC_{50} (μM)
secobarbital	8
pentobarbital	18
amobarbital	26
butabarbital	40
phenobarbital	70
barbital	400
methohexital	>> 1000
hexobarbital	>> 1000

and hexobarbital) showed relatively weak inhibitory activity, which is in accordance with the notion that their physiological antidepressant activity derives primarily from demethylated metabolites (26). Non-sedative barbituric acid had very little or no inhibitory activity.

The interaction of the enkephalinase with the barbiturate secobarbital was reversible, and removal of the barbiturate by dialysis completely restored the enzymatic activity. The kinetics of the interaction is of a mixed noncompetitive-competitive type, with K_I^S of 2 x 10^{-5}M and K_I^I of 6 x 10^{-5}M (25). Thus, secobarbital interacts with the unoccupied enzyme and with the enzyme substrate complex according to different kinetic constants.

The inhibition of enkephalinase by the barbiturates was not dependent upon its association with the membranes. More than 75% of the enzyme could be released into the high speed supernatant on the addition of 1% Triton X-100 (12). We found that the detergent-treated enzyme was inhibited by barbiturates to the same extent as the membrane-associated enzyme.

The barbiturates are valuable as a tool to distinguish and characterize the brain enzymatic activities which hydrolyze enkephalin. Further experiments are needed to determine whether the barbiturates inhibit enkephalinase *in vivo*, and whether this inhibition results in an increased accumulation of non-degraded enkephalin in the synaptic clefts.

REFERENCES

1. Pert, C.B., Pert, A., Chang, J.K. and Fong, B.T.W. (1976) Science 194, 330-332.

2. Belluzzi, J.D., Grant, N., Garsk, V., Sarantakis, D., Wise, C.D. and Stein, L. (1976) Nature 260, 625-626.

3. Meek, J.L., Yang, H.Y.T. and Costa, E. (1977) Neuropharmacol. 16, 151-154.

4. Craves, F.B., Law, P.Y., Hunt, C.A. and Loh, H.H. (1978) J. Pharmacol. Exp. Ther. 206, 492-506.

5. Dupont, A., Cusan, L., Garon, M., Alvarado-Urbina, G. and Labrie, F. (1977) Life Sci. 21, 907-914.

6. Roemer, D., Buescher, H.H., Hill, R.C., Pless, J., Bauer, W., Cardinaux, F., Closse, A., Hauser, D. and Huguenin, R. (1977) Nature 268, 547-549.

7. Vogel, Z. and Altstein, M. (1977) FEBS Letters 80, 332-336.

8. Vogel, Z. and Altstein, M. (1979) FEBS Letters 98, 44-48.

9. Barclay, R.K. and Phillips, M.A. (1978) Biochem. Biophys. Res. Commun. 81, 1119-1123.

10. Knight, M. and Klee, W.A. (1978) J. Biol. Chem. 253, 3843-3847.

11. Malfroy, B., Swerts, J.P., Guyon, A., Rocques, B.P. and Schwartz, J.C. (1978) Nature 276, 523-526.

12. Vogel, Z. and Altstein, M. (1979) in Endogenous and Exogenous Opiate Agonists and Antagonists, (Way, E.L. ed.), Pergamon Press, New York, p.353.

13. Gorenstein, C. and Snyder, S.H. (1979) Life Sci. 25, 2065-2070.

14. Malfroy, B., Swerts, J.P., Llorens, C. and Schwartz, J.C. (1979) Neurosci. Lett. 11, 329-334.

15. Jones, D.H. and Matus, A.I. (1974) Biochim. Biophys. Acta 356,276-287

16. Vogel, Z. and Altstein, M. (1980) in Endogenous Peptides and Centrally Acting Drugs, (Series Progr. Biochem. Pharmac.) (Levi, R., Heldman, E., Vogel, Z. and Gutman, Y., eds.) AG Karger, Basel, Vol.16 (in press).

17. Fournie-Zaluski, M.C., Perdrisot, R., Gacel, G., Swerts, J.P., Roques, B.P. and Schwartz, J.C. (1979) Biochem. Biophys. Res. Commun. 91, 130-135.

18. Vogel, Z. and Altstein, M. (1977) Israel J. Med. Sci. 13, 943.

19. Blumberg, S., Vogel, Z. and Altstein, M. (1980) Submitted for publication.

20. Nishino, N. and Powers, J.C. (1978) Biochemistry 18, 2846-2850.

21. Erenprise, S., Comaty, J.E. and Myles, S.B. (1978) in Characteristics and Function of Opioids, (Van Ree, J.M. and Terenius, L. eds.), Elsevier, Amsterdam, pp. 417-418.

22. Takagi, H., Shiomi, H., Ueda, H. and Amano, H. (1979) Eur. J. Pharmacol. 55, 109-111.

23. Vivante, A.F., Kau, F.F. and Belford, J. (1954) J. Pharmacol. Exp. Ther. 111, 436-446.

24. Furst, Z., Folders, F.F. and Knoll, J. (1977) Life Sci. 20, 921-926.

25. Altstein, M., Mittman, S. and Vogel, Z. (1980) Submitted for publication.

26. Maynert, E.W. (1972) in Drills Pharmacology in Medicine, (DiPalma, J.R., ed.), McCgraw-Hill Book Co., New York, Fourth Edition, p. 250.

EXCITABLE MEMBRANES AND CYTOSKELETON

Neurotransmitters and their Receptors
Edited by U.Z. Littauer, Y. Dudai, I. Silman,
V.I. Teichberg and Z. Vogel

The Voltage-Dependent Sodium Channel as a Drug Receptor

M. Lazdunski, M. Balerna, J. Barhanin, R. Chicheportiche, M. Fosset
C. Frelin, Y. Jacques, A. Lombet, J. Pouyssegur, J.F. Renaud,
G. Romey, H. Schweitz, J.P. Vincent
*Centre de Biochimie du CNRS, Faculté des Sciences, Parc Valrose,
06034 Nice Cedex, France*

The voltage-dependent sodium channel is a drug receptor for a variety of specific neurotoxins. The paper describes the properties of interaction of the following toxins with their receptors : tetrodotoxin, veratridine, batrachotoxin, grayanotoxin, pyrethroids and scorpion and sea anemone toxins. Three types of approaches have been used in this work : (i) binding of radiolabeled toxins, (ii) toxin-stimulated $^{22}Na^+$ flux through the Na^+ channel and (iii) electrophysiology including voltage-clamp of neuroblastoma cells. The main results include (i) the determination of the number of toxin binding sites, of the number of families of sites for the different toxic compounds, of the properties of interaction between these different families; (ii) the demonstration that there also exist silent Na^+ channels, i.e. channels which cannot be activated electrically but which can be activated chemically by the toxins; these structures are present in fibroblasts; (iii) the fact that these neurotoxins are very useful tools to study the differentiation of the Na^+ channel.

Recent progress in the analysis of the molecular mechanism of the Na^+ channel have made a large use of a series of neurotoxins which can specifically interfere either with the selectivity filter or with the gating system of the channel. The selectivity filter is the structure which defines the cationic specificity of the channel; the gating system is involved in the voltage-dependent opening and closing steps of the sodium ionophore.

Tetrodotoxin interactions with the Na^+ channel : the tetrodotoxin receptor - Tetrodotoxin (TTX) and saxitoxin (STX) are the two important toxins blocking at or near the selectivity filter of the sodium channel. The biochemical analysis of the structural and functional properties of the sodium channel was started with the introduction of tritiated TTX by HAFEMAN (1). Unfortunately it is extremely difficult to be sure that [^{3}H]TTX prepared by this technique is pure (2) and it is nearly impossible to incorporate a specific radioactivity higher than 1 Ci/mmol. [^{3}H]Saxitoxin has been introduced by RITCHIE and his colleagues (2). It is a very useful ligand to study the Na^+ channel (2). However there are two difficulties with this toxin : the first one is that it is not commercially available and the second is that it dissociates rapidly from its receptor.

Because the densities of sodium channels are low in excitable membranes, there is a great need for TTX samples of high specific radioactivity for their titration. It has been our purpose to make derivatives of TTX which would have a toxic activity similar to TTX itself and which would be of a high specific radioactivity. At the same time, the experience acquired in the chemical modification of TTX, has been used to synthesize a series of photoactivable affinity derivatives of the toxin.

Fig. 1 schematically indicates some chemical modifications of TTX which have given useful toxin derivatives (3,4). The only place in which the toxin can be modified with a minimum loss of biological activity is on carbons in position 6 and 11. Oxidations to form a keto or an aldehyde group allow coupling of the TTX molecule to an RNH_2 molecule. For example, one of the derivatives used in binding studies comes from a covalent association between a TTX and a radioactive glycine moiety. Glycine can be replaced by a variety of other amino acids such as lysine, β-alanine and by ethylenediamine. [^{3}H]gly-TTX for example can be obtained at a specific radioactivity near 45 Ci/mmol that is nearly 100 times higher than usual samples of [^{3}H]TTX prepared according to HAFEMAN. [^{3}H]gly-TTX binds well to pure axonal membranes prepared from crab nerves according to BALERNA et al. (5). The Scatchard plot corresponding to the binding is linear, indicating a single family of binding sites and the dissociation constant of the [^{3}H]gly-TTX-receptor complex is 3.2 nM, nearly identical to the dissociation constant of the TTX-receptor complex measured by electrophysiological techniques (6). The capacity of binding of these pure membranes is 10 ± 2 pmol of receptor per mg of membrane protein. A dissociation constant of 9 nM was found for the [^{3}H] gly-TTX-receptor complex in synaptosomes, the binding capacity being in that case of 1.8 ± 0.2 pmol of receptor per mg of membrane protein. Comparative binding data have been obtained (4) with TTX, TTX-derivatives and STX to axonal membranes and to the receptor in a solubilized form either from axonal membranes or from *Electrophorus* membranes. The receptor solubilized from axonal membranes forms a more stable complex with toxins and toxin derivatives than the receptor solubilized from the electric organ membranes. The most kinetically stable complexes are formed with the sodium channel in axonal membranes and have half-lives of more than 10 min at 0° (t 1/2 = 43 min for the [^{3}H]gly-TTX-receptor complex using crab axonal membranes).

Fig. 1 shows that photoactivable derivatives of TTX (the azido group is the photoactivable function) can be prepared; they form reversible complexes with the TTX receptor in the dark and give an irreversible block of the Na^+ channel after UV irradiation (3,7).

Derivatives of TTX can be used to analyse the solubilization and some of the elementary molecular properties of the Na^+ channel. The TTX receptor from axonal membranes can easily be solubilized in 0.8% Lubrol WX and it retains 60 to 80% of its binding activity for labeled TTX. To keep an active form of the TTX receptor it is necessary to protect it before, during, and after the solubilization by maintaining a medium containing 40 nM TTX. The TTX-receptor complex is much more stable during detergent treatment than the free receptor itself. The estimated molecular weight of the TTX receptor from crab axonal membranes determined by gel filtration is 250,000 ± 20,000. It is in satisfactory agreement with the molecular weight estimated by LEVINSON and ELLORY using the radiation inactivation technique (8). An important purification of the Na^+ channel can be obtained using DEAE cellulose and ultrogel chromatographies. However the instability of the Na^+ channel makes it difficult to carry its purification to completion.

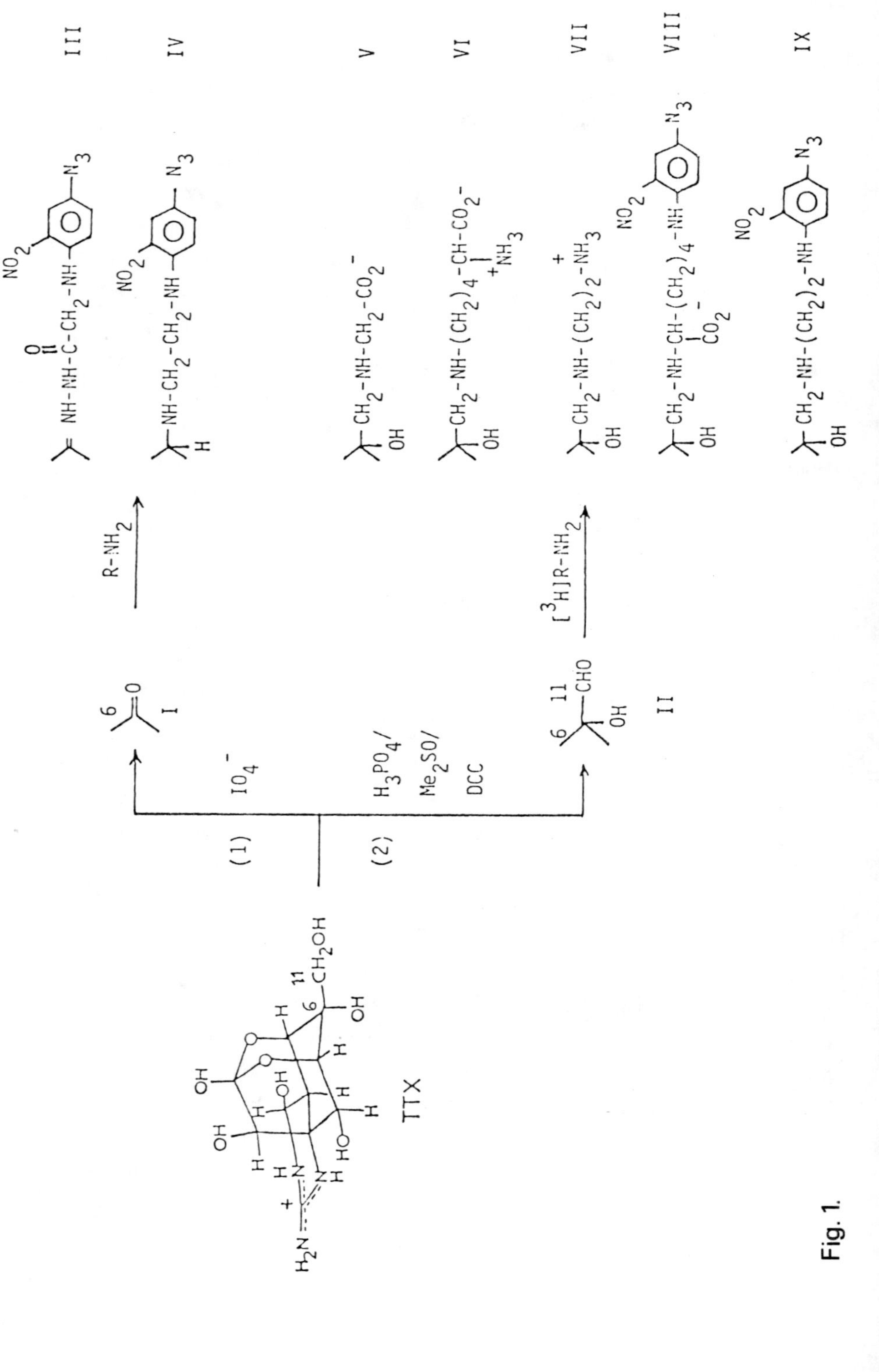
TTX
(1) IO4-
(2) H3PO4/ Me2SO/ DCC
I
II
R-NH2
[3H]R-NH2
III
IV
V
VI
VII
VIII
IX

Fig. 1.

Fig. 1. Derivatives of TTX, useful for binding assays and irreversible blocking of the Na^+ channel. TTX oxidations were performed with sodium periodate (pathway 1) or dimethylsulfoxide-dicyclohexylcarbodiimide (pathway 2). The derivatives were obtained by coupling these two oxidized derivatives of TTX (I or II) with [^{3}H]glycine (V), [^{3}H]lysine (VI), [^{3}H]ethylenediamine (VII), N-(2-nitro-4-azidophenyl)ethylenediamine (IV, IX) or N-(2-nitro-4-azidophenyl)lysine (VIII) by reductive amination with sodium cyanoborohydride or with 2-nitro-4-azidophenyl-glycine hydrazide to form stable hydrazone (III). Derivatives V to IX can be obtained at a high specific radioactivity.

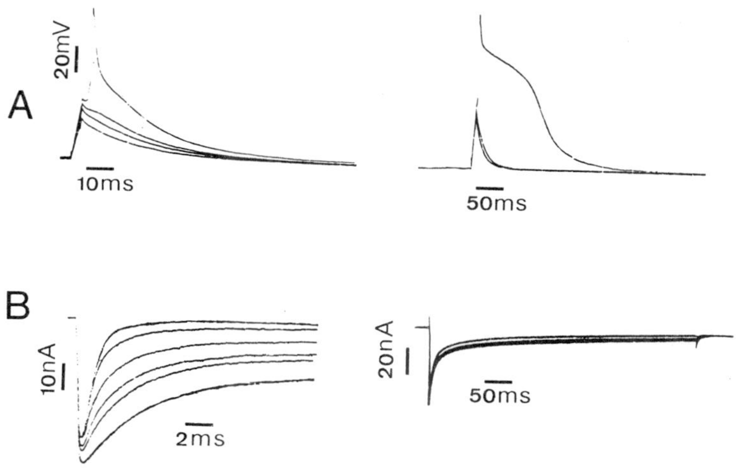

Fig. 2. A. Effect of ATX_{II} on the action potential of NIE115 neuroblastoma cells. Left : Control action potentials. Right : 5 min after the application of 1 μM ATX_{II}. B. Voltage-clamp analysis of ATX_{II} action on the inward Na^+ current. Left : Time-course of the effect of 1 μM ATX_{II} on Na^+ current during 80 mV depolarizing pulses from a holding potential of -100 mV. Successive recordings (arrow) were taken at 20 sec intervals after ATX_{II} application. Note that ATX_{II} decreases the inactivation rate of Na^+ current without affecting the activation rate. Current scale : 10 nA; time scale : 2 msec. Right : Same experiment but with a different time scale : 50 msec. Note that the Na^+ current decline exhibits a fast and a slow phase instead of a single fast phase in the control (initial left record). Current scale : 20 nA.

Toxin interactions with the gating system and their use for the analysis of the structure-function relationship of the action potential Na^+ channel - A variety of toxic compounds alter the gating system of the Na^+ channel. There are first "small" molecules like veratridine, veratridine-like compounds (batrachotoxin, aconitine, etc...) and grayanotoxins which alter both the activation and the inactivation of the Na^+ channel (9), pyrethroïd-type molecules which inhibit the sodium inactivation (10). None of these toxic compounds prevents binding of TTX or STX to the sodium channel. There are two distinct sites of action on the gating system for these different toxins. One site is specifically recognized by veratridine, batrachotoxin, aconitine and grayanotoxins, another one is recognized by molecules of the pyrethroïd family (11). There are also polypeptide toxins like scorpion and sea anemone (ATX) toxins. A large part of the following presentation will deal with the sea anemone toxins. The sequences of four sea anemone toxins are currently known (12-15). These toxins are small proteins cross-linked with disulfide bridges which have respectively 46, 47, 27 and 49 aminoacids. The chemical analysis of structure-function relationships of ATX_{II}, the most abundant toxin from Anemonia sulcata indicates the essentiality of Arg_{14}. Voltage-clamp analysis of their action on crustacean giant axons, on myelinated fibers and on neuroblastoma cells has shown that these polypeptide neurotoxins selectively slow down the inactivation of the sodium channel (16) (Fig. 2). They do not alter the activation process or the functioning of the potassium channel. The mode of action of sea anemone toxins and scorpion toxins is similar but not identical. Scorpion toxins which are small polypeptide toxins also decrease the rate of inactivation of the Na^+ channel (17). The electrophysiological approach shows that these polypeptide toxins have the following properties of binding : (i) They associate with the gating system and have no interaction with the selectivity filter of the sodium channel (ii) Their receptor site is on the external face of the excitable membrane (iii) Their receptor site is distinct from the veratridine and the pyrethroïd sites.

The information collected with these toxins with the only use of the voltage-clamp technique is important. It suggests (i) that the two "gates" h and m which control the opening and closing events of the sodium channel correspond to independent conformational changes. Polypeptide toxins alter h and leave m unchanged (ii) that the molecular component which constitutes the h gate spans the membrane: it is accessible to polypeptide toxins from the outside and can be destroyed by protease application to the inside of the excitable membrane (18). The action of sea anemone toxins like that of scorpion toxins is not limited to the axonal membrane. ATX_{II} stimulates the release of radioactive neurotransmitter from preloaded synaptosomes at toxin concentrations between 5 and 500 nM (19). This stimulating effect like the one produced by scorpion toxins (20) is completely suppressed by TTX. ATX_{II} also interacts with the cardiac cell membrane; its primary site of action is the Na^+ channel but as a consequence of this interaction the toxin induces a strong positive inotropic effect (21).

ATX_{II} and scorpion toxin II from the venom of *Androctonus australis Hector* have been radiolabeled with iodine and their binding properties to the sodium channel of synaptosomes have been studied (22). These binding data are presented in Fig. 3. Both toxins can obviously be used to selectively label the sodium channel. The main properties of these associations are the following : (i) The polypeptide toxin which displays the highest affinity for the sodium channel is the scorpion toxin; (ii) The scorpion toxin association is potential-dependent. Binding is suppressed in synaptosomes depolarized by high K^+ concentrations or by veratridine in the presence of 140 mM Na^+. Conversely the association of ATX_{II} is not influenced by the synaptosomal potential; (iii) Stoechiometries of association are very different for the two polypeptide toxins; the maximal stoechiometry of binding of the scorpion toxin being 10 times less than the stoechiometry of binding of ATX_{II} which is itself of the same order of magnitude as the stoechiometry of binding of TTX to the Na^+ channel in synaptosomes (19); (iv) ATX_{II} displaces the binding of the radiolabeled scorpion toxin, but the scorpion toxin is unable to displace the binding of $[^{125}I]ATX_{II}$. This work indicates (i) the respective stoechiometry of TTX and ATX_{II} receptors in the sodium channel : each sodium channel comprises one TTX receptor at its selectivity filter for two ATX_{II} receptors at the level of its gating system (ii) that if the scorpion

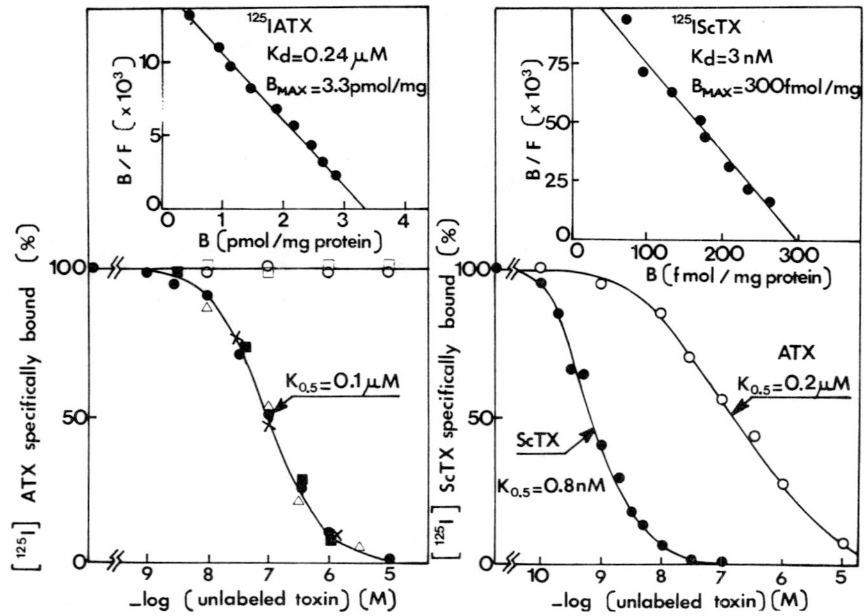

Fig. 3. Binding properties of [^{125}I]labeled sea anemone and scorpion toxins to rat brain synaptosomes, 20°, pH 7.4. Insets. Scatchard plots for the association of the sea anemone toxin (ATX), left, and the scorpion toxin (ScTX), right. Main panels. Left : Displacement of [^{125}I]ATX$_{II}$ (8 nM) by unlabeled ATX$_{II}$ from its association with its receptor. (●) Ringer with 140 mM choline, (■) Ringer with 140 mM Na^+, (X) Ringer with 140 mM K^+, (△) Ringer with 140 mM Na^+ and veratridine 0.1 mM. Absence of displacement of [^{125}I]ATX$_{II}$ by scorpion toxins from Androctonus australis Hector (□) and Leiurus quinquestriatus (○). Right : Displacement of 0.2 nM [^{125}I]scorpion toxin II (Androctonus australis Hector) by unlabeled scorpion toxin and ATX$_{II}$ in Ringer with 140 mM choline.

toxin binds at the same site as ATX_{II} it only recognizes the small proportion of sodium channels which are in the "polarized" conformation.

ATX_{II} also interacts with neuroblastoma cells. Again the toxin selectively acts by slowing down the inactivation of the channel (23). Photoaffinity derivatives of ATX_{V} have been synthesized, they irreversibly prolong the action potential (Fig. 4).

The analysis of the toxin stimulation of radioactive sodium fluxes in neuroblastoma cells in culture has been shown to be a fruitful approach to study the functional properties of the sodium channel (24). ATX_{II} alone stimulates $^{22}Na^{+}$ uptake in neuroblastoma cells. This stimulation is completely abolished by 100 nM TTX. The half-maximal effect is observed at 0.2 μM ATX_{II} and maximal stimulation is about 2.5-fold. Veratridine is also known to increase the Na^{+} permeability of the neuroblastoma cell membrane by chemically activating the sodium channel (25). Veratridine and ATX_{II} have a synergistic action on the action potential Na^{+} ionophore which is abolished by 100 nM TTX (24). The dose-response curve obtained with ATX_{II} is greatly modified when veratridine concentrations are increased. Veratridine reveals high and low affinity sites for ATX_{II} (24).

A synergy of action has been shown both by electrophysiological and by $^{22}Na^{+}$ influx techniques (i) between veratridine (or batrachotoxin or dihydrograyanotoxin) and scorpion toxins or ATX_{II} (ii) between veratridine (or batrachotoxin or dihydrograyanotoxin) and pyrethroïds (iii) between polypeptide neurotoxins and pyrethroïds (24, 21,11). An example of this synergy between the different toxins is presented in Fig. 5. All these results taken together show that there exist at least four types of toxin binding sites on the Na^{+} channel (i) one type of sites for TTX and STX, (ii) one type of sites at least for polypeptide toxins from scorpion or sea anemone venoms, (iii) one type of site for batrachotoxin, veratridine, dihydrograyanotoxin, (iv) one type of site for pyrethroïds.

$^{22}Na^{+}$ flux studies with neuroblastoma cells have suggested (24) the existence of both functional and silent channels in these cells, silent Na^{+} channels being defined as channels which cannot be activated electrically but which can be activated with neurotoxins which alter the functioning of the gating system.

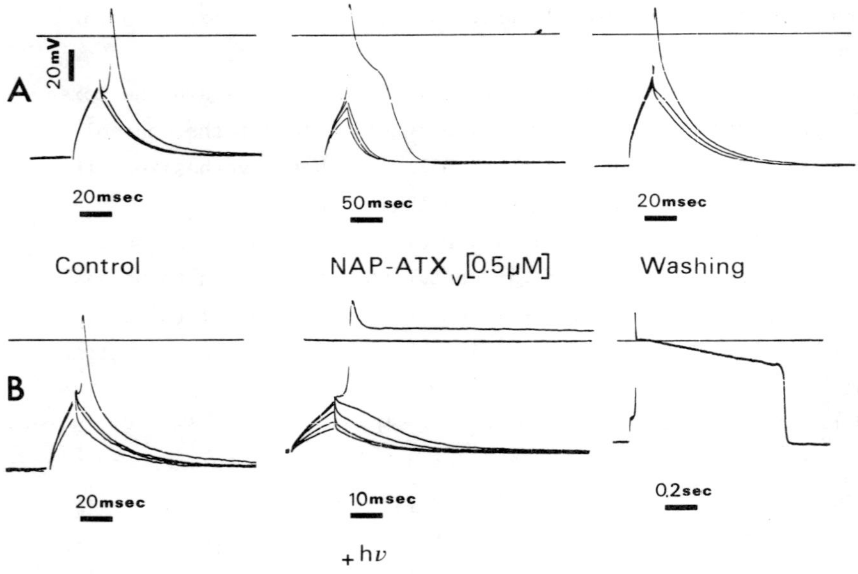

Fig. 4. Irreversibility of NAP-ATX$_V$ action by photoirradiation. A. Left : Control action potential from NIE115 neuroblastoma cell. Middle : 5 min after 0.5 μM NAP-ATX$_V$ application in the dark. Right : Complete reversibility after a 10 min washing period with the toxin-free Earle solution. B. Left : Control action potential. Middle : After 5 min incubation in the dark with 0.5 μM NAP-ATX$_V$, the cells were irradiated with 50 flashes of visible light. Note that the effect of the toxin is more pronounced after photoirradiation than in the dark. Right : Persistence of the NAP-ATX$_V$ effect after a 15 min washing period.

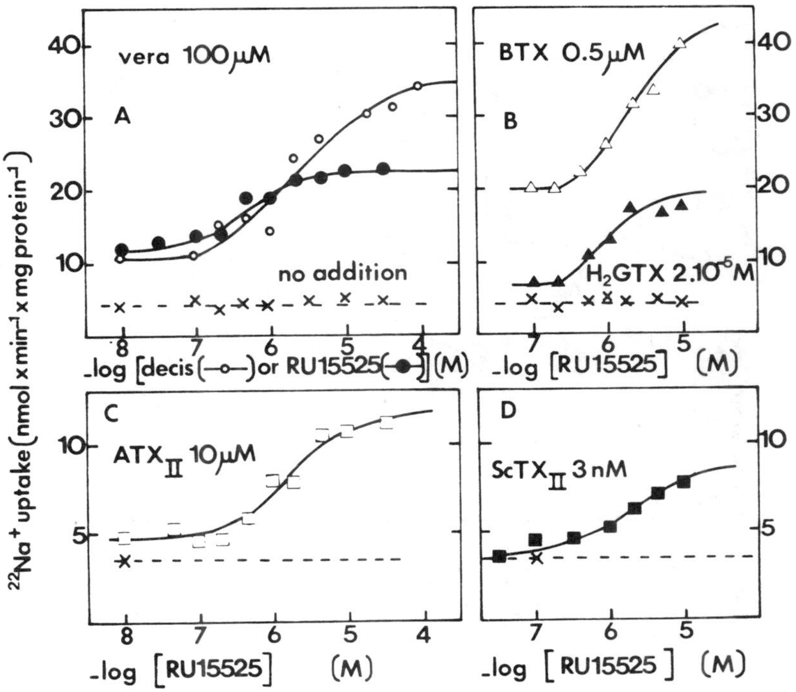

Fig. 5. Synergistic effects of pyrethroids and other toxins acting on the gating system of the Na^+ channel. A. Dose-response curve for Decis and RU 15525 in the absence (X) and in the presence (○,●) of 100 μM veratridine. B. Dose-response curve for RU 15525 in the absence (X) and in the presence of 20 μM dihydrograyanotoxin II (▲) or 0.5 μM batrachotoxin (△). C. Dose-response curve for RU 15525 in the absence (X) and in the presence (□) of 10 μM ATX_{II}. D. Dose-response curve for RU 15525 in the absence (X) and in the presence (■) of 3 nM $ScTX_{II}$.

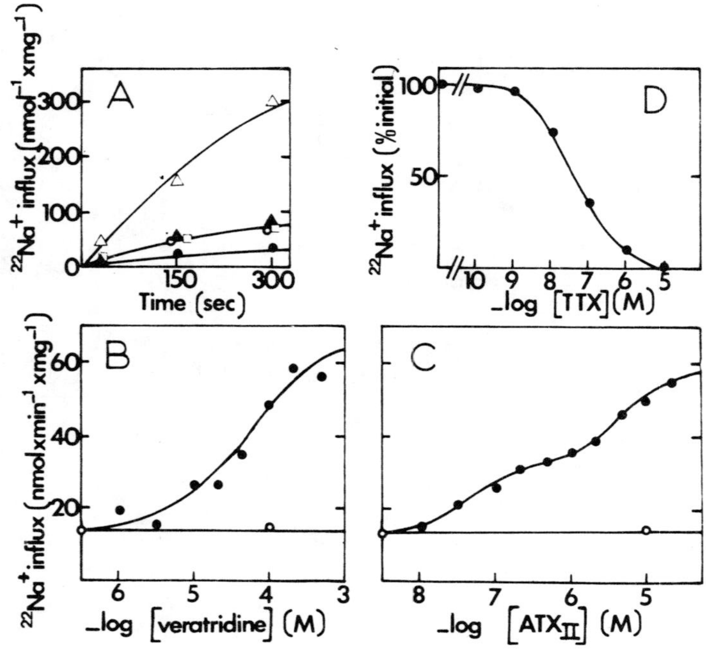

Fig. 6. Stimulation of $^{22}Na^+$ influx into CCl39 fibroblasts by veratridine and sea anemone toxin II. Inhibition of the toxin-stimulated influx by tetrodotoxin. A. Kinetics of $^{22}Na^+$ influx into cells have been measured without toxins (●,○) or in the presence of 10 μM ATX_{II} (▲), 100 μM veratridine (□) or 10 μM ATX_{II} + 100 μM veratridine (△). Experiments were performed in the presence of 0.5 mM ouabain to block Na^+ efflux catalyzed by the (Na^+,K^+)ATPase, except in (●). B. Dose-response curves for the effect of veratridine on the initial rate of $^{22}Na^+$ influx were determined in the absence (○) or the presence of of 10 μM ATX_{II} (●). Ouabain was present at a concentration of 0.5 mM. C. Dose-response curves for the effect of ATX_{II} determined in the absence (○) or the presence of veratridine (100 μM) (●). Ouabain was present at a concentration of 0.5 mM. D. Inhibition by tetrodotoxin of the stimulating effect induced by the mixture of ATX_{II} (10 μM) and veratridine (100 μM) on the initial rate of $^{22}Na^+$ influx in the presence of 0.5 mM ouabain.

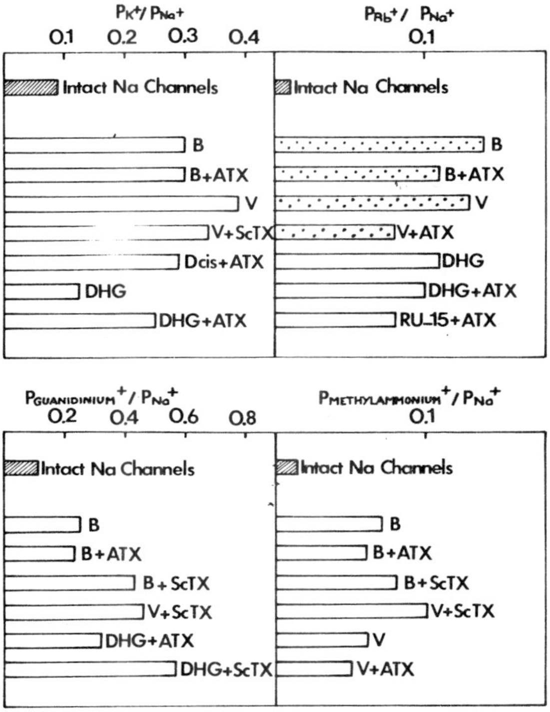

Fig. 7. Relative permeabilities to sodium of toxin-activated fast sodium channels from neuroblastoma (□) and skeletal muscle cells (⊡) Neuroblastoma (NIE115) or chick embryo skeletal muscle cells were preincubated for 15 min with toxin in 140 mM choline chloride, sodium-free Earle solution buffered with 25 mM Hepes-Tris pH 7.4. Initial rates of cation uptake were determined after 1 min in 130 mM choline chloride sodium-free Earle solution supplemented with 10 mM of the desired cation, toxins, 0.5 mM ouabain and $^{22}Na^+$, $^{42}K^+$, $^{86}Rb^+$ [^{14}C]guanidinium or [^{14}C]methylammonium. The toxin stimulated TTX-sensitive Na^+ influx determined on replicate cultures to yield permeability ratio. Toxins used were : 1 μM batrachotoxin (B), 100 μM dihydrograyanotoxin (DHG), 10 nM Androctonus australis Hector toxin (ScTX), 100 μM pyrethroids (RU 15525 and Decis), 100 μM veratridine (V) in experiments using muscle cells and 10 μM veratridine in experiments using neuroblastoma. ATX_{II} was used at 10 μM in experiments using muscle cells and neuroblastoma in the presence of pyrethroids and 1 μM in all other experiments.

TABLE I

A COMPARATIVE STUDY BETWEEN C_9 AND NEUROBLASTOMA CELLS: PROPERTIES OF ASSOCIATION OF SEA ANEMONE TOXIN II AND VERATRIDINE WITH THE Na^+ IONOPHORE AND THEIR EFFECTS ON THE $^{22}Na^+$ INFLUXES

The maximum Na^+ permeability (P_{Na^+} (max)) is related to the maximum $^{22}Na^+$ influx (J_{Na^+} (max)), the external Na^+ concentration $[Na^+]_0$ and the membrane potential (V) by the Goldman equation

$$J_{Na^+}(\max) = P_{Na^+}(\max) \times [Na^+]_0 \frac{F}{RT} \frac{V}{e^{VF/RT} - 1};$$

$[Na^+]_0$ = 140 mM and the mean value of V is −5 mV for both C_9 cells and neuroblastoma cells in the presence of saturating concentrations of veratridine and sea anemone toxin II (unpublished data).

	C_9 cells	Neuroblastoma cells
Unstimulated $^{22}Na^+$ influx (insensitive to tetrodotoxin)	30 nmol · min^{-1} · mg^{-1} of protein	15 nmol · min^{-1} · mg^{-1} of protein
$^{22}Na^+$ influx stimulated by a saturating concentration of sea anemone toxin II (tetrodotoxin inhibitable)	30 nmol · min^{-1} · mg^{-1} of protein	23 nmol · min^{-1} · mg^{-1} of protein
$^{22}Na^+$ influx stimulated by a saturating concentration of veratridine (tetrodotoxin inhibitable)	60 nmol · min^{-1} · mg^{-1} of protein	80 nmol · min^{-1} · mg^{-1} of protein
$^{22}Na^+$ influx stimulated by a mixture of veratridine and sea anemone toxin II at saturating concentrations (tetrodotoxin inhibitable), J_{Na^+} (max)	500 nmol/min per mg protein	147 nmol/min per mg of protein
Membrane area S	13.2 cm^2 · mg^{-1} of protein	11.2 cm^2 · mg^{-1} of protein
P_{Na^+} (max)	$4.9 \cdot 10^{-6}$ cm · S^{-1}	$1.7 \cdot 10^{-6}$ cm · S^{-1}
$K_{0.5}$ (sea anemone toxin II)	0.038 µM	0.15 µM
$K_{0.5}$ (veratridine)	86 µM	44 µM
$K_{0.5}$ (scorpion toxin)	scorpion toxin II : 5 nM	scorpion toxin I : 0.25 nM
$K_{0.5}$ (tetrodotoxin)	0.5 µM	5 nM

TABLE II

EFFECT OF VERATRIDINE AND SEA ANEMONE TOXIN II ON Na^+ INFLUX IN VARIOUS FIBROBLAST CELL TYPES

$^{22}Na^+$ uptake was measured as described in the legend for Fig. 6, in the presence of 0.5 mM ouabain (basal) or 100 μM veratridine + 10 μM sea anemone toxin II for the toxin-stimulated influx. Figures in brackets represent the toxin-stimulation factor when cells were arrested by serum deprivation.

Cell type	Origin	5 min $^{22}Na^+$ uptake nmol/mg protein		Stimulation x fold
		Basal	Veratridine + sea anemone toxin	
CC139	Chinese Hamster lung fibroblast (ATCC)	72	570	7.9
CHL-V 79	Chinese Hamster lung fibroblast (ATCC)	88	95	1.1 (2.1)
CHO	Chinese Hamster ovary (Toronto's strain)	67	190	2.8 (4.7)
FR3T3	Fisher rat fibroblast	16	154	9.6
FR3T3-PY	Fisher rat polyoma-transformed	67	132	2
CEF	Secondary chick embryo fibroblast	67	93	1.4
NIE115	Neuroblastoma	46	320	7

It has been demonstrated in this laboratory that some cells have all their Na^+ channels in the silent form. For example one of our cell lines, C9, has a resting potential of -50mV but it is unable to generate action potentials. The cell membrane, however, has receptors for TTX, pyrethroïds, batrachotoxin, veratridine, ATX_{II} and the scorpion toxin. Although the membrane is not electrically excitable, the whole machinery of the Na^+ channel is present and can be chemically activated. The gating system toxins are able to generate a stimulation of $^{22}Na^+$ influx with properties very similar to those observed with neuroblastoma cells. The comparative properties of toxin interactions with neuroblastoma and C9 cells are presented in Table I. The membrane of this non-impulsive cell is not excitable in the absence of toxins probably because the kinetics of the gating system are not adequate (26). The application of ATX_{II} chemically activates the Na^+ channel and generates an electrical signal.

The Na^+ channel has been identified in fibroblasts as shown in Fig. 6 and Table II. In fibroblasts Na^+ channels are activated neither by veratridine alone nor by ATX_{II} alone but they are activated by the mixture of the two neurotoxins.

Toxins which alter the gating system, change the selectivity of the Na^+ channel - Although neither veratridine, batrachotoxin, dihydrograyanotoxin, ATX_{II}, scorpion toxin nor pyrethroïds alter the interaction of TTX with its receptor, all these toxins drastically change the selectivity of the channel for monovalent cations as shown in Fig. 7. All these toxins tend to decrease the selectivity of the channel. Similar type of conclusions have been made by electrophysiological techniques using aconitine (27) and batrachotoxin (28).

The first conclusion from this observation is that the selectivity filter and the gating system are not independent entities. It has been known for a long time that changing permeant monovalent cations does not alter the gating kinetics of the Na^+ channel (29). Clearly, the reverse is not true, changing the gating kinetics with neurotoxins does change the ionic selectivity of the channel. As there are several closed conformations of the Na^+ channel (the resting form, the inactivated form for example), it is clear now that there are also several open forms of the channel.

Use of neurotoxins for the analysis of developmental properties of the action potential sodium channel - The experiments with chick embryo cardiomyocytes in culture following $^{22}Na^+$ entry stimulated by ATX_{II} or veratridine through the TTX-inhibitable Na^+ channel (30,31) gave useful information concerning the development of the fast sodium channel. The sodium channel in young hearts (2- to 4-day-old) is slow, tetrodotoxin-insensitive and activated-inactivated at a low membrane potential (32). In contrast, the Na^+ channels of cells in older hearts (5-day-old) are fast and tetrodotoxin-sensitive. However, when heart cells of these old chick embryo are grown in monolayer cultures, it has been demonstrated that the fast Na^+ channels revert back to slow channels generating an action potential that is not blocked by tetrodotoxin. Although TTX has no effect on the action potential (33) of cardiac cells in monolayer cultures, the TTX receptor i.e. one important part of the Na^+ channel machinery is present in the plasma membrane of the cell with an excellent affinity for TTX; veratridine and sea anemone receptors are also present in the membrane (30,31). Veratridine stimulates $^{22}Na^+$ influx in these cardiac cells in a way similar to the one observed with neuroblastoma cells. ATX_{II} has a synergistic action with veratridine as for nerve cells. In other words the Na^+ ionophore in embryonic heart cells in monolayer cultures is in a form which dces not respond to electrical depolarization to generate a TTX-sensitive action potential. The question is to know in this case why is this channel in the silent form. The most probable interpretation at present is that the inactivation ("h" system in the HODGKIN-HUXLEY terminology) of the Na^+ channel is faster than the activation ("m" system). If this is really the case, even if the selectivity filter has the adequate properties, the Na^+ channel ionophore will never permit the generation of an action potential. The appearance of a TTX-sensitive action potential during the development of the cardiac cell should then correspond to a slowing down of the inactivation process as compared to the activation step. It has been shown in this laboratory (21,34) that with cardiac cells in culture, if one applies ATX_{II} which selectively alters the inactivation of the Na^+ channel, one then observes an action potential which is considerably prolonged, the prolongation induced by ATX_{II} being completely abolished by TTX.

In conclusion, it is clear now that the use of a variety of neurotoxins has already permitted and will permit in a near future to make important progress in the understanding at the molecular level of the structure-function relationships of the sodium channel.

ACKNOWLEDGMENTS

This work was supported by the Centre National de la Recherche Scientifique, the Délégation Générale à la Recherche Scientifique et Technique and the Institut National de la Santé et de la Recherche Médicale.

REFERENCES

1. HAFEMAN, D.R. 1972. Biochim.Biophys.Acta 266 : 548-556.

2. RITCHIE, J.M. & R.B. ROGART. 1977. Rev.Physiol.Biochem. Pharmacol. 79 : 1-50.

3. CHICHEPORTICHE, R., M. BALERNA, A. LOMBET, G. ROMEY & M. LAZDUNSKI. 1979. J.Biol.Chem. 254 : 1552-1557.

4. CHICHEPORTICHE, R., M. BALERNA, A. LOMBET, G. ROMEY & M. LAZDUNSKI. 1980. Eur.J.Biochem. 104 : 617-625.

5. BALERNA, M., M. FOSSET, R. CHICHEPORTICHE, G. ROMEY & M. LAZDUNSKI. 1975. Biochemistry 14 : 5500-5511.

6. COLQUHOUN, D. & J.M. RITCHIE. 1972. Mol.Pharmacol. 8 : 285-292.

7. BALERNA, M., R. CHICHEPORTICHE, A. LOMBET, G. ROMEY & M. LAZDUNSKI. to be published.

8. LEVINSON, S.L. & J.C. ELLORY. 1973. Nature (London) New Biol. 245 : 122-123.

9. ULBRICHT, W. 1969. Ergeb.Physiol.Biol.Chem.Exp.Pharmakol. 61 : 18-71.

10. WANG, C.M., T. NARAHASHI & M. SCUKA. 1972. J.Pharmacol.Exp. Ther. 182 : 442-449.

11. JACQUES, Y., G. ROMEY, M.T. CAVEY, B. KARTALOVSKI & M. LAZDUNSKI. 1980. Biochim.Biophys.Acta in press.

12. WUNDERER, G. & M. EULITZ. 1978. Eur.J.Biochem. 89 : 11-17.

13. WUNDERER, G., H. FRITZ, E. WACHTER & W. MACHLEIDT. 1976. Eur.J. Biochem. 68 : 193-198.

14. MARTINEZ, G., C. KOPEYAN, H. SCHWEITZ & M. LAZDUNSKI. 1977. FEBS Lett. 84 : 247-252.

15. TANAKA, M., M. HANIU, K.T. YASUNOBU & T.R. NORTON. 1977. Biochemistry 16 : 204-208.

16. ROMEY, G., J.P. ABITA, H. SCHWEITZ, G. WUNDERER & M. LAZDUNSKI. 1976. Proc.Natl.Acad.Sci.USA 73 : 4055-4059.

17. ROMEY, G., R. CHICHEPORTICHE, M. LAZDUNSKI, H. ROCHAT, F. MIRANDA & S. LISSITZKY. 1975. Biochem.Biophys.Res.Commun. 64 : 115-121.

18. AMSTRONG, C.M., F. BENZANILLA & E. ROJAS. 1973. J.Gen.Physiol. 62 : 375-391.

19. ABITA, J.P., R. CHICHEPORTICHE, H. SCHWEITZ & M. LAZDUNSKI. 1977. Biochemistry 16 : 1838-1844.

20. ROMEY, G., J.P. ABITA, R. CHICHEPORTICHE, H. ROCHAT & M. LAZDUNSKI. 1976. Biochim.Biophys.Acta 448 : 607-619.

21. ROMEY, G., J.F. RENAUD, M. FOSSET & M. LAZDUNSKI. 1980. J.Pharmacol.Exp.Ther. in press.

22. VINCENT, J.P., M. BALERNA, J. BARHANIN, M. FOSSET & M. LAZDUNSKI. 1980. Proc.Natl.Acad.Sci.USA 77 : 1646-1650.

23. ROMEY, G. & M. LAZDUNSKI. to be published.

24. JACQUES, Y., M. FOSSET & M. LAZDUNSKI. 1978. J.Biol.Chem. 252 : 7383-7392.

25. CATTERALL, W.A. & M. NIRENBERG. 1973. Proc.Natl.Acad.Sci.USA 70 : 3759-3763.

26. ROMEY, G., Y. JACQUES, H. SCHWEITZ, M. FOSSET & M. LAZDUNSKI. 1979. Biochim.Biophys.Acta 556 : 344-353.

27. MOZHAYEVA, G.N., A.P. NAUMOV, Y.A. NEGULYAEV & E.D. NOSYREVA. 1977. Biochim.Biophys.Acta 446 : 461-473.

28. KHODOROV, B.I. & S.V. REVENKO. 1979. Neuroscience 4 : 1315-1330.

29. HILLE, B. 1971. J.Gen.Physiol. 58 : 599-619.

30. DE BARRY, J., M. FOSSET & M. LAZDUNSKI. 1977. Biochemistry 16 : 3850-3855.

31. FOSSET, M., J. DE BARRY, M.C. LENOIR & M. LAZDUNSKI. 1977. J.Biol.Chem. 252 : 6112-6117.

32. SPERELAKIS, N. & K. SHIGENOBU. 1972. J.Gen.Physiol. 60 : 430-453.

33. SPERELAKIS, N. & A.J. PAPPANO. 1969. J.Gen.Physiol. 53 : 97-114.

34. ROMEY, G., J.F. RENAUD & M. LAZDUNSKI. to be published.

Neurotransmitters and their Receptors
Edited by U.Z. Littauer, Y. Dudai, I. Silman,
V.I. Teichberg and Z. Vogel

Optical Methods to Elucidate Electrophysiological Parameters

A. Grinvald*, W.N. Ross*, I. Farber*, D. Saya*, A. Zutra*, R. Hildesheim*, U. Khunt*, M. Segal** and Y. Kimhi*

**Department of Neurobiology and **Department of Isotope Research, The Weizmann Institute of Science, Rehovot, Israel*

ABSTRACT

Optical methods to monitor electrical activity were developed for mammalian neurons. Most of the experiments were carried out on monolayer cultures of neuroblastoma cells. Preliminary experiments were done with rat hippocampal slices.

For transmission experiments we have found a membrane potential probe which has satisfactory sensitivy: WW 401, a merocyanine rhodanine derivative. A 10x10 array of photodiodes was positioned in the real magnified image formed by a microscope objective. It was used to detect voltage changes simultaneously from many points along the arborization of cultured neurons. Action potentials were detected from the cell body with a signal-to-noise ratio of 20:1 without signal-averaging. With averaging, signals could be detected from every diode on which the image of the cell or its processes fell.

A He-Ne laser was stabilized for fluorescence experiments. It was focused onto a small spot and changes in fluorescence from cells stained with an oxonol dye (WW 802) were monitored with a phototube. Action potentials were detected without signal-averaging even from 5 μm processes or growth cones of these cells. Fluorescence proved to be by far more sensitive; up to 7% change in fluorescence for 100 mV membrane potential change, two orders of magnitude larger relative to the absorption change. Different sites on the same cell could be examined by changing the position of the cell relative to the laser microbeam. A conduction velocity of 0.2 m/sec in the 7 μm process was determined by the simultaneous measurement of the action potential in the cell body, with an electrode, and a remote growth cone with the laser microbeam.

The same type of transmission measurements was to detect simultaneous activity from hundred of neurons in rat hippocampal slices.

INTRODUCTION

The ability to measure electrical responses from neuronal arborization or from the growth cone, may provide a powerful tool for solving important questions in neurobiology. Examples include studies of the regional localization of ionic channels or receptors and the passive and active electrical properties of complex dendritic arborizations.

In most cases intracellular techniques are nearly impossible to use for recording from small processes. Extracellular recordings have sometimes been tried. For example, the propagation of action potentials in the processes of dissociated neurons has been examined (1,2,3). The extracellular technique, however, is inadequate when studying graded potentials (4) or regional variation in the form of the action potential (5,6).

Recently, optical methods for measuring membrane potential using voltage-sensitive dyes have been developed by Cohen and coworkers (7-10) and Waggoner and colleagues (11). These dyes act as molecular transducers which transform changes in membrane potential into changes of optical properties of stained neurons (i.e., changes in absorption, fluorescence, birefringence, light scattering (8)). For recent reviews see Cohen *et al.* (12), Cohen and Salzberg (13), and Waggoner (11). Theoretical aspects are discussed elsewhere (8,14).

Changes in transmission and fluorescence of these dyes are relatively small. Therefore it is imperative to select dyes with the greatest sensitivity and to design the optimum apparatus. About 1000 dyes have been screened on squid giant axons (7,8). A few of these are sensitive enough to be used to record the neuronal activity of several invertebrate central nervous systems (15). However, Ross and Reichart (16) reported that there was a species-specific difference in the optical response of a number of absorption dyes. The best probes for squid axons gave at least 5 times smaller responses and a different action spectrum when tested on dissociated cells from vertebrate neuronal preparations. We have confirmed these results and screened additional dyes on two lines of neuroblastoma cells. We have found a merocyanine-rhodanine (WW 401) which can be used to record even from processes when averaging is permitted.

Waggoner and Grinvald (14) pointed out that, theoretically, fluorescence changes could be much greater than transmission changes. This prediction should be realized in practice in a monolayer culture where background fluorescence from non-relevant binding sites is minimal. Indeed, in similar cases investigators have found large fractional changes in fluorescence during electrical activity (17,18). However, the low level of light emission made the signal-to-noise ratio of these fluorescence signals no better than those from transmission, when standard illumination was used.

We have implemented a stabilized He-Ne laser as a light source. Using this laser, and an oxonal dye (WW 802), we have recorded action potentials from growth cones and processes of neuroblastoma cells without signal-averaging. The techniques which we developed were used not only to measure conduction velocity in the processes but also to measure space constants, rectification and regional variations in electrical parameters (19-23), properties which are not accessible with conventional techniques.

In preliminary experiments (24) we were able to monitor optically heterogeneous electrical activity, in different portions of rat HPC slices, in response to electrical stimulation.

MATERIALS AND METHODS

Cell cultures: Mouse neuroblastoma clone NIE-115 and the glioma neuroblastoma hybrid cells NG-108-15 were originally obtained from Dr. M. Nirenberg. The NIE-115 cells and the NG-108-15 cells were grown as described by Kimhi *et al.* (25) and Yavin and Zutra (26).

Electrophysiology: For physiological experiments the culture medium was changed just before use to a solution of DMEM (Cat.# H-21, Gibco) adjusted to 5.4mM K^+, 4.1mM Ca^{+2}, 120mM Na^+, 10mM glucose, 20mM sucrose and 10mM HEPES buffer adjusted to pH 7.4. Total osmolarity was 340 mOs.

Cells were impaled with microelectrodes filled with 3M KCl and stimulated through a bridge circuit in the WPI 701 electrometer. The electrodes were controlled by M-103 Narishige hydraulic micromanipulators mounted on the moveable stage. With this arrangement the cell could be moved relative to the fixed microbeam while maintaining a stable electrode penetration. The criteria for mature healthy cells were a resting potential lower than 50 mV and action potential larger than 40 mV. Optical and electrophysiological experiments were done at 37°C.

Staining with voltage-sensitive probes: Staining solutions were freshly prepared before each experiment. Usually, the dye (e.g. WW 401) was directly dissolved in saline. In others (e.g. WW 802) the stock solution of dye in ethanol was evaporated before adding saline. The final concentration of ethanol was less than 0.5% and control experiments established that it had no significant effect on the optical signals or electrical parameters of these cells.

For absorption experiments cells were stained for 5 minutes with 0.04-4mM dye and then washed twice in physiological medium. When low concentrations of dye were used, the dye was left in solution during the experiment. For fluorescence experiments concentrations of 5-50μM dye were typically used. The dye in solution was usually much less fluorescent than the membrane-bound dye and therefore it was possible to leave it in during the measurements without increasing the background fluorescence intensity.

Dyes are available from Dr. A.S. Waggoner (Dept. of Chemistry, Amherst College), from other sources cited in reference (8) or from us.

Apparatus: The prototype of the computer-controlled optical apparatus was developed in Dr. Cohen's laboratory and is described in detail elsewhere (15,22). Transmission and fluorescence experiments were done on an apparatus built around a Zeiss Universal Microscope rigidly mounted on a vibration isolation table (Fig. 1).

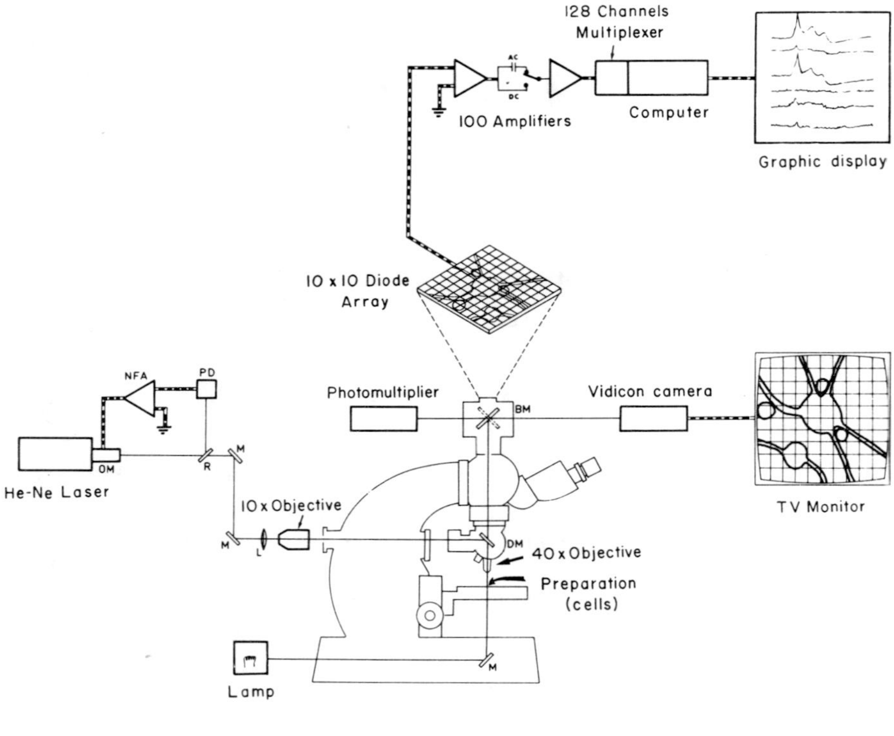

Fig. 1. Schematic diagram of the computer-controlled optical apparatus used to record activity from many targets. (See text for details). Traces showing activity detected by the optical monitor were displayed on an interactive graphic display terminal. In parallel, the preparation was viewed by a vidicon camera. An enlarged 10x10 matrix was superimposed with the monitor screen, where each square corresponded to an individual photodetector element. Thus, traces showing electrical activity displayed on the graphic terminal could be assigned to individual cells or cell processes.

RESULTS

Search for sensitive transmission probes: About 30 voltage sensitive probes were tested, and one of them WW 401 (see the structure in Figure 2) was 2-3 times more sensitive than any other dye we have tested. NIE-115 and NG-108-15 cells stained with 0.4mM WW 401 gave normal electrical responses (27) when stimulated with an intracellular microelectrode (See Fig. 2A, bottom trace). During the action potential there was a decrease in transmitted intensity at 690±15 nm which could easily be detected without averaging (Fig. 2A, top). Inspection of this figure shows that the change in intensity closely follows the time-course of the action potential. Experiments with 0.04mM WW 401 gave similar signals of about one-half the size shown in Fig. 2A. WW 401 is as sensitive on these cells as the best dyes on invertebrate neurons. No difference was detected in the optical signals from NIE-115 or NG-108-15 cells.

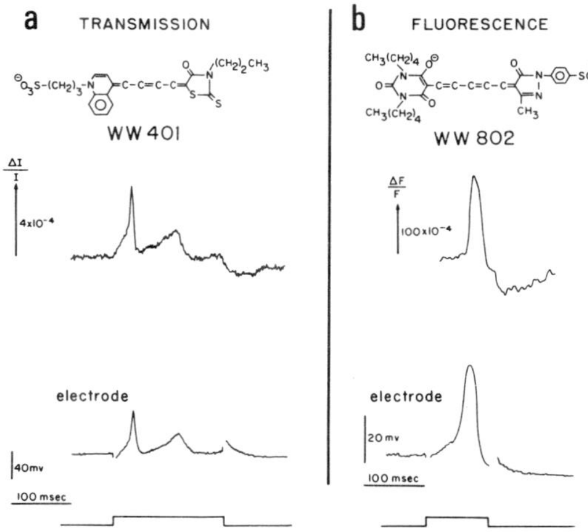

Fig. 2. Transmission and fluorescence signals from stained NIE-115 neuroblastoma cells detected without signal averaging. A) Change in transmission recorded by a square photodiode positioned over the image of a 45x45 μm area in the center of a 120 μm diameter cell stained with 0.2mM WW 401. The simultaneous electrical measurement is shown below. The shape of the undershoot following the action potential is distorted in the optical record because of the AC capacitor, which had a time-constant of 100 msec. Wavelength was 690±15 nm. The filter of the optical amplifier has a time-constant of 0.7 msec. The structure of WW 401 is shown on the top. The arrow shows increase in absorption. B) Change in fluorescence from a 90 μm diameter cell stained with 30μM WW 802 and stimulated with a microelectrode in the soma (top). The fluorescence was excited by a 120 μm diameter laser-microbeam. Excitation light was blocked by a Schott RG 665 post filter. The fluorescence intensity was corrected for bleaching by dividing the experimental curve by an exponential function. The time constant of the exponential bleaching was estimated from the first and the last point of the experimental curve. The arrow shows increase in fluorescence.

The action spectrum for the transmission signal was tri-phasic: between 510-600 nm and between 730-780 nm there was an increase in transmission while the change at 600-730 nm was larger and in the opposite direction. The action spectrum on squid axons was monophasic, i.e. there was an increase in transmission at all wave lengths.

Small transmission changes with the same triphasic spectrum were also obtained with the dye WW 375 except that the sensitivity was only about 20% of the value obtained with WW 401. These changes with WW 375 were similar to those observed with dissociated neurons from the rat and chick (16), suggesting that neuroblastoma cells are a good model system for evaluating the effect of voltage-sensitive dyes on cultured vertebrate neurons.

Screening for sensitive fluorescence probes: About 25 fluorescent voltage-sensitive probes were tested. The best results were obtained with the barbituric pyrazolone oxonols, a family of fluorescent dyes which was recently designed and synthesized (28).

Fluorescence was observed from the membranes of NIE-115 or NG-108-15 cells stained with 5μM of the oxonal dye WW 802 (See Fig. 2B for structure). When tested with a microelectrode these cells had normal electrical properties. Under the fluorescence microscope the cells clearly showed a bright fluorescent ring indicating that the dye does not penetrate live neurons quickly.

The action spectrum for the fluorescence signal of WW 802 peaks at 630 nm, thus allowing us to excite the fluorescence with the 632.8 nm line of the stabilized 50 mW He-Ne laser. A 90 μm cell was impaled with a microelectrode and was positioned in the center of the 120 μm laser microbeam. The shutter was turned on for 300 msec and the cell electrically stimulated. Following electrical stimulation there was an increase of 1-5% in the fluorescence intensity. In addition, the fluorescence intensity decreased monotonically due to bleaching. This decrease could be "approximated" by an exponential with a time constant of 100-300 msec depending upon the intensity of the beam. After computer correction for the exponential bleaching the fluorescence records clearly followed the time course of the electrically recorded action potential (Fig. 2B).

Simultaneous recording of activity from many targets in the field: The large absorption signals obtained from the soma with WW 401 suggested that this dye could be used to record from small processes. A large NIE-115 cell with 5 major processes was positioned in the center of the field, dyed with WW 401, and stimulated repetitively with a microelectrode in the soma. The records in Fig. 3 show that transmission changes were detected simulataneously in all photodiodes on which an image of any part of the cell fell. The signals from the processes were noisier than those from the soma since there was less membrane area under these diodes. However, it is clear that the propagation of the action potential can be followed along any of the processes. The signals from several diodes over a single process could be combined in the computer to give a signal with improved S/N. Examples of this procedure are shown in Fig. 4A. In some records (in other experiments) it seemed that there was a difference in the form of the action potential recorded in different parts of the cell. We are currently pursuing experiments to examine the regional membrane specialization which might be responsible for these variations in signal shape.

Electrical activity in the processes: Large fluorescence signals were also obtained from the processes of these cultured cells (Fig. 4B). These signals could be observed in a single sweep, unlike the absorption signals from the processes which required signal averaging. In these experiments, the laser microbeam was reduced to a diameter of 30 μm. The excitation light intensity was increased by a factor of about 10 relative to the cell body experiments. The increased intensity led to the good S/N ratio shown in the figure. However, under this condition, significant bleaching occurs with the present fluorescent probe. In the above experiment the bleaching during 100 msec was about 6% whereas the signal was 4%. Under such circumstances, the approximate exponential correction may be inadequate to restore a fluorescence record which faithfully represents the potential change.

Conduction velocity in a process and electrical responses in the growth cone: By moving the position of a cell relative to the laser spot recordings could be made from several positions along a process. Measurements shown in Fig. 5, for example, allow us to estimate the conduction velocity of the action potential in a process. There was a noticeable delay of 1.6 msec between the fluorescence record of the action potential in the cell body and the fluorescence record of the action potential in

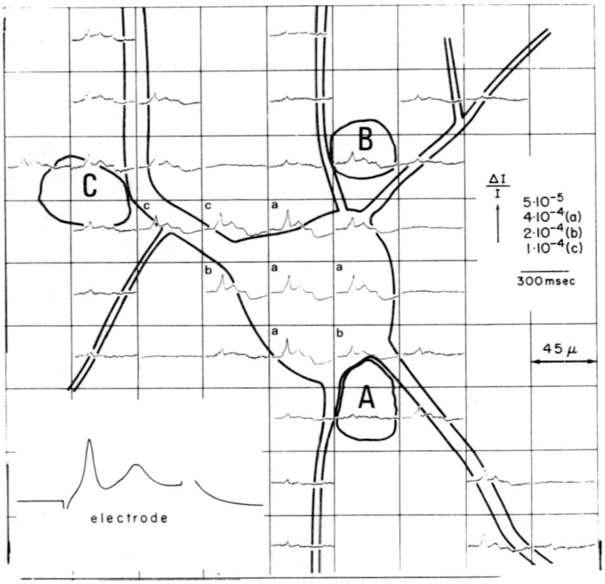

Figure 3: Simultaneous transmission changes recorded by a 10x10 photodetector array positioned over the real magnified image of a stained NIE-115 neuroblastoma cell. Each square shows the area that a diode detected light from (45x45 μm). Traces in the individual boxes show the optically detected electrical activity. 50 sweeps were averaged. Some records which are not from the cell or its processes are shown at high gain to show the noise level. Occasionally, as in C there is a large signal over another small cell in the field. It is possible that these cells were electrically coupled to the stimulated cell or the large cell extended a process under the little cell which was not visible. In this figure the outline of the cell is positioned with respect to the array to an accuracy of about 10 μm. The gain of the optical recordings is usually $5x10^{-5}$ as shown on the scale, but different records may have different gains. A letter in the top right corner of each square indicates the appropriate scale.

the growth cone. By measuring the length of the process, a conduction velocity of 0.2 m/sec was calculated. Control experiments (as in Fig. 2B) showed that there was no significant difference between the electrically and optically detected action potential when measured at the same point.

Studies of regional specializations of electrical properties of space constants and rectification are described elsewhere (19,20,22). Detection of Ca^{2+} action potentials in the processes of neuroblastoma cells is reported (21,23).

An example of the type of optical records obtained from rat hippocampal slices (30) in our preliminary experiments (24) is depicted in Fig. 6.

DISCUSSION OF THE METHODOLOGY

The results presented here show that available dyes and optical technology are adequate to detect action potentials from cultured neurons without signal-averaging using either transmission or fluorescence. The signal to noise ratio should also permit the detection of 5-10 mV synaptic potentials without averaging. When averaging is feasible then this sensitivity is sufficient to detect 0.5 mV synaptic potentials in cell bodies of 25 μm diameter.

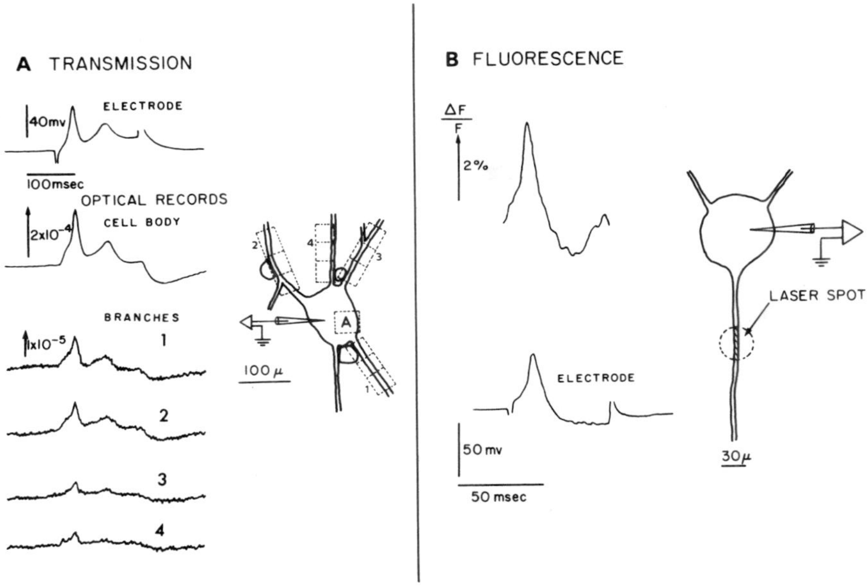

Figure 4: Transmission and fluorescence recordings from processes. A) Transmission: The records from the several diodes over each process shown in Fig. 3 have been combined in the computer to improve the S/N of the traces. The top trace shows the electrically recorded action potential. The middle trace is the optical record from a single diode over the cell body (detector A). B) Fluorescence: Single sweep records from a 5 μm process. Spot diameter about 30 μm. The fluorescence record may be a slight distortion of the true potential change due to the approximate bleaching correction. Only 1 sweep was needed for this fluorescence signal while 50 responses were averaged in the transmission experiment.

Comparison between transmission and fluorescence techniques: An advantage of the absorption mode is that photodiodes can be used as the detectors. Photodiodes are cheap and can be manufactured in almost any shape. For example, we found it useful to use a 10x10 array in these experiments in order to simultaneously detect from many parts of a cell.

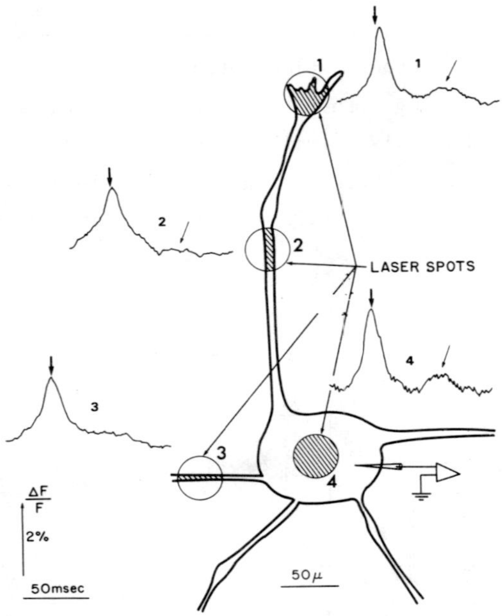

Figure 5: Fluorescence changes measured during stimulation of a stained NIE-115 cell at several points on the growth cone, processes, and cell-body. Each trace is the average of four sweeps. For each record the stage was adjusted to position the appropriate point under the laser microbeam which had a diameter of about 30 μm. Records were taken in the order of 1,2,3,4. The arrows on each record indicate the time of the peak of the action potential as recorded with an electrode in the cell body. There is a greater delay at points further away from the cell body. Conduction velocity along a process is calculated from records 1 and 4 to be 0.2 meter /sec.

In other kinds of experiments the array can be used to detect activity from many neurons simultaneously (15). However, photodiodes are not adequate for fluorescence detection, because the dark current of a photodiode-amplifier combination is larger than the shot noise of the fluorescence. Simultaneous recording from many targets in fluorescence can be done by the use of several light-guides which are coupled to individual photomultipliers. Such a solution was described using individual photodiodes by Salzberg et al. (10).

The main advantage of fluorescence is that it is much more sensitive than absorption, especially for a small target. In the experiments reported here, the change in intensity is typically 5-7% for 100 mV potential

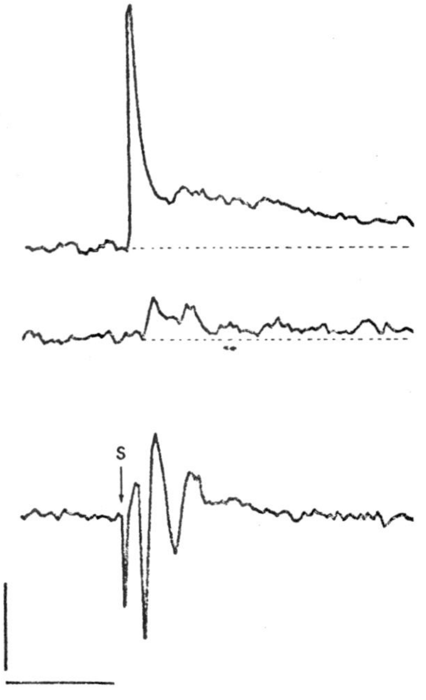

Figure 6: A correlation between electrical and optical recording of responses to afferent stimulation in rat hippocampal slice. Hippocampal slices were prepared according to Segal (30). Electrical recording was made from 4M NaCl filled glass pipettes in the pyramidal layer of region CA1 of the hippocampus. A bipolar stimulating electrode was placed in stratum radiation and activated the Schaffer collateral system. Calibration 25 msec and 5 mV. Top two traces, optical recording, bottom trace, electrical recording. The peak of the response in the first trace is delayed by 0.8 msec relative to the stimulus artefact. Single sweep (averaging was not used).

change in a neuroblastoma cell compared with 0.04%/100 mV for transmission.

By examining other analogs of WW 401 or completely different compounds, it may be possible to find more sensitive absorption dyes. Waggoner and Grinvald (14) have argued, however, that the present level of sensitivity is already close to the theoretical maximum (if extensive binding is not desirable because of pharmacological effects). However, unlike the absorption case, the theoretical upper limit to fluorescence sensitivity is still far away and one may expect that future design and synthesis efforts, will improve the sensitivity as well as minimize photodynamic damage and the bleaching (14).

The important parameter for evaluating these dyes is the signal to noise ratio for detecting physiological events. Since the fluorescence intensity is typically four orders of magnitude less than the transmitted intensity, the shot-noise is 100 times worse. In the past this fact has cancelled the advantage of the greater fluorescence sensitivity. In our laser experiments we have increased the light intensity at 630 nm by a factor of a 10-100 compared to that achievable with a tungsten-halogen bulb. At this intensity the noise level is about 10^{-3} and action potentials can be detected with a S/N better than in transmission. The major source of noise is the laser instabilities. Future improvements can be expected with better stabilization technique. However, the increased intensity used in the present fluorescence experiments accelerates the rate of photodynamic damage and dye bleaching. More recently the light level was significantly reduced, yet the signal to noise ratio is still satisfactory (23).

Signals from processes: Action potentials can be detected with about equal sensitivity from neuronal somata using transmission or fluorescence. However, fluorescence is the preferred technique for small processes. A single sweep fluorescence record from 5 μ branch has a signal to noise ratio which is 3 times better than the transmission record obtained after 50 sweeps were averaged (see Fig. 4). When the area of the photodetector is bigger than the area of the target transmission measurements are more difficult. The signal to noise ratio from a 5 μ cell detected with a photodetector covering a 50 μm diameter spot will be reduced by a factor of 10. The size of the photodetector is not important in fluorescence experiments when only dye bound to the target is fluorescent and there are no other cells in the field.

Current limitations and future prospects:

Pharmacological effects: In fluorescence experiments with WW 802, 5 μM of purified dye had no significant effects on the resting potential and the detailed shape of the action potential. However, 50 μM caused a narrowing of the action potential and disappearance of the slow after depolarization (27). In transmission experiments with 0.4 mM WW 401 we did not detect any significant effects, yet 10 times higher dye concentration reversibly hyperpolarized the membrane by 5 mV.

It is expected that large amounts of probe molecules bound to the cell will modify membrane properties. However our experience in other systems suggests that these difficulties may be obviated by the choice of the right probe and by lowering the concentration (15). It is pertinent to mention in this respect that theoretically, in transmission, the S/N depends linearly on the concentration of dye, C, while in fluorescence it increases with the $\sqrt{C}$ (14).

Bleaching and photodynamic damage: In absorption experiments photodynamic damage (8,30) is not a significant problem. Constant illumination at 690 nm for one minute caused only a slight broadening of the action potential in a cell which was being stimulated at a rate of 1/sec. There was no change in the resting potential.

Constant illumination does bleach the dye which then reduces the signal size. After 2 minutes the signal is one-half the original amplitude. However, the cells can be restained to regain the original signals with no effect on the cell electrical parameters.

In fluorescence experiments the higher light intensities accelerate both bleaching and photodynamic damage. In order to minimize these effects, successful experiments are best carried out with short light pulses (100-300 msec). In this case 4-10 sweeps can be sampled future significant damage occurs.

It seems likely that better fluorescent probes can be designed. For example, some styryl dyes cause smaller photodynamic damage by a factor of 10 (e.g. NK 2345) (8). Photodynamic damage can be reduced by 100-1000 fold when the measurement is carried out in oxygen free saline (8). Whenever photodynamic damage is disturbing, one can alternately perfuse the cells with oxygen free and oxygen enriched solutions. Frequently, negligible interference with the physiological state of the system could be obtained if the appropriate conditions are used.

CONCLUSIONS

The experiments show that both fluorescence and transmission can be used to record from the somata and processes of cultured neurons. While future improvements are expected, currently available dyes and techniques are adequate to investigate a wide variety of problems in the neurobiology of cultured cells. Examples include the regional specialization of ionic channels, receptors and the study of the patterns of synapse formation in populations of neurons. These problems would be much more difficult to investigate using conventional electrophysiological techniques. The preliminary results obtained in brain slices suggest that the technique may be useful to study the pharmacology of local circuits in the mammalian brain.

ACKNOWLEDGEMENTS

We would like to thank L.B. Cohen for a generous loan of equipment, Alan Waggoner for dyes. Supported in part by grant # NS 274-79 from USPHS a grant from the Muscular Dystrophy Association, and a grant from the U.S.-Israel Binational Science Foundation, Jerusalem, Israel.

REFERENCES

1. Okun, L.M. (1972). Isolated dorsal root ganglion neurons in culture: cytological maturation and extension of electrically active processes. J. Neurobiology 3, 111-151.

2. Scoot, B.S., Engelberg, V.E. and Fischer, K.C. (1969). Morphological and electrophysiological characteristics of dissociated chick embryonic spinal ganglion cells in culture. Expl. Neurology 23, 230-248.

3. Varon, S. and Raiborn, C. (1971). Excitability and conduction in neurons of dissociated ganglionic cell-cultures. Brain Research 30, 83-98.

4. Bader, C.R., Macleish, P.R. and Schwartz, E.A. (1979). A voltage clamp study of the light response in solitary rods of the tiger salamander. J. Physiol. 296, 1-26.

5. Dichter, M.A. & Fischbach, G.D. (1977). The action potential of chick dorsal root ganglion neurons maintained in cell culture. J. Physiol. 267, 281-298.

6. Willard, A.L. (1980). Electrical excitability of outgrowing neurites of embryonic neurons in cultures of dissociated neural plate of Xenopus laevis. J. Physiol. 301, 115-128.

7. Cohen, L.B., Salzberg, B.M. Davila, H.V., Ross, W.M., Landowne, D., Waggoner, A.S. and Wang, C.H. (1974). Changes in axon fluorescence during activity; molecular probes of membrane potential. J. Memb. Biol. 19, 1-36.

8. Ross, W.N., Salzberg, B.M., Cohen, L.B., Grinvald. A., Davila, H.V., Waggoner, A.S. and Wang, C.H. (1977). Changes in Absorption, Fluorescence, Dichroism and Birefringence in stained axons: optical measurement of membrane potential. J. Mem. Biol. 33, 141-183.

9. Grinvald, A., Salzberg, B.M. and Cohen, L.B. (1977). Simultaneous recording from several neurons in an invertebrate central nervous system. Nature 268, 140.

10. Salzberg, B.M., Grinvald, A., Cohen, L.B., Davila, H.V. and Ross, W.N. (1977). Optical recording of neuronal activity in an invertebrate central nervous system; simultaneous monitoring of several neurons. J. Neurophysiol. 40, 1281-1291.

11. Waggoner, A.S. (1979). Dye indicators of membrane potential. Ann. Rev. Biophys. Bioeng. 8, 47-68.

12. Cohen, L.B., Salzberg, B.M. and Grinvald, A. (1978). Optical methods for monitoring neuron activity: Ann. Rev. of Neurosci. 1, 171-182.

13. Cohen, L.B. and Salzberg, B.M. (1978). Optical measurement of membrane potential. Rev. Physiol. Biochem. Pharm., 83, 35-88.

14. Waggoner, A.S. and Grinvald, A. (1977). Mechanisms of rapid optical changes of potential sensitive dyes. Ann. N.Y. Acad. Sci. 303, 217-242.

15. Grinvald, A., Cohen, L.B., Lesher, S. and Boyle, M. (1980). Simultaneous monitoring of activity of many neurons in Invertebrate CNS: Localization of neurons participating in behavioral responses. Submitted.

16. Ross, W.N. and Reichardt, L.B. (1979). Species specific effects on the optical signals of voltage sensitive dyes. J. Membrane Biol. 48, 343-356.

17. Oetliker, H., Baylor, S.M. and Chandler, W.K. (1975). Simultaneous changes in fluorescence and optical retardation in single muscle fiber during activity. Nature 257, 693-696.

18. Vergara, J. and Bezannilla, F. (1976). Fluorescence changes during electrical activity in frog muscle. Nature 259, 684-259.

19. Ross, W.N., Grinvald, A., Farber, I. and Waggoner, A.S. Optical detection of electrical responses from processes of neuroblastoma cells in monolayer culture. Biophys. J. in press (Abstract).

20. Grinvald, A. and Farber, I. The minilaser microelectrode: Determination of conduction velocity in processes of neuroblastoma cells utilizing fluorescent voltage sensitive probes. Biophys. J. in press (Symposium lecture).

21. Grinvald, A. and Farber, I. The "mine laser microelectrode". Detection of calcium spikes in processes and growth cones of neuroblastoma cells, utilizing fluorescent voltage sensitive probes. Soc. for Neurosci. (1980) in press.

22. Grinvald, A., Ross, W.N. and Farber, I. Detection of regional variation in electrical properties of single neurons by simultaneous optical recording from multiple sites. Submitted to Proc. Natl. Acad. Sci., U.S.A.

23. Grinvald, A. and Farber, I. The minilaser microelectrode; Detection of Ca^{2+} channels sustaining action potentials in the neurites of neuroblastoma cells. Submitted for publication.

24. Grinvald, A. and Segal, M. Optical measurements of electrical activity from rat hippocampal slices (in preparation).

25. Kimhi, Y., Palfrey, C., Spector, I., Barak, Y. and Littauer, U.Z. (1976). Maturation of neuroblastoma cells in the presence of dimethyl-sulfoxide. Proc. Natl. Acad. Sci., USA. 73, 462-466.

26. Yavin, E. and Zutra, A. (1979). Translocation and turnover of phospholipids analogs in plasma membrane-derived vesicles from cell cultures. Biochim. Biophys Acta 553, 424-437.

27. Moolenaar, W.H. and Spector, I. (1978). Ionic currents in cultured mouse neuroblastoma cells under voltage clamp conditions. J. Physiol. 278, 265-286.

28. Grinvald., A., Kamino, K., Lesher, S. and Cohen, L.B. (1978). Larger fluorescence and birefringence signals for optical monitoring of membrane potential. Biophys. J. 21, 82a. (Abstract)

29. Pooler, J. (1972). Photodynamic alteration of sodium currents in lobster axons. J. Gen. Physiol. 60, 367-387.

30. Segal, M. (1980). The active of serotonin in the rat hippocampal slice. J. Physiol. in press.

Neurotransmitters and their Receptors
Edited by U.Z. Littauer, Y. Dudai, I. Silman,
V.I. Teichberg and Z. Vogel

Control of Tubulin Expression in the Developing Nervous System

U.Z. Littauer, A. de Baetselier, I. Gunzburg and I. Gozes

Department of Neurobiology, The Weizmann Institute of Science, Rehovot, Israel

ABSTRACT

Our studies show that there is no change in the level and rate of synthesis of tubulin during morphological differentiation of mouse neuroblastoma cells. This would imply that the assembly of neuroblastoma microtubules that are necessary for neurite outgrowth proceed from a pre-existing pool of tubulin. Studies on the level and rate of synthesis of tubulin in developing rat brain led to similar conclusions. Maximal levels of cytoplasmic tubulin were found in newborn rats while brain neurons differentiate postnatally. Thus, large pools of tubulin are formed prior to neuronal differentiation. Moreover, by about day 10 after birth there is a progressive decrease in the level and rate of synthesis of tubulin until the rat reaches adulthood. It was also possible to show that the decline in the level and rate of synthesis of tubulin results from a decrease of the corresponding mRNA species, suggesting a diminution in the absolute requirement for these proteins during brain development. Brain maturation, myelination and synapse formation is paralleled by an increase in the particulate tubulin fraction. It was shown by several criteria that tubulin is also associated with presynaptic and synaptic vesicle membranes. It appears that the α-tubulin is an integral membrane protein, whereas most of the β-tubulin can be easily dissociated from these membranes.

Despite the overall decrease in tubulin synthesis during brain maturation more tubulin mRNA species are expressed in the mature than in the prenatal brain. In adult brain, tubulin displays extensive microheterogeneity and several non-identical isotubulins exhibiting different isoelectric points but similar molecular weights have been identified. Brain tubulin microheterogeneity is developmentally determined, increasing from five to six components (isotubulins 1-6) in the prenatal rat brain to nine components in the mature brain (isotubulins 1-9). Mature brain mRNA, when translated *in vitro*, directed the synthesis of five tubulin forms, namely isotubulins 1, 3, 4 (or 5), 6 and 7. The mRNA species coding for isotubulins 3 and 7 could be partially separated on formamide-sucrose gradients while in the absence of formamide, the mRNA species directing the synthesis of isotubulins 1, 4 (or 5) and 6 showed differences in mobility. It therefore appears that brain mRNA may consist of five different species coding for distinct isotubulins. Moreover, a marked age-dependent enhancement in the relative translation of mRNA coding for isotubulin 7, which is not apparent among the translation products directed by the prenatal mRNA, was detected. Thus, some of the age-dependent increase in tubulin microheterogeneity might be controlled at the mRNA level.

To gain further insight at the control of tubulin gene expression, we have recently constructed several recombinant plasmids which contain cDNA nucleotide sequences hybridizable with brain tubulin and actin mRNAs.

INTRODUCTION

Microtubules are present in all eukaryotic cells and have a variety of structural and dynamic roles in cell shape, division, motility, transport and secretion. Models have been proposed which suggest that changes in the organization of the cytoplasmic microtubules alter the mobility and distribution of membrane surface receptors. Microtubules are highly abundant in nerve processes: their number per axon and per length increases with development. Axon outgrowth and axoplasmic transport are also thought to depend on microtubule integrity (1).

PRE-EXISTING POOL OF TUBULIN IS UTILIZED FOR MICROTUBULES FORMATION DURING NEURITE OUTGROWTH OF NEUROBLASTOMA CELLS

We have initially focused our attention on the maturation of mouse neuroblastoma cells in culture as a model system to study the role of tubulin in neurite extension. These cells can be induced to differentiate and express many of the properties of mature neurons, such as neurotransmitter synthesis (2), the possession of an electrically excitable membrane (3,4) and the development of a neurite network (5). To achieve extensive expression of these properties cells have been treated with various agents such as aminopterin (6,7) or dibutyryl cAMP (8-10). We have shown that a highly differentiated population of neuroblastoma cells can be obtained by the addition of dimethyl sulfoxide or hexamethylene bisacetamide to the growth medium (11-16). Under these conditions a high level of electrical and morphological differentiation is attained. The transition from round, actively dividing cells to morphologically differentiated cells is characterized by the appearance of an abundant number of long neurites that contain high concentrations of microtubules (17,18). These conclusions are supported by visualizing the neurite microtubules using indirect immunofluorescence with anti-tubulin antibodies (B. Geiger, unpublished observations). The extension of neurites is assumed to depend on the integrity of the microtubules. This is inferred from the sensitivity of this process to low temperatures and its inhibition by colchicine or vinblastine (5). All of these treatments are known to prevent tubulin assembly. We have asked whether the formation of these long neurites requires an increased rate of tubulin synthesis. It was found that the level and rate of synthesis of tubulin does not change during morphological differentiation of mouse neuroblastoma cells and is about 12% of the total soluble proteins (12,18,19). This would imply that assembly of neuroblastoma microtubules, that is necessary for neurite outgrowth, proceeds from a preexisting pool of tubulin. In that respect it is interesting to note that the level of tubulin in rat glioma C6 cells is 4-5 times lower than in mouse neuroblastoma cells.

DECREASE IN LEVELS AND RATE OF SYNTHESIS OF TUBULIN IN DEVELOPING RAT BRAIN

Studies of the level and rate of synthesis of tubulin in developing rat brain led to similar conclusions to that obtained with neuroblastoma cells. The concentration of tubulin is much higher in central nervous system cells as compared to other tissues. It was further shown that the relative amount of soluble tubulin increases during prenatal brain development, thereafter decreasing in the postnatal stage. The time period in which this decrease occurs, varies in different animals and corresponds to the maturation process of the brain from the respective animal (20-22). In our studies rats were chosen as a model system. In this animal a crucial period in brain maturation appears to occur from birth until about 21 days. Although this process varies for each brain region the maturation of most brain neurons takes place postnatally. The amount of tubulin in postnatal developing rat brain was determined as a function of age by three independent methods. In the first method soluble extracts were resolved by electrophoresis in $NaDodSO_4$-polyacrylamide gels, and the amount of tubulin was determined by densitometric scanning of the Coomassie Brilliant Blue stained gels. In another method the $[^3H]$colchicine-binding activity of the extracts was measured (23). Similar results were obtained by both methods and were in agreement with radioimmune quantitation in which aliquots were tested for their capacity to compete with $[^{125}I]$ tubulin for binding to anti-tubulin antibodies (24). These studies showed that the amount of tubulin in the soluble fraction increases after birth and levels off at the age of 10-15 days, whereas the total protein content is still increasing. It therefore appears that a high pool of tubulin is synthesized prior to the termination of neuronal differentiation. Moreover, by about day 10 after birth there is a progressive decrease in the rate of synthesis and level of soluble brain tubulin until the rat reaches adulthood. Thus, while the percentage of tubulin in the soluble fraction is about 33% between day 0 and 10 after birth, it then decreases to 20% between day 10 and 15 (12,23,24). It is obvious that the complexity of the various brain cell types allows one to draw only tentative conclusions from this phenomenon. One possibility is that the decrease in tubulin content may be related to the transient redundancy in the number of brain connections which has been observed during early brain maturation and which is followed by a marked reduction in the number of neuronal contacts (25). We were also able to show that the decline in the level and rate of synthesis of tubulin results from a decrease of the corresponding mRNA species, suggesting a diminution in the absolute requirement for these proteins during brain development (26,12,19,27).

THE α-SUBUNIT OF TUBULIN IS PREFERENTIALLY ASSOCIATED WITH PRESYNAPTIC AND SYNAPTIC VESICLE MEMBRANES

Tubulin is not only confined to the cytoplasm, as it is found to be associated with various membranes (28-32). During brain development there is a marked increase in the particulate brain proteins, paralleled by an increase in the particulate tubulin and reaches a value of about 50% of the total cellular tubulin (23). Some of the particulate tubulin is associated with the myelin membrane (31)and several investigators have suggested (33,34) that a contractile system may be involved in the neurosecretory processes. A necessary condition for the elucidation of such mechanisms would be the presence of contractile proteins as intrinsic constituents of the presynaptic membranes and synaptic vesicles. Tubulin and actin have been identified as major constituents in these structures (35-39). A striking feature is the observation that the α- and β-tubulin subunits differ in their association with brain presynaptic membranes (38) as well as synaptic vesicle membranes (39). It appears that the α-subunit is an integral membrane protein, whereas most of the β-subunit can be easily dissociated from these membranes. The finding of tubulin in the presynaptic and synaptic vesicle membranes may point to the existence of microtubules in this region in which the α-tubulin subunit serves as nucleation site for the assembly of microtubules. Alternatively the tighter association of the α-tubulin with these membranes may indicate a non-microtubular structure. The membrane-associated tubulin functions, perhaps, by ways other than polymerization into microtubules and thus pharmacological agents affecting microtubule assembly will not necessarily interfere with its presumptive role in synaptic transmission.

TUBULIN MICROHETEROGENEITY IS DEVELOPMENTALLY DETERMINED

The microtubule subunit protein, tubulin, is a heterodimer composed of two polypeptides, α and β, both of which show microheterogeneity (40-44). The question therefore arises as to whether changes occur in the proportions of the multiple forms of tubulin upon assumption of different roles within the nerve cell. It was shown in our laboratory (45,46) as well as by others (47-49) that brain tubulin is highly heterogeneous. Thus, by isoelectric focusing we were able to resolve nine distinct tubulin species from mature rat brain (under different isoelectric conditions it appears that adult brain tubulin may be resolved into eleven forms). The extensive tubulin microheterogeneity seems to be more prominent in the brain as compared to tubulin from other tissues such as spleen or liver (Figure 1). Tubulin from neuroblastoma cells (NIE-115) as well as neuroblastoma x glioma hybrid cells (NG108-15) are also less heterogeneous and

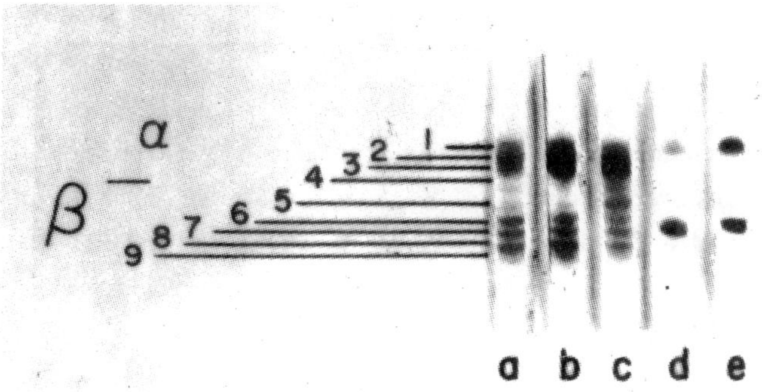

Fig. 1: Isoelectric focusing of tubulin from various brain areas, liver and spleen.
Tubulin was purified from 30 day-old rats by vinblastine precipitation and subjected to isoelectric focusing on polyacrylamide gels as described (46). Tubulin from: (a) cerebellum; (b) cerebrum; (c) medulla oblongata; (d) liver; (e) spleen.

contain two major subunits and several minor components (50,51). Two-dimensional gel electrophoresis of tubulin from adult rat brain established that the α-subunit consists of isotubulins 1-4 while the β-subunit is composed of isotubulins 5-9. Analysis of protease cleavage products showed a close similarity in the overall distribution of the peptide chains derived from each of the nine brain tubulin forms, indicating a structural homology between the isotubulins and eliminating the possibility of non-tubulin contaminants. However, several minor differences in the distribution pattern of the cleavage peptides were also evident. It was noted that the cleavage peptides of isotubulin 5 closely resemble those from bands 1-4 (α-tubulin), although it migrates as β-tubulin when resolved by two-dimensional gel electrophoresis. Band 5 also differs from isotubulin 1-4 in its inability to undergo *in vitro* tyrosylation. In addition, several control experiments indicated that the tubulin microheterogeneity does not arise from artifactual proteolysis (46). All the above results suggest the existence in the adult rat brain of multiple non-identical tubulin species exhibiting different isoelectric points, but similar molecular weights.

The distribution of the various isotubulins changes during development of rat brain (46,49,51,52). Thus, tubulin from prenatal brain displays five to six components (isotubulins 1-6) while nine forms (isotubulins 1-9) are evident in the isoelectric focusing pattern of tubulin from mature brain (46,51,52). With the development of the brain, the proportion of isotubulin 6 decreases and in particular the microheterogeneity of the β-subunit becomes more extensive with the appearance of isotubulins 7, 8 and 9. The question therefore arises as to whether these changes occur within the same cells upon assumption of different roles during brain maturation, or alternatively, that the increase in tubulin microheterogeneity reflects variations in the brain cell-population during brain development. In an attempt to answer this we have examined tubulin microheterogeneity in homogenous cell populations of cloned cells which were derived from both neuronal and glial origin. We have also examined changes of tubulins in a neuroblastoma-glioma somatic cell hybrid. Our results show that isotubulin patterns in various mouse neuroblastoma cell lines(NIE-115, NI8TG-2) are almost identical to each other. The rat glioma cell line (C6BU-1) showed a slightly different pattern. Each of these cells contained two major isotubulins and several minor components. It is in the latter tubulin forms that differences in the two cell lines are evident. The differences observed between the various cultures did not result from species specificity; mouse brain tubulin showed the same isotubulin pattern as that of rat brain (50). Isotubulins of the hybrid cells displayed an intermediate pattern of that found in the parental cell lines. These results suggest that the expression of isotubulins in a hybrid cell is not activated or suppressed in the cell hybrids unlike expression of other proteins.

The above results suggest that the changes in patterns of isotubulin observed in the developing brain could be affected by the changes in the heterogeneous cell population of the brain. The dissimilarity in the distribution of isotubulins isolated from various brain regions is also in accord with this hypothesis (51,52). However, multiple tubulin forms can be found in a single neuron (53). Single isolated neurons were grown in long-term primary cultures of dissociated cells from the rat superior cervical ganglion. Tubulin purified from such a single sympathetic neuron exhibited an isotubulin pattern similar for tubulin purified from brain. The possibility that changes in microenvironment, hormone action etc. can bring about shifts in the relative amounts of different tubulin forms during brain maturation remains open. Moreover, we have recently observed significant changes in tubulin microheterogeneity following diBUcAMP induced differentiation of NG108-15 hybrid cells.

USE OF RECOMBINANT PLASMIDS CONTAINING RAT BRAIN TUBULIN IN STUDYING BRAIN DEVELOPMENT

It was shown above that the reduction in the relative synthesis of tubulin during brain cell maturation is paralleled by a decrease in the *in vitro* translation activity of brain tubulin mRNA. On the other hand, the number of tubulin forms increases during postnatal brain development. In order to test whether some of these changes occur at the mRNA level we have translated mature mRNA in a reticulocyte lysate cell-free system. The mRNA directed the *in vitro* synthesis of five tubulin forms namely isotubulins 1, 3, 4 (or 5), 6 and 7. The mRNA species coding for isotubulins 3 and 7 could be partially separated on formamide-sucrose gradients while in the absence of formamide the mRNA species directing the synthesis of isotubulins 1, 4 (or 5) and 6 showed differences in mobility. It therefore appears that brain mRNA may consist of five different species coding for distinct isotubulins. Moreover, a marked age-dependent enhancement in the relative translation of mRNA coding for isotubulin 7, which is not apparent among the translation products directed by the prenatal mRNA, was detected. Thus, some of the age-dependent increase in tubulin microheterogeneity might be controlled at the mRNA level. We therefore conclude that despite the overall decrease in total tubulin synthesis more tubulin mRNA species are expressed in the adult than in the newborn brain (52).

One of the main conclusions from our present work is the finding that some of the developmentally controlled changes in the proportion of the brain specific isotubulins are mediated by parallel or preceding changes in the proportions of the mRNAs coding for these proteins. The changes in the functional level of isotubulin specific mRNAs could be a result of gene amplification, regulation of their rate of transcription, changes in transport through nuclear membrane or may be a post-transcriptional event. To distinguish between these mechanisms, homogenous DNA probes specific to the nucleotide sequences of tubulin mRNA chains have been synthesized. We have constructed several recombinant plasmids which contain nucleotide sequences hybridizable with brain tubulin and actin mRNAs. In brief, brain mRNA was isolated and fractionated by sucrose gradient centrifugation. The enriched tubulin mRNA fractions served as template for the synthesis of single-stranded cDNA using the enzyme reverse transcriptase. The single-stranded cDNA was converted to double-stranded cDNA by DNA-polymerase I. After treatment with S_1 nuclease, tails of oligo(dC) were added with terminal transferase. The tailed DNA was inserted by annealing into Pst_1 site of pBR 322 plasmid which was tailed in turn with oligo(dG). The advantage of using dG:dC tails, is the preservation of the Pst_1 site; thus, the original insert can be excised and recovered from the plasmid. The recombinant plasmid was used to transform competent *E.coli* χ 1776 cells. Over two thousand independent bacterial clones resistant to tetracycline but sensitive to ampicillin were isolated. These bacterial clones were screened by colony hybridization, for plasmids containing brain-specific nucleotide sequences. The clones were hybridized *in situ* with ^{32}P-labeled cDNA complementary to total mRNA from brain or total mRNA from liver. The selection procedure rests on the observation that brain mRNA is about 30-fold more enriched for tubulin sequences than that of liver mRNA. Over a hundred clones were selected by this procedure and the plasmid DNA was isolated from each of these clones by CsCl density equilibrium centrifugation. The various DNA preparations were immobilized on nitrocellulose filters and used to isolate the mRNA sequences which hybridize to the recombinant plasmid DNA. The hybridized-selected RNAs were then eluted and translated in a cell-free system in order to identify their encoded polypeptide. Figure 2 shows an autoradiograph of [^{35}S]methionine-labeled polypeptides separated by SDS-polyacrylamide gel electrophoresis. The cDNA clones specific for tubulin is evident. The [^{35}S]methionine product was further identified by two-dimensional gel electrophoresis and isoelectric focusing gels (54).

It is hoped that the availability of pure probes for brain specific proteins will now enable us to study further the molecular control of nerve cell differentiation.

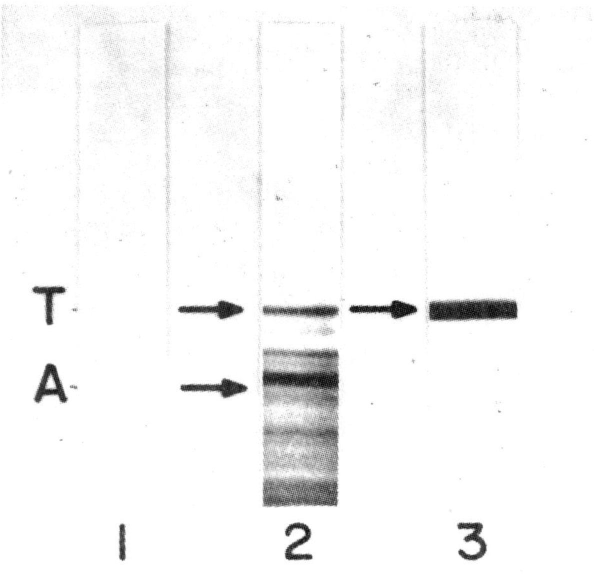

Fig. 2: Selection and *in vitro* translation of mRNA hybridized to DNA from a tubulin clone. Autoradiogram of [^{35}S]methionine labeled proteins synthesized in nuclease-treated reticulocyte lysate extracts and separated by electrophoresis on polyacrylamide slab gel containing 5-15% polyacrylamide gradient and 0.1% SDS. Synthesis of [^{35}S] labeled proteins directed: 1) by background mRNA nonspecifically bound to uncloned parent pBR 322 plasmid; 2) by total brain poly(A)$^+$ RNA; 3) by mRNA that was selected by plasmid No. 25 DNA containing tubulin-specific nucleotide sequences.

ACKNOWLEDGEMENT

This work was supported in part by a grant (to U.Z.L.) from the U.S.-Israel Binational Science Foundation (BSF), Jerusalem.

REFERENCES

1. Shelanski, M.L. and Feit, H. (1972). The Structure and Function of the Nervous Tissue, Vol. 6 (Bourne, G.E., Ed.), pp. 47-48, Academic Press, New York.

2. Amano, T., Richelson, E. and Nirenberg, M. (1972). Proc.Natl.Acad.Sci. USA 69, 258-263.

3. Nelson, P.G., Ruffner, B.W. and Nirenberg, M.W. (1969). Proc.Natl. Acad.Sci.USA 64, 1004-1010.

4. Spector, I., Palfrey, C. and Littauer, U.Z. (1975). Nature 254, 121-124.

5. Seeds, N.W., Gilman, A.G., Amano, T. and Nirenberg, M.W. (1970). Proc. Natl.Acad.Sci.USA 66, 160-167.

6. Peacock, J., Minna, J., Nelson, P.G. and Nirenberg, M.W. (1972). Exp. Cell Res. 73, 367-377.

7. Spector, I., Kimhi, Y. and Nelson, P.G. (1973). Nature 246, 124-126.

8. Fumarski, P., Silverman, D.J. and Lubin, M. (1971). Nature 233, 413-415.

9. Richelson, E. (1973). Nature [New Biol.] 242, 175-177.

10. Chalazonitis, A. and Greene, L.A. (1974). Brain Res. 72, 340-345.

11. Kimhi, Y., Palfrey, C., Spector, I., Barak, Y. and Littauer, U.Z. (1976). Proc.Natl.Acad.Sci.USA 73, 462-466.

12. Littauer, U.Z., Schmitt, H. and Gozes, I. (1976). J.Natl.Cancer Inst. 57, 647-651.

13. Littauer, U.Z., Palfrey, C., Kimhi, Y. and Spector, I. (1978). Natl. Cancer Inst. Monogram 48, 333-337.

14. Littauer, U.Z., Giovanni, M.Y. and Glick, M.C. (1980). J.Biol.Chem., in press.

15. Palfrey, C. and Littauer, U.Z. (1976). Biochem.Biophys.Res.Commun. 72, 209-215.

16. Palfrey, C., Kimhi, Y., Littauer, U.Z. Reuben, R.C. and Marks, P.A. (1977). Biochem.Biophys.Res.Commun. 76, 937-942.

17. Olmsted, J.B., Carlson, K., Klebe, R., Ruddle, F. and Rosnbaum, J. (1970). Proc.Natl.Acad.Sci.USA 65, 129-136.

18. Morgan, J.L. and Seeds, N.W. (1975). J.Cell Biol. 67, 136-145.

19. Schmitt, H. (1976). Brain Res. 115, 165-173.

20. Dutton, G.R. and Barondes, S. (1969). Science 166, 1637-1638.

21. Bamburg, J.R., Shooter, E.M. and Wilson, L. (1973). Biochemistry 12, 1476-1482.

22. Fellous, A., Francon, J., Virion, A. and Nunez, J. (1975). FEBS Lett. 57, 5-8.

23. Schmitt, H., Gozes, I. and Littauer, U.Z. (1977). Brain Res. 121, 327-342.

24. Gozes, I., Littauer, U.Z., Geiger, B. and Fuchs, S. (1977). FEBS Lett. 73, 109-114.

25. Changeux, J.P. and Danchin, A. (1976). Nature 264, 705-712.

26. Gozes, I., Schmitt, H. and Littauer, U.Z. (1975). Proc.Natl.Acad. Sci.USA 72, 701-705.

27. Gozes, I., Walker, M.D., Kaye, A.M. and Littauer, U.Z. (1977). J.Biol. Chem. 252, 1819-1825.

28. Bhattacharyya, B. and Wolff, J. (1975). J.Biol. Chem. 250, 7639-7646.

29. Bhattacharyya, B. and Wolff, J. (1976). Nature 264, 576-577.

30. Estridge, M. (1977). Nature 268, 60-63.

31. Gozes, I. and Richter-Landsberg, C. (1978). FEBS Lett. 95, 169-172.

32. Zisapel, N. and Littauer, U.Z. (1979). Eur.J.Biochem. 95, 51-59.

33. Berl, S., Puszkin, W. and Nicklas, J. (1973). Science 179, 441-446.

34. Blitz, A.L. and Fine, R.E. (1974). Proc.Natl.Acad.Sci.USA 71, 4472-4476.

35. Kornguth, S.E. and Sunderland, E. (1975). Biochim.Biophys.Acta 393, 100-114.

36. Mahler, H.R., Wang, Y.J., De Blas, A. and Crawford, G. (1977). In: Mechanisms, Regulation and Special Function of Protein Synthesis in the Brain (Robert et al., eds.), pp.205-220, Elsevier/North-Holland Biomedical Press, Amsterdam, New York.

37. Kelly, P.T. and Cotman, C.W. (1978). J.Cell Biol. 79, 173-183.

38. Gozes, I. and Littauer, U.Z. (1979). FEBS Lett. 99, 86-90.

39. Zisapel, N., Levi, M. and Gozes, I. (1980). J.Neurochem. 34, 26-32.

40. Feit, H., Slusarek, L. and Shelanski, M.L. (1971). Proc.Natl.Acad. Sci. USA 68, 2028-2031.

41. Witman, G.B., Carlson, K. and Rosenbaum, J.L. (1972). J.Cell Biol. 54, 540-555.

42. Feit, H. and Shelanski, M.L. (1975). Biochem.Biophys.Res.Commun. 66, 920-927.

43. Bibring, T., Baxandall, J., Denslon, S. and Walker, B. (1976). J.Cell Biol. 69, 301-312.

44. Kobayashi, Y. and Mohri, H. (1977). J.Mol.Biol. 116, 613-617.

45. Gozes, I. and Littauer, U.Z. (1977). In: Proc. 6th Intl.Soc.Neurochemistry (Sourkes, T.L. and Clausen, J., eds.), p. 121.

46. Gozes, I. and Littauer, U.Z. (1978). Nature 276, 411-413.

47. Marotta, C.A., Harris, J.L. and Gilbert, J.M. (1978). J.Neurochem. 30, 1431-1440.

48. Nelles, L.P. and Bamburg, J.R. (1979). J.Neurochem. 32, 477-489.

49. Dahl, J.L. and Weibel, V.J. (1979). Biochem.Biophys.Res.Commun. 86, 822-828.

50. Gozes, I., Saya, D. and Littauer, U.Z. (1979). Brain Res. 171, 171-175.

51. Gozes, I. and Littauer, U.Z. (1980). Scan.J.Immunol., Suppl., in press.

52. Gozes, I., de Baetselier, A. and Littauer, U.Z. (1980). Europ.J. Biochem. 103, 13-20.

53. Gozes, I. and Swendner, K.J. (1980). Cold Spring Harbor Meeting on: Forms of Microtubular Organization in Cells.

54. Ginzburg, I., de Baetselier, A., Walker, M., Behar, L., Lehrach, H., Frischauf, A.M. and Littauer, U.Z., in preparation.

Neurotransmitters and their Receptors
Edited by U.Z. Littauer, Y. Dudai, I. Silman,
V.I. Teichberg and Z. Vogel

Screening of the Protease Plasminogen Activator in the Developing Mouse Brain

Hermona Soreq[+] and Ruth Miskin*

Depts. of Neurobiology[+] and Biochemistry, The Weizmann Institute of Science, Rehovot, Israel*

Abstract

The developing mouse brain was found to express high specific activity of the serine protease Plasminogen Activator (PA). Analysis of the electrophoretic mobility of the enzyme revealed two subspecies, which migrated as a major band of the molecular weight of 60,000 and a minor one of 35,000 with no developmental variations. In five out of six brain regions that were tested the specific activity was found to change with the development and appeared to be higher during periods of cell proliferation and migration. These findings suggest that Plasminogen Activator plays a role in the development of the mouse brain. The possibility of the enzyme involvement in cell migration and/or tissue remodeling in the brain is discussed.

Results and Discussion

During early brain development cell proliferation is followed by massive cell migration and tissue remodeling (1). Although the anatomical and histological changes that accompany these processes have been extensively characterized, the molecular mechanisms underlying these changes are poorly understood. Evidence which has accumulated in recent years suggests a strong correlation between processes associated with tissue rearrangement and/or cell migration and the synthesis of the protease Plasminogen Activator (PA) in several adult and embryonic mammalian tissues. It was suggested that the plasminogen activation system operates as a means of general extracellular proteolysis, that functions in cell repositioning and reorganization of tissues during periods of development (For review see 2). We therefore initiated a systematic study of PA in the premature mouse brain to examine its possible involvement in brain development.

Generally, the mouse brain continues to develop during the first three postnatal weeks, but each brain region has a different timing and rate of development (3). We therefore tested PA activity in homogenates prepared from different regions of the developing and the mature mouse brain. PA activity was assayed as plasminogen dependent fibrinolysis (Fig. 1), calibrated as Urokinase (UK) Ploug units and expressed as specific activity.

Fig. 1.

PLASMINOGEN ACTIVATOR DEPENDENT FIBRINOLYSIS

Plasminogen activators are a group of serine proteases of high specificity. They convert the inactive Zymogen plasminogen into plasmin, a trypsin-like protease of broad specificity. Plamsin is a potent fibrinolytic protease, that digests insoluble fibrin (the blood clot) into soluble peptides. This reaction is exploited to assay PA activity.

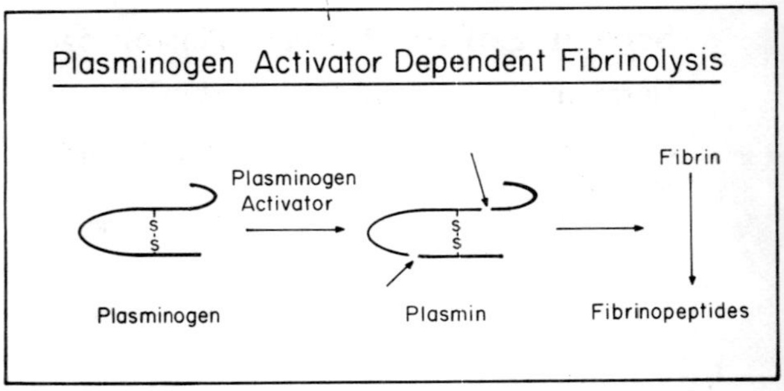

Three different patterns of PA specific activity were observed: 1. In the cerebral cortex, which is fully differentiated at birth , PA activity is at a consistently low level of about 0.9 ploug units per mg protein. 2. In the cerebellum, where extensive cell proliferation and migration occur during early postnatal life (4), PA activity is relatively high at birth, at a level of 3,3 Units/mg Protein, and it begins to decline at the third postnatal week concomitantly with the stabilization of the total cerebellar protein content. A decreasing pattern, from 3,2 U/mg at birth to 1.1 U/mg in adulthood, is also found in the brain stem. 3. A more complex pattern was observed in the hippocampus and the hypothalamus, where PA activity appears as two distinct peaks during the first and the third postnatal weeks and then decreases; the latter peak of PA activity appears in the thalamus as well (Table 1).

The electrophoretic mobility of PA activity from mouse brain was compared to PA from other sources by a zymographic technique applied following SDS-polyacrylamide gel electrophoresis according to Granelli-Piperno and Reich (7). In homogenates prepared from mature whole mouse brain a major band of 60,000 and a minor band of 35,000 molecular weight were observed. The major band comigrated with the apparent PA from mouse neuroblastoma N18 TG, while the minor band comigrated with Rat urine PA. Other mouse organs revealed the same two species, in addition to other PA mobilities (Fig. 2). A prolonged incubation of a mixutre of the liver extract, containing the 35,000 band, with the Neuroblastoma extract, containing the 60,000 band, did not affect the migration pattern, suggesting that the different mobilities of PA species did not result merely from a proteolytic digestion during the preparation and storage of the homogenates.

Table 1. PA levels in Developing Mouse Brain Regions

Age, days postnatal	0	5	10	15	20	25	120
Mouse brain region			Urokinase, Units/mg protein				
Cerebral cortex	0.9	0.9	0.9	1.1	1.0	0.9	0.7
Cerebellum	3.3	2.8	2.6	2.3	1.3	1.7	1.1
Brain stem	3.2	2.8	2.7	2.6	2.8	2.0	1.1
Hippocampus	1.8	3.0	3.6	2.6	3.5	2.4	2.6
Thalamus	1.0	0.9	0.9	2.7	4.3	2.4	2.2
Hypothalamus	0.9	3.3	2.2	2.9	3.0	2.5	2.1

Legend to Table 1.

C 57 BL/6J mice were sacrificed by cervical dislocation; brain was removed, the olfactory balb was discarded and remaining tissue was dissected on ice. Homogenates were prepared from dissected regions of 10 brains per sample in 10 volumes per weight of 0.5% Triton X-100. Protein concentration was determined according to Lowry et al. (5). PA activity was determined within one week of sample preparation as previously described (6) but in the presence of human plasminogen. No activity could be detected in the absence of plasminogen, indicating an absolute plasminogen dependence of the activity tested.

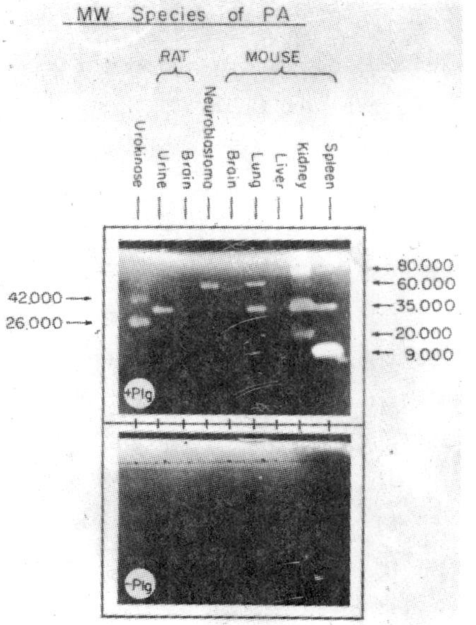

Fig. 2.

MOLECULAR WEIGHT SPECIES OF PA

Equal volumes of homogenates (10 volumes: weight) prepared from various mouse and rat organs were electrophoretically separated in 10% SDS-polyacrylamide gels. Washed gels were incubated on fibrin underlays for 24 hrs at 37° (7). Undigested fibrin was stained by Coomassie Brilliant Blue: White bands represent enzyme activity.

Analysis of homogenates from various brain regions of mature and newborn mice revealed similarly migrating bands of 60,000 and 35,000 at the same relative intensities observed in whole brain homogenates with no apparent developmental variations.

A quantitative determination of PA activity in the various tissue homogenates is presented in Fig. 3.

Fig. 3.

PA ACTIVITY IN DIFFERENT MOUSE ORGANS

Homogenates (10 volumes: weight) were prepared in 0.5% Triton X-100 from organs of mature perfused mice. Protein concentration was determined according to Lowry et al. PA activity was assayed as plasminogen dependent fibrinolysis. Columns represent the relative specific activity of PA as compared with brain homogenate. (100% = 1.8 UK U/mg).

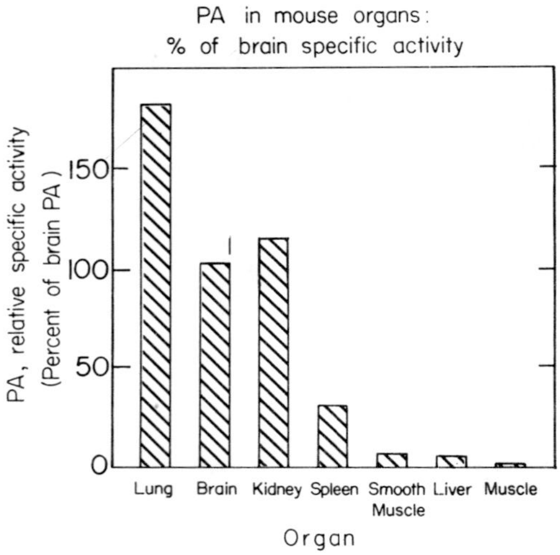

In order to further localize the varying PA activities to specific areas within the analyzed brain regions, we applied a fibrin overlay analysis (8) to creostat brain sections prepared from perfused mouse brain. Prominent PA activity was observed in certain subregions of such sections, while other areas had little or no activity. In the histochemical analysis of creostat sections from a 17 days old mouse brain, high activity was localized around the cortical menings of the cerebrum and the cerebellum, in agreement with earlier findings obtained by staining of fibrin underlays (9). The thalamic region showed the highest activity, as expected from the homogenate assay at this age (see Table 1). Within the cerebral cortex, the corpus callosum exhibited high activity as compared with the main mass of the cortical cell layers, and a section through the hippocampus revealed high PA activity at or close to the neural cell bodies layers (data not shown). The histochemical analysis therefore confirmed data that were obtained by the homogenate assay and provided additional information regarding the localization of PA in specific cell layers within the tested brain regions.

The findings presented in this communication suggest that Plasminogen Activator may play a role in the development of the mouse brain. The possibility of the enzyme participation in migration of nerve cells during the remodeling of the brain tissue is under investigation.

We thank Prof. U. Littauer for encouraging and helpful discussions and Mr. Y. Yarimi for skillful handling of mice. This research was supported by grants from United-States-Israel Binational Science Foundantion (BSF), Jerusalem, Israel (to R.M) and from the Israeli commission for basic research (to H.S.).

REFERENCES

1. Jacobson, M. (1970) Differentiation, growth and maturation of Neurons. in: Developmental Neurobiology. Holt, Rinehart and Winston, Inc. PP. 107-195.

2. Reich, E. (1978) in: Biological Markers of Neoplasia: Basic and Applied Aspects, Ruddon ed., Elsevier North Holland, Inc. pp. 491-500.

3. Benjamins, J.A. and McKhan, G.M. (1976) Development, Regeneration, and Aging. in: Basic Neurochemistry, Siegel et al., eds. Little Brown, Boston. pp. 365-387.

4. Palay, S.L. and Chan-Palay, V. (1974) Cerebellar Cortex, Cytology and Organization. Springer-Verlag, Berlin, Heidelberg, New York.

5. Lowry, O.H., Rosenbrough, N.J., Farr, A.L. & Randall, R.J. (1951) Protein measurement with the Folin Phenol reagent. J. Biol. Chem. 193, 265-275.

6. Wilson, E.L. and Reich, E. (1979) Modulation of Plasminogen Activator Synthesis in Chick Embryo Fibroblasts by Cyclic Nucleotides and Phorbol Myristate Acetate. Cancer Res. 39, 1579-1586.

7. Granelli-Piperno, A. and Reich, E. (1978) A study of Proteases and Protease-Inhibitor. Complexes in Biological Fluids. J. Exp. Med. 148, 223-234.

8. Miskin, R., Easton, T.G. and Reich, E. (1978) Plasminogen Activator in Chick Embryo Muscle Cells: Induction of Enzyme by RSV, PMA and Retinoic Acid. Cell 15, 1301-1312.

9. Takashima, S., Koga, M. and Tanaka, K. (1969) Fibrinolytic activity of human brain and cerebrospinal fluid. Br. J. Exp. Path. 50, 533-539.

Neurotransmitters and their Receptors
Edited by U.Z. Littauer, Y. Dudai, I. Silman,
V.I. Teichberg and Z. Vogel

Mechanism of Mammalian Toxicity of the Pyrethroids

A. Gray, T.A. Connors and J. Rickard

MRC Toxicology Unit, Woodmansterne Road,

Carshalton, Surrey, England

Abstract

The synthetic pyrethroids are a recently developed group of extremely potent insecticides. Their insecticidal potency and mammalian toxicity are both dependent on the isomeric configuration at various chiral centres, but not all compounds which have the correct configuration for insecticidal activity are neurotoxic to mammals. The toxicity of these compounds has been shown to be directly on the central nervous system. It is suggested that the differences in toxicity of the isomers are due to the selective interaction of toxic pyrethroid isomers with stereospecific receptors within the central nervous system of mammals.

Cismethrin and bioresmethrin

The synthetic pyrethroids are a recently developed group of extremely potent insecticides. The insecticidal activity of these compounds is dependent on the (1R)-configuration of the chiral carbon in the C1 position of the cyclopropane ring, irrespective of their *cis*- or *trans*-orientation across the ring. However, in mammals the (1R,*cis*)-isomers are always more toxic than their *trans* analogues. although, as in insects, both (1S)-isomers are non-toxic.

	LD50(ng/Insect) A. stephensi (Mosquito)	IV LD50 to Rats (mg/kg)
CIS METHRIN. (IR,CIS) 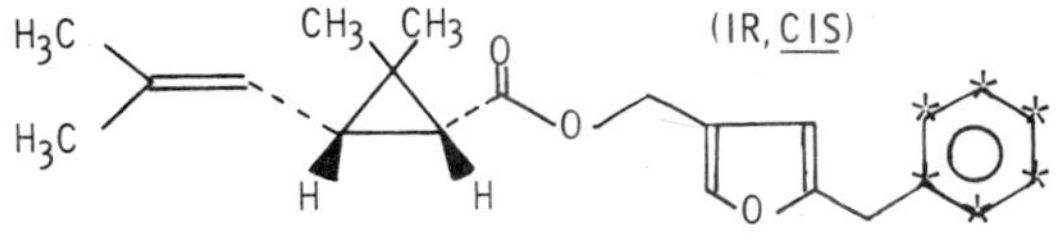	0.64	5
BIORESMETHRIN (IR,TRANS) 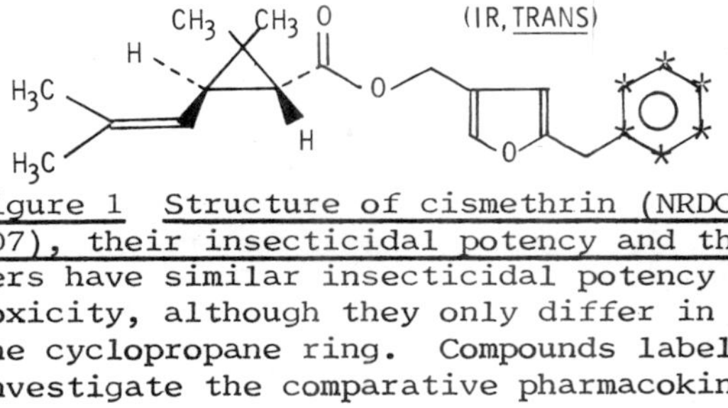	0.95	500

Figure 1 Structure of cismethrin (NRDC 119) and bioresmethrin (NRDC 107), their insecticidal potency and their toxicity. These two isomers have similar insecticidal potency but widely different mammalian toxicity, although they only differ in their configuration at C3 of the cyclopropane ring. Compounds labelled with ^{14}C (*) were used to investigate the comparative pharmacokinetics of these two isomers.

The synthetic pyrethroid resmethrin (1), [5-benzyl-3-furylmethyl-(1RS,cis,trans)-chrysanthemate] has two chiral centres (C1 and C3 of the cyclopropane ring) and hence four isomers, of which only the two 1R-isomers shown in Figure 1 have insecticidal activity. The mammalian toxicity of bioresmethrin is at least 100 fold less than that of cismethrin, and even this toxicity is now considered to be due to small amounts of cis-isomer impurity (1-5%) in the bioresmethrin (2). Pharmacokinetic investigations were initiated to compare the distribution of these two isomers after intravenous administration to rats at equimolar doses (2.5 mg/kg). Cismethrin at this dose causes mild tremors (3) within 1 to 2 minutes of dosing and these continue for up to 30 minutes. The concentrations of these two isomers were followed in a number of tissues. Values for blood and brain are shown in Figures 2 and 3.

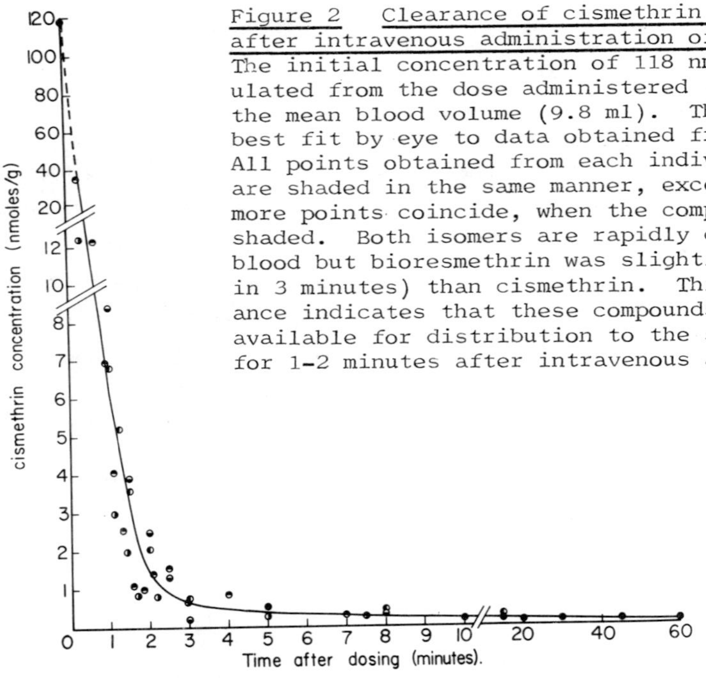

Figure 2 Clearance of cismethrin from rat blood after intravenous administration of 2.5 mg/kg
The initial concentration of 118 nmol/g was calculated from the dose administered (1109 nmol) and the mean blood volume (9.8 ml). The curve is the best fit by eye to data obtained from 4 animals. All points obtained from each individual animal are shaded in the same manner, except when two or more points coincide, when the complete symbol is shaded. Both isomers are rapidly cleared from blood but bioresmethrin was slightly slower (99% in 3 minutes) than cismethrin. This rapid clearance indicates that these compounds are only available for distribution to the site of action for 1-2 minutes after intravenous administration.

The entry of both isomers into the central nervous system (CNS) was extremely rapid, the maximum concentration being achieved within 2 minutes after intravenous dosing. The clearance of both parent isomers from the CNS was much slower (Figure 3) than from other tissues examined and there was no evidence of any accumulation of metabolites in the CNS.

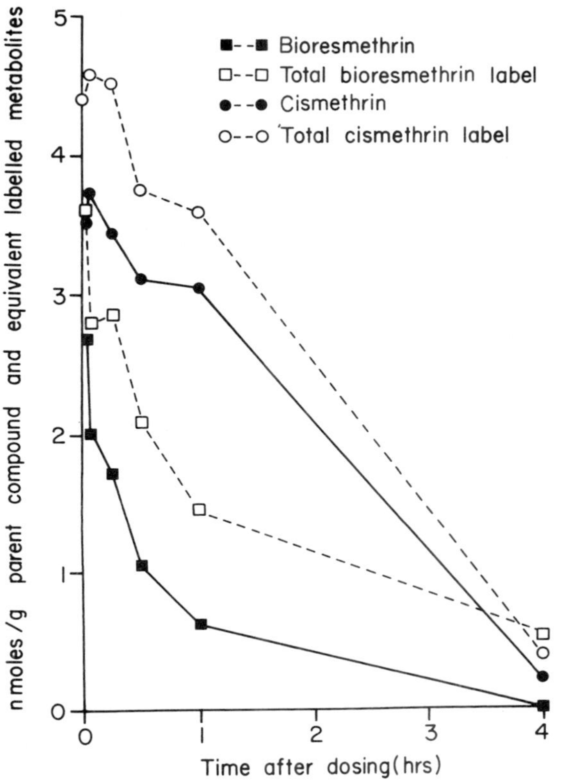

Figure 3 Concentration of cismethrin and bioresmethrin in the brain after intravenous administration of 2.5 mg/kg to rats. The difference between parent compound concentration and total label is largely accounted for by the efficiency of the extraction and analysis methods. Bioresmethrin concentrations are slightly less than those of an equimolar dose of cismethrin and decrease more rapidly. In agreement with previous work (4), signs of toxicity were only observed in cismethrin dosed animals which had brain concentrations of parent compound exceeding 3.5 nmol/g. Bioresmethrin concentrations can exceed this level without causing toxicity (4).

Administration of cismethrin into the lateral ventricles of the brain or into the spinal cord, at doses which would achieve similar concentrations of the compound in the CNS, cause the same symptoms as observed after intravenous administration. The onset of tremors after intraventricular administration of cismethrin was delayed for about 15 minutes whilst after intraspinal injection the symptoms occurred within 2 to 5 minutes indicating that cismethrin may act directly on spinal cord rather than in the brain.

Decamethrin

Decamethrin [S-α-cyano-3-phenoxybenzyl-(1R,cis)-3-(2,2-dibromovinyl)-2,2-dimethylcyclopropanecarboxylate], the most potent pyrethroid insecticide yet developed (5) is a single isomer having the most active configuration at each optical centre including the S-configuration of the cyano group which is essential for insecticidal potency (Figure 4). In mammals decamethrin is approximately twice as toxic (Figures 1 and 4) as cismethrin and causes toxicity quite distinct from the resmethrin type of pyrethroid (6).

DECAMETHRIN
(S - α - cyano, IR - Cis)

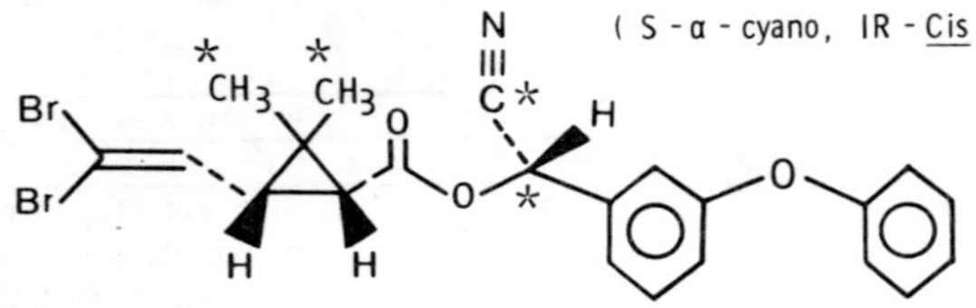

LD50 (ng/Insect) A. stephensi (Mosquito)	IV LD50 to Rats (mg/kg)
0.036	3

Figure 4 The structure of decamethrin, its insecticidal potency and mammalian toxicity. Decamethrin, labelled with ^{14}C (*), was used to study the comparative pharmacokinetics of this pyrethroid with that of cismethrin.

The CNS concentrations of decamethrin which are achieved at the time the signs of toxicity are present are 1/10th of those of an equally toxic dose of cismethrin. Intraspinal or intraventricular administration of doses which result in similar CNS concentrations of decamethrin produce some symptoms equivalent to those seen after intravenous administration.

The neurotoxicity of the pyrethroids both to mammals and insects is very dependent on their stereochemical configuration suggesting that a stereospecific receptor(s) must exist in the CNS, possibly within the spinal cord, that is responsible for pyrethroid toxicity. These receptors may be associated with the control of the sodium channel as it has been shown that the pyrethroids prolong the transient increase in sodium permeability in nerve preparations after excitation (7).

References

1. Elliott, M., Farnham, A.W., Janes, N.F., Needham, P.H. and Pearson, B.C. (1967) Nature, 213, 493-494.

2. Gray, A.J. and Connors, T.A. (1980) Pesticide Science, In Press.

3. Verschoyle, R.D. and Barnes, J.M. (1972) Pesticide Biochemistry and Physiology, 2, 308-311.

4. White, I.N.H., Verschoyle, R.D., Moradian, M.H. and Barnes, J.M. (1976) Pesticide Biochemistry and Physiology, 6, 491-500.

5. Elliott, M., Farnham, A.W., Janes, N.F., Needham, P.H. and Pulman, D.A. (1974) Nature, 248, 710-711.

6. Ray, D.E. and Cremer, J.E. (1979) Pesticide Biochemistry and Physiology, 10, 333-340.

7. Vijverberg, H.P.M. and Van den Bercken, J. (1979) European Journal of Pharmacology, 58, 501-504.

Author Index